The Unofficial Guide to Prescribing

EDITION
2

The Unofficial Guide to Prescribing

Series and Volume Editor
Zeshan Qureshi BM, BSc (Hons), MSc, MRCPCH, FAcadMEd, MRCPS (Glasg)
Paediatric Registrar, London Deanery, London, UK

Volume Editors
Ali B.A.K. Al-Hadithi MB Bchir, MA (Cantab), MRCP (UK), AFHEA, PGCert (Med Ed)
Clinical Research Training Fellow
University of Cambridge, Cambridge, UK;
Cambridge University Hospitals NHS Foundation Trust, Cambridge, UK

Simon R.J. Maxwell BSc, MB, ChB, MD, PhD, FRCP, FRCPE, FHEA, FBPhS
Professor
Clinical Pharmacology Unit
University of Edinburgh
Edinburgh, Scotland, UK

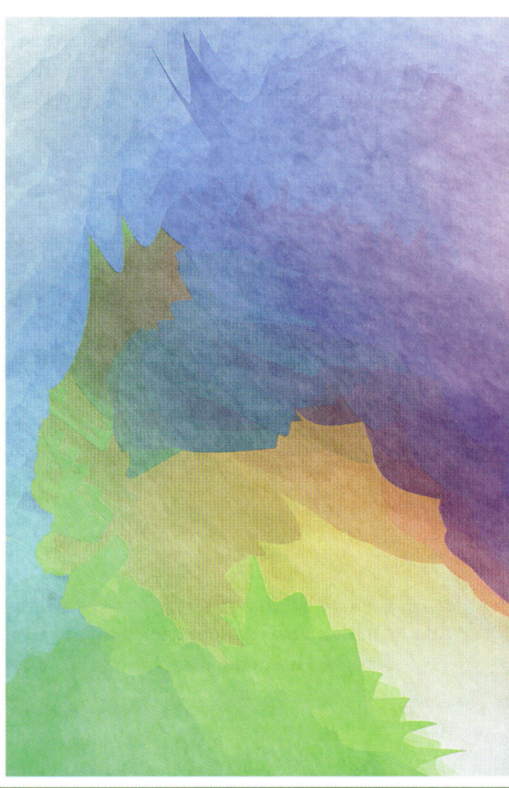

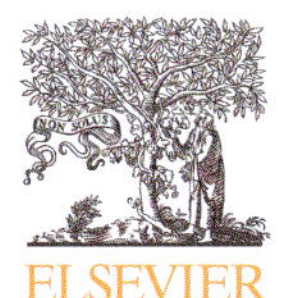

ELSEVIER

For accessibility purposes, images in electronic versions of this book are accompanied by alt text descriptions provided by Elsevier. For more information, see https://www.elsevier.com/about/accessibility.

Publisher's note: *Elsevier* takes a neutral position with respect to territorial disputes or jurisdictional claims in its published content, including in maps and institutional affiliations.

First edition 2014

Notice

Practitioners and researchers must always rely on their own experience and knowledge in evaluating and using any information, methods, compounds or experiments described herein. Because of rapid advances in the medical sciences, in particular, independent verification of diagnoses and drug dosages should be made. To the fullest extent of the law, no responsibility is assumed by Elsevier, authors, editors or contributors for any injury and/or damage to persons or property as a matter of products liability, negligence or otherwise, or from any use or operation of any methods, products, instructions, or ideas contained in the material herein.

ISBN: 978-0-443-11345-1

Content Strategist: Alexandra Mortimer
Content Project Manager: Tapajyoti Chaudhuri
Design: Hitchen Miles
Marketing Manager: Deborah J. Watkins

Printed in India

Last digit is the print number: 9 8 7 6 5 4 3 2 1

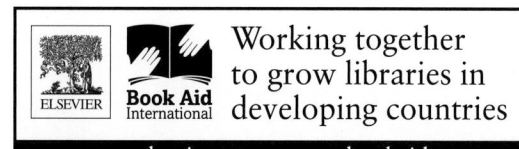

Ali would like to dedicate this book to his family, Bara, Suhair, Ahmed and Miriam, for their continuous support.

Ali B.A.K. Al-Hadithi

Contents

Series Editor's Foreword, ix

Preface, xi

How to Use This Book, xiii

Acknowledgements, xvii

Abbreviations, xix

Contributors, xxiii

1 Introduction to Prescribing, 1
Simon R.J. Maxwell

2. Cardiology, 31
Simon R.J. Maxwell

3. Respiratory Medicine, 63
Simon R.J. Maxwell

4. Gastroenterology, 91
Ali B.A.K. Al-Hadithi

5. Neurology, 121
Ali B.A.K. Al-Hadithi

6. Endocrinology, 157
Ali B.A.K. Al-Hadithi

7. Obstetrics and Gynaecology, 209
Samuel Lockley, Matthew G. Wood

8. General Surgery, 239
Ali B.A.K. Al-Hadithi

9. Paediatrics, 269
Alexandra Richards, Zeshan Qureshi

10. Additional Important Scenarios, 307
Ali B.A.K. Al-Hadithi

Index 337

Series Editor's Foreword

The Unofficial Guide to Medicine is not just about helping students study, it is also about allowing those who learn to take back control of their own education. Since its inception, it has been driven by the voices of students, and through this, democratised the process of medical education, blurring the line between learners and teachers.

Medical education is an evolving process, and the latest iteration of our titles has been rewritten to bring them up to date with modern curriculums, after extensive deliberation and consultation. We have kept the series up to date, incorporating new guidelines and perspectives from a wide range of students, junior doctors and senior clinicians. There is greater consistency across the titles,more illustrations, and through these and other changes, I hope the books will now be even better study aids.

These books though are a process of continual improvement. By reading this book, I hope that you not only get through your exams but also consider contributing to a future edition. You may be a student now, but you are also the future of medical education.

I wish you all the best with your future career and any upcoming exams.

Zeshan Qureshi
November 2022

Preface

The book is designed to take the theoretical knowledge of medical school and apply it to real-life practical situations. When a 55-year-old man with a new diagnosis of Hodgkin lymphoma is confused and has a sodium of 118, what do you do? When a 17-year-old girl is unresponsive with a blood glucose of 1.8, what do you do?

Prescribing is a major challenge for students because of its volume and complexity, and the need to gather experience. It is the thing that new graduates fear the most and feel least prepared for, and it's the commonest thing new graduates do which directly affects patient safety and can produce clinical errors.

The Unofficial Guide to Prescribing, much like its OSCE companion, will take you through the practical steps of how you assess, investigate and manage each individual patient, with a focus on prescribing, specifically what you prescribe, and how you prescribe it, with clear examples of generic drug charts showing you how the prescriptions would look in real life.

The book is aimed not just at medical students but also junior doctors, nursing staff, pharmacists and all those involved in prescribing and hospital care of patients. This book aims to empower you to excel at dealing with emergencies and handling complex prescribing scenarios.

We wish you all the best in any upcoming examinations and your future career.

How to Use This Book

Each scenario is broken down into the following:

- The scenario as it might present itself to you within hospital practice.
- **Initial ABCDE assessment of the patient**—divided into three sections: (a) how you will assess each parameter: 'airway', 'breathing', 'circulation', 'disability', 'exposure'; (b) what the assessment findings are in the scenario; and (c) what immediate management is required.
- **Initial investigations**—what tests are needed to allow you to ascertain: (a) the diagnosis; (b) the severity of the condition; and (c) any complications that have arisen. The results of any suggested tests are given.
- **Initial management**—what needs to be done to stabilise the patient, and to start treating the initial diagnosis.
- **Reassessment**—whether the treatment has been effective, or whether there is a need to escalate treatment or consider an alternative diagnosis.
- **Handing over the patient**—summarising the findings and your involvement to either the specialist, or to your colleague who is taking over responsibility for the patient.
- **Further treatment**—what needs to be done to ensure this patient is optimally managed. This includes other treatments outstanding and who else might need to be involved.

PRESCRIBING

Throughout the text are 'Prescribe' alerts that tell you exactly what needs to be prescribed. We have emphasised drug classes rather than individual drugs because of the variability in prescribing practice. Individual drugs are given merely as practical examples, and we have used a variety of drugs within the same broad area (e.g. dalteparin and enoxaparin for thromboprophylaxis) to illustrate different reasonable approaches to the same prescribing challenge.

This is followed by the prescription charts as they would look in these cases. The aim is to show you exactly what will need to be produced in practical prescribing, rather than just theoretically. Please note that prescription charts vary between hospitals. There may also be specialist charts available for oxygen, blood products, anticoagulants, insulin and certain IV infusions.

The blank prescription charts on the following pages can be photocopied freely for studying and examination preparations.

PRESCRIPTION AND ADMINISTRATION RECORD

Standard Chart

Hospital/Ward:	Consultant:	Name of Patient:
Weight:	Height:	Hospital Number:
If re-written, date:		D.O.B.:
DISCHARGE PRESCRIPTION Date completed:-	Completed by:-	

OTHER MEDICINE CHARTS IN USE	
Date	Type of Chart

PREVIOUS ADVERSE REACTIONS This section must be completed before any medicine is given		Completed by (sign & print)	Date
None known ☐			
Medicine/Agent	Description of Reaction		

CODES FOR NON-ADMINISTRATION OF PRESCRIBED MEDICINE

If a dose is not administered as prescribed, initial and enter a code in the column with a circle drawn round the code according to the reason as shown below. **Inform the responsible doctor in the appropriate timescale.**

1. Patient refuses
2. Patient not present
3. Medicines not available – CHECK ORDERED
4. Asleep/drowsy
5. Administration route not available – CHECK FOR ALTERNATIVE
6. Vomiting/nausea
7. Time varied on doctor's instructions
8. Once only/as required medicine given
9. Dose withheld on doctor's instructions
10. Possible adverse reaction/side effect

ONCE-ONLY

Date	Time	Medicine (Approved Name)	Dose	Route	Prescriber – Sign + Print	Time Given	Given By

OXYGEN	Start Date	Start Time	Route Mask (%)	Route Prongs (L/min)	Prescriber – Sign + Print	Administered by	Stop Date	Stop Time

Name:

Date of Birth:

REGULAR THERAPY

PRESCRIPTION	Date → / Time ↓													

Medicine (Approved Name)		Time													
Dose	Route	6													
Notes	Start Date	8													
Prescriber – sign + print		12													
		14													
		18													
		22													

Medicine (Approved Name)		Time													
Dose	Route	6													
Notes	Start Date	8													
Prescriber – sign + print		12													
		14													
		18													
		22													

Medicine (Approved Name)		Time													
Dose	Route	6													
	Start Date	8													
Prescriber – sign + print		12													
		14													
		18													
		22													

Medicine (Approved Name)		Time													
Dose	Route	6													
	Start Date	8													
Prescriber – sign + print		12													
		14													
		18													
		22													

Medicine (Approved Name)		Time													
Dose	Route	6													
Notes	Start Date	8													
Prescriber – sign + print		12													
		14													
		18													
		22													

Medicine (Approved Name)		Time													
Dose	Route	6													
Notes	Start Date	8													
Prescriber – sign + print		12													
		14													
		18													
		22													

FLUID PRESCRIPTION CHART

Hospital/Ward:	Consultant:	Name of Patient:
		Hospital Number:
Weight:	Height:	D.O.B:

Date/ Time	FLUID / ADDED DRUGS	VOLUME / DOSE	ROUTE	RATE	PRESCRIBER – SIGN AND PRINT

Acknowledgements

We would like to acknowledge the hard work of the contributors to the first edition of the book, including ShiYing Hey, Tobias Hunt, Matthew M.Y. Lee, Emily R. McCall-Smith, Constantinos A. Parisinos, Mark A. Rodrigues, Matthew Sims, Matthew Harris and Anatole V. Wiik.

Abbreviations

ABG	arterial blood gas
ABPA	allergic bronchopulmonary aspergillosis
ACE	angiotensin-converting enzyme
ACR	albumin–creatinine ratio
ACS	acute coronary syndrome
ADR	adverse drug reaction
A&E	accident and emergency
AF	atrial fibrillation
AKI	acute kidney injury
ALP	alkaline phosphatase
ALT	alanine transaminase
AMP	adenosine monophosphate
AMT/AMTS	abbreviated mental test/score
AP	anteroposterior
APTT	activated partial thromboplastin time
ARB	angiotensin receptor blocker
ARDS	acute respiratory distress syndrome
AS	aortic stenosis
AST	aspartate aminotransferase
ATN	acute tubular necrosis
AV	arteriovenous
AVM	arteriovenous malformation
AVPU	A = alert, V = voice, P = pain, U = unresponsive
AXR	abdominal radiograph
BBB	bundle branch block
BBB	blood–brain barrier
BD	bis die (twice daily)
BE	base excess
β-hCG	beta-human chorionic gonadotropin
BM	blood glucose
BNF	British National Formulary
BNFC	British National Formulary for Children
BP	blood pressure
BiPAP	bilevel positive airway pressure
CABG	coronary artery bypass graft
CAP	community-acquired pneumonia
CBD	common bile duct
CCF	congestive cardiac failure
CCU	coronary care unit
CDS	clinical decision support
CF	cystic fibrosis
CHM	Commission on Human Medicines
CIWA-Ar	Clinical Institute Withdrawal Assessment for Alcohol, revised
CKD	chronic kidney disease
COPD	chronic obstructive pulmonary disease
CPAP	continuous positive airway pressure
CPR	cardiopulmonary resuscitation
CMV	cytomegalovirus
CNS	central nervous system
CR	capillary refill
CrCl	creatinine clearance
CRP	C-reactive protein
CRT	capillary refill time
CSF	cerebrospinal fluid
CT	computerised tomography
CTG	cardiotocograph
CTPA	computed tomographic pulmonary angiography
CURB 65	C = Confusion, U = Urea, R = Respiratory Rate, B=Blood Pressure, 65 = Age 65
CV	cardiovascular
CVP	central venous pressure
CVS	cardiovascular system
CXR	chest radiograph
DH	drug history
DIC	disseminated intravascular coagulation
DOIS	distal intestinal obstruction syndrome
DKA	diabetic ketoacidosis
DMARD	disease-modifying antirheumatic drug
DOAC	direct acting oral anticoagulant
DoTS	dose, timing and susceptibility
DVLA	Driver and Vehicle Licensing Agency
DVT	deep vein thrombosis
ECG	electrocardiogram
ECST	European Carotid Surgery Trial
EEG	electroencephalography
EFNS	European Federation of Neurological Societies
eGFR	estimated glomerular filtration rate
EMA	European Medicines Agency
EMC	Electronic Medicines Compendium
ENT	ear, nose and throat
ERCP	endoscopic retrograde cholangiopancreatography
ESR	erythrocyte sedimentation rate
FBC	full blood count
FEV_1	forced expiratory volume in 1 second
FFP	fresh frozen plasma
FT4	free T4
FVC	forced vital capacity
GABA	gamma-aminobutyric acid
GAD	generalised anxiety disorder
GB	gall bladder disease
GCS	Glasgow Coma Scale
GFR	glomerular filtration rate
GGT	gamma-glutamyl transferase
GI	gastrointestinal
GMAWS	Glasgow Modified Alcohol Withdrawal Scale
GMP	guanosine monophosphate
GORD	gastroesophageal reflux disease
GP	general practitioner
GPCR	G-protein-coupled receptor
G6PD	glucose-6-phosphate dehydrogenase

GRACE	Global Registry of Acute Cardiac Events
G&S	group and save
GSL	general sales list
GTCS	generalised tonic–clonic seizures
GTN	glyceryl trinitrate
GU	genitourinary
HAS	human albumin solution
HB	heart block
HCG	human chorionic gonadotrophin
HDL	high-density lipoprotein
HDU	high dependency unit
HELLP syndrome	H = haemolysis, EL = elevated liver enzymes, LP = low platelets
HER2+	human epidermal growth factor receptor 2-positive
HHFNC	humidified high-flow nasal cannula
HHFNO	humidified high-flow nasal oxygen
HHS	hyperosmolar hyperglycaemic state
HONK	hyperosmolar nonketotic coma
HR	heart rate
HRT	hormone replacement therapy
HS	heart sounds
HVS	high vaginal swab
Hx	history
IBD	inflammatory bowel disease
ICS	inhaled corticosteroid
ICU	intensive care unit
IHD	ischaemic heart disease
IM	intramuscular
INH	inhaled
INN	International Nonproprietary Name
INR	international normalised ratio
ITP	idiopathic thrombocytopenic purpura
ITU	intensive therapy unit
IV	intravenous
IVI	intravenous infusion
IVIg	intravenous immunoglobulin
JVP	jugular venous pressure
LABA	long-acting beta-agonist
LAD	left anterior descending
LAMA	short-acting muscarinic antagonist
LCX	left circumflex artery
LDL	low-density lipoprotein
LFT	liver function test
LLETZ	large loop excision of the transformation zone
LMP	last menstrual period
LMW	low molecular weight
LMWH	low-molecular-weight heparin
LP	lumbar puncture
LRTI	lower respiratory tract infection
LV	left ventricular
LVF	left ventricular failure
LVH	left ventricular hypertrophy
LVSD	left ventricular systolic dysfunction
MAOIs	monoamine oxidase inhibitors
MAU	medical admissions unit
MCV	mean cell volume
MHRA	Medicines and Healthcare products Regulatory Agency
MI	myocardial infarction
MO	marginalis obtusis
MOH	major obstetric haemorrhage
MMSE	Mini-Mental State Examination
MRI	magnetic resonance imaging
MRSA	methicillin-resistant *Staphylococcus aureus*
MST	morphine sulphate tablets
MSU	midstream urine
NAC	*N*-acetyl cysteine
NASCET	North American Symptomatic Carotid Endarterectomy
NBM	nil by mouth
NCA	nurse-controlled analgesia
NEB	nebulised
NG	nasogastric
NIF	negative inspiratory force
NJ	nasojejunal
NICE	National Institute for Health and Care Excellence
NIV	noninvasive ventilation
NMDA	*N*-methyl-D-aspartate
NP	nasopharyngeal
NPA	nasopharyngeal aspirate
NPIS	National Poisons Information Service
NSAID	nonsteroidal antiinflammatory drug
NSTEMI	non-ST elevation myocardial infarction
NTD	neural tube defects
NYHA	New York Heart Association
OCP	oral contraceptive pill
OD	omni die (once daily)
PA	postero-anterior
PCA	patient-controlled analgesia
PCI	percutaneous coronary intervention
PCR	protein–creatinine ratio
PE	pulmonary embolism
PEF	peak expiratory flow
PIL	Patient Information Leaflet
PMH	past medical history
PO	per oram (orally)
POM	prescription-only medication
PPHN	persistent pulmonary hypertension of the newborn
PPI	proton pump inhibitor
PR	per rectum
PRN	pro re nata (when required)
PT	prothrombin time
PV	per vaginam (by vagina)
QDS	quater die sumendus (four times daily)
RCA	right coronary artery
RCC	red cell concentrate
RDS	respiratory distress syndrome
RR	respiratory rate
RSV	respiratory syncytial virus
RUL	right upper lobe
RCX	right circumflex artery
SABA	short-acting β2 agonist
SAMA	short-acting muscarinic antagonist
SBP	spontaneous bacterial peritonitis
SBR	serum bilirubin
SC	subcutaneous
SCBU	special care baby unit
SFH	symphysis–fundal height
SHO	Senior House Officer
SIADH	syndrome of inappropriate antidiuretic hormone

SIRS	systemic inflammatory response syndrome
SL	sublingual
SLE	systemic lupus erythematosus
SmPCs	Summary of Product Characteristics
SNRI	serotonin norepinephrine reuptake inhibitor
SOB	shortness of breath
SR	sinus rhythm
SR	sustained release
SSRI	selective-serotonin reuptake inhibitor
STAT	statim (immediately)
STEMI	ST elevation myocardial infarction
SVC	superior vena cava
SVT	supraventricular tachycardia
TA-GvHD	transfusion-associated graft vs host disease
TB	tuberculosis
TIA	transient ischaemic attack
TDS	ter die sumendus (three times daily)
TED	thromboembolism deterrent
TENS	transcutaneous electrical nerve stimulation
TFT	thyroid function test
THR	total hip replacement
TPMT	thiopurine methyltransferase
TIPSS	transjugular intrahepatic portosystemic shunt
TOP	topical
TPMT	thiopurine *S*-methyl transferase
TPN	total parenteral nutrition
TRALI	transfusion-related acute lung injury
TSH	thyroid stimulating hormone
TTO	to take out
tx	treatment
UC	ulcerative colitis
U&E	urea and electrolyte
UKTIS	UK Teratology Information Service
U/L	units per litre
USS	ultrasound
UTI	urinary tract infection
VBG	venous blood gas
VSD	ventricular septal defect
VTE	venous thromboembolism
VWD	von Willebrand disease
WBC	white blood cell
WCC	white cell count
WHO	World Health Organization

Contributors

SERIES AND VOLUME EDITOR

Zeshan Qureshi, BM, BSc (Hons), MSc, MRCPCH, FAcadMEd, MRCPS (Glasg)
Paediatric Registrar
London Deanery
London, UK

VOLUME EDITORS

Ali B.A.K. Al-Hadithi, MB Bchir, MA (Cantab), MRCP (UK), AFHEA, PGCert (Med Ed)
Clinical Research Training Fellow
University of Cambridge
Cambridge, UK;
Cambridge University Hospitals NHS Foundation Trust
Cambridge, UK

Simon R.J. Maxwell, BSc, MB, ChB, MD, PhD, FRCP, FRCPE, FHEA, FBPhS
Professor
Clinical Pharmacology Unit
University of Edinburgh
Edinburgh, Scotland, UK

AUTHORS

Samuel Lockley, MA, MBChB, MRCOG
Consultant Obstetrician and Gynaecologist
Walsall Healthcare NHS Trust
Walsall, UK

Alexandra Richards, MBBCh, BSc
Senior Resident Medical Officer
Sydney Children's Hospital Network;
Conjoint Associate Lecturer
Discipline of Paediatrics and Child Health
University of New South Wales

Matthew G. Wood, BM, MRCOG
Consultant Obsterician and Gynaecologist
The Shrewsbury and Telford Hospitals
NHS Trust, UK

Introduction to Prescribing

1

Simon R.J. Maxwell

Chapter Outline

The Characteristics of a Good Prescriber
Basic Principles of Clinical Pharmacology
Adverse Drug Reactions
Drug Interactions
Medication Errors
Rational Prescribing
Prescribing for Patients With Special Requirements
Getting Information About Medicines
Writing a Prescription
Prescribing Intravenous (IV) Fluids
Monitoring Drug Therapy

THE CHARACTERISTICS OF A GOOD PRESCRIBER

Prescribing is an essential skill for most doctors and is the major tool used to restore or preserve the health and quality of life of their patients. Prescribing is also associated with significant risks related to adverse drug reactions (ADRs) and interactions, often caused by inappropriate prescribing, as well as prescribing errors. Prescribing effectively and safely represents a significant intellectual challenge that combines knowledge, judgement and skills, and can be subdivided into 10 basic components (Fig. 1.1).

The important characteristics of good prescribers include:

- Being clear about the reasons for prescribing a medicine and seeking to establish an accurate diagnosis whenever possible (although this may often be difficult).
- Taking into account the patient's medication history before prescribing by obtaining an accurate list of current and recent medications as well as prior ADRs.
- Taking into account other variables that might alter the benefits and risks of treatment (e.g. physiological changes with age and pregnancy, or impaired kidney, liver or heart function).
- Taking into account the patient's ideas, concerns and expectations; seeking to form a partnership with the patient when selecting treatments, and making sure that they understand and agree with the reasons for taking the medicine.
- Selecting effective, safe and cost-effective medicines individualised for the patient and choosing the optimal formulation, dose, frequency, route of administration and duration of treatment.
- Adhering to national guidelines and local formularies where appropriate, and knowing where to find reliable information to inform prescribing decisions.
- Writing unambiguous legal prescriptions using the correct documentation and being aware of common factors that cause medication errors.
- Knowing how to monitor the beneficial and adverse effects of medicines and modifying the prescription appropriately as a result of this information.
- Communicating and documenting prescribing decisions clearly with patients and professional colleagues and being able to counsel patients about their medicines.
- Prescribing within the limitations of their knowledge, skills and experience.

It is an increasing challenge for junior prescribers to acquire these skills and put them into practice in the face of growing pressures related to the increasing number of drugs available, the greater complexity of treatment regimens taken by individual patients ('polypharmacy') and the greater number of elderly and vulnerable patients being treated. The following sections review in more detail some of the knowledge and skills that form the basis of good prescribing.

BASIC PRINCIPLES OF CLINICAL PHARMACOLOGY

Clinical pharmacology is the study of the way that drugs act on and are handled by the human body and it is the science that underpins rational prescribing. It can be divided into two fundamental concepts (Fig. 1.2):

- Pharmacodynamics: the study of 'what the drug does to the body'
- Pharmacokinetics: the study of 'what the body does to the drug'

Both have an important influence on the way in which an individual responds to a prescribed drug and provide an understanding of why there is so much potential interindividual variation in the response to the same prescription.

PHARMACODYNAMICS

Drugs act to restore normal function in diseased cells and tissues by acting on receptors or other target

PATIENT History - examination - investigations				
1	Make a diagnosis	Knowledge	Judgement	Skill
2	Establish the therapeutic goal	Knowledge	Judgement	Skill
3	Choose the therapeutic approach	Knowledge	Judgement	Skill
4	Choose the drug	Knowledge	Judgement	Skill
5	Choose the dose, route and frequency	Knowledge	Judgement	Skill
6	Choose the duration of therapy	Knowledge	Judgement	Skill
7	Write the prescription	Knowledge	Judgement	Skill
8	Inform the patient	Knowledge	Judgement	Skill
9	Monitor the drug effects	Knowledge	Judgement	Skill
10	Review/alter the prescription	Knowledge	Judgement	Skill

Fig. 1.1 **The subcomponents of the prescribing process.** The process of prescribing can be conveniently divided into 10 subcompetencies, each of which involves a mix of knowledge, judgement and skills. A 'prescription' is sometimes referred to more specifically as a 'medication order'. Steps 2 and 3 should try to take the patient's views into consideration to establish a therapeutic partnership. A drug is a single chemical substance that has pharmacological effects on the body and is administered as a 'medicine', a formulation containing one or more drugs mixed with other ingredients.

molecules in the affected organ (Table 1.1). Binding to target receptors exerts a biological effect, either by initiating new events (e.g. smooth muscle contraction, synthesis of new proteins) or by blocking the actions of endogenous substances (e.g. neurotransmitters, hormones).

Formation of the drug–receptor complex is usually reversible and the proportion of receptors occupied (and thus the response) is directly related to the concentration of the drug. This reversibility means that prescribers usually have to plan a series of repeated drug administrations to achieve the desired therapeutic outcome. Some drug–receptor interactions are so strong that they are effectively irreversible (e.g. aspirin acting at the enzyme cyclo-oxygenase). The extent of the reversibility is determined by the strength of the chemical bond that is formed, often referred to as the 'affinity' of the binding. Differences in affinity mean that some drug ligands may show 'selectivity' for different types of receptors and allow them to be further divided into 'subtypes'. For example, adrenoceptors can be subtyped into α, β_1 and β_2, on the basis of their binding and responsiveness to the endogenous agonists, adrenaline and noradrenaline. Agonist or antagonist drugs that are considered to be 'selective' for one receptor subtype can still produce significant effects at other subtypes if a high enough dose is given. For instance, 'cardioselective' beta-blocking drugs have antianginal effects on the heart (β_1) but may cause bronchospasm in the lung (β_2) and are absolutely contraindicated for asthmatic patients.

Dose–Response Relationships

The relationship between the concentration of the drug to which tissues are exposed and the response that is achieved can be plotted on a dose–response

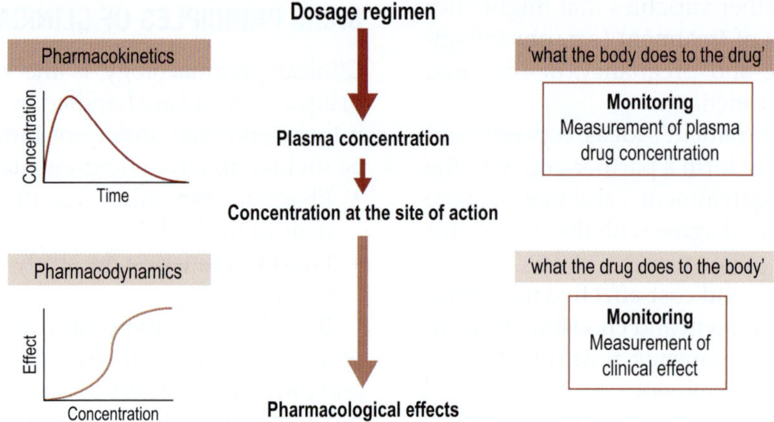

Fig. 1.2 **Relationship between pharmacodynamics and pharmacokinetics.** Basic pharmacodynamic studies involve exposing cells or tissues to varying doses (concentrations) of a drug and observing the response to describe a 'dose–response' curve. For prescribers, the situation is more complex, because tissue drug exposure depends on how effectively drug molecules are absorbed into the body, distributed to their site of action and subsequently eliminated from the body by metabolism and excretion. These processes are known collectively as pharmacokinetics and are described by plotting drug concentration over time.

Table 1.1 Drug Targets

DRUG TARGET RECEPTORS	DESCRIPTION	EXAMPLE
Channel-linked receptors	Receptor binding opens a channel, making the cell membrane permeable to specific ions	Nicotinic acetylcholine receptor
G-protein-coupled receptors (GPCRs)	Receptor binding leads to interaction with a family of closely related 'G-proteins' that are coupled to intracellular enzyme activation (or the opening of an ion channel). Secondary messenger systems include the enzymes, adenylate cyclase and guanylate cyclase, which generate cyclic AMP and cyclic GMP, respectively	Muscarinic acetylcholine receptor β-Adrenoceptors Dopamine receptors Serotonin receptors Opioid receptors
Kinase-linked receptors	Receptor binding is linked to activation of an intracellular protein kinase that triggers a cascade of phosphorylation reactions	Insulin receptors
DNA-linked receptors	These are located in the cell nucleus ('nuclear receptors') where binding promotes or inhibits signals to synthesise new proteins, which may take hours or days to produce a biological effect	Steroid receptors Thyroid receptors Vitamin D receptors
Other Targets		
Voltage-sensitive ion channels	Drugs can alter the conductance of these channels that are required to allow the transmission of depolarisation in excitable tissues	Na^+ channels blocked by local anaesthetics (e.g. lidocaine)
Enzymes	Drugs interfere with the active site of the enzyme that catalyses biochemical reactions involved in the production of key mediators of physiological processes	Cyclo-oxygenase (e.g. aspirin) Angiotensin-converting enzyme (ACE) (e.g. ramipril) Xanthine oxidase (e.g. allopurinol)
Transporter proteins	Specialised proteins that carry ions or molecules across cell membranes	Serotonin reuptake transporter (e.g. fluoxetine)

AMP, Adenosine monophosphate; *GMP*, guanosine monophosphate.

curve. When the relation between drug dose (x-axis) and drug response (y-axis) is plotted on a base 10 logarithmic scale, this produces a sigmoidal dose–response curve (Fig. 1.3). Progressive increases in the drug dose (which for most drugs is proportional to the plasma drug concentration) produce increasing response, but this occurs over a relatively narrow part of the overall concentration range; further increases in drug dose beyond this range produce little extra effect. The clinical implication of this relationship is that simply increasing drug dose may not result in any further beneficial effects for patients and may cause adverse effects.

When drugs are used in clinical practice, the prescriber is unable to construct a careful dose–response curve for each individual patient. Therefore, most drugs are licensed for use within a recommended dose range that is expected to be close to the top of the dose–response curve for most patients. This ensures that most patients will achieve a good clinical response without the need for frequent review and dose increases. However, this means that it is sometimes possible to achieve the desired therapeutic response at doses towards the lower end of the recommended range.

Agonists and Antagonists

Agonists are drugs that bind to a receptor and initiate a biological response (e.g. adrenaline causing an increase in heart rate via β_1-adrenoreceptors in the heart). Other examples of agonists in clinical use include opioid analgesics (μ-opioid receptor), benzodiazepines (gamma-aminobutyric acid type A ($GABA_A$)), and sumatriptan ($5\text{-}HT_{1D}$ and $5\text{-}HT_{1B}$).

Antagonists are drugs that bind to a receptor but do not initiate any biological response. Their importance is that they can block the effect of agonists (e.g. atenolol antagonising the effect of adrenaline at β_1 adrenoreceptors in the heart).

'Competitive antagonists' will lead to a shift in the agonist dose–response curve to the right because higher agonist concentrations are now required to achieve a given percentage receptor occupancy (and therefore effect). Their effect can be overcome by giving the agonist at a sufficiently high concentration (i.e. it is surmountable). Examples of competitive antagonists used in clinical practice are atenolol (β_1-adrenoceptors), atropine (muscarinic M2), naloxone (μ-opioid), losartan (angiotensin-AT_1) and ranitidine (histamine-H_2).

'Noncompetitive' antagonists inhibit the effect of an agonist in ways other than direct competition for receptor binding with the agonist (e.g. by affecting the secondary messenger system). This makes it impossible to achieve maximum response even at very high-agonist concentration. Examples include the action of ketamine at *N*-methyl-D-aspartate (NMDA) receptors. Irreversible antagonists can be considered as a particular form

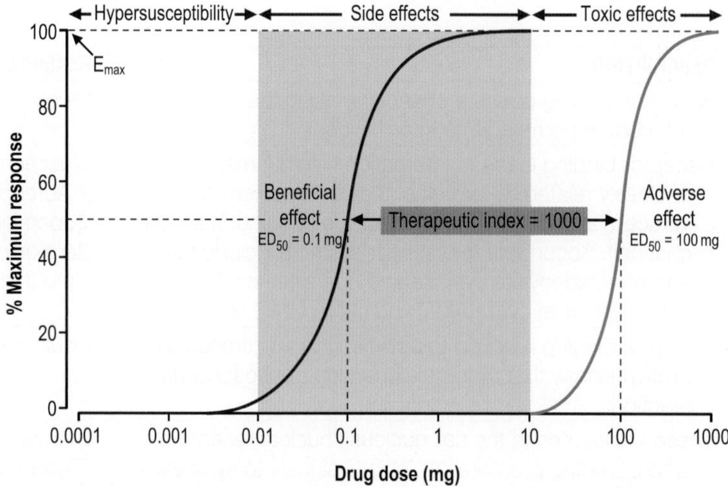

Fig. 1.3 **Dose–response curve.** A plot of drug response in relation to changes in drug dose on a $\log_{10}$ scale. The *purple curve* represents this relationship for the beneficial therapeutic effect of this drug. The maximum response on the curve is referred to as the E_{max} and the dose (or concentration) producing half this value ($E_{max}/2$) is the ED_{50} (or EC_{50}). Clinical responses that might be plotted in this way include change in heart rate, blood pressure, gastric pH or blood glucose. It is possible to plot a curve for the adverse effects of drugs, which are also usually dose related. The *grey curve* illustrates the relationship for the most important adverse effect of this drug. This requires much higher doses to become manifest. The relationship between the ED_{50} for the adverse effects and beneficial effects is known as the 'therapeutic index'. This nominal figure is an expression of how much margin there is for prescribers when choosing a dosage that will provide beneficial effects without also causing adverse effects. Adverse effects that occur at doses beyond the therapeutic range *(purple box)* are normally called 'toxic effects', while those occurring within it and below it are known as 'side effects' and 'hypersusceptibility effects', respectively. The therapeutic index in this example is calculated as 100/0.1=1000.

of noncompetitive antagonist characterised by antagonism that persists even after the antagonist drug has been removed because of irreversible binding to the receptor (e.g. phenoxybenzamine at α_1-adrenoceptors). Similar irreversible binding occurs at other target molecules (e.g. aspirin at cyclo-oxygenase, omeprazole at proton pumps) and requires synthesis of new target proteins before normal function is restored.

Efficacy and Potency

'Efficacy' is the term used to describe the maximum response that a drug can achieve when all available receptors or binding sites are occupied. This is equivalent to E_{max} on the dose–response curve.

'Therapeutic efficacy' is a term used to describe the maximum response of drugs that produce the same therapeutic effects on the body but do so via different pharmacological mechanisms (e.g. loop diuretics have greater therapeutic efficacy as natriuretics than thiazide diuretics).

'Potency' is a term used to describe the amount of a drug required for a given response (i.e. more potent drugs produce biological effects at lower doses).

Therapeutic Index

The adverse effects of drugs are usually dose related in a similar way to the beneficial effects, although the dose–response curve for significant adverse effects is normally found to the right (see Fig. 1.3). The ED_{50} points for each curve indicate that the ratio between the doses that have similar proportionate effects on the two outcomes is 100/0.1 = 1000. This ratio is known as the 'therapeutic index'. In reality, drugs have multiple potential adverse effects but the concept of therapeutic index is usually reserved for those requiring dose reduction or discontinuation. For most drugs, the therapeutic index is greater than 100, but there are some notable exceptions with therapeutic indices less than 10, which are in common use (e.g. digoxin, warfarin, insulin, phenytoin, opioids). The challenge for prescribers is to titrate doses carefully to establish the dose for individual patients that maximises benefits but avoids adverse effects.

Desensitisation and Withdrawal

Desensitisation refers to the situation where the response to a drug diminishes when it is given continuously or repeatedly. The response may be restored by increasing the dose of the drug, but in some cases, the tissues may become completely refractory.

'Tachyphylaxis' describes desensitisation that occurs very rapidly, sometimes due to depletion of chemicals that may be necessary for drug action (e.g. a stored neurotransmitter).

'Tolerance' describes a more gradual loss of response to a drug that occurs over days or weeks, which may be due to changes in receptor numbers or the development of counter-regulatory physiological changes that offset the actions of the drug (e.g. activation of the sympathetic and renin–angiotensin systems in response to vasodilator or diuretic therapy).

When desensitisation arises because of chemical, hormonal and physiological changes that offset the actions of a drug, discontinuation may allow these

Table 1.2 Drugs Associated With Desensitisation and Withdrawal Effects

DRUG	SYMPTOMS AND SIGNS
Alcohol	Anxiety, panic, paranoid delusions, hallucinations, agitation, restlessness, confusion, tremor, tachycardia, ataxia, reduced consciousness, disorientation, seizures
Benzodiazepines	As for alcohol
Opioids	Anxiety, lacrimation, rhinorrhoea, sneezing, yawning, abdominal cramping, leg cramping, nausea, vomiting, diarrhoea, dilated pupils, photophobia, insomnia, autonomic hyperactivity (tachypnoea, hyperreflexia, tachycardia, sweating, hypertension, hyperthermia)
Selective serotonin reuptake inhibitors	Dizziness, sweating, nausea, insomnia, tremor, confusion, nightmares
Corticosteroids	Weakness, fatigue, decreased appetite, weight loss, nausea, vomiting, diarrhoea, abdominal pain, hypotension, hypoglycaemia
Nitrates	Chest pain, dyspnoea, palpitations
Clonidine	Hypertensive crisis
Cannabinoids	Insomnia, irritability, decreased appetite, shakiness and, less often, sweating and chills

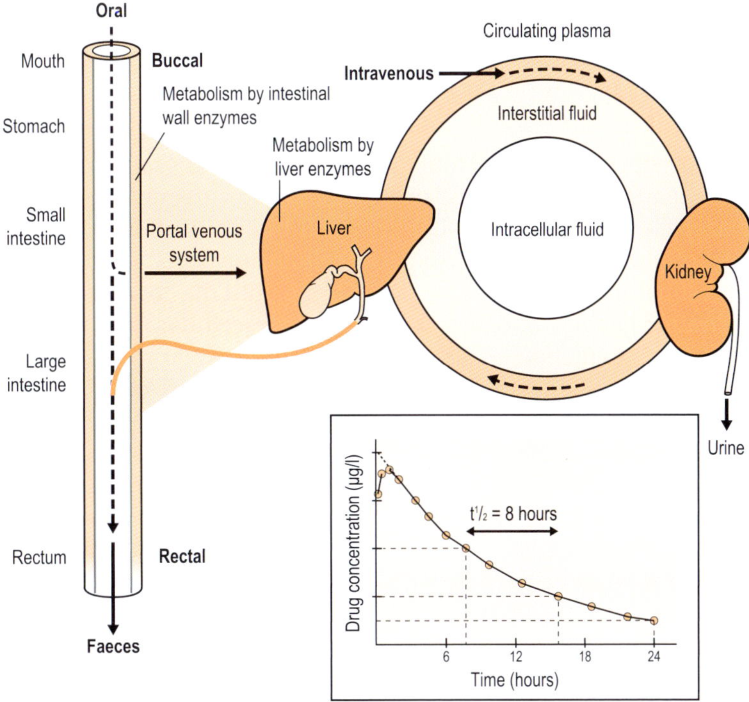

Fig. 1.4 **Pharmacokinetics summary.** A simple view of the main phases of pharmacokinetics. Most drugs are taken orally. Drug molecules are subsequently absorbed from the intestinal lumen, enter the portal venous system and are conveyed to the liver, where they may be subject to first-pass metabolism. Those passing through unchanged enter the systemic circulation, from which they may diffuse out into the surrounding interstitial fluid and into the intracellular fluid. Drug that remains in circulating plasma will be continuously exposed to the possibility of liver metabolism and renal excretion. These processes will lead to the elimination of all of the drug with time *(inset graph)* unless further doses are administered. First-pass metabolism is avoided if drugs are administered via the buccal or rectal mucosa, or parenterally (e.g. by intravenous injection).

changes to cause rebound 'withdrawal effects'. Examples of drugs associated with desensitisation and withdrawal effects are shown in Table 1.2.

PHARMACOKINETICS

Pharmacokinetics is the study of the rate and extent to which drugs are absorbed into the body and distributed to the body tissues, and the rate and pathways by which drugs are eliminated from the body by metabolism and excretion (Fig. 1.4). An understanding of these four processes is important for prescribers because they form the basis on which the optimal dose regimen is chosen and explain the majority of the inter-individual variation in the response to drug therapy.

The term 'bioavailability' describes the proportion of the dose that reaches the systemic circulation unscathed.

Drug Absorption

Absorption is the process by which drug molecules gain access to the bloodstream from the site of drug administration. The rate and extent of drug absorption depend on the route of administration (see Fig. 1.4). The 'enteral' routes of absorption are those that involve administration via the gastrointestinal tract:

- *Oral (ORAL or PO)* administration is the commonest route because it is simple, convenient and can readily be used by patients to self-administer their medicines. For successful oral administration, it is necessary that the medicine is swallowed, the drug survives exposure to gastric acid, avoids unacceptable food binding, is absorbed across the small bowel mucosa into the portal venous system and survives metabolism by gut wall or liver enzymes ('first-pass metabolism'). Therefore, absorption is usually incomplete following oral administration
- *Buccal and sublingual (SL)* administration enables rapid absorption into the systemic circulation without the uncertainties associated with the oral route (e.g. organic nitrates for angina pectoris, triptans for migraine, opioid analgesics)
- *Rectal (PR)* administration is useful when the oral route is compromised because of nausea and vomiting or unconsciousness (e.g. diazepam in status epilepticus).

The 'parenteral' routes of administration avoid absorption via the gastrointestinal tract:

- *Intravenous (IV)* administration enables all of a dose reliably to enter the systemic circulation, without any concerns about absorption or first-pass metabolism (i.e. the dose is 100% bioavailable), and rapidly achieves a high-plasma concentration. It is the ideal route to use when treating very ill patients where rapid, certain effect is critical to outcome (e.g. benzylpenicillin for meningococcal meningitis)
- *Intramuscular (IM)* administration is usually easier to achieve than the IV route (e.g. adrenaline for acute anaphylaxis) but absorption is unpredictable and depends on muscle blood flow
- *Subcutaneous (SC)* administration is ideal for drugs that require parenteral administration, are absorbed well from SC fat and might ideally be injected by patients themselves (e.g. insulins, low-molecular-weight heparins).

Other common routes of administration include:

- *Inhaled (INH)* administration allows drugs to be delivered directly to a target in the respiratory tree, usually the small airways (e.g. salbutamol and beclometasone for asthma). The most common mode of delivery is the metered-dose inhaler but its success depends on some degree of manual dexterity and timing. Patients who find these difficult may use a 'spacer' device to improve drug delivery. A special mode of inhaled delivery is via a 'nebulised' (NEB) solution created by using pressurised oxygen or air to break up solutions and suspensions into small aerosol droplets that can be directly inhaled from the mouthpiece of the nebuliser and is often used in emergency treatment
- *Transdermal* administration, often via a transdermal patch, can enable a drug to be absorbed through the skin and into the circulation (e.g. oestrogens, nicotine, nitrates, opioids)
- *Topical (TOP)* administration involves direct application to the site of action (e.g. skin, eye, ear). This has the advantage of achieving sufficient concentration at this site while minimising systemic exposure and the risk of unwanted adverse effects elsewhere.

Drug Distribution

Distribution is the process by which drug molecules move from their site of absorption into the bloodstream and then enter the extracellular fluid (and potentially cells) in various tissues around the body, including the site of action. The rate and extent at which distribution occurs will depend upon the drug's molecular size and lipid solubility, and the extent to which it binds reversibly to plasma proteins. Most drug molecules diffuse passively across capillary walls down a concentration gradient into the extracellular (interstitial) fluid surrounding organs and tissues. There they will bind reversibly with target molecules and other cellular proteins. Distribution to the tissues will continue until the concentration of free drug molecules in the extracellular fluid and (if the drug can enter cells) the intracellular space is equal to the concentration in the plasma and equilibrium is achieved. The movement of drug molecules will then reverse, because the plasma drug concentration begins to fall as those that remain in the blood are subject to elimination by metabolism or excretion. This reverse movement of the drug away from the tissues will be prevented if further drug doses are administered and absorbed into the plasma.

Volume of Distribution

The apparent volume of distribution (V_d) is the volume that a drug appears to have distributed into shortly following IV injection. It is calculated from the equation $C_0 = D/V_d$, where D is the amount of drug given and C_0 is the initial plasma concentration. Drugs that are highly bound to plasma proteins may have a low V_d < 10 L (e.g. warfarin, aspirin), while those that diffuse into the extracellular fluid but have low lipid solubility do not enter cells and may have a V_d between 10 and 30 L (e.g. gentamicin, amoxycillin). It is an 'apparent' volume because drugs that are lipid soluble and highly tissue bound may have a V_d > 100 L (e.g. digoxin, amitriptyline). Drugs with a larger V_d have longer 'half-lives', take longer to achieve 'steady state' after regular administration, are more likely to require a 'loading dose' if an early clinical effect is important (e.g. digoxin, amiodarone) and take longer to eliminate after administration is stopped.

Drug Metabolism

Metabolism is the process by which drugs are structurally altered from a lipid-soluble form suitable for absorption and distribution to a water-soluble form that is necessary for excretion. There are two phases of drug metabolism. 'Phase I metabolism' involves oxidation, reduction or hydrolysis to make drug molecules suitable for phase II reactions or for excretion.

- *Phase I metabolism.* Oxidation is the commonest form of phase I reaction and involves chiefly members of the cytochrome P450 family of membrane-bound enzymes in the smooth endoplasmic reticulum of the liver cells. Phase I metabolism typically renders drugs pharmacologically inactive but is sometimes necessary to activate 'prodrugs' (e.g. clopidogrel, codeine). The activity of phase I enzymes can be increased by enzyme inducing drugs (e.g. rifampicin, phenytoin, carbamazepine), a process that reduces the bioavailability of other P450 substrates and takes several days to occur. Conversely, some drugs are enzyme inhibitors (e.g. fluconazole, clarithromycin, ciprofloxacin, omeprazole) that rapidly increase the plasma concentration of other P450 substrates as soon as they are co-administered. These phenomena are the basis of some important drug interactions.
- *Phase II metabolism.* This involves combining phase I metabolites with an endogenous substrate (e.g. glucuronidation, sulphation, methylation) to form an inactive conjugate that is much more water soluble. This is necessary to enable excretion because lipid-soluble metabolites will simply diffuse back into the body. Most conjugates are pharmacologically inactive but a notable exception is morphine 6-glucuronide.

Drug Excretion

Excretion is the process by which drugs and their metabolites are removed from the body. They may leave in the urine, bile, faeces or expired air. Renal excretion is the main route of elimination for low molecular weight drugs (<300 Da) and their metabolites if they are sufficiently water soluble to avoid reabsorption from the renal tubule. For some drugs, active secretion from capillaries into the proximal tubule, rather than glomerular filtration, is the predominant mechanism of excretion (e.g. methotrexate, penicillin). Faecal excretion is the preferred route of elimination for larger-molecular-weight drugs, including those that are excreted in the bile after conjugation with glucuronide in the liver, and any drugs that are not absorbed. Some drugs or metabolites that are excreted in the bile are sufficiently lipid soluble to be reabsorbed through the gut wall and return to the liver via the portal vein (see Fig. 1.4). This recycling is known as the 'entero-hepatic circulation' and can significantly prolong the residence of drugs in the body. 'Clearance' is the term used to describe the volume of plasma that is completely cleared of drug per unit time (expressed as mL/min) and is usually the result of either hepatic metabolism or renal excretion, or a combination of both.

Concentration–Time Relationships

For most drugs, elimination is a high-capacity process that does not become saturated, even at high dosage. Within this range, the rate of elimination is proportional to the amount of drug in the body (i.e. the higher the drug concentration the faster the rate of elimination). This results in so-called 'first-order kinetics' where a constant fraction of the drug remaining in the body is eliminated in a given time and the decline in concentration over time is exponential (Fig. 1.5). The importance of this relationship to prescribers is that it means the effect of increasing doses on plasma concentration is predictable—a doubled dose leads to a doubled concentration at all time points. Half-life ($t_{½}$) is the time taken for the plasma concentration of a drug eliminated by first-order metabolism to halve. For a few drugs in common use (e.g. phenytoin, salicylates, alcohol), elimination capacity is exceeded (saturated) within the therapeutic range of dosage resulting in 'zero-order (saturable) kinetics', where a constant amount of the drug remaining in the body is eliminated in a given time. If the rate of administration exceeds the maximum rate of elimination, the drug will accumulate progressively leading to serious toxicity.

Repeated Doses

For most drugs, it is necessary to maintain therapeutic effect beyond the first dose, often for several days (e.g. antibiotics) or even for months or years (e.g. antihypertensives, lipid-lowering drugs). This requires prescribers to plan a regimen of repeated doses, indicating the size of each individual dose, the frequency of dose administration and the overall duration of treatment. When doses are repeated, the drug will progressively accumulate in the body and its eventual plasma concentration will be considerably higher than that after a single dose (Fig. 1.6). Accumulation will continue until a 'steady state' is reached because the rate of elimination has increased to equal the rate of administration. It takes five half-lives to achieve a plasma concentration that is 97% of the steady-state level (irrespective of the dosing interval). This is important for prescribers because it means that the effects of a new prescription, or dose titration, for a drug with a long half-life (e.g. digoxin—36 hours) may not be known for a few days. In these circumstances, the target plasma concentration can be achieved safely before five half-lives have elapsed by giving an initial 'loading dose' that is much larger than the maintenance dose, and equivalent to the amount of drug required in the body at steady state (see Fig. 1.6). This achieves a peak plasma concentration close to the plateau concentration, which can then be maintained by successive maintenance doses.

The steady state achieved by regular drug administration actually involves fluctuations in drug

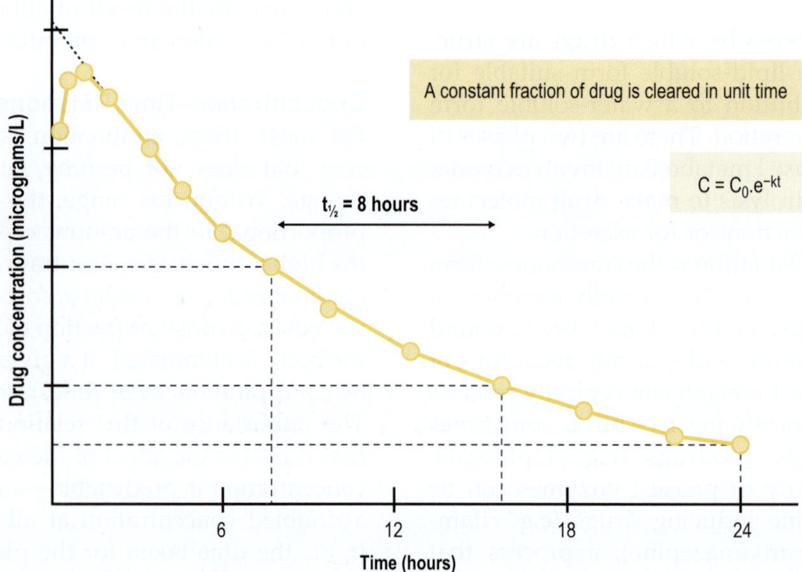

Fig. 1.5 First-order kinetics. The decline of drug concentration with time when elimination is a first-order process. The time period required for the plasma drug concentration to halve (half-life, $t_{½}$) remains constant throughout the elimination process. K = elimination rate constant, e = base of the natural logarithm, C_0 = concentration at time zero, t = time.

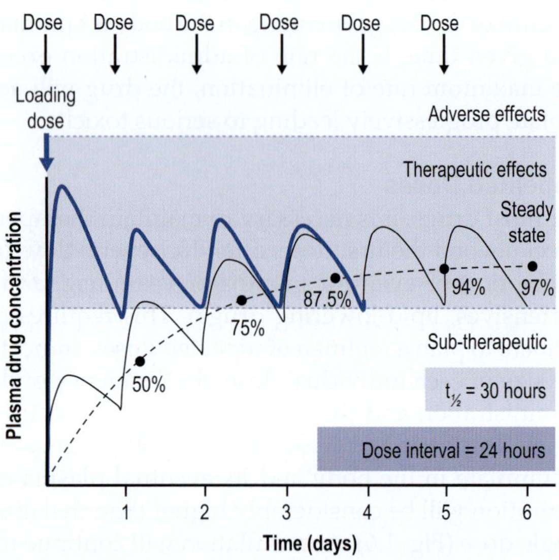

Fig. 1.6 Repeated drug doses. The plasma drug concentration rises after successive daily oral doses. The drug's half-life is 30 hours so each successive dose is administered at a time when there is still drug present in the body. The peak, average and trough concentrations steadily increase as drug accumulates in the body. Steady state is reached after approximately five half-lives when the concentration of drug in the body is sufficient to mean that the rate of elimination (the product of concentration and clearance) is equal to the rate of drug absorption (the product of rate of administration and bioavailability). The long half-life means that it takes 6 days for steady state to be achieved and, for most of the first 3 days of treatment, plasma drug concentrations are below the therapeutic range. This problem can be overcome if a larger loading dose is used to achieve the quantity of drug in the body at steady state more rapidly. It still requires five half-lives to get to steady state but therapeutic concentrations are present for most of this period.

concentration between peaks just after administration and troughs just prior to the next administration. Recommended dosing regimens are chosen to keep the troughs in the effective range while the peaks are not high enough to cause adverse effects. The dose interval is a compromise between convenience for the patient and a constant level of drug exposure. More frequent administration (25 mg four times daily) achieves a smoother plasma concentration profile than 100 mg once daily but is much more difficult to sustain. For drugs with short half-lives that would need frequent administration, a solution is the use of 'modified-release' formulations. These allow drugs to be more slowly absorbed from the gastrointestinal tract and provide a smoother plasma concentration profile, which is especially important for drugs with a low therapeutic index (e.g. levodopa, verapamil, morphine).

INTERINDIVIDUAL VARIATION

The recommendations of how to prescribe drugs safely and effectively (e.g. dose, route, frequency, duration) for specific indications are based on average dose–response data derived from observations in many individuals. Prescribers can never be certain about the response for particular patients that they treat. However, much of the variability in response is predictable and good prescribers are able to anticipate it and adjust their prescriptions accordingly to maximise the chances of benefit and minimise harm. Different responses may be due to several factors:

- *Pharmacodynamic variation* arises when an equivalent drug concentration results in a different response because of varying receptor number and structure, receptor-coupling mechanisms and physiological changes in target organs resulting from differences in genetics, age and health. For example, the beneficial natriuresis produced by the loop diuretic furosemide is often significantly reduced at a given dose in patients with renal impairment while confusion caused by opioid analgesics is more likely in the elderly.

- *Pharmacokinetic variation* arises when the drug concentrations achieved by equivalent doses vary and is a much more important cause of the interindividual variation in drug responses encountered in clinical practice. For example, when given at equivalent dosages, patients with renal impairment have higher steady-state concentrations of renally excreted drugs (e.g. aminoglycosides) and patients with advanced liver disease have a similarly increased exposure to drugs normally eliminated by hepatic metabolism (e.g. verapamil).
- *Pharmacogenetic variation* arises because of genetic polymorphisms that influence both the pharmacodynamic response and pharmacokinetic handling of drugs. The impact of genetics on the response to specific drugs ('pharmacogenetics') is gradually being uncovered and will eventually enable prescribers to identify in advance the good responders and those who will suffer adverse effects. This move towards 'personalised medicine', based on genetic testing, has the potential to improve the benefit–risk ratio of the drugs that we already have but also to improve the chances of drug discovery (many drugs are lost in development because they cause an unacceptable rate of adverse effects in average unselected patient groups).

Important examples of variations in drug responses are given in Table 1.3. The uncertain outcome of drug therapy for individual patients emphasises the need for prescribers to monitor the effects of treatment (see later).

ADVERSE DRUG REACTIONS

The decision to prescribe a drug always involves a judgement of the balance of therapeutic benefit and risk of an adverse outcome. Both prescribers and patients tend to focus on the former but a truly informed prescribing decision requires consideration of both.

DEFINITION

An ADR is a response to a medicinal product that is noxious and unintended. The reaction is usually experienced following the administration of a drug, or combination of drugs, under normal conditions of use and is suspected to be related to the drug. ADRs can be conveniently divided into those that occur at concentrations beyond the normal therapeutic range ('toxic effects'), those that occur at concentrations in the therapeutic range (side effects) and those that occur at concentrations less than the therapeutic range (hypersusceptibility effects) (see Fig. 1.3). ADRs are important because they reduce the quality of life for patients, cause diagnostic confusion, undermine the confidence of patients in their healthcare and consume scarce healthcare resources because of the need for extra care of patients and litigation costs.

PREVALENCE

ADRs are a common cause of illness and account for around 3% of consultations in primary care and 7% of emergency admissions to hospital, and affect around 15% of hospital inpatients. Many 'disease' presentations are eventually attributed to ADRs, emphasising the importance of always taking a careful drug history from all patients (Box 1.1). ADRs appear to be increasing in prevalence due to the increasing age and vulnerability of patients, polypharmacy (higher risk of drug interactions) and the increasing trend towards self-medication (over-the-counter preparations, herbal or traditional medicines and medicines obtained from internet pharmacies). Retrospective analyses of ADRs have shown that around half could have been avoided if the prescriber had taken more care in anticipating the potential hazards of drug therapy. Non-steroidal anti-inflammatory drug (NSAID) use alone accounts each year for many thousands of emergency admissions as a result of upper gastrointestinal bleeding, additional cardiovascular events and acute kidney injury. In many cases, the patients were at increased risk due to their age, interacting drugs (e.g. aspirin, warfarin, angiotensin-converting enzyme (ACE) inhibitors, diuretics) or a past history of relevant organ damage (e.g. peptic ulcer disease). Drugs that commonly cause ADRs are listed in Table 1.4 and well-recognised risk factors for the occurrence of ADRs in Box 1.2.

FREQUENCY OF ADRS

Prescribers and their patients ideally want to know the frequency with which ADRs occur for a specific drug. Although this may be well characterised for common ADRs observed in carefully conducted clinical trials, it is less clear for rarely reported ADRs where the total number of reactions and patients exposed is not known. The words used to describe frequency are often misinterpreted by patients but the generally agreed meanings of descriptors found in product literature are very common (10% or more patient exposures result in an ADR), common (1%–10%), uncommon (0.1%–1%), rare (0.01%–0.1%) and very rare (0.01% or less).

CLASSIFICATION

ADRs have traditionally been classified into two major groups:

- *Type A ('Augmented') ADRs* are predictable from the known pharmacodynamic effects of the drug and are dose dependent, common (detected early in drug development) and usually mild (e.g. constipation caused by opioids, hypotension caused by antihypertensives).
- *Type B ('Bizarre') ADRs* are not predictable and are not obviously dose dependent in the therapeutic range, rare (remaining undiscovered until post-licensing)

Table 1.3 Examples of Intraindividual Variation Leading to Altered Drug Response

Pharmacodynamic Variation	
Increased sensitivity to drug action	Individuals may experience greater effects (beneficial or adverse) to a drug because their tissues or organs respond more effectively (e.g. the antihypertensive effect of ACE inhibitors is increased in dehydrated patients who have an activated renin–angiotensin system, confusion in response to opioid analgesics is more likely in elderly patients)
Reduced sensitivity to drug action	Individuals may be less likely to respond to some drugs (e.g. antihypertensive effect of ACE inhibitors patients with reduced glomerular filtration rate are less responsive to thiazide diuretics)
Pharmacokinetic Variation	
Age	Drug metabolism may be enhanced in young children and becomes less effective with advancing age. Drug excretion is reduced in old age because of the decline in renal function
Sex	Women have a greater proportion of body fat than men, meaning that the volume of distribution and half-life of lipid-soluble of drugs are increased
Body weight	Patients with increased body mass index (BMI) have a greater proportion of body fat, meaning that the volume of distribution and half-life of lipid-soluble drugs are increased. Larger patients with a normal BMI have larger body compartments into which drugs are distributed and may require larger doses
Hepatic function	Drug metabolism depends largely on isoenzymes of the cytochrome P450 system. Metabolism may be reduced in those patients with significant hepatic disease or those taking drugs that inhibit the enzymes (e.g. cimetidine, ciprofloxacin). Metabolising capacity may be increased as enzymes are induced following exposure to drugs (e.g. alcohol, carbamazepine, rifampicin, ritonavir) or herbs (e.g. St John's wort)
Renal function	Many drugs and their metabolites depend on renal excretion for elimination from the body (e.g. lithium, digoxin, gentamicin). Renal function declines with age and a variety of diseases, which may lead to drug accumulation
Gastrointestinal function	The extent of absorption depends on the absorptive capacity of the intestinal mucosa, which may be reduced in disease (e.g. Crohn's disease, coeliac disease) or after surgical resection
Food	Food in the stomach delays gastric emptying and reduces the rate of drug absorption. Some food constituents bind to drugs and reduce the extent of absorption
Alcohol	Regular alcohol consumption stimulates liver enzyme synthesis, while binge drinking may temporarily inhibit drug metabolism
Drugs	Drug–drug interactions have the potential to cause marked variation in the pharmacokinetic handling of drugs (see Table 1.5)
Pharmacogenetic Variation	
Affecting pharmacodynamic response	Trastuzumab has increased effectiveness in women with breast cancer expressing the human epidermal growth factor receptor 2-positive ($HER2^+$) Oxidant drugs (e.g. the antimalarials chloroquine and primaquine) are more likely to induce haemolysis in patients with glucose-6-phosphate dehydrogenase deficiency (G6PD)
Affecting pharmacokinetic handling	Individuals vary in their capacity to acetylate drugs and those who do so poorly may be exposed to increased adverse effects (e.g. isoniazid, hydralazine) Variations in several cytochrome P450 enzymes can alter the metabolism of many drugs: codeine undergoes oxidation (CYP2D6) to its more active metabolite morphine and so this variation may alter effectiveness and toxicity Decreased inactivation of suxamethonium (succinylcholine) during anaesthesia in those who have plasma pseudocholinesterase deficiency leads to prolonged paralysis of respiratory muscles and sometimes persistent apnoea requiring mechanical ventilation until the drug can be eliminated by alternate pathways (around 1 in 1500 people)

ACE, Angiotensin-converting enzyme.

and often severe. Patients who experience type B reactions are generally 'hypersusceptible' because of unpredictable immunological or genetic factors (e.g. anaphylaxis caused by penicillin, isoniazid causing peripheral neuropathy in poor acetylators).

This simple classification has shortcomings and a more detailed classification based on dose (see Fig. 1.3), timing and susceptibility (DoTS) is now used by those analysing ADRs in greater depth. The AB classification can be extended further as a reminder of some other types of ADR:

- *Type C ('Chronic/continuous') ADRs* occur only after prolonged continuous exposure to a drug (e.g. osteoporosis caused by corticosteroids).
- *Type D ('Delayed') ADRs* are delayed until after drug exposure, making diagnosis difficult (e.g.

Box 1.1 How to Take a Drug History

INFORMATION FROM THE PATIENT

- Current prescribed drugs including formulations (e.g. modified-release tablets), doses, routes of administration, frequency and timing, duration of treatment
- Medications that are often forgotten (e.g. contraceptives, over-the-counter drugs, herbal remedies, vitamins)
- Drugs that have been taken in the recent past and reasons for stopping
- Previous drug hypersensitivity reactions, their nature and time course (e.g. a rash, anaphylaxis)
- Previous ADRs, their nature and time course (e.g. muscle aches with simvastatin)
- Adherence to therapy (e.g. 'are you taking your medication regularly?')

INFORMATION FROM THE GENERAL PRACTITIONER OR PHARMACIST

- Current list of medications
- Previous ADRs

INFORMATION FROM THE MEDICAL RECORD

- Previous prescriptions and their indications
- Previous ADRs

INSPECTION OF MEDICINES

- Drugs and their containers (e.g. blister packs, bottles, vials) should be inspected for name, dosage and the number of dosage forms taken since dispensed as a guide to adherence

ADR, Adverse drug reaction.

malignancies that may emerge after immunosuppressive treatment such as azathioprine post-transplantation).

- *Type E ('End of treatment') ADRs* occur after abrupt drug withdrawal (see Table 1.2).

REPRODUCTIVE ADRS

A teratogen is a substance with the potential to affect the development of the fetus in the first 10 weeks of intrauterine life, leading to congenital abnormalities. Important drugs that are known to be teratogens include warfarin, phenytoin, sodium valproate, lithium, retinoids, statins and antithyroid drugs. The thalidomide disaster in the early 1960s highlighted the risk of teratogenicity and led to mandatory testing of all new drugs. Congenital defects in a live infant or aborted fetus should always lead to the suspicion of an ADR and a list of drug exposures should be sought. Drugs known to have important effects later in pregnancy include ACE inhibitors (renal agenesis), tetracyclines (teeth discolouration), NSAIDS (circulatory development) and opioids (neonatal respiratory depression).

DETECTING ADRS

Many type A ADRs become apparent early in the development of a new drug. However, simple mathematics

Table 1.4 Drugs That Are Common Causes of ADRs Seen in Clinical Practice

DRUG OR DRUG CLASS	IMPORTANT ADRS
ACE inhibitors (e.g. lisinopril)	Renal impairment, hyperkalaemia
Antibiotics (e.g. amoxycillin)	Nausea, diarrhoea
Anticoagulants (e.g. warfarin, heparin, apixaban)	Bleeding
Antipsychotics (e.g. haloperidol)	Falls, sedation, confusion
Aspirin	Gastrotoxicity (dyspepsia, gastrointestinal bleeding)
Benzodiazepines (e.g. diazepam)	Drowsiness, falls
Beta-blockers (e.g. atenolol)	Cold peripheries, bradycardia, lethargy
Calcium-channel blockers (e.g. amlodipine)	Ankle oedema
Digoxin	Nausea, anorexia, bradycardia
Insulin	Hypoglycaemia
Diuretics (e.g. furosemide, bendroflumethiazide)	Dehydration, electrolyte disturbance (hypokalaemia, hyponatraemia), hypotension, renal impairment
NSAIDs (e.g. ibuprofen)	Gastrotoxicity (dyspepsia, gastrointestinal bleeding) Renal impairment
Opioid analgesics (e.g. morphine, oxycodone)	Nausea, vomiting, confusion, constipation
Statins (e.g. atorvastatin)	Myalgia

ACE, Angiotensin-converting enzyme; *ADR,* adverse drug reaction; *NSAID,* non-steroidal antiinflammatory drug.

dictates that, at the time of licensing, rarer but potentially serious (type B) ADRs may remain undiscovered because of the limited number of human subjects exposed. 'Pharmacovigilance' is the process of detecting and evaluating ADRs in order to help prescribers (and patients) to be better informed about the risks of drug therapy. Drug regulatory agencies may respond to this information by restricting the prescribing indications of licensed medicines, altering the recommended dose range, adding special warnings and precautions for prescribers in product literature or withdrawing the product from the market.

ADRs can be detected in various ways. Common ADRs will become apparent during clinical trials undertaken with healthy volunteers and patients during drug development. Rarer ADRs may be identified later (after licensing) by voluntary reporting of suspected reactions using systems such as the 'Yellow Card' scheme that was set up in the UK in response to the thalidomide tragedy. Important weaknesses are

Box 1.2 Risk Factors for Adverse Drug Reactions

PATIENT RISK
- Elderly age (e.g. low physiological reserve)
- Neonates (e.g. uncertainty over pharmacokinetics)
- Polypharmacy (e.g. drug interactions)
- Genetic predisposition (see Table 1.3)
- Hypersensitivity/allergy (e.g. beta-lactam antibiotics)
- Diseases altering pharmacokinetic handling (e.g. hepatic or renal impairment)
- Diseases enhancing adverse pharmacodynamic responses (e.g. bladder instability)
- Adherence problems (e.g. related to cognitive impairment)

DRUG RISK
- Steep dose–response curve (e.g. insulin)
- Low therapeutic index (e.g. anticoagulants)
- Known to commonly cause ADRs (e.g. cytotoxic drugs)

PRESCRIBER RISK
- Poor understanding of principles of clinical pharmacology
- Poor knowledge of the prescribed drug
- Poor knowledge of the patient
- Inadequate instructions and warnings provided to patients
- Inadequate monitoring arrangements planned

ADR, Adverse drug reaction.

the low reporting rates (only 3% of all ADRs and 10% of serious ADRs are ever reported) and the inability to quantify risk (because the ratio of ADRs to prescriptions is unknown).

The increased availability of routinely collected data by modern healthcare systems means that, in the future, identifiable data on prescriptions might be linked to healthcare events (e.g. hospitalisation, operations, new clinical diagnoses) to become a powerful tool for assessing both the harms and benefits of drugs.

SUSPECTING AN ADR

Every prescriber will be responsible for prescriptions that cause ADRs and will see patients experiencing ADRs caused by prescriptions written by others. It is often difficult to be certain whether a suspected ADR is, in fact, caused by a drug because the 'reaction' may be a manifestation of the disease for which it was prescribed or may have another cause. Features that should raise suspicion of an ADR and the need to respond by stopping the medicine, reducing the dose and, in some cases, reporting include:

- The patient expresses concern that a drug has harmed them.
- Abnormal clinical measurements are made (e.g. blood pressure, blood glucose) or laboratory results reported (e.g. abnormal liver or renal function) while on drug therapy.
- New treatments that could be used to treat an ADR (e.g. omperazole, allopurinol, laxatives) have been started.
- The patient is vulnerable to experiencing ADRs (e.g. elderly, renal or hepatic disease).
- The drug has a narrow therapeutic index (e.g. digoxin, warfarin).
- The temporal relationship between the exposure to the drug and the onset of symptoms is reasonable.
- There is evidence of dose-relatedness of the suspected reaction.
- The reaction subsides when the drug is withdrawn ('de-challenge').
- The reaction returns when the drug is restarted ('re-challenge').

PREVENTION OF ADRS

Prescribers can minimise the occurrence of ADRs by being aware of risk factors for ADRs (see Box 1.2), adopting a rational approach to prescribing, counselling patients carefully about important warning signs, careful monitoring of treatment and improved communication with patients and other healthcare professionals.

DRUG INTERACTIONS

A drug interaction occurs when the administration of one drug alters the clinical effects of another. This may result in an increase or decrease in either the beneficial or harmful effects of the second drug. Although the number of potential interacting drug combinations is very large, only a small number are relevant in clinical practice (Table 1.5). Drug interactions are more likely when the affected drug has a low therapeutic index, a steep dose–response curve or a single mechanism of elimination.

PHARMACODYNAMIC INTERACTIONS

These occur when the administration of a second drug produces additive, synergistic or antagonistic effects by acting at the same drug target (e.g. a receptor or enzyme) or physiological system (e.g. electrolyte excretion, heart rate) as the first. Pharmacodynamic interactions are more common in clinical practice than pharmacokinetic interactions.

PHARMACOKINETIC INTERACTIONS

These occur when the administration of a second drug alters the concentration of the first at its site of action because of changes in the way the first drug is handled. The *rate* of absorption of drugs may be slowed by other drugs that either delay (e.g. anticholinergic drugs) or enhance (e.g. prokinetic drugs) gastric emptying. The *extent* of absorption can be influenced by second drugs that bind to form insoluble complexes or chelates (e.g. aluminium-containing antacids binding with ciprofloxacin, iron salts binding with tetracyclines). There are many drugs that rely on metabolism by different isoenzymes of cytochrome P450 (CYP) in the liver, especially 3A4, 2D6, 2C9, 2C19 and 1A2 for

Table 1.5 Common Pharmacodynamic and Pharmacokinetic Interactions

MECHANISM	INTERACTING DRUGS: OBJECT DRUG	INTERACTING DRUGS: PRECIPITANT DRUG	RESULT
Pharmacokinetic			
Reduced metabolism (CYP3A4)	simvastatin	grapefruit juice	Myopathy
	warfarin	clarithromycin	Enhanced anticoagulation
Reduced metabolism (CYP2C19)	phenytoin	omeprazole	Phenytoin toxicity
Reduced metabolism (xanthine oxidase)	azathioprine	allopurinol	Azathioprine toxicity
Reduced metabolism (monoamine oxidase)	catecholamines	monoamine oxidase inhibitors	Hypertensive crisis due to monoamine toxicity
Increased metabolism (induction)	ciclosporin	St John's wort	Loss of immunosuppression
Reduced renal elimination	lithium	diuretics	Lithium toxicity
	methotrexate	NSAIDs	Methotrexate toxicity
Pharmacodynamic			
Direct antagonism at the same receptor	salbutamol	atenolol	Inhibits the bronchodilator effect
Direct potentiation at the same organ system	benzodiazepines	alcohol	Increased sedation and risk of falls
	ACE inhibitors	NSAIDs	Increased risk of renal impairment
Indirect potentiation	digoxin	diuretics	Digoxin toxicity enhanced because of hypokalaemia
	warfarin	aspirin NSAIDs	Increased risk of bleeding because of gastrotoxicity and antiplatelet effects

ACE, Angiotensin-converting enzyme; *NSAID*, non-steroidal antiinflammatory drug.

their elimination. Interacting drugs have the potential either to increase the rate of metabolism by inducing the formation of more CYP isoenzyme (e.g. phenytoin, rifampicin) or decrease metabolism by inhibiting isoenzyme activity (e.g. clarithromycin, cimetidine, grapefruit juice). Enzyme induction effects usually take at least a few days to manifest because of the need to synthesise the new CYP enzyme while the effects of enzyme inhibition may be rapid. Some interactions occur because a second drug alters the renal clearance of the first. Drugs that reduce glomerular filtration rate (GFR) include ACE inhibitors and NSAIDs. This can reduce the clearance and increase the plasma concentration of many drugs, including some with a low therapeutic index (e.g. digoxin, lithium, gentamicin).

AVOIDING DRUG INTERACTIONS

The risk of drug interactions grows as patients are progressively prescribed more medicines (polypharmacy). Prescribers can avoid the consequences of drug–drug interactions by taking a careful drug history (see Box 1.1) before prescribing additional drugs, only prescribing for clear indications and taking special care when prescribing drugs with a narrow therapeutic index (e.g. warfarin). If concomitant prescribing of an interacting drug is unavoidable, good prescribers will anticipate the potential risk and provide special warnings for the patient as well as arranging for appropriate monitoring of either the clinical effects (e.g. blood sugar) or plasma concentration (e.g. lithium).

MEDICATION ERRORS

A medication error is any *preventable* event that may cause or lead to inappropriate medication use or patient harm while the medication is in the control of the healthcare professional or patient. Medication errors are usually classified on the basis of which stage of the medication process they occur (prescribing, dispensing, preparation, administration or monitoring). They can also be categorised on the basis of the harm they cause, the healthcare professional involved or whether they involve commission or omission. A prescribing error occurs when, as a result of a prescribing decision or prescription writing process, there is a significant reduction in the probability of treatment being timely and effective or increase in the risk of harm, when compared with generally accepted practice. Prescribing errors are very common. Recent UK studies suggest that 7% to 9% of hospital prescriptions contain an error, mostly perpetrated by relatively junior doctors (who write most of the prescriptions).

TYPES AND CAUSES OF PRESCRIBING ERRORS

Common types of prescribing error in hospitals include omission of medicines (especially failure to prescribe regular medicines at the point of admission or discharge, i.e. 'medicines reconciliation'), dosing errors, unintentional prescribing and poor use of documentation (Table 1.6). The causes of prescribing errors can be conveniently divided into those that

Table 1.6 Types of Hospital Prescribing Error

ERROR TYPE	APPROXIMATE % OF TOTAL
Omission on admission	30
Underdose	10
Overdose	10
Strength or dose missing	5
Omission on discharge	5
Administration times incorrect or missing	5
Duplication	5
Product or formulation not specified	5
Incorrect formulation	5
No maximum dose	5
Unintentional prescribing	3
No signature	2
Clinical contraindication	1
Incorrect route	1
No indication	1
IV instructions incorrect or missing	1
Drug not prescribed but indicated	1
Drug continued for longer than needed	1
Route missing	1
Start date incorrect or missing	1
Others, including drug interaction, controlled drug requirements incorrect/missing, daily dose divided incorrectly, allergy, failure to discontinue after ADRs, premature discontinuation, failure to respond to monitoring	2

ADR, Adverse drug reaction; *IV*, intravenous.

relate to the individual prescriber and those relating to the system in which they work (Box 1.3). It is now recognised that most errors result from a combination of both. Hospitals increasingly encourage reporting of errors within a 'no blame culture' so that they can be subject to 'root cause analysis' using Human Error Theory. Resource constraints mean that prescribers will always work in suboptimal circumstances, emphasising the need for rigorous training and attention to detail when prescribing, which will enable them to cope with these shortcomings more effectively.

RESPONDING TO ERROR

All prescribers make errors. When an error occurs, the prescriber should take action to protect the patient's safety with remedial treatment (e.g. reverse the effects of an opioid with naloxone) and appropriate monitoring arrangements. The event should be recorded in the notes, the patient and other healthcare staff should be informed, and the error should be reported so that others can learn from it.

Box 1.3 Causes of Hospital Prescribing Errors

SYSTEMS FACTORS

- Working hours of prescribers
- High patient workload
- Poor teamwork
- Lack of supervision
- Inadequate provision of clinical information
- Relaxed attitude towards prescribing
- Distractions
- Lack of decision support
- Poor checking routines (e.g. clinical pharmacy)
- Poor reporting and reviewing of incidents

PRESCRIBER FACTORS

Lack of Knowledge

- Principles of clinical pharmacology
- Common drugs
- Common diseases
- Workplace systems and routine

Inadequate Skills

- Drug history
- Obtaining information to support prescribing
- Communicating with patients and colleagues
- Numeracy and calculations
- Prescription writing

Suboptimal Attitudes

- Coping with risk and uncertainty
- Monitoring of prescribing
- Checking routines
- Overconfidence

PREVENTION OF PRESCRIBING ERRORS

The responsibility for reducing errors rests with both prescribers and those responsible for the systems in which they work. Prescribers can reduce the risk of error by being knowledgeable about the drugs they prescribe (e.g. indications, contraindications, common interactions, adverse effects), knowing the patients they are treating (e.g. comorbidities that might be relevant to the choice or dose of a medicine), taking an accurate drug history (see Box 1.1), writing legible and accurate prescriptions, calculating drug doses accurately, communicating clearly with colleagues and monitoring the effects of their prescriptions. They should also recognise the limitations of their competence and be able to ask for help when they are exceeded. Systems-based approaches aim to improve the safety of the systems in which prescribers work. Clinical pharmacists can play a critical role in helping to prevent errors and identify them before patients are harmed. This may be by review of prescription charts, improving medicines reconciliation at the point of admission and discharge from hospital and by 'medication use reviews', which provide an opportunity to educate patients, ensure better understanding of and adherence to prescriptions and identify medication errors related to misinterpretation and poor communication. *Electronic prescribing systems*, often combined with clinical decision support (CDS), also have a key future role in helping prescribers to choose the optimal prescription, taking into account patient-specific data (e.g. clinical history, drug history) and provide warnings that prevent potential errors.

RATIONAL PRESCRIBING

Prescribing should be based on a rational approach to the series of challenges highlighted in Fig. 1.1.

MAKING A DIAGNOSIS

Prescribing should ideally be based on a confirmed diagnosis. However, in clinical practice, many prescriptions have to be written based on the balance of probability, taking into account a range of differential diagnoses (e.g. antibiotics for a presumed urinary tract infection). The less certain the diagnosis, the more important it is that the impact of the treatment is monitored.

ESTABLISHING THE THERAPEUTIC GOAL

The goals of treatment are often clear, particularly when relieving unpleasant symptoms (e.g. pain, nausea, constipation). Sometimes the goal is less obvious to the patient, especially when the goal is prevention of future events (e.g. ACE inhibitors to prevent hospitalisation and extend life in chronic heart failure). Prescribers should try to establish the therapeutic goal because it will be a measure against which they will judge the success or failure of treatment.

CHOOSING THE THERAPEUTIC APPROACH

For many clinical problems, drug therapy is not mandated. A fundamental question that all prescribers must address is whether, having taken the potential benefits and harms into account, drug therapy is in the patient's interest and is superior to no treatment or one of a range of alternative approaches (e.g. physiotherapy, psychotherapy, surgery).

CHOOSING A DRUG

For most clinical indications (e.g. hypertension, depression), there will be more than one drug available. Although prescribers will often have guidance about which represents the rational choice for the average patient, they may still need to think about whether this is the optimal choice for their specific patient. Factors that may influence the choice of a particular drug include:

- *Pharmacokinetic considerations.* Patients may find some formulations easier to swallow than others or may be vomiting and require parenteral administration. Drugs that are extensively metabolised should be avoided in severe liver disease (e.g. opioid analgesics). Similarly, drugs that depend on renal excretion for elimination (e.g. digoxin, aminoglycoside antibiotics) should be avoided in renal disease if suitable alternatives exist.
- *Efficacy.* Prescribers will normally choose drugs with the greatest efficacy in achieving the goals of therapy (e.g. proton pump inhibitors rather than histamine-2 receptor antagonists). However, other factors such as convenience, safety or expense may lead to the choice of a less efficacious drug.
- *Disease variables.* The choice of an antibiotic should be based on the known or suspected sensitivity of the infective organism (e.g. trimethoprim for a urinary tract infection). Disease and/or symptom severity may also be an important influence on the choice of drug (e.g. analgesia) or the route of therapy (IV versus oral therapy in severe pneumonia).
- *Comorbidities.* The choice of drug may take account of coexisting diseases if they present either an indication or contraindication to therapy. A hypertensive patient who also has left ventricular impairment might be prescribed a beta-blocker, although the latter would be contraindicated if they have asthma.
- *Avoiding adverse effects or interactions.* Prescribers should be wary of choosing drugs that are more likely to cause adverse effects (e.g. cephalosporins rather than alternatives for patients allergic to penicillin) or worsen coexisting conditions (e.g. beta-blockers as treatment for angina in patients with asthma). They should also avoid giving combinations of drugs that might interact, either directly or indirectly (see Table 1.5)
- *Cost-effectiveness.* Prescribers should choose the cheaper drug if two drugs are of equal efficacy and safety. Even if cost is not a concern for the individual patient, unnecessary expenditure will ultimately limit choices for other prescribers and patients.

CHOOSING A DOSAGE REGIMEN

Prescribers have to choose a dose, route and frequency of administration (dosage regimen) that will achieve a steady-state drug concentration that provides sufficient exposure of the target tissue without producing toxic effects at other tissues. Recommendations made by manufacturers are based on observations in the average patient but the optimal regimen that will maximise the benefit/harm ratio for an individual patient is never certain. Rational prescribers treat each prescription as a clinical trial and gather sufficient information to amend it if necessary. They should be aware of the following general principles:

- *Dose and frequency.* Prescribers should generally start with a low dose and titrate this upwards as necessary. This cautious approach is particularly important if patients are likely to be more sensitive to adverse pharmacodynamic effects (e.g. confusion or postural hypotension in the elderly), have altered pharmacokinetic handling (e.g. renal or hepatic impairment) or when using drugs with a low therapeutic index (e.g. benzodiazepines, lithium, insulin). Exceptions to this approach are drugs where a rapid high concentration is critical (e.g. antibiotics, glucocorticoids, carbimazole). Indeed, some drugs have to be started with a loading dose to hasten the achievement of steady-state concentrations (e.g. digoxin, warfarin, amiodarone) (see Fig. 1.6). Convenience for the patient should be considered when timing doses (e.g. giving morning medications at a similar time) and, on the ward, convenience for the nursing staff should be considered (e.g. avoiding prescribing medications to be given during nursing handover times).

- *Dose titration*. The dose should be increased slowly, monitoring the therapeutic effect at regular intervals and looking for adverse effects. It is important to remember that the shape of the dose–response curve (see Fig. 1.3) means that dose titration may produce little added therapeutic effect and might increase the chances of toxicity.
- *Route*. A particular route of administration may be favoured in certain circumstances. Seriously ill patients may require a particular route for rapid assured action (e.g. IV rather than SC insulin for diabetic ketoacidosis, IV rather than oral furosemide for acute left ventricular failure). Patients who are vomiting will require parenteral therapy (e.g. for analgesia or antiemetics). Nitrates undergo significant first-pass metabolism and are often given via the buccal or SL route. Bronchodilators are usually given via inhalation rather than other routes to maximise the effect on the target tissues while minimising systemic exposure. Patients who are having prolonged seizures can be given diazepam PR rather than IV for ease of administration.
- *Frequency*. Less frequent doses are more convenient for patients but imply greater fluctuation between peaks and troughs in drug concentration (see Fig. 1.6). This is relevant if the peaks are associated with adverse effects (e.g. dizziness with antihypertensives) or the troughs are associated with troublesome loss of effect (e.g. antiparkinsonian drugs). These problems can be addressed by splitting the dose between the morning and evening or by choosing a modified-release formulation, if available.
- *Formulation*. Some formulations are easier to ingest for some patients, notably children (e.g. elixirs). It should be noted that the bioavailability of the same drug may vary between formulations and is very important when writing repeat prescriptions for drugs with a low therapeutic index (e.g. lithium, phenytoin, theophylline).
- *Duration*. Some drugs require a single dose (e.g. thrombolysis for pulmonary embolus) while others may require short courses (e.g. antibiotics). For many drugs, the duration will be largely at the prescriber's discretion depending on response and disease progression (e.g. analgesics, antidepressants, glucocorticoids).

WRITING A PRESCRIPTION

The ultimate goal of the planning above is writing an accurate and legible prescription so that the drug will be dispensed and administered as planned (see later).

INFORMING THE PATIENT

Patients are important partners in rational prescribing decisions and should, wherever possible, be involved in making the previously mentioned choices. However, in many cases, they are happy to delegate this task to the prescriber. Nevertheless, it is important that they are provided with sufficient information to understand the choice that has been made on their behalf, what to expect from the treatment and any measures that must be undertaken to enhance the safety or effectiveness of the treatment (Table 1.7). Patients who have received such information are likely to have improved adherence to treatments, more confidence in prescribers and greater satisfaction with healthcare services.

Table 1.7 What Patients Need to Know About Their Medicines

The reason for taking the medicine, which will reinforce the goals of treatment
How the medicine works
How to take the medicine—may be important for the effectiveness (e.g. inhaled salbutamol in asthma) and safety of treatment (e.g. alendronate for osteoporosis)
What benefits to expect
What adverse effects might occur—common and mild effects that may be transient and might not require discontinuation as well as serious effects that might influence the patient's consent
Precautions that improve safety—symptoms to report, monitoring that will be required and potentially important drug interactions
When to return for review—either for routine review or because of adverse effects

MONITORING TREATMENT EFFECTS

Rational prescribing requires some monitoring for the beneficial and adverse effects of treatment to establish that the balance remains in favour of a positive outcome and supports continued treatment (see later).

STOPPING DRUG THERAPY

Long-term treatments should be reviewed at regular intervals to assess whether the risk–benefit balance is still favourable and whether the goals of treatment are still valued by the patient. Elderly patients often wish to reduce their medication burden and may prefer to make compromises around the original goals of long-term preventative therapy to achieve this.

PRESCRIBING FOR PATIENTS WITH SPECIAL REQUIREMENTS

RENAL DISEASE

Patients with renal impairment are usually identified by prescribers because the routine biochemistry suggests a low estimated glomerular filtration rate (eGFR; <60 mL/min) based on their serum creatinine, age, and sex, and this group will include a large proportion of elderly patients. If a drug (or an active metabolite) is eliminated predominantly by the kidneys, it will tend to accumulate and so the maintenance dose must be reduced. For some drugs, renal impairment makes patients more sensitive to their beneficial or adverse pharmacodynamic effects. It is important to remember that the eGFR calculation is unreliable at extremes of body weight and may overestimate true GFR in patients with rapidly declining renal function in acute kidney injury (AKI). Drugs that require extra caution in patients with renal disease are listed in Table 1.8.

HEPATIC DISEASE

The liver has a large excess capacity for drug metabolism and liver disease has to be advanced before drug dosages need to be reduced. Prescribers may be alerted to patients who may have impaired metabolism because they present with clinical signs such as jaundice, ascites, hypoalbuminaemia, malnutrition or encephalopathy, or because they have significantly deranged liver biochemistry. There are no quantitative tests of hepatic drug metabolising capacity; prescribers have to be vigilant for the possibility of altered drug metabolism and monitor the therapeutic response and potential adverse effects. Drugs that require extra caution in patients with hepatic disease are listed in Table 1.8.

ELDERLY PATIENTS

Elderly patients are more vulnerable to adverse effects because of reduced drug elimination (due largely to impaired renal function allowing accumulation of drugs), increased sensitivity of target organs to drug effects (e.g. brain, kidney) and interactions as a result of polypharmacy. The dosage regimens of many drugs need to be adjusted to avoid toxicity with lower starting doses and more cautious dose titration. Drugs that require particular care are listed in Table 1.8.

The elderly may also fail to derive maximum benefit from drugs because of difficulties with adherence to the treatment regimen. Swallowing is difficult for many older people because some tablets and capsules can adhere to the oesophageal mucosa. Cognitive impairment means that many patients forget their medicines or get confused about when to take them. These problems can be overcome by simplifying the regimen, providing automatic or remote reminders and supplying medicines in pill organisers (e.g. dosette boxes or calendar blister packs).

WOMEN WHO ARE PREGNANT OR BREASTFEEDING

Prescribing in pregnancy should be avoided, if possible, because of the potential risk to the developing fetus. Pregnant women sometimes require treatment for either a preexisting problem (e.g. diabetes, asthma) or for problems that arise during pregnancy (e.g. morning sickness, hypertension). Around one-third of women take a medicine at least once during pregnancy, some of whom take drugs during the first trimester (excluding iron, folic acid and vitamins). Commonly used drugs are simple analgesics, antibacterial drugs and antacids.

Pharmacokinetic handling of drugs is altered in pregnancy. Vomiting in the early stages may reduce the effectiveness of drugs administered by the oral route. The plasma albumin concentration falls during pregnancy and the albumin-bound fraction of drugs may be reduced (e.g. the unbound fraction of phenytoin increases during pregnancy and total plasma phenytoin concentrations fall). GFR increases significantly during pregnancy and drugs that are excreted by the kidneys (e.g. lithium, atenolol) are cleared more quickly.

Teratogenesis is damage to the fetus in the critical period from 2 to 8 weeks of gestation when important organ systems are developing. For a list of common teratogens, see Table 1.8. This risk means that all drugs should be avoided at this time unless the benefit to the mother greatly outweighs the risk to the fetus. It follows that prescribers should always use drugs for which some record of safety has been established and use them at the lowest dose for the shortest time possible.

Some drugs may have important effects later in pregnancy (e.g. tetracycline stains teeth), at delivery (e.g. salbutamol and nifedipine have a tocolytic effect) and in the neonatal period (e.g. opioid analgesics can depress respiration in the neonate either after transfer from the placental circulation or via breast milk).

CHILDREN

Prescribing for children presents significant challenges because of the many differences from the more familiar setting of adult medicine. Some of the more important are:

- *Medicine taking*. Younger children may find it harder to take medicines than adults and a liquid formulation is often more acceptable than tablets or capsules. An oral syringe (see later) should be used for accurate measurement and controlled administration of an oral liquid medicine. The unpleasant taste of an oral liquid can be disguised by flavouring. Dental hygiene should be optimal for those receiving sugar-containing medicines and sugar-free alternatives should be provided whenever possible.
- *Adherence*. Factors that contribute to poor adherence are difficulties with medicine taking, poor instructions, concerns about lack of efficacy or adverse effects and lack of parental support.
- *Pharmacokinetics*. The pharmacokinetic handling of medicines may be less predictable than with adults and is not solely proportional to the reduced body size. Children have a higher proportion of body water than adults, affecting drug distribution. Metabolism is immature in the early months (especially in preterm neonates) but rises rapidly to exceed adult metabolism in the later stages of

Table 1.8 Drugs That Require Extra Caution in Special Patient Groups

DRUG	POTENTIAL PROBLEMS
Renal Disease	
ACE inhibitors and ARBs	Renal impairment, hyperkalaemia
Metformin	Lactic acidosis
Spironolactone	Increased risk of hyperkalaemia
NSAIDs	Impaired renal function
Sulfonylureas	Hypoglycaemia
Insulin	Hypoglycaemia
Aminoglycosides (e.g. gentamicin)	Reduced clearance
Vancomycin	Reduced clearance
Digoxin	Reduced clearance
Lithium	Reduced clearance
Atenolol	Reduced clearance
Allopurinol	Reduced clearance
Cephalosporins	Reduced clearance
Methotrexate	Reduced clearance
Opioids (e.g. morphine)	Reduced clearance
Hepatic Disease	
Warfarin	Increased risk of bleeding
Metformin	Lactic acidosis
Chloramphenicol	Bone-marrow suppression
NSAIDs	Gastrointestinal bleeding, fluid retention
Sulfonylureas	Hypoglycaemia
Benzodiazepines	Coma
Phenytoin	Reduced metabolism
Rifampicin	Reduced metabolism
Propranolol	Reduced metabolism
Warfarin	Reduced metabolism
Diazepam	Reduced metabolism
Opioids (e.g. morphine)	Reduced metabolism
Elderly	
Digoxin	Increased risk of toxicity because of diuretic-induced hypokalaemia and renal impairment favouring accumulation
Antihypertensive drugs	Falls due to reduced baroreceptor function
Central nervous system depressant drugs (e.g. antidepressants, hypnotics, sedatives, tranquillisers)	Increased sensitivity of the brain to inhibitory effects and reduced elimination
Warfarin	Increased risk of bleeding from intra- and extracranial sites
NSAIDs	Increased risk of adverse effects on renal function and gastrotoxicity
Pregnancy	
Alcohol	Teratogenic
Warfarin	Teratogenic
Cytotoxic drugs	Teratogenic
ACE inhibitors	Teratogenic
Corticosteroids	Teratogenic
Antiepileptics	Teratogenic
Retinoids (e.g. isotretinoin)	Teratogenic
Tetracyclines	Enter and stain growing teeth and bones
Beta-blockers	Low birth weight
Sulfonylureas	Neonatal hypoglycaemia
Opioid analgesics	Neonatal respiratory depression
Penicillin	Excreted in breast milk may cause penicillin hypersensitivity
Opioid analgesics	Neonatal respiratory depression

ACE, Angiotensin-converting enzyme; *ARBs*, angiotensin receptor blockers; *NSAID*, non-steroidal antiinflammatory drug.

childhood. Particular caution is needed in the neonatal period (first 28 days of life) and doses should always be calculated with care.
- *Pharmacodynamics*. The pharmacodynamic response to medicines may differ.
- *Medication error*. Appropriate doses of drugs vary considerably with age. Many paediatric doses are determined by a weight-based calculation, and some are based on body surface area, introducing the chances of a serious dosing error. Great care should be taken therefore in making measurements of height and weight, documenting calculations and having them independently checked. Other doses are based on age ranges.
- *Consent*. Younger children may be unable to give informed consent to treatment and this will involve a parent or guardian.
- *Unlicensed medicines*. Many paediatric prescriptions are for medicines being used outside their licence. Prescribing medicines that are unlicensed or being used outside their marketing authorisation increases the professional responsibility and liability of prescribers, who should be able to justify and feel competent in using such medicines.
- *Information*. Few medicines are developed specifically for children and so the evidence base for the beneficial and adverse effects is more limited. Reliable background information and reference materials are available in the British National Formulary for Children (BNFC) and other international equivalents. Most paediatric units also have a Drug & Therapeutics committee that will be responsible for developing and making available guidelines to support prescribers.

RACE AND ETHNICITY

In general, prescribing should be done independently of race or ethnicity. It is not a good proxy marker for genetic or other markers relevant to pharmacodynamics, pharmacokinetics or pharmacogenomics. Some UK prescribing protocols include ethnicity in treatment algorithms. Newer angiotensin II receptor blockers (ARBs) are recommended in preference to angiotensin-converting enzyme (ACE) inhibitor in those of Black African or Afro-Caribbean family origin in the 2022 NICE hypertension guideline. The 2023 NICE obesity guideline gives a lower BMI threshold for starting the drug Liraglutide (32.5 kg/m^2 instead of 35 kg/m^2) for members of 'minority ethnic groups known to be at equivalent risk of the consequences of obesity at a lower BMI than the white population'. Such protocols remain controversial and may change in the future, especially as genetic testing becomes cheaper and personalised medicine becomes more common. There has been a trend to remove race and ethnicity from physiological calculators, like for example its recent removal from eGFR calculations from NICE guidelines. Race and ethnicity should not in general be considered relevant for prescribing practice, and where it is currently used, the evidence base is limited and practice varies.

GETTING INFORMATION ABOUT MEDICINES

Prescribers need reliable sources of information to support safe and effective prescribing. There are a number of important paper and electronic sources available as well as the support of drug information and clinical pharmacy services run by most large hospitals.

BRITISH NATIONAL FORMULARY (BNF)

The BNF (www.bnf.nice.org.uk) is the most important drug information reference source for doctors (and all other prescribers) in the UK. The BNF provides important carefully reviewed monographs about commonly prescribed medicines, but also contains limited information about over-the-counter remedies, herbal medicines, nutraceuticals and unlicensed products. It is designed to be a practical reference source for busy doctors rather than exhaustive in its coverage. The BNF is a joint publication of the Royal Pharmaceutical Society of Great Britain and the British Medical Association and is steered by the Joint Formulary Committee. It uses reliable evidence, national guidelines for best practice, emerging safety issues and the input of experienced clinicians to provide independent advice on the most effective and safest drug and dose selection for patients. The BNF provides relatively little detail on some areas of specialist practice such as obstetrics, malignant disease and anaesthesia. It is available in paper format, online and as an electronic application viewable on smart phones and tablet computers. More recently, the BNF for Children (www.bnfc.nice.org.uk) has been created, which provides drug information specific to paediatric patients.

The BNF and BNFC contain the following sections:
- *General prescribing guidance*. This provides general guidance about practical considerations for prescribers including legal and regulatory considerations, adherence, licensed and unlicensed medicines, excipients, sugar-free and extemporaneous formulations, appropriate drug-naming systems, prescription writing requirements, emergency supply of medicines, controlled drug prescribing and drug dependence, ADRs and the 'Yellow Card scheme'. It also covers prescribing for specific patients such as paediatric patients, renal and hepatic impairment, pregnancy and breastfeeding, palliative care, the elderly, medical emergencies and the treatment of poisoning as well as specific advice for dentists and other nonmedical prescribers
- *Guidance on specific medicines*. The BNF and BNFC are no longer organised by body system to reflect the increased complexity of medicines use and the fact that most users now access them in a searchable electronic format. Each drug monograph follows the same pattern (indications and

dose, contraindications, cautions, safety warnings issued by the Medicines and Healthcare Products Regulatory Agency (MHRA), relevant guidance issued by the National Institute for Health and Care Excellence (NICE), interactions, side-effects, pregnancy, breastfeeding, renal impairment, hepatic impairment, monitoring requirements, treatment cessation, directions for administration, patient and carer advice, generic and proprietary medicinal forms). Preparations are listed by approved name and there is also information about drug formulation, dose of active ingredient, pack size, net price and cautionary advisory labels required. Proprietary brands include manufacturer name, formulation-specific information and available strengths. Compound preparations include manufacturer name, formulation-specific information and basic price. In addition to this information, there are a series of symbols, keys and numbers, which provide information about the drug's legal classification (prescription-only medication (POM), general sales list (GSL), Controlled Drug schedules 1–4), drugs considered less suitable for prescribing and drugs for which all suspected adverse reactions should be reported (denoted by a black triangle)
- *Treatment summaries*. The BNF and BNFC provide an easily searchable list of treatment summaries covering around 200 common medical conditions with hyperlinks to the relevant monographs for the drug mentioned.

OTHER INFORMATION RESOURCES FOR PRESCRIBERS

The BNF and BNFC are the first point of reference for UK prescribers, but other key reference resources for more depth or specialist information include:
- *Medicines Complete*. This is an online gateway providing access to several important medicines information resources including the BNF and BNFC, Martindale: The Complete Drug Reference, The Injectable Drugs Guide, Stockley's Interaction Checker and various clinical calculators. www.medicinescomplete.com
- *National Institute for Health and Care Excellence (NICE)*. NICE provides access to the BNF, BNFC, Clinical Guidelines and Clinical Knowledge Summaries relating to the presentation, investigation and management of many conditions. www.nice.org.uk
- *Electronic Medicines Compendium (EMC)*. EMC is a compendium of the Summary of Product Characteristics (SmPCs) and Patient Information Leaflets (PILs) approved by the regulatory authorities in the UK (MHRA) and Europe (European Medicines Agency (EMA)). https://www.medicines.org.uk/emc
- *Drug Safety Update*. A monthly electronic bulletin from the MHRA that provides the most up-to-date advice to support the safer use of medicines. www.mhra.gov.uk/Publications/Safetyguidance/DrugSafetyUpdate/index.htm

WRITING A PRESCRIPTION

A prescription is a means by which a prescriber communicates their intended plan of treatment to the pharmacist who dispenses a medicine and a nurse (or patient) who administers it. It should be precise, accurate, clear and legible. The two main kinds of prescription are those written, dispensed and administered in hospital and those written by a general practitioner (GP), dispensed at a community pharmacy and self-administered by the patient. The information supplied must include:
- The date
- Identification of the patient
- The name of the drug
- The formulation
- The dose
- The frequency of administration
- The route and method of administration
- The amount to be supplied (GP only)
- Instructions for labelling (GP only)
- The prescriber's signature

HOSPITAL PRESCRIBING

Although GP prescribing is increasingly electronic, in many hospitals, prescribing continues to be based around the Prescription and Administration Record (the 'drug chart'). There are many variations in use but most contain the following sections (Fig. 1.7):
- *Basic patient information*. Identifies the prescription with the correct patient and will usually include name, age, date of birth, hospital number and address. These details are often 'filled in' using a sticky addressograph label, which introduces the real possibility of serious error.
- *Previous adverse reactions/allergies*. Communicates important patient safety information based on a careful drug history or the medical record.
- *Other treatment charts*. Notes any other hospital prescription documents that contain current prescriptions being received by the patient (e.g. anticoagulants, insulin, oxygen, fluids)
- *Once-only therapy*. For prescribing medicines to be used infrequently such as single-dose prophylactic antibiotics and other preoperative medications.
- *Regular therapy*. For prescribing medicines to be taken for a number of days or continuously, such as a course of antibiotics, antihypertensive drugs, antiparkinsonian drugs, etc.
- *'As-required' therapy*. For prescribing medicines for symptomatic relief, usually to be administered at the discretion of the nursing staff (e.g. antiemetics, analgesics).

Some examples of poor prescribing are shown in Fig. 1.8.

(A)

PRESCRIPTION AND ADMINISTRATION RECORD

Standard Chart

Hospital/Ward: W26 **Consultant:** MAXWELL	**Name of Patient:** JOHN SMITH
Weight: 78 kg **Height:** 1.84 m	**Hospital Number:** WGH5522589
If re-written, date: 14.2.24	**D.O.B.:** 16.10.64
DISCHARGE PRESCRIPTION **Date completed:-** **Completed by:-**	

OTHER MEDICINE CHARTS IN USE		**PREVIOUS ADVERSE REACTIONS** This section must be completed before any medicine is given		Completed by (sign & print)	Date
Date	Type of Chart	None known ☐			
		Medicine/Agent	Description of Reaction		
14.2.24	WARFARIN	PENICILLIN	SERIOUS REACTION (HOSPITALIZED) AGE 15	SJ S.JONES	14.2.24
		CEFALEXIN	RASH (DISCONTINUED)	SJ S.JONES	14.2.24

CODES FOR NON-ADMINISTRATION OF PRESCRIBED MEDICINE

If a dose is not administered as prescribed, initial and enter a code in the column with a circle drawn round the code according to the reason as shown below. **Inform the responsible doctor in the appropriate timescale.**

1. Patient refuses
2. Patient not present
3. Medicines not available – CHECK ORDERED
4. Asleep/drowsy
5. Administration route not available – CHECK FOR ALTERNATIVE
6. Vomiting/nausea
7. Time varied on doctor's instructions
8. Once only/as required medicine given
9. Dose withheld on doctor's instructions
10. Possible adverse reaction/side effect

(B)

ONCE-ONLY

Date	Time	Medicine (Approved Name)	Dose	Route	Prescriber – Sign + Print	Time Given	Given By
14.2.24	16.00	MORPHINE	5 mg	IV	S.JONES	16.20	ST
14.2.24	16.00	GLYCERYL TRINITRATE	500 micrograms	SL	S.JONES	16.10	SL
14.2.24	16.00	METOCLOPRAMIDE	10 mg	IV	S.JONES	16.20	ST

Fig. 1.7 **Example prescriptions.** (A) Front page of a Prescription and Administration Record. The correct identification of the patient is critical to reducing the risk of an administration error. This record also clearly identifies other prescription charts in use and previous adverse reactions to drugs in order to alert prescribers and reduce the risk of repeated exposure. Note also the codes employed by the nursing staff to indicate reasons why drugs may not have been administered. (B) 'Once-Only Therapy' box. This area is used for prescriptions for drugs that are unlikely to be repeated on a regular basis. Note that the prescriber has written the names of all drugs legibly in block capitals and signed and written their name clearly. The nurse who administered the prescription has signed to confirm that the dose has been administered.

GENERAL CONSIDERATIONS BEFORE PRESCRIBING

A fundamental principle of rational prescribing, deserving of consideration prior to writing any prescription, is that, on the balance of probability, the patient has a significantly greater chance of deriving benefit from the prescribed medication than being harmed. This judgement depends on knowledge of four important areas:

- the clinical and medication history, including previous adverse reactions
- the clinical diagnosis

(C)

PRESCRIPTION		Time		14/02/24	15/02/24	16/02/24	17/02/24	18/02/24	19/02/24	20/02/24	21/02/24				
Medicine (Approved Name) AMOXICILLIN		6													
		(8)		X	DK	RB	RB	DK		X	X	X	X	X	X
Dose 500 mg	Route ORAL	12													
Notes For 5 days: stop 20.2.24	Start Date 14.02.24	(14)		X	DK	RB	RB			X	X	X	X	X	X
Prescriber – sign + print S.JONES		18													
		(22)		X	DK	RB	RB			X	X	X	X	X	X
Medicine (Approved Name) AMLODIPINE		6													
		(8)		X	DK	RB									
Dose 5 mg	Route ORAL	12													
Notes	Start Date 14.02.24	14													
		18													
Prescriber – sign + print S.JONES		22													
Medicine (Approved Name) LISINOPRIL		6													
		(8)		X	DK	RB	RB	DK							
Dose 20 mg	Route ORAL	12													
Notes Review renal function on 16.2.24	Start Date 14.02.24	14													
		18													
Prescriber – sign + print S.JONES		22													

(Amlodipine entry crossed through:) DISCONTINUED DUE TO PERSISTENT ANKLE OEDEMA SM S.MAXWELL 16.02.24

(D) **AS REQUIRED THERAPY**

Prescription				
Medicine (Approved Name) PARACETAMOL		Date	16.2.24	
		Time	11.15	
Dose and Frequency 1 g 4-HOURLY	Route ORAL	Dose	1 g	
Notes For pain Maximum 4 g/24 h	Start Date 16.02.24	Initials	DK	
Prescriber – sign + print S.JONES		Date		
		Time		
Medicine (Approved Name) GLYCERYL TRINITRATE		Dose		
		Initials		
Dose and Frequency 500 micrograms	Route SL	Date		
Notes FOR CARDIAC ISCHAEMIA	Start Date 16.02.24	Time		
		Dose		
Prescriber – sign + print S.JONES		Initials		

Fig. 1.7 cont'd (C) 'Regular Therapy' box. This area is used for prescriptions for drugs that are going to be given regularly. Note the use of the notes box to communicate additional important information and the care with which the prescription for amlodipine has been cancelled with a clear explanation provided. (D) 'As Required Therapy' box. These prescriptions leave the administration of the drug to the discretion of the nursing staff. Note the clarity with which the indications for administration have been stated and, in the case of paracetamol, the importance of stating a maximum daily dose.

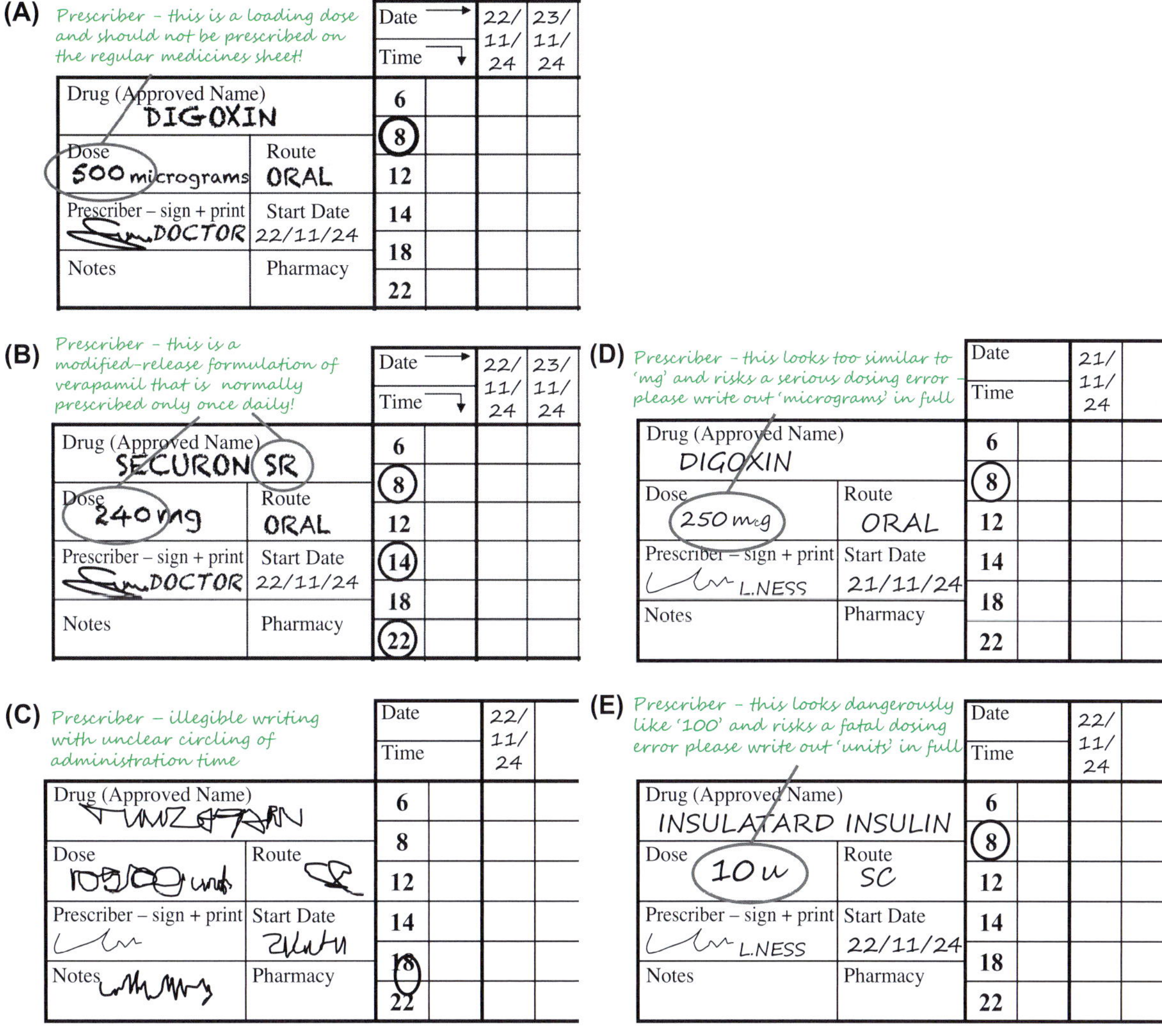

Fig. 1.8 Examples of prescription errors. (A) Digoxin loading dose prescribed as regular medication. (B) Modified-release preparation of verapamil given three times daily instead of as a once-daily dose. (C) An illegible prescription, with unclear circling of time. (D) Ambiguous units of digoxin: mcg and mg are easily confused. (E) Ambiguous units of insulin: u and 0 are easily confused.

- relevant patient and clinical factors that might influence drug action (e.g. age, pregnancy, renal and hepatic impairment)
- familiarity with the medicine to be prescribed.

Uncertainty in any of these areas is likely to increase the chances of adverse outcomes. Table 1.9 provides a more general list of 'high-risk moments' for prescribers.

There are many excellent resources, such as the BNF, that support rational prescribing but none can anticipate the many clinical problems that individual prescribers face on a day-to-day basis. Having taken the previously mentioned factors into account, if doubt remains about the wisdom of prescribing, it may be appropriate to seek a more experienced opinion, if available. Patient consent is usually assumed when prescribing on hospital wards but there may be circumstances where this should be obtained specifically (e.g. high risk of adverse events, prescribing a medicine outside its licensed indication).

WRITING THE PRESCRIPTION

Prescribers should follow some basic rules when using a paper prescription chart:

- A written prescription is a form of communication between the person prescribing a medicine (usually a doctor) and the person who dispenses and administers the medicine (usually a nurse in a hospital). The ultimate requirement for that communication is that it is clear and unambiguous. Handwriting remains an important reason why this objective is sometimes not met. For that reason, all drug names should be written in block capitals with black pen to maximise legibility. Particular care should be taken around the legibility of numbers and dosage units although the latter should follow standard abbreviations and do not need to be written in capitals. Supplementary notes should be written clearly (in upper or lower case) in the spaces provided or in close proximity to the prescription if insufficient space is available.

Table 1.9 High-Risk Prescribing Moments

SITUATION	RESPONSE
Trying to amend an active prescription (e.g. altering the dose/timing)	*Always avoid and start again*
Writing up drugs in the immediate presence of more than one prescription chart or set of notes	*Avoid*
Diverting attention in the middle of completing a patient's prescription(s)	*Avoid*
Prescribing 'high-risk' drugs (e.g. anticoagulants, opioids, insulin, sedatives)	*Ask for help if necessary*
Prescribing parenteral drugs	*Take extra care*
Rushing prescribing (e.g. during a busy ward round)	*Avoid*
Prescribing unfamiliar drugs	*Ask for help if necessary*
Transcribing multiple prescriptions from an expired chart to a new one	*Take extra care*
Writing prescriptions solely based on information from another source such as a referral letter, which may contain errors and medicines that may be the cause of the patient's illness	*Review the justification for each as if it is a new prescription* *Seek corroborating evidence of current prescriptions*
Writing or recording prescriptions at the point of transfer of care (because these will become the patient's regular medication for the immediate future and may not be reviewed)	*Take extra care*
Calculating drug doses	*Ask for an independent calculation*
Prescribing sound-alike or look-alike drugs (e.g. chlorphenamine and chlorpromazine)	*Take extra care*

- Clear and unambiguous labelling of the prescription chart with the details of the intended recipient should be the starting point for all prescriptions (see Fig. 1.7A). Essential identifying details such as the patient's name, hospital number and date of birth (and age if under 12 years) should be written on every sheet. The patient's weight and height may be required to calculate safe doses for many drugs with narrow therapeutic indices.
- Special instructions to guide safe and effective administration of the medicine or subsequent monitoring arrangements should be highlighted in the relevant 'Notes' box on the prescription chart (see Fig. 1.7C). There is often insufficient room to provide all of the information and prescribers should feel able to write notes within the drug administration area of the chart as long as this is done clearly and does not impinge on the administration record completed by the nursing staff.
- Most drugs that have to be given by IV infusion will be prescribed using a dedicated IV drug infusion chart (this should be indicated on the main chart). However, it remains common for some drugs that have to be given regularly by IV infusion (rather than as a bolus injection) to be written up on the standard 'regular medicines' section of the prescription chart (e.g. IV vitamin B supplements, some IV antibiotics). When prescribing an IV infusion, it is important to highlight the total dose and the intended duration of the infusion. The prescription may also indicate the diluent, but since most common fluids are created prepared based on wards based on IV protocols, this is often omitted by the prescriber.
- The drug sensitivities/allergies box (see Fig. 1.7A) should be checked and further details of the drug history obtained if there are any doubts about its accuracy.
- *Medicine names*. Use the generic International Nonproprietary Name (INN) rather than brand name (e.g. write 'SIMVASTATIN', not 'ZOCOR'). The only exception to this rule comes when there is variation in the properties of different brands (e.g. modified-release preparations of drugs such as lithium, theophylline, phenytoin and nifedipine) or when the drug is a combination product with no generic name (e.g. Kliovance and other hormone preparations). Do not use abbreviations of drug names (e.g. write 'ISOSORBIDE MONONITRATE' not 'ISMN').
- *Dose*. Write the drug dose clearly. The only acceptable abbreviations are 'g' and 'mg'. 'Micrograms' must always be written in full, never as 'μg', nor 'mcg', nor 'ug'. 'Units' (with regard to insulin, heparin, etc.) must always be written in full. Avoid decimal points (e.g. use 500 mg not 0.5 g). If a decimal point cannot be avoided, always put a '0' in front of it (e.g. '0.5 micrograms' not '.5 micrograms'). It is not necessary to use a decimal point if the number is a round number (e.g. '7 mg' not '7.0 mg'). For liquid preparations, write the dose in mg. The only exceptions when 'mL' can be written are if the product is a combination product (e.g. Gaviscon liquid), or if the strength is not expressed by weight (e.g. adrenaline 1 in 1000). Use numbers (e.g. 1 or 'one') to denote use of a sachet or enema. Always include the dose of inhaled drugs (e.g. beclometasone) in addition to stating '2 puffs', as strengths can vary. For some drugs, a maximum dose may need to be stated (e.g. colchicine in gout).

- *Route and method of administration*. Widely accepted abbreviations for route of administration are: intravenous—'IV'; intramuscular—'IM'; subcutaneous—'SC'; sublingual—'SL'; per rectum—'PR'; per vagina—'PV'; nasogastric—'NG'; inhaled—'INH'; and topical—'TOP'. Never abbreviate 'ORAL' to 'O' (some hospitals will accept abbreviation to 'PO'). Never abbreviate 'INTRATHECAL'. Care should be taken in specifying 'RIGHT' or 'LEFT' for eye drops and ear drops. It may be necessary to specify the method of giving a medicine intravenously (e.g. as a single undiluted bolus injection, as an infusion in a small volume of saline over a few minutes or in a larger volume over a longer period of time, giving the precise rate of flow if necessary).
- *Frequency*. Indicate the frequency of administration clearly. For example: furosemide 40 mg PO once daily; amoxicillin 250 mg PO three times a day. Widely accepted latin abbreviations for dose frequency are: once daily—'OD'; twice daily—'BD'; three times daily—'TDS'; and four times daily—'QDS'. The hospital chart usually requires specific times to be identified for regular medicines that coincide with nursing drug rounds.
- *Instructions*. Space is provided for notes on important administration advice not detailed elsewhere (e.g. whether a medicine should be taken with food, type of inhaler device used and anything else that the drug dispenser should know). It is also important to state here the times for taking peak or trough plasma levels for drugs requiring therapeutic monitoring. If a course of treatment is for a known time period, cross off subsequent days when the medicine is not required. For example, for a 5-day course of antibiotics, put a cross in the administration boxes from the sixth day to 'gate' the prescription (see Fig. 1.7C) and/or in the 'instructions' section write the 'stop date' for the drug. Similarly, if a drug is not to be given every day, cross off the days it is not required (e.g. alendronic acid and methotrexate usually have a once-weekly schedule).
- *Prescriber identification*. Prescribers should sign and print their name clearly so that they can be identified by colleagues. The prescription should be dated.
- *Discontinuation*. When a prescription is stopped, this should be clearly marked. One way of doing this is illustrated here: a vertical line could be drawn at the point of discontinuation, horizontal lines through the remaining days on the chart and diagonal lines through the prescription details and administration boxes. Sign and date this action and consider writing a supplementary note to inform colleagues about this action. The underlying details should remain legible (see Fig. 1.7C).
- *'As-required' medicines*. Provide exact instructions as to the maximum frequency (e.g. 'not more often than four-hourly'). Prescribers should always note the indication, frequency, minimal time interval between doses and maximum dose in any 24-hour period (see Fig. 1.7D).

OTHER CONSIDERATIONS AFTER PRESCRIBING

There are a number of important considerations that follow an initial prescription. The patient should be provided with relevant information about the medicine (see Table 1.7). When medicines are initiated (or discontinued), an entry should be placed in the patient record to justify these decisions, as this provides valuable information for other colleagues involved in the patient's care. This is especially important for drugs that require therapeutic monitoring (e.g. digoxin, lithium), for drugs prescribed outside their licensed use or for those discontinued because of adverse effects. It is a basic principle that a prescription will be followed by some sort of judgement as to its success or failure, typically based on a clinical or laboratory measurements, so that appropriate changes can be made if necessary (e.g. ineffective medicines stopped or substituted).

HOSPITAL DISCHARGE ('TO TAKE OUT') MEDICINES

Most patients will be prescribed a short course of their medicines at discharge to last until they can visit their GP. This prescription is particularly important because it usually informs about future therapy at the point of transfer of prescribing responsibility. Great care is required to ensure that this list is accurate and that any hospital medicines to be stopped are not inadvertently included or are identified as short duration (to be specified). It is also important that any significant ADRs experienced in hospital are recorded and that any specific monitoring or review is identified.

HOSPITAL ELECTRONIC PRESCRIBING

Although most hospital prescriptions have been handwritten on paper inpatient medication charts, the last two decades have seen increasing deployment of electronic prescribing systems. These systems largely remove many of the problems of illegibility and ambiguity often seen with paper prescribing and enforce many of the rules outlined earlier. It also enables multidisciplinary teams to prescribe, order and administer medicines to patients by electronic means, and provides an audit trail attributable to each healthcare professional and each drug.

Important advantages for prescribers are:

- Allowing routine protocols to be prescribed accurately (e.g. postoperative pain relief, venous thromboprophylaxis, oxygen) by using standard templates.
- Avoiding the need to transcribe medicines from one chart to another.
- Removing the problem of 'missing charts' by ensuring the medication record is visible at all times and from multiple locations around the hospital.
- Preventing 'specialised charts' being forgotten by linking them together.

- Ensuring that administration of critical medicines (e.g. antibiotics, antiparkinsonian medicines) is not missed because overdue administrations are automatically flagged.
- Improving the process of medicines reconciliation at transfers of care.

When combined with the electronic health record containing contextualised data about patients (age, eight, height, previous adverse reactions, comorbidities and other prescriptions), prescribers can benefit from the assistance of additional CDS. This helps to promote better choices of drug treatment and avoid—or at least reducing—the risk of medication errors. Examples of errors that are reduced include the prescribing of drugs that are contraindicated because of:

- known hypersensitivity (e.g. penicillin allergy)
- preexisting conditions (e.g. verapamil in the presence of heart failure)
- age (e.g. aspirin for children)
- weight (e.g. reduced paracetamol dose when body mass is less than 50 kg)
- pregnancy (e.g. tetracyclines, warfarin)
- therapeutic duplication (e.g. opioids, laxatives, calcium channel blockers)
- drug–drug interactions (e.g. atenolol and verapamil, clarithromycin and simvastatin)
- drug–disease interactions (e.g. NSAIDs in renal impairment)

Many of these problems will be signalled by 'alerts' that are generated for the attention of the prescriber. There may be interruptive, demanding immediate response before the prescription can be completed, or noninterruptive where any response is at the discretion of the prescriber. A major problem for prescribers is 'alert fatigue', where excessive numbers of alerts are increasingly ignored. This highlights the importance of focusing alerting on the most significant issues rather than highlighting every minor potential problem.

While reductions in prescribing errors have been identified in most studies, it has become clear that the move to selecting key information (e.g. patient identity, drug name, drug dose, route and frequency) from drop-down menus or predictive text, and use of 'defaults', also introduces the possibility of serious errors that would be less likely when such actions require more time and active contribution from the prescriber.

GENERAL PRACTICE PRESCRIBING

Most of the general hospital prescribing advice discussed earlier is equally applicable to general practice (GP) prescribing. Important additional issues relevant to GP prescribing are:

- *Formulation*. The prescription needs to carry information about the formulation for the dispensing community pharmacist (e.g. tablets or oral suspension).
- *Amount to be supplied*. In a hospital, the pharmacist will organise this. Elsewhere prescribers should specify the required quantity of medicine, either as the precise number of tablets or the duration of treatment. Creams and ointments should be specified in grams and lotions in millilitres.
- *Controlled drugs*. Prescriptions for 'controlled' drugs (e.g. opioid analgesics) are subject to additional legal requirements. In the UK, they must contain the address of the patient and prescriber (not necessary on most hospital forms), the form and the strength of the preparation and the total quantity of the preparation or number of dose units in words and figures.
- *Repeat prescriptions*. A large proportion of GP prescribing involves 'repeat prescriptions' for chronic conditions. These are often generated automatically although the prescriber remains responsible for ensuring that the benefit-to-harm ratio is still favourable at the time of each repeat.

PRESCRIBING INTRAVENOUS (IV) FLUIDS

Hospital prescribers not only have to prescribe medicines but frequently are called on to prescribe IV fluids for patients for whom the enteral route is not available. The patients include those who simply require their hydration maintained (e.g. nil by mouth around the time of surgery), those who have to have specific fluid losses replaced (e.g. vomiting, diarrhoea) and those who required significant established losses to be replaced before either of these options need to be considered (e.g. resuscitation of patients who are severely dehydrated after a prolonged period of fluid losses and/or poor fluid intake).

NORMAL FLUID REQUIREMENTS

The normal fluid requirements for a healthy adult are around 25–30 mL/kg/day (2400 mL/day for an 80 kg adult). This might typically consist of water that is drunk (1200 mL) and water in food (1000 mL), to which around 200 mL is added by cellular respiration. Balance is maintained because around 1400 mL of water is lost in urine, 100 mL in faeces and 900 mL by breathing and perspiration. A significant reduction in fluid intake can be accommodated by producing a lower volume of more concentrated urine. When providing IV fluid maintenance, a simple rule of thumb is that a typical adult will have a daily requirement of 25–30 mL/kg of water, approximately 1 mmol/kg/day of potassium, sodium and chloride and approximately 50 to 100 g/day of glucose to limit starvation ketosis.

MAKING AN ASSESSMENT OF FLUID REQUIREMENTS

When assessing fluid requirements, prescribers should consider:

- the average daily requirement for fluids and electrolytes
- the likely composition of any fluid losses (e.g. vomiting, burns)

- the presence of medical conditions that may affect fluid distribution or increase the risk of fluid overload (e.g. heart failure, renal impairment, respiratory failure, brain injury).

Approximate fluid requirements can be calculated based on the previous rough estimates for noncritical patients. For postsurgical and critical care patients, fluid volumes should ideally be based on haemodynamic measures. Intravascular volume status can be measured more accurately using invasive techniques such as a central venous catheter to monitor central venous pressure.

TYPES OF FLUIDS

There are four basic types of fluids (Table 1.10). They differ in their constituents, electrolyte content and the clinical situations for which they are prescribed:

- *Resuscitation fluids*. These are used to resuscitate patients suffering shock due to hypoxia, septicaemia or blood loss. They are given rapidly and must be isotonic with blood.
- *Maintenance fluids*. These are used to supply daily requirements of water and electrolytes (notably potassium) in patients who cannot receive fluids by mouth. They may also provide some of the body's energy requirements.
- *Replacement fluids*. These are used to correct fluid and electrolyte balance after specific fluid losses, for example due to diarrhoea, vomiting or gastric aspiration and sweating as a result of fever.
- *Parenteral nutrition fluids*. These are used to fulfil the patient's requirements for fluid, electrolytes and nutrition when the enteral route is unavailable or not functioning. Malnutrition delays a patient's recovery from illness and impairs wound healing after surgery. The nutrient and electrolyte content of parenteral nutrition will usually be reviewed and adjusted on a daily basis by a specialist nutrition team. The prescriber often prescribes this fluid as 'TPN' (total parenteral nutrition) with a volume and rate of administration.

Table 1.10 Types of Intravenous Fluids

TYPE OF FLUID	EXAMPLES
Resuscitation fluids	Sodium chloride 0.9% (9 mg/mL or 154 mmol/L sodium) Blood Fresh frozen plasma (FFP) Compound sodium lactate solution (e.g. Hartmann's solution, Ringer's lactate) (130 mmol/L sodium) Plasma substitutes (e.g. dextran, gelatin)
Maintenance fluids	Sodium chloride 0.9% with/without potassium Glucose 5% with/without potassium (50 g/L glucose) Glucose 4%/sodium chloride 0.18% ('dextrose saline') solutions with/without potassium Compound sodium lactate solution (Hartmann's solution, Ringer's lactate)
Replacement fluids	Sodium chloride (various strengths) with/without potassium Glucose (various strengths) with/without potassium
Parenteral nutrition	Available for administration through a central or a peripheral intravenous line with its tip lying in a large vein. These vary in their content of nitrogen, carbohydrates, lipids and electrolytes. They may also contain trace elements and vitamins

PRESCRIBING AN IV FLUID

IV fluids are usually prescribed on a hospital parenteral drug administration chart (Fig. 1.9). This document details the medicine(s) to be administered parenterally to a patient, usually by IV or SC infusion, and the diluent fluid into which they should be diluted. In some institutions, this may form an integral part of the inpatient chart or it may be a totally separate document. IV fluids are not usually prescribed on the main inpatient drug administration chart, but if drugs are included within the fluid, these must be cross-referenced to the main chart.

The parenteral drug administration chart may be used to prescribe:

- IV fluids (crystalloids and colloids)
- blood and blood products
- IV drugs (short or continuous infusions)
- parenteral nutrition
- SC fluids
- SC infusions (such as syringe pumps)

The chart is also a record of administration of the drug by nursing staff. It may include space to record the product batch number and start and end time of the infusion, and the total amount given to the patient is also recorded. The infusion chart may be accompanied by patient monitoring charts to minimise patient risk (e.g. fluid balance chart to check for fluid overload; timings of IV cannula insertion; progress of an infusion to ensure it is being administered correctly at the prescribed rate).

The risks associated with IV drug infusions are significant and so the application of the general rules of accurate prescribing previously outlined is extremely important. When prescribing IV fluids, details that must be clear are:

- Date of (administration of) the prescription
- Route of administration (usually IV or SC)
- Type of line (e.g. arterial or IV)
- Total volume to be administered
- Rate of administration
- Approved generic name of the fluid
- Approved generic name of any drug additive
- Any relevant additional information (e.g. 'monitor ECG', 'maintain systolic BP >100 mmHg')

FLUID PRESCRIPTION CHART

Hospital/Ward: REI SURGICAL	Consultant: MR WALKER	Name of Patient: JAKE SMITH
		Hospital Number: J345600
Weight: 75 kg	Height: 1.8 m	D.O.B: 5/3/1952

Date/ Time	FLUID / ADDED DRUGS	VOLUME / DOSE	ROUTE	RATE	PRESCRIBER – SIGN AND PRINT
2/9/24 19.30	SODIUM CHLORIDE 0.9%	500 mL	IV	OVER 15 MIN	J. Meyer JOHN MEYER
2/9/24 19.45	SODIUM CHLORIDE 0.9%	500 mL	IV	125 mL/H	J. Meyer JOHN MEYER
	POTASSIUM CHLORIDE (KCL)	20 mmol			

Fig. 1.9 Hospital intravenous fluid prescription chart.

MONITORING FLUID THERAPY

The beneficial and adverse effects of fluid therapy can be assessed by clinical signs (e.g. improved urine output, reduced heart rate, reduced capillary refill time, skin turgor), biochemical measurements (e.g. serum sodium, potassium, urea and creatinine) and more subjective features (e.g. thirst, general well-being). Daily weighing of the patient is probably the best short-term method of monitoring overall fluid status but provides no information about fluid distribution. Prescribers must also consider possible confounding factors. Urine output may remain low for 24 hours after surgery despite adequate fluid therapy as a normal response to injury. Diuretic therapy maintains urine output irrespective of the patient's fluid status.

POTENTIAL COMPLICATIONS OF FLUID THERAPY

Possible complications of fluid therapy include:

- *Fluid overload.* Fluid overload is a serious risk in patients with impaired cardiac function, renal failure or hepatic failure. All tend to be in a salt- and water-retaining state and are vulnerable to complications such as pulmonary oedema. Great care must be taken, especially when prescribing sodium chloride-containing fluids.
- *Biochemical abnormalities.* Prescribers should take care to assess the needs of the patient and monitor electrolytes. Hypokalaemia is a particular danger if patients are given too much fluid without potassium.
- *Allergic reactions.* These are a rare but important concern in patients who are given some synthetic plasma substitutes.
- *Haemodilution.* Large volumes of fluid may lead to haemodilution and a fall in haemoglobin, although this will usually correct itself over a few days as the fluid load is excreted.
- *Dilutional coagulopathy.* Large volumes of IV fluids may cause an apparent dilutional coagulopathy. Large volumes of some plasma substitutes can increase the risk of bleeding through depletion of coagulation factors.

MONITORING DRUG THERAPY

The outcome of a prescription, even if it is optimal and based on best evidence, is never certain for individual patients because of the pharmacodynamic and pharmacokinetic variables discussed previously. Prescribers should try to measure the effects of the drug, beneficial and harmful, to inform decisions about dose titration (up or down) or discontinuation of treatment. Monitoring can be achieved subjectively by asking the patient about their symptoms or more objectively by measuring the actual clinical effect. Alternatively, if the pharmacodynamic effects of the drug are difficult to assess then it may be possible to measure the plasma drug concentration on the basis that it will be closely related to the effect of the drug (see Fig. 1.2).

CLINICAL AND SURROGATE ENDPOINTS

The optimal approach to monitoring is to assess the clinical endpoints directly (e.g. control of ventricular rate in a patient with atrial fibrillation). The drug dosage can be titrated to achieve the desired heart rate. Sometimes, this is impractical because the clinical endpoint is a future event that cannot be detected until it is inevitable or irreversible (e.g. prevention of cardiovascular events by statins) or because it cannot be assessed at a time that allows it to be used as a guide for therapy (e.g. treating a chest infection with antibiotics). In these circumstances, it may be possible to select a surrogate endpoint that will serve to predict success or failure in achieving the desired outcome. The surrogate end point may be either:

- *Directly related to the clinical endpoint* by being an obligatory intermediate step in the pathophysiological process (e.g. serum cholesterol as a surrogate for myocardial infarction); or
- *Indirectly related to the clinical endpoint* because, although it indicates the progress of the pathophysiology, it is not a key factor in progression to the clinical endpoint (e.g. serum C-reactive protein as a surrogate marker for resolution of inflammation).

When the surrogate marker is a biological characteristic, it is termed a 'biomarker'.

PLASMA DRUG CONCENTRATION

'Therapeutic drug monitoring' is the term usually applied to the monitoring using plasma drug concentration. Three criteria must be met if plasma concentration is to be a useful marker for clinical endpoints:

- Clinical endpoints and other pharmacodynamic (surrogate) effects are difficult to monitor. If either were available, they would be preferable to a more 'remote' marker like plasma drug concentration.
- The relationship between plasma concentration and clinical effects is predictable. If this relationship is unpredictable then the drug concentration will be a poor predictor of clinical benefit or toxicity. Among antiepileptic drugs, phenytoin is exceptional in having a good correlation between its plasma concentration and clinical effects.
- The therapeutic index is low. For drugs with a high therapeutic index, any variability in plasma concentrations is likely to be irrelevant. Knowledge of the dosage alone may be sufficient to predict whether the plasma concentration is within the therapeutic range.

Some examples of drugs that fulfil these criteria are listed in Table 1.11. Measurement of plasma drug concentration can help when planning the next dose (e.g. gentamicin), assessing inadequate response (e.g. antiepileptics) or the likelihood a drug is causing an adverse effect (e.g. digoxin). The timing of the sample

Table 1.11 Drugs Commonly Monitored by Plasma Drug Concentration

DRUG	HALF-LIFE (HOURS)	MEASUREMENT
Digoxin	36	Samples should be taken at least 6 hours postdose to confirm the clinical impression of toxicity or nonadherence but not clinical effectiveness (better assessed by heart rate)
Gentamicin	2	Measure predose trough concentration to ensure that accumulation leading to nephrotoxicity and ototoxicity is avoided
Lithium	24	Samples should be taken 12 hours postdose
Phenytoin	24	Measure predose trough concentration to ensure that accumulation is avoided
Theophylline	6	Samples should be taken 6 hours postdose
Vancomycin	6	Measure predose trough concentration to assess likely clinical efficacy and ensure that accumulation and the risk of nephrotoxicity is avoided

has to take into account the rises and falls during the dosage interval (see Fig. 1.6). Measurements made during the initial absorption and distribution phases will be unpredictable because of the rapidly changing concentration. Therefore, samples are usually taken at the end of the dosage interval (a 'trough' or 'predose' concentration). This measurement has to await the attainment of steady state (five half-lives after the introduction of the drug or any change to the dosage regimen). A 'target range' is provided for most drugs and is based on average thresholds for therapeutic benefit and toxicity. Interindividual variability means that these can only be used as a guide. For instance, a patient who describes symptoms that could be consistent with toxicity but has a concentration in the top half of the target range should still be suspected of suffering toxic effects.

FURTHER READING

BPS Assessment. An interactive e-learning portal aimed primarily at medical students containing learning sessions divided into principles of clinical pharmacology, drugs, therapeutics and prescribing skills. Additional features are an online student formulary, prescribing simulator and library of resources for prescribers in training. There are also links to information about the UK Prescribing Skills Assessment. Available at https://www.bpsassessment.com/

British National Formulary (BNF). The BNF is the key reference resource for all UK prescribers with a guide to currently available formulations, with notes on dosages, uses, adverse effects and interactions; chapters on prescribing, especially in renal failure, in liver disease, in pregnancy and during breastfeeding, and appendices on drug interactions and IV additives. Available at https://bnf.nice.org.uk/

British National Formulary for Children (BNFC). The BNFC is a key reference resource to help healthcare professionals prescribe, monitor, supply and administer medicines for childhood disorders. Covering neonates to adolescents, BNFC includes key clinical and pharmaceutical information. Available at https://bnfc.nice.org.uk/

Interactive Clinical Pharmacology. An interactive learning site designed to increase understanding of important and sometimes difficult concepts and principles in clinical pharmacology. Available at https://www.icp.org.nz/

UK Teratology Information Service (UKTIS). The UKTIS provides a national service on all aspects of reproductive toxicity of medication, vaccines, chemical and radiological exposure in pregnancy and prior to pregnancy. Available at https://uktis.org/

TOXBASE. TOXBASE is run by the National Poisons Information Service (NPIS) for health professionals in the UK and contains information on approximately 14,000 products, together with generic advice on the management of poisoning. Available at https://www.toxbase.org/

The Cochrane Collaboration. The Cochrane Collaboration is a leading international collaboration to promote the accessibility of evidence-based reviews—around 7500 systematic reviews so far—published online in The Cochrane Library. Available at https://www.cochrane.org/

Food and Drug Administration (FDA). The US regulator of medicines, devices and other biological products. Available at https://www.fda.gov/

Medicines and Healthcare products Regulatory Agency (MHRA). The major regulator of medicines in the UK and home of the Yellow Card pharmacovigilance system. Available at https://www.gov.uk/government/organisations/medicines-and-healthcare-products-regulatory-agency

National Prescribing Curriculum. A series of interactive cases designed for Australian students learning to prescribe. Available at https://www.nps.org.au/cpd/npc-modules

Therapeutic Guidelines. Therapeutic Guidelinesis a leading source of independent, evidence-based, practical treatment advice to assist Australian practitioners with decision making at the point-of-care. Available at https://www.tg.org.au/

Good Practice in Prescribing and Managing Medicines. Guidance advice from the UK medical regulator (General Medical Council) about standards for prescribing and managing medicines. Available at https://www.gmc-uk.org/professional-standards/professional-standards-for-doctors/good-practice-in-prescribing-and-managing-medicines-and-devices

NICE Guidelines. NICE makes recommendations to the UK NHS on new and existing medicines, treatments and procedures for treating and caring for people with specific diseases and conditions. Available at https://www.nice.org.uk/guidance

NICE Guideline CG174. Intravenous fluid therapy in adults in hospital. Available at https://www.nice.org.uk/guidance/cg174

World Health Organization. Essential Medicines and Pharmaceutical Policies. A list of key policies related to medicines availability worldwide. Available at https://www.who.int/health-topics/medicines/#tab=tab_1

Cardiology

2

Simon R.J. Maxwell

Chapter Outline

Station 2.1: Acute Pericarditis
Station 2.2: Acute Left Ventricular Failure
Station 2.3: Acute Coronary Syndrome
Station 2.4: Bradycardia
Station 2.5: Tachycardia
Station 2.6: Warfarin Prescribing

STATION 2.1: ACUTE PERICARDITIS

You are an emergency department junior doctor. Your next patient is Jason Anderson (date of birth (DOB) 22/03/95), a 29-year-old man, who has come in with chest pain. He says he has felt generally unwell over the last few days with a fever, muscle aches and a sore throat. Today, he developed sharp retrosternal chest pain radiating to his neck. The pain is worsened by movement and breathing. Please assess Mr Anderson and start appropriate management.

Patient Details

Name:	Jason Anderson
DOB:	22/03/95
Hospital number:	2203959943
Weight:	75 kg
Height:	1.8 m
Consultant:	Dr Chang
Hospital/Ward:	RIE Ward 6
Current medications:	None
Allergies:	None
Admission date:	19/10/24

Initial Differential Diagnosis of Sharp Chest Pain

- Cardiac: Acute pericarditis, acute coronary syndrome, angina
- Respiratory: Pneumothorax, pneumonia, pulmonary embolism
- Gastrointestinal (GI): Oesophageal pain (e.g. spasm, reflux), gastric pain, biliary pain
- Other: Musculoskeletal chest pain (e.g. costochondritis, rib fracture), shingles

Acute Pericarditis Management

- Non-steroidal antiinflammatory drugs (NSAIDs) (+gastric protection)
- Colchicine
- Pericardiocentesis and drainage may be required if a large pericardial effusion is present

INITIAL ASSESSMENT

AIRWAY

- Assess the patency of the airway.

'The patient is maintaining a patent airway.'

No additional airway support required.

BREATHING

- Assess respiratory rate, oxygen saturations and work of breathing. Palpate for chest wall tenderness. Percuss; hyperresonance suggests a pneumothorax, dullness to percussion suggests pleural effusion or pneumonia. Auscultate for air entry and additional sounds (e.g. wheeze, crepitations).

'Respiration rate (RR) 12/min, oxygen saturations are 97% on air. No chest wall tenderness. The chest is resonant throughout. Good air entry is heard bilaterally with no wheeze or crackles.'

No respiratory support required.

CIRCULATION

- Assess haemodynamic stability by measuring heart rate (HR), blood pressure (BP) and capillary refill time (CRT).
- Perform a cardiovascular examination. A pericardial friction rub points to pericarditis. Muffled heart sounds, a raised jugular venous pressure (JVP) and hypotension point to cardiac tamponade.

'Heart rate (HR) 78 bpm regular, blood pressure (BP) 128/64 mmHg, capillary refill time (CRT) <2 seconds. The JVP is not elevated. Cardiovascular system (CVS) examination shows normal heart sounds (HS) with a pericardial friction rub. No murmurs.'

Obtain intravenous (IV) access and send off bloods.

For patients with chest pain, ask a colleague to perform an electrocardiogram (ECG) while you perform your clinical assessment.

DISABILITY

- Assess the patient's conscious level, using AVPU (Is the patient Alert? If not, do they respond to Verbal or Painful stimuli? Or are they Unresponsive?). Check glucose levels.

'The patient is alert. Blood glucose 6.9 mmol/L.'

EXPOSURE

- Expose the patient and perform a full examination (while maintaining the patient's dignity). In particular, look at the throat for evidence of upper respiratory tract infection and the chest wall for signs of shingles. Measure the temperature.

'Temperature is 37.2°C. There is mild erythema in his throat with some palpable cervical lymph nodes. The rest of the examination is normal.'

Causes of Acute Pericarditis

- Viral
- Acute myocardial infarction
- Autoimmune disease, e.g. rheumatoid arthritis or systemic lupus erythematosus (SLE)
- Uraemia
- Malignant disease
- Bacterial or tuberculosis (TB) infection (rare in UK)
- Rheumatic fever (rare in UK)

ECG Changes in Acute Pericarditis

- Initially concave anterior and inferior ST elevation
- ST segments will return to baseline over the next couple of weeks with T wave inversion developing
- PR depression
- ECG returns completely to baseline usually after a few months

INITIAL INVESTIGATIONS

- **Bloods**: Full blood count (FBC), urea and electrolyte (U&Es), erythrocyte sedimentation rate (ESR), C-reactive protein (CRP) (Table 2.1). Look for evidence of inflammation. Troponin is used as a marker of myocardial damage (elevated in ≈50% with pericarditis) but may also help differentiate from acute coronary syndrome (ACS). U&Es will show elevated urea in uraemic pericarditis.
- **ECG**: Classical finding is widespread 'saddle-shaped' ST elevation with upwards concavity in I, II, aVF, aVL and V3–6. PR depression is virtually diagnostic of pericarditis. Helps distinguish from myocardial infarction.

Table 2.1 Mr Anderson's Blood Test Results

PARAMETER	VALUE	NORMAL RANGE (UNITS)
Haemoglobin	140 g/L	Men: 135–180 (g/L) Women: 115–160 (g/L)
WCC	**18.3 × 10^9/L**	**3.2–11.0 (×10^9/L)**
Neutrophil	**9.4 × 10^9/L**	**1.9–7.7 (×10^9/L)**
Lymphocyte	**8.2 × 10^9/L**	**1.3–3.5 (×10^9/L)**
Platelet	350 × 10^9/L	120–400 (×10^9/L)
ESR	**48 mm/h**	**Men: (Age in years)/2 (mm/h) Women: (Age in years + 10)/2 (mm/h)**
CRP	**63 mg/L**	**0–10 (mg/L)**
Urea	5.5 mmol/L	2.5–6.7 (mmol/L)
Creatinine	80 µmol/L	70–130 (µmol/L)
eGFR	>60 mL/min	>60 (mL/min)
Sodium	140 mmol/L	135–145 (mmol/L)
Potassium	4.2 mmol/L	3.5–5.0 (mmol/L)
Troponin	0.01 µg/L	0–0.1 (µg/L)

Data in bold signifies results that are outside the normal laboratory range.
CRP, C-reactive protein; *CXR*, chest radiograph; *eGFR*, estimated glomerular filtration rate; *ESR*, erythrocyte sedimentation rate; *WCC*, white cell count.

- **Chest radiography (CXR)**: Can range from normal to the classic water-bottle-shaped heart seen with pericardial effusions. Helps exclude differential diagnoses such as pneumothorax and pneumonia.
- **Echocardiogram**: Will show pericardial effusions (present in 10% of cases of pericarditis) and tamponade if present—although tamponade should be diagnosed clinically. It will also demonstrate concomitant heart disease, such as left ventricular wall motion abnormalities seen post-myocardial infarction.

'Bloods show an elevated WCC (18.3 × 10^9/L), ESR (48 mm/h) and CRP (63 mg/L). Troponin and U&Es are normal. ECG shows widespread concave ST elevation and PR depression. CXR shows mild cardiomegaly, with clear lungs and no pneumothorax. The echocardiogram shows a small pericardial effusion.'

INITIAL MANAGEMENT

- This patient has acute pericarditis, most likely secondary to a viral infection.
- **Airway support:** Airway patent in this case, with no intervention required.
- **Supplementary oxygen:** If oxygen saturation is <94%.
- **NSAID:** Ibuprofen is preferred due to its side effect profile and large dose range (300–800 mg PO 6–8 hourly depending on severity).
- **Colchicine:** Can be used in combination with NSAIDs or as a monotherapy as a second-line treatment. Dose is 0.5 mg PO twice daily (BD) or once daily (OD) for patients <70 kg.

- **Additional analgesia:** Use the World Health Organization pain ladder, starting at the most appropriate level.
- **Gastric protection:** Should be considered in all patients starting NSAIDs particularly those at increased risk of gastrotoxicity such as the elderly or those treated over an extended period.
- **Thromboembolic risk assessment:** This should be considered but, in a potential pericardial effusion, avoid anticoagulation due to risk of haemorrhagic transformation of the effusion.

Prescribe (see Figs 2.1 and 2.2)

Antiinflammatory:
- IBUPROFEN 400 mg PO STAT then TDS

Gastric protection:
- OMEPRAZOLE 20 mg PO OD

Analgesia:
- CO-CODAMOL 30/500 2 tablets STAT then 2 tablets PO QDS

Mechanical thromboembolic prophylaxis:
- ANTIEMBOLISM STOCKINGS TOP

Corticosteroids are not routinely used in acute pericarditis. They are reserved for patients with connective tissue disease, autoimmune or uraemic pericarditis. Corticosteroids may also be helpful in recurrent pericarditis and in patients who are refractory to NSAIDs and colchicine.

Complications of Acute Pericarditis

- Recurrence
- Pericardial effusion
- Cardiac tamponade
- Constrictive pericarditis

REASSESSMENT

- After receiving some ibuprofen and co-codamol, the patient is reassessed.

'Mr Anderson looks more comfortable. He still has chest pain but it is not as severe. His observations remain stable and his clinical examination is unchanged.'

FURTHER TREATMENT

- **Tapered dose of NSAIDs:** As the patient recovers. Patients with viral pericarditis usually take a few days or weeks to recover.
- **Pericardiocentesis:** Mandatory in patients with cardiac tamponade (hypotension, raised JVP, muffled heart sounds and pulsus paradoxus). It should be considered in patients with possible bacterial or neoplastic pericarditis. It is optional in patients with large or recurrent pericardial effusions or patients with small pericardial effusions in whom the other tests have been inconclusive (allows identification of underlying aetiology of the effusion).

HANDING OVER THE PATIENT

'Mr Anderson is a 29-year-old man with acute viral pericarditis. He presented with sharp chest pain on a background of an upper respiratory tract infection. He is haemodynamically stable. Investigations are in keeping with viral pericarditis and there is a small pericardial effusion, confirmed on echocardiogram. He has commenced ibuprofen, co-codamol and gastric protection.

He has been reviewed by the cardiology registrar and will be admitted to the cardiology ward overnight for observations with a view to discharge tomorrow and plans for a repeat echocardiogram in a couple of days to ensure the pericardial effusion is not enlarging. He requires a pain review later this evening.'

STATION 2.2: ACUTE LEFT VENTRICULAR FAILURE

You are the junior doctor on the hospital-at-night team. One of the nurses fast-bleeps you to see an 84-year-old woman, Mrs Margaret Jenkins (DOB 20/08/40), who has become acutely breathless and is coughing up pink frothy sputum. She was admitted last night with a 4-day history of diarrhoea and dehydration. She has been given 4 litres of fluid over the last 12 hours.

She was diagnosed with moderate left ventricular systolic dysfunction (LVSD) during a previous admission to hospital 2 weeks ago following an episode of collapse. During that admission, she was started on an angiotensin-converting enzyme (ACE) inhibitor, a beta-blocker and furosemide, all of which have been withheld so far because of her dehydration.

Patient Details

Name:	Margaret Jenkins
DOB:	20/08/40
Hospital number:	2008406547
Weight:	58 kg
Height:	1.5 m
Consultant:	Dr Ross
Hospital/Ward:	LGH Ward 45
Current medications:	Enoxaparin 40 mg SC OD (started on admission) 0.9% sodium chloride 500 mL (with 20 mmol potassium chloride) 125 mL/h (started on admission) Ramipril 1.25 mg PO OD (withheld) Bisoprolol 1.25 mg PO OD (withheld) Furosemide 40 mg PO BD (withheld)
Allergies:	Clarithromycin (rash)
Admission date:	21/10/24

Initial Differential Diagnosis of Acute Dyspnoea

- Cardiac: myocardial infarction (MI), pulmonary oedema, cardiac tamponade
- Respiratory: asthma, pneumothorax, pulmonary embolism (PE), pneumonia
- Anaphylaxis
- Inhaled foreign body
- Metabolic acidosis

Acute Left Ventricular Failure (LVF) Initial Management Summary

- Sit the patient upright
- Oxygen (for hypoxaemia)
- Loop diuretic
- Nitrate (in some circumstances)
- Morphine (no longer used routinely)

INITIAL ASSESSMENT

AIRWAY

- Assess patency of the airway.

'There is a large amount of frothy pink secretions coming from the patient's mouth and you hear a strange choking noise.'

You clear the patient's airway using suction and the airway noises clear.

BREATHING

- Sit the patient up.
- Assess respiratory rate, oxygen saturations and work of breathing.
- Perform a respiratory examination—particularly looking for use of accessory muscles and bibasal crackles on auscultation.

'RR is 34/min, oxygen saturation is 82% on room air. There is no history of COPD. Mrs Jenkins is using her accessory muscles. There are coarse bibasal crackles.'

Start the patient on oxygen at a rate of 15 L/min via a nonrebreather mask (unless there is a known history or suspicion of CO_2 retention). Perform an arterial blood gas (ABG) and request an urgent portable CXR.

CIRCULATION

- Assess haemodynamic status by measuring HR, BP, CRT and urine output.
- Perform a cardiovascular examination, looking at the JVP, listening to the heart for murmurs, e.g. ventricular septal defect (VSD) or mitral regurgitation, and additional heart sounds. Feel for hepatomegaly or ascites, and check for peripheral oedema around the ankles or over the sacrum in bed-bound patients.

'The patient is tachycardic at 150 bpm, with a BP of 152/90 mmHg and CRT of 3 seconds. She looks distressed and is sweating profusely. The JVP is raised—so much so that the earlobe is "wiggling". There is a third heart sound on auscultation. Mrs Jenkins has pitting oedema of both legs to the knees.'

Stop the IV fluids (which have precipitated acute heart failure) and treat for pulmonary oedema with oxygen and furosemide. Nitrates (e.g. glyceryl trinitrate IV infusion) may be given in specific circumstances such as concomitant myocardial ischaemia or severe hypertension. Consider morphine (with an antiemetic drug) if there is pain or severe distress, but there is increasing evidence that its use is associated with dose-dependent adverse effects and worse outcomes. Perform an ECG looking for any precipitating causes for the LVF such as arrhythmias, left ventricular hypertrophy (LVH) (secondary to hypertension) or ischaemia. Obtain IV access and take bloods. Insert a urinary catheter, if not already in place, to allow accurate assessment of fluid balance.

Prescribe (see Figs 2.3–2.5)

High-flow oxygen:
- 15 L/min of OXYGEN (via a NONREBREATHER MASK)

Loop diuretic:
- FUROSEMIDE 40 mg IV STAT

CONSIDER PRESCRIBING

Nitrate:
- GLYCERYL TRINITRATE IV infusion starting at a rate of 20–25 micrograms/minute and titrate upwards as appropriate

Analgesia/venodilator:
- MORPHINE 1 to 10 mg (titrate to response) IV STAT

Antiemetic:
- METOCLOPRAMIDE 10 mg IV STAT

STOP

IV fluids

DISABILITY

- Assess the patient's Glasgow Coma Scale (GCS) or AVPU and check the blood glucose.

'The patient is GCS 14 (E4, M6, V4). Blood glucose is 4.0 mmol/L.'

EXPOSURE

- Expose the patient while ensuring you maintain her dignity.
- Examine the abdomen (although this can also be part of the CVS examination).
- Check the temperature.

'Abdominal examination is unremarkable. Temperature is 35.9°C.'

LVF is most commonly caused by ischaemic heart disease, but it can also be due to hypertension, cardiomyopathy or aortic/mitral valve disease.

Cardiomegaly on CXR is defined as a cardiothoracic width ratio >50% (compare the transverse diameter of the heart with the transverse diameter of the lungs). This is only an accurate sign if seen on a PA (postero-anterior) CXR.

INITIAL INVESTIGATIONS

- **CXR:** Look for the typical features of LVF, although the radiographic changes can lag behind the clinical picture. Features of pulmonary oedema on chest X-ray are 'bat's wing' shadowing, pleural effusions, Kerley B lines, cardiomegaly and upper lobe blood flow diversion. Look for other causes of acute dyspnoea, such as consolidation or pneumothorax.
- **ECG:** Look for ischaemic changes indicating an MI which may have caused the LVF, or arrhythmias, such as fast atrial fibrillation (AF), which can cause or be a consequence of LVF.
- **ABG:** This will likely show hypoxia. Initially, the $PaCO_2$ might be low due to hyperventilation but may rise later due to reduced gas exchange. Look to see if the patient is acidotic, as this is important in determining whether continuous positive airway pressure (CPAP) (type 1 respiratory failure) or bilevel positive airway pressure (BiPAP) (type 2 respiratory failure) is required. Remember patients with renal failure may already have a metabolic acidosis, and therefore could be acidotic with a normal $PaCO_2$ as well as with type 2 respiratory failure. Indeed, a metabolic and respiratory acidosis might exist together.
- **Echocardiogram:** An important investigation to be performed early. This may demonstrate the cause of heart failure, e.g. LVSD or aortic stenosis (AS), which would guide decisions about later treatment, e.g. ACE inhibitor/beta-blocker for LVSD, surgery for AS.
- **Bloods:** FBC, U&Es, liver function tests (LFTs), thyroid function tests (TFTs), CRP (Table 2.2). Look for evidence of infection by doing an FBC and CRP. Look for anaemia as this may exacerbate heart failure. Check U&Es (because you will be treating the patient with diuretics and an ACE inhibitor) and look at the LFTs, which may be deranged if there is hepatic congestion in right heart failure. Check blood glucose for diabetes. Troponin may be high if an MI has precipitated the LVF; however, it may be difficult to interpret as it can be raised by LVF itself. Thyroid function tests should be done, as thyroid disease can aggravate or mimic heart failure.

'CXR shows cardiomegaly, upper lobe venous diversion, pleural effusions, with fluid in the horizontal fissure, and Kerley B lines. ECG shows sinus tachycardia. Bloods show a normal FBC, urea 6.8 mmol/L, creatinine 156 µmol/L, eGFR 58 mL/min, Na 140 mmol/L, K 4.2 mmol/L. TFTs are in progress. LFTs are normal. ABG on air shows type 1 respiratory failure, with a PaO_2 8.1 kPa, $PaCO_2$ 4.9 kPa, pH 7.35, HCO_3^- 24 mmol/L.'

Table 2.2 Mrs Jenkins' Blood Test and Arterial Blood Gas Results

PARAMETER	VALUE	NORMAL RANGE (UNITS)
Haemoglobin	150 g/L	Men: 135–180 (g/L) Women: 115–160 (g/L)
WCC	10.2 × 10^9/L	3.2–11.0 (×10^9/L)
Neutrophil	6.1 × 10^9/L	1.9–7.7 (×10^9/L)
Lymphocyte	3.2 × 10^9/L	1.3–3.5 (×10^9/L)
Platelet	200 × 10^9/L	120–400 (×10^9/L)
CRP	4 mg/L	0–10 (mg/L)
Urea	**6.8 mmol/L**	**2.5–6.7 (mmol/L)**
Creatinine	**156 µmol/L**	**70–130 (µmol/L)**
eGFR	**58 mL/min**	**>60 (mL/min)**
Sodium	140 mmol/L	135–145 (mmol/L)
Potassium	4.2 mmol/L	3.5–5.0 (mmol/L)
Bilirubin	5 µmol/L	3–17 (µmol/L)
ALT	20 IU/L	5–35 (IU/L)
ALP	57 IU/L	30–300 (IU/L)
pH	7.35	7.35–7.45
PaO_2	**8.1 kPa on air**	**>10.0 (kPa) on air**
$PaCO_2$	4.9 kPa	4.7–6.0 (kPa)
HCO_3^-	24 mmol/L	22–26 (mmol/L)

Data in bold signifies results that are outside the normal laboratory range.
ABG, Arterial blood gas; *ALP*, alkaline phosphatase; *ALT*, alanine transaminase; *CRP*, C-reactive protein; *CXR*, chest radiograph; *ECG*, electrocardiogram; *eGFR*, estimated glomerular filtration rate; *FBC*, full blood count; *LFT*, liver function test; *TFT*, thyroid function test; *WCC*, white cell count.

INITIAL MANAGEMENT

- **Posture:** Simple but important—sit the patient up to reduce venous return to the heart.
- **Oxygen:** Should be given to treat hypoxaemia when oxygen saturation is <90%, which is associated with an increased short-term mortality. Oxygen should not be given if the patient is not hypoxaemic, as it can cause vasoconstriction and reduced cardiac output. Consider CPAP for early refractory hypoxia.
- **Loop diuretic:** Treat with furosemide. If the patient is diuretic naïve and has normal renal function, then 40 mg IV initially is adequate. If the patient is already on diuretics or has renal failure, then higher doses may be needed, e.g. 50 to 100 mg IV. Doses above 50 mg must be given by IV infusion and at a rate no faster than 4 mg/min. Elderly people, especially if they have a low body weight, will also require a dose reduction. Diuretics will cause immediate vasodilation as well as the delayed diuresis.

- **Nitrates:** Consider giving a glyceryl trinitrate IV infusion immediately providing the systolic BP is >100 mmHg. Start at a rate of 20 to 25 micrograms/minute and titrate upwards by 20 to 25 microgram/minute increments at 15- to 30-minute intervals until the desired effect is obtained. Common side effects are headache and hypotension. The nitrate will act as a venodilator, which is intended to reduce preload on the heart.
- **Morphine:** Opioids are no longer given routinely but should be considered when there is pain or distress. They have the added benefit of causing venodilatation and reducing preload on the heart. Titrate 1 to 10 mg in 1-mg increments according to response. Reduce the dose if the patient is elderly, frail or has a history of respiratory disease. Don't forget to prescribe a prophylactic antiemetic with it, for example, metoclopramide 10 mg IV. Monitor respiratory rate while giving morphine.
- **Monitor urine output:** Insert a catheter. This will demonstrate whether a good diuresis has occurred. Start a fluid balance chart.
- If the patient has evidence of bronchospasm, treat with a salbutamol nebuliser, e.g. 5 mg, which will improve work of breathing and improve oxygen saturation.
- **Deep vein thrombosis (DVT) prophylaxis:** As per local protocol, to be given to patients not already being anticoagulated, who have no contraindications.
- **Consider early high-dependency unit (HDU)/intensive therapy unit (ITU) referral:** The patient may need central venous pressure (CVP) monitoring, or ventilation support (CPAP for type 1 respiratory failure, or BiPAP for type 2 respiratory failure).

Prescribe (see Figs 2.3–2.5)

Loop diuretic:

- FUROSEMIDE 60 mg IV OD and 40 mg IV OD (total 100 mg in 24 h)
  Ensure appropriate thromboprophylaxis

REASSESSMENT

- Repeat the ABCDE process.

'Mrs Jenkins does not appear to be much better. She is still producing secretions and is now requiring airway support with a nasopharyngeal airway device. RR is now 36/min. Oxygen saturations are 93% on 15 L oxygen. There are still loud bibasal crackles. HR is 125 bpm and BP is 98/66 mmHg. The peripheries are clammy with a CRT of 3 seconds. Cardiac examination is unchanged. Mrs Jenkins has passed approximately 10 mL of urine over the last 45 minutes. The nurse is worried about managing her on the ward as they have other patients who require their attention.'

You need to speak with ITU urgently. The patient has had a poor response to the initial treatment. In severe or resistant cases, patients will require more invasive monitoring (e.g. CVP) and may require support with inotropes or an intraaortic balloon pump, particularly as she is now hypotensive. Obviously, this is something that a junior doctor will not be required to deal with, but it is useful to know what further treatment may be available.

When you're working night shifts, you will often be given a pile of fluid charts for patients who are on IV fluids. While it can be time consuming to assess every individual patient, this scenario highlights the importance of regular fluid reviews and the dangers of excessive fluid administration to frail, elderly patients.

When Doing a Fluid Review:

- Look at the fluid chart to calculate the fluid balance.
- Check the observations and recent U&E results.
- Examine the patient—look at the CRT, look for dry mucous membranes, check the JVP, listen to the heart and lungs and look for peripheral oedema.

HANDING OVER THE PATIENT TO ITU

'My name is Emma Smith and I'm the Foundation Year 1 (FY1) doctor covering the wards tonight. I'd like to discuss a patient with you, whom I'd like you to review please.

The patient is Mrs Jenkins, an 84-year-old woman, who has developed acute pulmonary oedema this evening, after treatment with IV fluids for the last 2 days. She is known to have a history of moderate LVSD but has no other significant medical history.

She has failed to improve significantly despite high-flow oxygen, furosemide and a glyceryl trinitrate infusion. Her current observations are oxygen sats 93% on 15 L oxygen, RR is 36/min, HR 125 bpm, BP 98/66 mmHg. She has a markedly elevated JVP, coarse bibasal crackles and bilateral pitting oedema. She has only passed 10 mL of urine in the last 45 minutes.

She was previously independent and had a good quality of life, and we feel that she would be a candidate for escalation of her care. I'm just about to repeat her ABG, but please could you review her urgently.'

When referring a patient to ITU, you should be able to give a bit of background about the patient's comorbidities and health status prior to the current illness. Was Mrs Jenkins living independently prior to admission or was she in a nursing home? Did she get out to socialise, or do her shopping or was she housebound with a package of care? Does she have any other chronic illnesses, for example chronic respiratory disease or end-stage cancer? These are all important factors in considering whether a patient is an appropriate candidate for intensive care treatment.

FURTHER MANAGEMENT

After 24 hours in ITU, Mrs Jenkins has improved and she is transferred to the ward for ongoing care.

- Closely monitor the patient's symptoms, signs and observations.
- Measure the fluid intake and output on daily fluid balance charts.
- Tailor ongoing treatment according to clinical response.
- Weigh the patient daily.
- Monitor U&Es daily. Diuretics can impair renal function and cause hypokalaemia, ACE inhibitors can impair renal function and cause hyperkalaemia.
- **Diuretics:** To relieve symptoms of fluid overload, tailor the dose to the patient's clinical need with careful review of renal function.
- **ACE inhibitors:** Recommended in all patients with heart failure and a reduced ejection fraction. This reduces the risk of future heart failure related hospitalisations and premature death. Start at a low dose and titrate up, monitoring U&Es after each increment. Note angiotension receptor blocker (ARB) can be used if ACE inhibitor not tolerated, usually due to a persistent cough.
- **Beta-blockers:** Once the episode of acute left ventricular failure has been stabilised. They are recommended for all patients with heart failure and reduced ejection fraction to reduce the risk of future heart failure-related hospitalisations and premature death. Titrate the dose up, monitoring HR and BP after each increment.
- **Mineralocorticoid (aldosterone) receptor antagonists, e.g. spironolactone or eplerenone:** Recommended for patients with class II to IV heart failure and persistent fluid overload despite the above treatment, as it again, reduces the risk of future heart failure-related hospitalisations and premature death.
- **Digoxin:** Now less frequently prescribed but may still be considered for patients with reduced ejection fraction and coexisting AF or patients with severe and resistant LVSD.
- Antiplatelet drugs (e.g. aspirin) and statin drugs should be considered for patients with atherosclerotic arterial disease.
- Sodium-glucose co-transporter 2 (SGLT2) inhibitors (e.g. dapagliflozin) should be considered for patients with symptomatic chronic heart failure.
- Causes of heart failure (e.g. coronary artery disease, arrhythmias, hypertension, cardiomyopathy) should be identified and managed. This may involve an angiogram, measuring BP or further blood tests, e.g. TFTs, ferritin, vitamin B_{12}
- Patient education is important—diagnosis and treatment should be discussed, as well as risk factor modification, diet and general lifestyle advice.
- Consider involving a specialist heart failure nurse for ongoing patient education and review in the community.
- Other issues to consider are the emergence of symptoms of depression or anxiety, vaccinations against influenza and pneumococcal infections and, if appropriate, advanced planning about care options in the event of future clinical deterioration.

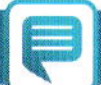

Prescribe (see Figs 2.3–2.5)

ACE inhibitor:
- RAMIPRIL 1.25 mg PO OD

Beta-blocker:
- BISOPROLOL 1.25 mg PO OD

New York Heart Association (NYHA) Functional Classification of Heart Failure Symptoms

Stage I: No limitation to activities

Stage II: Slightly limited physical activity—no symptoms at rest but ordinary physical activity may cause symptoms

Stage III: Marked limitation of physical activity, less than ordinary physical activity causes symptoms, with no symptoms at rest

Stage IV: Unable to carry out any physical activity, and symptoms present at rest

STATION 2.3: ACUTE CORONARY SYNDROME

You are the junior doctor covering the evening shift on the medicine of the elderly ward. One of the nurses asks you to come and urgently assess Mr John Drummond (15/10/52), a 72-year-old man, who was admitted 14 days ago with cellulitis. He has been recovering well and was due to be discharged tomorrow. The nurse tells you he is complaining of central crushing chest pain. On your arrival, Mr Drummond looks clammy and grey, and is clutching a sick bowl.

Patient Details

Name:	John Drummond
DOB:	15/10/52
Hospital number:	1510521543
Weight:	72 kg
Height:	1.86 m
Consultant:	Dr James
Hospital/Ward:	KGH Ward 26
Current medications:	Enoxaparin 40 mg SC OD (started on admission for thromboprophylaxis)
Allergies:	None known
Admission date:	8/10/24

Initial Differential Diagnosis of Chest Pain

- Cardiac: ACS or angina, pericarditis, aortic dissection
- Respiratory: Pneumonia, PE, pneumothorax
- GI: Gastroesophageal reflux disease (GORD)
- Musculoskeletal: Costochondritis, trauma

Initial Management of Non-ST Elevation (NSTEMI) Acute Coronary Syndrome

- Oxygen (if hypoxaemic)
- Morphine (with antiemetic)
- Nitrates
- Aspirin
- Fondaparinux sodium (or unfractionated heparin if there is a high bleeding risk or significant renal impairment)
- Assess 6-month mortality using a risk scoring system (e.g. Global Registry of Acute Cardiac Events (GRACE))
- Second antiplatelet agent with choice depending on risk stratification: clopidogrel for low-risk patients being managed conservatively (or those with higher bleeding risk), ticagrelor or prasugrel for high-risk patients having angiography and percutaneous coronary intervention (PCI)
- Cardiac monitoring

Management of ST Elevation (STEMI) Acute Coronary Syndrome

- Patients with ST elevation ACS should be considered for early reperfusion therapy (if presenting within 12 hours of symptom onset). If PCI cannot be performed within 120 minutes of diagnosis, they should be considered for immediate thrombolysis.
- Treatment is otherwise similar as for non-ST elevation ACS (prasugrel is the preferred second antiplatelet agent for patients undergoing a primary PCI unless there is a high bleeding risk).
- Contraindications to thrombolysis include intracranial tumour, aortic dissection, pericarditis, stroke or GI/genitourinary (GU) bleed within the last 3 months, major surgery/biopsy/trauma/head injury within the last 6 weeks, bleeding diathesis, prolonged cardiopulmonary resuscitation (CPR) (>10 minutes), impaired GCS following cardiac arrest, pregnancy and neurosurgery within the last year.

INITIAL ASSESSMENT

AIRWAY

- Assess patency of the airway.

'The airway is patent.'

No further airway support required.

BREATHING

- Assess respiratory rate, oxygen saturations and work of breathing.
- Perform a respiratory examination—particularly listening out for bibasal crackles suggesting left ventricular failure.

'RR 30/min, oxygen saturations are 92%. On auscultation the chest sounds clear.'

Given these, you put the patient on high-flow oxygen via a nonrebreather mask (providing there is no history of chronic obstructive pulmonary disease (COPD)) and maintain the SpO_2 >94%.

CIRCULATION

- Assess haemodynamic status by measuring HR, BP and CRT.
- Perform a cardiovascular examination, looking for a raised JVP indicating right heart failure, any murmurs or extra heart sounds (e.g. a third heart sound may be heard in congestive cardiac failure (CCF)) and bibasal crackles or peripheral oedema also indicating LVF or CCF.
- Perform an ECG and attach the patient to continuous cardiac monitoring.

'HR is 122 bpm, BP is 110/70 mmHg, CRT is 4 seconds and the peripheries feel cold and clammy. CV examination reveals a normal JVP, HS I + II + no added sounds. ECG shows a sinus tachycardia with 3 mm ST depression in leads II, III and aVF.'

Obtain IV access and take bloods. Treat for non-ST elevation ACS.

Prescribe (see Figs 2.6–2.7)

HIGH-FLOW OXYGEN:
- 15 L/min (via a NON-REBREATHER MASK)

Antiplatelet:
- ASPIRIN 300 mg PO STAT and CLOPIDOGREL 300 mg PO STAT

Gastric protection alongside antiplatelets:
- LANSOPRAZOLE 30 mg PO STAT

LMWH or Factor Xa inhibitor:
- FONDAPARINUX 2.5 mg SC STAT

Analgesia:
- MORPHINE 1 to 10 mg IV (titrate to response) STAT, with METOCLOPRAMIDE 10 mg IV STAT

Nitrates:
- GLYCERYL TRINITRATE 800 micrograms (2 sprays) SL STAT

STOP

Enoxaparin (thromboprophylaxis dose)

- ACS encompasses ST-elevation MI, non-ST-elevation MI and unstable angina. Patients who have ST elevation (>1 mm in two or more adjacent limb leads, or >1 mm in two or more adjacent chest leads) should be taken for primary PCI treatment immediately to reperfuse the ischaemic myocardium.

The ECG should be repeated after 10 minutes to look for any evolving changes.

DISABILITY

- Assess the patient's GCS or AVPU level, and check blood glucose.

'Mr Drummond is GCS 15 and his blood glucose is 8 mmol/L.'

EXPOSURE

- Expose the patient looking for any further abnormalities, and don't forget to check the legs for any signs of a DVT. Check the temperature.

'Temperature is 36.5°C, and examination is otherwise normal.'

Myocardial ischaemia can sometimes be secondary to anaemia, e.g. due to an acute GI bleed (in which case anticoagulant treatment would be contraindicated). It can be easy to overlook these things during a stressful situation!

INITIAL INVESTIGATIONS

- **ECG:** The initial investigation. Infarction: ST elevation. Ischaemic change: ST depression. T-wave flattening, inversion or becoming biphasic. Q-wave changes are seen later on—look for 'pathological' Q waves which are >1 mm wide and >2 mm deep.
- **CXR:** This should be portable if the patient is unstable. Look for acute LVF secondary to MI, cardiomegaly—which may indicate chronic cardiovascular disease, or widening of the aorta indicating a possible dissection as well as any pulmonary causes for the pain.
- **Bloods:** Perform a baseline troponin, FBC, U&Es, lipid profile and glucose (Table 2.3). Lipid profile must be done within the first 12 hours, after this the result can be inaccurate. A 12-hour troponin would be needed subsequently.

Table 2.3 Mr Drummond's Blood Test Results

PARAMETER	VALUE	NORMAL RANGE (UNITS)
Haemoglobin	150 g/L	Men: 135–180 (g/L) Women: 115–160 (g/L)
WCC	8.3 × 10^9/L	3.2–11.0 (×10^9/L)
Neutrophil	4.8 × 10^9/L	1.9–7.7 (×10^9/L)
Lymphocyte	22.7 × 10^9/L	1.3–3.5 (×10^9/L)
Platelet	250 × 10^9/L	120–400 (×10^9/L)
Urea	6.1 mmol/L	2.5–6.7 (mmol/L)
Creatinine	80 µmol/L	70–130 (µmol/L)
Sodium	140 mmol/L	135–145 (mmol/L)
Potassium	4.4 mmol/L	3.5–5.0 (mmol/L)
eGFR	>60 mL/min	>60 (mL/min)
Troponin	**1 µg/L**	**0–0.1 (µg/L)**
Total cholesterol	**7.9 mmol/L**	**3.9–5.5 (mmol/L)**
HDL cholesterol	1.5 mmol/L	0.9–1.9 (mmol/L)
LDL cholesterol	**5.8 mmol/L**	**1.5–4.4 (mmol/L)**
Glucose	5.5 mmol/L	3.5–5.5 (mmol/L) (fasting)

Data in bold signifies results that are outside the normal laboratory range.
ECG, Electrocardiogram; *eGFR*, estimated glomerular filtration rate; *FBC*, full blood count; *HDL*, high-density lipoprotein; *LDL*, low-density lipoprotein; *U&E*, urea and electrolyte; *WCC*, white cell count.

- **ABG:** Only if clinically indicated (e.g. other diagnosis suspected) as it can cause damage to the radial arteries which may be required for PCI.

'The portable chest X-ray shows cardiomegaly; however, it is unchanged compared with his admission X-ray. On a repeat ECG you see, in addition to the ST changes, T-wave flattening in the inferior leads. Bloods have shown an initial troponin of 1.0 µg/L, with a normal FBC and U&Es, total cholesterol of 7.9 mmol/L (LDL 5.8 mmol/L) and a random glucose of 5.5 mmol/L.'

INITIAL MANAGEMENT

When a patient presents with chest pain that is characteristic of myocardial ischaemia, the patient's individual risk of further cardiovascular events should be calculated. This can then be used to guide clinical management. An example is the GRACE score. This takes into account age, BP, HR, ECG changes, creatinine, presence of heart failure and troponin to estimate whether a patient is at high, intermediate or low risk. Several online calculators are available for calculating the GRACE score. The GRACE score in this case is 148. This equates to a probability of death within 6 months of 19%.

- **Oxygen:** Evidence suggests that routine administration of oxygen does not alter the outcome during an MI; however, it should be considered if the SpO_2 level is <94%, or if the patient is acutely breathless.
- **Cardiac rhythm monitoring:** Monitor for any arrhythmias which can occur in association with myocardial ischaemia.
- **Morphine:** Give 1 to 10 mg IV and titrate to achieve adequate pain control.
- **Antiemetic:** Usually metoclopramide 10 mg IV (caution as this can cause dystonic reactions, especially in young females).
- **Nitrates:** Start with glyceryl trinitrate spray 800 micrograms (two sprays) SL, but if pain continues after three sublingual doses, the patient may require a glyceryl trinitrate infusion. Remember to check that the systolic BP is >100 mmHg.
- **Aspirin:** 300 mg to chew (this is often already given by ambulance crew—so double check before giving this).
- **Clopidogrel**: 300 mg PO would be given in this case, 300 to 600 mg in ST elevation ACS. Other options include ticagrelor 180 mg or prasugrel 60 mg (for patients undergoing PCI).
- **Gastric protection:** Alongside antiplatelets, proton pump inhibitors (PPIs) should be prescribed to reduce GI side effects. Examples include lansoprazole and omeprazole.
- **Fondaparinux/low-molecular-weight heparin (LMWH):** fondaparinux 2.5 mg SC (if the patient is not undergoing angiography within the next 24 hours, there is not a high bleeding risk and renal function is adequate) or unfractionated heparin (if

patient is undergoing angiography within the next 24 hours or has renal impairment).

- **Reperfusion therapy:** Patients presenting with non-ST elevation ACS will normally undergo inpatient angiography ± PCI. This should be done as soon as possible if haemodynamically unstable or at high risk, otherwise it should be within 96 hours.
- **Call for help!** Speak with your senior early on and involve the on-call cardiologist. Patients who are having angiography and PCI may require complex decisions to be made regarding optimal antiplatelet therapy, fondaparinux and heparin. Many will also receive a glycoprotein IIb/IIIa receptor antagonist (e.g. abciximab, eptifibatide) while in the catheter laboratory.
- **Blood glucose control:** Patients with ACS and a glucose of >11.0 mmol/L should have intensive blood glucose control with an insulin sliding scale regimen. This should be continued for at least 24 hours.

Examiners will sometimes ask you to localise the region of the infarct by looking at the ECG leads where ST-segment abnormalities occur:

- Inferior infarct (right coronary artery (RCA) or right circumflex artery (RCX)): leads II, III and AVF
- Anterior infarct (left anterior descending (LAD)): leads V_2–V_6
- Lateral infarct (left circumflex artery (LCX) or marginalis obtusis (MO)): leads I, II and AVL, V_5 and V_6
- Posterior infarct (RCX): there are no posterior ECG leads, so this is diagnosed by looking for reciprocal changes in V_1–V_2. Look for ST depression (>2 mm), tall R waves and tall T waves.

REASSESSMENT

- Always start from the top and repeat the ABCDE process.
- Check to see that Mr Drummond has been given all of the medications you prescribed.
- Assess his pain score—all patients should be kept pain-free if possible.
- Don't forget to explain to him and his family what is going on and what will happen next.

'On approaching Mr Drummond, he looks much better. Airway is patent and RR is now 14/min. Oxygen saturations were 100% on 15 L/min oxygen; this was reduced and he is now maintaining an SpO_2 level of 94% on 2 L. The chest is still clear and HS remain normal. HR is 80 bpm and BP is 101/62 mmHg. He is no longer cold and clammy and says that he is pain free.'

Note that Mr Drummond is slightly hypotensive. This is likely to be secondary to the nitrate and morphine and it should be monitored closely.

It is now 8:55 pm and you are due to finish your shift at 9:00 pm.

Don't be afraid to hand over patients—especially after a busy shift like this! You need to make sure you get your rest between shifts, and if you are tired or hungry you are more likely to make mistakes. If the patient is stable, ensure nurses know when to contact you, and then go to a handover meeting. If you are worried about leaving the patient, then you can always bleep a doctor from the night team to come up and receive handover on the ward.

HANDING OVER THE PATIENT

'Mr Drummond is a 72-year-old man who was recently treated for cellulitis. Today he has had a non-ST elevation ACS.

He presented tonight with chest pain and associated autonomic symptoms. ECG has confirmed an inferior non-ST elevation ACS and he has been treated initially with oxygen, glyceryl trinitrate, aspirin, clopidogrel and fondaparinux. He has required 7 mg of IV morphine.

Investigations have shown an initial troponin rise to 1.0 µg/L. His observations are now stable—BP is 101/62 mmHg, HR 80 bpm, RR 14/min, SpO_2 94% on 2 L O_2 and temp 36.5°C. GRACE score is 148. He is now pain free.

The cardiology registrar is on his way to review him and he has agreed to transfer Mr Drummond to CCU thereafter. Please could you review him within 1 hour and perform a 12-hour troponin at 07.00.'

COMPLICATIONS OF ACUTE CORONARY SYNDROME

- **Recurrent ischaemia:** Treat with further morphine, nitrates and a nitrate infusion if required. Patients with recurrent ischaemia after non-ST elevation ACS may need urgent PCI and consideration of a GIIA/IIIB antagonist if not already given.
- **Arrhythmias**: Mr Drummond presented with a sinus tachycardia. This was likely to be secondary to anxiety or pain in his case, but it can also be a sign of acute LVF secondary to MI. Heart block is common after infarction to the inferior territory of the heart—temporary pacing may be required if the patient is symptomatic or haemodynamically compromised by it, but it usually resolves spontaneously. Complete heart block occurring after an anterior MI has a poorer prognosis, is unlikely to resolve and permanent pacing is generally necessary. Other arrhythmias after MI include AF, ventricular ectopics, VF and VT.
- **Heart failure:** Look for shortness of breath, raised JVP, crackles or tachycardia. Repeat the CXR. An isolated raised JVP may indicate right ventricular infarction. Acute LVF may also occur after mitral valve papillary muscle or ventricular septal rupture. This has a poor prognosis and emergency cardiac surgery may be needed.
- **Pericarditis:** May occur initially, directly due to inflammation from the MI, or 2–12 weeks later, as a probable autoimmune type reaction, known as 'Dressler's syndrome'.
- **Thromboembolism:** May be secondary to a mural thrombus, AF or prolonged immobility, e.g. from bed rest.

FURTHER MANAGEMENT

- **Aspirin:** 75 mg per day should be continued indefinitely.
- Patients who are unable to tolerate aspirin can be given clopidogrel alone.
- **Clopidogrel (or ticagrelor or prasugrel):** Usually combined with aspirin for 12 months after a non-ST elevation ACS.
- **Continue fondaparinux/LMWH:** Up to 8 days or until hospital discharge.
- **Assess LV function:** Echocardiogram in all patients who have had an MI.
- Ensure that the patient is also on an ACE inhibitor and a beta-blocker, both of which should be continued indefinitely (unless there are adverse effects).
- **Statins:** Should also be given to all patients with acute myocardial infarction. This should normally be a 'high-intensity' statin dosage, e.g. atorvastatin 40 to 80 mg OD or rosuvastatin 20 to 40 mg. The treatment target is to achieve a greater than 40% reduction in non-high-density lipoprotein cholesterol (HDL-C) levels. Failure to achieve this might be due to poor adherence.
- **Screen for hypertension:** Based on the hospital observations and, if necessary, using home BP or ambulatory monitoring, after discharge.

Prescribe (see Figs 2.6–2.7)

Oxygen:

- 2 L/min via NASAL CANNULAE

LMWH/Factor Xa inhibitor:

- FONDAPARINUX 2.5 mg SC OD

Antiplatelet therapy:

- ASPIRIN 75 mg PO OD and CLOPIDOGREL 75 mg PO OD

ACE inhibitor:

- RAMIPRIL 2.5 mg PO OD to be titrated

Beta-blocker:

- BISOPROLOL 1.25 mg PO OD to be titrated

Statin:

- ATORVASTATIN 40 mg PO OD

Gastric protection alongside antiplatelets:

- LANSOPRAZOLE 30 mg PO OD

STOP

High-flow oxygen

Prior to discharge, Mr Drummond should be:

- given information about his diagnosis
- offered cardiac rehabilitation
- have a clear plan for outpatient medical review
- given lifestyle advice, e.g. smoking cessation, healthy eating.

STATION 2.4: BRADYCARDIA

You are a junior doctor working in the emergency department. You are asked urgently to review Mr Jack Lewis (DOB 03/08/50), a 74-year-old man, brought in by ambulance, who fainted on his way to the toilet. He is now conscious but is bradycardic and feels lightheaded. The patient describes how he accidently took three of his 10 mg bisoprolol tablets this morning instead of one. He is not on any other medications.

Patient Details

Name:	Jack Lewis
DOB:	03/08/50
Hospital number:	0308506874
Weight:	75 kg
Height:	1.88 m
Consultant:	Dr Jones
Hospital/Ward:	JDH Medical Ward
Current medications:	Bisoprolol 10 mg PO OD (for angina)
Allergies:	None known
Admission date:	19/10/24

Initial Differential Diagnosis of a Bradycardia

- Drug causes: Potassium or sodium channel blockers, beta-blockers, digoxin, calcium channel blockers, opioids
- Inferior myocardial infarction
- Electrolyte abnormalities: Hyper- or hypokalaemia, hyper- or hypocalcaemia
- Hypothyroidism
- Hypothermia
- Infection
- Athletes

Bradycardia Management

- Adverse features present: Atropine sulfate ± adrenaline ± pacing
- No adverse features present: Observe and monitor
- Correct underlying cause if possible

INITIAL ASSESSMENT

AIRWAY

- Assess patency of the airway. Can the patient maintain their own airway—particularly if they have reduced consciousness?

'The airway is not obstructed. The patient is able to maintain their own airway.'

No intervention is currently required; however, this needs to be reassessed regularly.

BREATHING

- Assess respiratory rate, oxygen saturations and work of breathing. Percuss for evidence of a pleural effusion, pneumonia or pneumothorax. Auscultate for air entry and additional sounds.

'RR 14/min, oxygen saturations are 95% on air. The chest is resonant throughout. Good air entry bilaterally with no crackles.'

No specific respiratory treatment is currently needed.

CIRCULATION

- Assess haemodynamic stability by measuring HR, BP, CRT (centrally and peripherally). Assess urine output.
- Perform a cardiovascular examination looking particularly for evidence of heart failure secondary to bradycardia.

'HR 35 bpm regular, BP 95/75 mmHg. CRT is 2 seconds. CV examination shows normal HS, with no murmurs. No clinical evidence of heart failure.'

Secure IV access and take bloods. Perform ECG. Supplementary IV fluids may be required.

DISABILITY

- Assess his conscious level, using AVPU (is the patient Alert? If not, do they respond to Verbal or Painful stimuli? Or are they Unresponsive?). Check glucose levels.

'He is alert, but slightly confused. Blood glucose is 6.6 mmol/L.'

EXPOSURE

- Check the patient's temperature. Expose the patient, and perform a quick assessment of the other systems.

'Mr Lewis's temperature is 37.0°C. The abdomen is soft and nontender. There is no evidence of any injury from the collapse. The rest of the examination is unremarkable.'

Ask a nurse or colleague to perform the ECG while you are assessing the patient.

INITIAL INVESTIGATIONS

- **ECG:** The most important investigation. Permits assessment of the HR and rhythm. May show heart block as underlying cause. May show abnormalities characteristic of specific electrolyte disturbances.
- **Bloods:** FBC, U&Es, Mg, calcium, TFT (Table 2.4). Look for evidence of anaemia; assess renal function, electrolytes and thyroid function.
- **CXR:** If concerned about infection or left ventricular failure.

'Hb 140 g/L, WCC 8.9 × 10^9/L, urea 5.7 mmol/L, creatinine 75 μmol/L, eGFR >60 mL/min. Sodium 135 mmol/L, potassium 4.3 mmol/L, calcium 2.4 mmol/L, magnesium 1.0 mmol/L. TFT is in progress. ECG shows a sinus bradycardia with a ventricular rate of 35 bpm, but no other changes.'

Table 2.4 Mr Lewis's Blood Test Results

PARAMETER	VALUE	NORMAL RANGE (UNITS)
Haemoglobin	140 g/L	Men: 135–180 (g/L) Women: 115–160 (g/L)
WCC	8.9 × 10^9/L	3.2–11.0 (× 10^9/L)
Neutrophil	5.8 × 10^9/L	1.9–7.7 (× 10^9/L)
Lymphocyte	2.8 × 10^9/L	1.3–3.5 (× 10^9/L)
Platelet	300 × 10^9/L	120–400 (× 10^9/L)
Urea	5.7 mmol/L	2.5–6.7 (mmol/L)
Creatinine	75 μmol/L	70–130 (μmol/L)
Sodium	135 mmol/L	135–145 (mmol/L)
Potassium	4.3 mmol/L	3.5–5.0 (mmol/L)
eGFR	>60 mL/min	>60 (mL/min)
Calcium	2.4 mmol/L	2.12–2.65 (mmol/L)
Magnesium	1.0 mmol/L	0.75–1.05 (mmol/L)

ECG, Electrocardiogram; *eGFR*, estimated glomerular filtration rate; *TFT*, thyroid function test; *WCC*, white cell count.

INITIAL MANAGEMENT

- This patient has a bradycardia, probably secondary to an overdose of beta-blockers, with an adverse presenting symptom of syncope.
- **Airway support:** The airway is patent in this case, with no intervention required.
- **Supplementary oxygen:** If saturations <94%. Not currently required.
- **Atropine sulfate:** 500 micrograms IV to increase the ventricular rate. Repeat doses may be necessary.
- **Senior help:** If the patient remains bradycardic, there are other medications, such as glucagon, adrenaline or isoprenaline and electrical therapies (temporary pacing), which can be tried; however, senior help should have arrived by this point.
- **Ensure appropriate thromboprophylaxis** although not always necessary for anticipated short admissions.

This patient is unwell and could deteriorate quickly. Be sure to get senior help early.

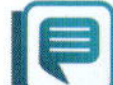

Not all patients with a bradycardia need treatment. If there are no adverse signs and no increased risk of asystole, then monitoring of the patient may be all that is required.

Prescribe (see Fig. **2.8**)

Antimuscarinic:

- ATROPINE 500 micrograms IV STAT followed by second dose if required

REASSESSMENT

- A second 500 microgram dose of atropine is given because the bradycardia remained. After this the patient is reassessed.

  'Mr Lewis looks better. He is maintaining his airway, RR 12/min, oxygen saturations are 96% on room air. HR 55 bpm, BP 116/84 mmHg. His peripheries are warm, and CRT<2 seconds. Repeat ECG shows sinus rhythm 50 bpm.'

FURTHER MANAGEMENT

- **Correct underlying cause:** In this case, the underlying cause is likely to be an overdose of beta-blockers. As it is several hours since the drugs were ingested, it is unlikely that activated charcoal or gastric lavage would have any benefit.
- **Monitor**: The patient should be transferred to a cardiac-monitored bed.

Potential Complications of Bradycardia

- Myocardial ischaemia
- Heart failure
- Renal failure
- Asystolic cardiac arrest

HANDING OVER TO THE WARD DOCTOR

'Mr Lewis is a 74-year-old man, who presented this morning with syncope and sinus bradycardia, secondary to an overdose of beta-blockers (which he has been on long term for hypertension). He is normally fit and well, and is on no other medication.

This morning he suddenly collapsed after probably taking three times his normal dose of bisoprolol. When initially assessed he was conscious but had a sinus bradycardia of 35 bpm, with a reduced BP. Bloods were unremarkable and the ECG showed sinus bradycardia.

The bradycardia responded to 1 mg of atropine, with his HR increasing to 50 bpm, and the BP is normalising as well. He is now stable.

He has been assessed by the medical registrar on call. He is to be transferred to a cardiac-monitored bed for observation. His beta-blocker has been withheld, and thyroid function tests need to be chased tomorrow.'

STATION 2.5: TACHYCARDIA

You are a junior doctor working in the Accident and Emergency Unit (A&E). Your next patient is Mr Benjamin Green (DOB 30/09/67), a 57-year-old man who has presented with palpitations and lightheadedness.

Patient Details

Name:	Benjamin Green
DOB:	30/09/67
Hospital number:	3009673361
Weight:	82 kg
Height:	1.92 m
Consultant:	Dr Jones
Hospital/Ward:	LDH Medical Ward
Current medications:	None
Allergies:	None known
Admission date:	19/10/24

Initial Differential Diagnosis of Palpitations

- Supraventricular tachycardia (SVT)
- Atrial fibrillation
- Atrial flutter
- Sinus tachycardia, e.g. pain/anxiety/thyrotoxicosis/phaeochromocytoma
- Ectopics

Tachycardia Management

- Sinus tachycardia: Treat the underlying cause
- Regular narrow complex tachycardia (e.g. atrial tachycardia, atrioventricular reentrant tachycardia, atrioventricular nodal reentrant tachycardia): Vagal manoeuvres ± adenosine
- Irregular narrow complex tachycardia (e.g. atrial fibrillation): Varies from patient to patient. Options include rate or rhythm control (with beta-blockers, calcium channel blockers or digoxin) and anticoagulation
- Regular broad complex tachycardia (e.g. VT, SVT with aberrancy): Amiodarone
- Irregular broad complex tachycardia (e.g. AF with conduction block, polymorphic VT): Seek expert help
- If there are significant adverse features (e.g. hypotension, hypoperfusion): Synchronised cardioversion ± amiodarone

INITIAL ASSESSMENT

AIRWAY

- Assess the patency of the airway.

  'The airway is not obstructed. The patient is able to maintain their own airway.'

No intervention is currently required but this should be reassessed regularly.

BREATHING

- Assess respiratory rate, oxygen saturation and work of breathing. Examine the chest, looking for evidence of infection.

  'RR 16/min, oxygen saturation is 97% on air. The chest is resonant throughout. Good air entry bilaterally with no crackles heard.'

Give supplementary oxygen if required to maintain oxygen saturations >94%.

CIRCULATION

- Assess haemodynamic stability by measuring HR, BP, CRT (centrally and peripherally). Assess urine output.
- Perform a cardiovascular examination looking particularly for evidence of heart failure and shock secondary to tachycardia.

'HR 188 bpm regular, BP 132/82 mmHg. Mr Green has warm peripheries with a CRT of <2 seconds. CV examination reveals normal HS, with no murmurs. No clinical evidence of heart failure.'

Secure IV access, take bloods and perform an ECG.

DISABILITY

- Assess his conscious level, using AVPU (is the patient Alert? If not, do they respond to Verbal or Painful stimuli? Or are they Unresponsive?). Check glucose levels.

'He is alert and orientated. Blood glucose is 6.5 mmol/L.'

EXPOSURE

- Check the patient's temperature. Expose the patient, and perform a quick assessment of the other systems, looking in particular for evidence of infection or thyrotoxicosis.

'Mr Green's temperature is 36.8°C. The abdomen is soft and nontender. The rest of the examination is unremarkable.'

The first question to ask is 'does this patient have any adverse features (e.g. syncope, shock, myocardial ischaemia or heart failure)?' If yes, then they are unstable and need urgent synchronised cardioversion ± amiodarone (as long as the patient does not have a sinus tachycardia—see previous box). If there are no adverse features then you have more time to make your assessment.

Ask a nurse or colleague to perform the ECG while you are assessing the patient.

INITIAL INVESTIGATIONS

- **ECG:** The most important investigation. Permits assessment of the cardiac rate and rhythm. Look for evidence of myocardial ischaemia, although this may be difficult to see with a rapid tachycardia.
- **Bloods:** FBC, U&Es, Ca, Mg, TFT, CRP (Table 2.5). Look for evidence of infection, assess renal function, electrolytes and thyroid function.

If infection is a possible precipitant, a septic screen may be indicated, including CXR, urinalysis and blood cultures.

Table 2.5 Mr Green's Blood Test Results

PARAMETER	VALUE	NORMAL RANGE (UNITS)
Haemoglobin	140 g/L	Men: 135–180 (g/L) Women: 115–160 (g/L)
WCC	9.2 × 10^9/L	3.2–11.0 (×10^9/L)
Neutrophil	4.9 × 10^9/L	1.9–7.7 (×10^9/L)
Lymphocyte	3.2 × 10^9/L	1.3–3.5 (×10^9/L)
Platelet	250 × 10^9/L	120–400 (×10^9/L)
Urea	5.7 mmol/L	2.5–6.7 (mmol/L)
Creatinine	78 µmol/L	70–130 (µmol/L)
Sodium	138 mmol/L	135–145 (mmol/L)
Potassium	4.4 mmol/L	3.5–5.0 (mmol/L)
eGFR	>60 mL/min	>60 (mL/min)
Calcium	2.5 mmol/L	2.12–2.65 (mmol/L)
Magnesium	1.0 mmol/L	0.75–1.05 (mmol/L)
CRP	4 mg/L	0–10 (mg/L)

CRP, C-reactive protein; *ECG*, electrocardiogram; *eGFR*, estimated glomerular filtration rate; *TFT*, thyroid function test; *U&E*, urea and electrolyte; *WCC*, white cell count.

'Hb 140 g/L, WCC 9.2 × 10^9/L, CRP is 4 mg/L. U&Es, Mg and Ca are normal. TFT is in progress. ECG shows a regular narrow complex tachycardia with a rate of 188 bpm. It does not have a saw-tooth appearance. There is no visible atrial activity on the ECG.'

INITIAL MANAGEMENT

- This patient has a narrow complex regular tachycardia, which is typical of a paroxysmal supraventricular tachycardia (SVT).
- There are no adverse features so synchronised cardioversion is not indicated.
- **Airway support:** The airway is patent in this case, with no intervention required.
- **Supplementary oxygen:** To maintain saturations >94%.
- **Vagal manoeuvres:** Vagal manoeuvres are used to increase vagal parasympathetic tone affecting the cardiac conduction system and are helpful in the diagnosis and treatment of various arrhythmias. Common vagal manoeuvres include carotid sinus massage, the Valsalva manoeuvre (forced exhalation against a closed glottis) and the diving reflex (breath-holding and cold water exposure of the face). Record an ECG while performing carotid sinus massage or Valsalva manoeuvres. This will terminate or slow around a third of SVTs. In atrial flutter, these manoeuvres will slow the ventricular rate, revealing the saw-tooth appearance of atrial flutter waves.
- **Adenosine:** If the tachycardia persists, give a rapid bolus of adenosine 6 mg IV through a large cannula in a large vein while recording an ECG. If there is no response, you can give up to two further 12 mg boluses 1 to 2 minutes apart. If the tachycardia persists, ask for senior advice.

- **Consider thromboprophylaxis:** Although this is not always necessary for anticipated short admissions.

 Adenosine is contraindicated in those with asthma, those taking dipyridamole or carbamazepine and patients with heart transplants. Use a calcium channel blocker (e.g. verapamil 2.5 mg IV over 2 minutes) instead.

 Adenosine can cause transient flushing and chest tightness—warn the patient before you give the bolus!

Prescribe (see Fig. 2.9)

ADENOSINE (over 2 seconds) 6 mg IV STAT

REASSESSMENT

- Vagal manoeuvres failed to terminate the tachycardia; 6 mg of adenosine was administered as a rapid bolus. The patient complains of chest tightness lasting 20 seconds. You then reassess the patient.

'Mr Green is maintaining his airway, RR 16/min, oxygen saturations are still 97% on air. HR 82 bpm, BP 124/76 mmHg. Respiratory and cardiac examinations are unremarkable. Repeat ECG shows sinus rhythm 82 bpm.'

FURTHER MANAGEMENT

- **Monitor:** The patient should be transferred to a cardiac-monitored bed.
- **Correct underlying cause**: Look for and correct any underlying cause. If episodes of SVT are frequent then prophylactic medication, such as verapamil or beta-blocker, or a catheter ablation may be required.

 **Potential Complications**

- Myocardial ischaemia
- Heart failure
- Syncope

HANDING OVER THE PATIENT

'Mr Green is a 57-year-old man with a first episode of SVT.

He presented with palpitations and light headedness. He did not display any adverse features and ECG demonstrated an SVT with a rate of 188 bpm. He did not respond to vagal manoeuvres but the SVT was terminated by 6 mg of adenosine. Repeat ECG confirms sinus rhythm of 82 bpm.

He is going to be reviewed later this evening by the medical registrar with a view to discharge. FBC, electrolytes and liver function are normal, but TFT results are to be chased'.

STATION 2.6: WARFARIN PRESCRIBING

Mr Jim Jackson (06/07/37) is an 87-year-old man who is admitted to hospital with shortness of breath and pleuritic chest pain shortly after returning from a visit to Australia. On examination, he is tachypnoeic, tachycardic and apyrexial. His BP is stable. His chest is clear and his chest X-ray is normal. ABG shows type 1 respiratory failure. A computed tomographic pulmonary angiography (CTPA) shows a PE. He has a history of investigations for unexplained GI bleeding. He is to be commenced on warfarin using an age-adjusted Fennerty regimen, with LMWH cover until his international normalised ratio (INR) has been therapeutic for 2 days.

Although warfarin has been used for six decades, its use as the first-line oral anticoagulant in most situations is now declining because of the availability of a new class of direct acting oral anticoagulants (DOACs) (e.g. dabigatran, rivaroxaban, apixaban). DOACs are as safe and effective as warfarin for most indications, but have the advantages of having set doses, not usually requiring regular INR monitoring, and having a faster onset and offset of action. An important disadvantage is that there is limited access to antidotes and so warfarin might have advantages for patients at higher risk of bleeding. Warfarin also remains the preferred anticoagulation option for patients with mechanical valves, rheumatic mitral valve disease, advanced renal failure, high-risk thrombophilias (e.g. antiphospholipid antibody syndrome) and some cancer patients.

Mr Jackson remains on the ward waiting for a package of care to be commenced following assessment by the occupational therapist.

FBC, U&Es and LFTs are normal and the INR is 1 at baseline. The target INR is 2.5, and the warfarin is to be given for 6 months. Given these data, prescribe the first dose of warfarin.

You will then be told subsequent INRs, and be asked to prescribe the next warfarin doses, and predict the maintenance dose.

Patient Details

Name:	Jim Jackson
DOB:	06/07/37
Hospital number:	0607371232
Weight:	60 kg
Height:	1.7 m
Consultant:	Dr James
Hospital/Ward:	HGH Ward 4
Current medications:	Enoxaparin 90 mg SC OD (started on admission for pulmonary embolism)
Allergies:	None known
Admission date:	10/11/24

The INRs are the following:

- Day 1: INR is 1
- Day 2: INR is 1.5

- Day 3: INR is 2.1
- Day 4: INR is 2.6

You check his INR twice over the next 7 days, and the results are 2.6 and 2.5 on 3 mg. You then recheck the week after and it is 2.4. He is ready to be discharged.

You arrange for him to have a further INR check the week after discharge at his general practice (GP) surgery.

 **Prescribe (see Fig. 2.10)**

Day 1: WARFARIN 6 mg PO
Day 2: WARFARIN 6 mg PO
Day 3: WARFARIN 3 mg PO
Day 4: WARFARIN 3 mg PO (continue this dose as the predicted maintenance dose, and discontinue heparin)

BACKGROUND INFORMATION

- Warfarin is a vitamin K antagonist, resulting in reduced production of coagulation factors II, VII, IX and X by the liver. This causes a prolongation of the INR and prothrombin time (PT).
- The anticoagulant effect takes 48 to 72 hours to work fully; therefore in acute thromboembolism, patients will need initial anticoagulation with treatment-dose LMWH, until the INR has been therapeutic for at least 2 days.
- The daily dose of warfarin varies between individuals depending on individual sensitivity. Factors such as diet, age, existing medications and other comorbidities can impact upon the anticoagulant response to warfarin (as assessed by the INR).
- Table 2.6 lists common indications for warfarin and target INRs.

INITIATING WARFARIN

- Assess patient adherence. Will they attend for regular blood tests? Will they be able to understand instructions regarding dose adjustment?
- Take a history—check for any history of liver disease, renal impairment, pregnancy, breastfeeding or haemorrhagic stroke. Is the patient prone to falls? (This can increase the risk of haemorrhage, particularly in the elderly.) The benefit/risk ratio should be assessed in every individual patient, and then reassessed each year.
- Check what other medications the patient is on and if they could interact with warfarin. Replace all potentially interacting drugs with alternatives if possible.
- Take baseline bloods—FBC, LFTs, U&Es and coagulation screen. This may reveal contraindications to warfarin, such as renal failure, a prolonged PT due to chronic liver disease or thrombocytopenia.
- All patients commencing warfarin should undergo 'warfarin counselling' prior to discharge. This can often be done by the ward pharmacist but is the responsibility of the prescriber to organise.
- Different hospitals will have different protocols regarding the initiation of warfarin. Hospital inpatients will often be rapidly 'loaded' with warfarin because their INR can be monitored daily. One such loading protocol is the Fennerty regimen. After its original publication in 1984, subsequent modifications have been published, which take account of the lower dose requirements for more elderly patients (Table 2.7).
- Patients being started on warfarin as outpatients under the supervision of the GP will undergo a slower initial regimen that requires less intensive monitoring.
- The indication for warfarin, intended duration of therapy and target INR should be recorded on the patient's drug chart.
- Patients should be given an anticoagulant therapy record booklet often called a 'yellow booklet'.

 Always ask a patient if they take any herbal or over-the-counter medications, as these too can interact with warfarin and have an effect on the INR.

Enzyme Inhibitors That *Increase* the Effects of Warfarin

Alcohol (acute use)
Allopurinol
Amiodarone
Azole antifungals (e.g. fluconazole, miconazole)
Cimetidine
Macrolide antibiotics (e.g. clarithromycin, erythromycin)
Penicillins (e.g. benzylpenicillin, phenoxymethylpencillin)
PPIs (e.g. omeprazole)
Quinolone antibiotics (e.g. ciprofloxacin, moxifloxacin)
Selective serotonin reuptake inhibitors (e.g. citalopram, fluoxetine)
Statins (e.g. simvastatin, rosuvastatin)
Sulfonamide antibiotics (e.g. sulfamethoxazole in co-trimoxazole)
Valproate

Enzyme Inducers That *Reduce* the Effects of Warfarin

Alcohol (chronic use)
Antiepileptics (e.g. carbamazepine, phenytoin)
Barbiturates
Griseofulvin
Rifampicin
St John's Wort

WARFARIN COUNSELLING

- **Adherence:** Take warfarin at the same time each day, usually 6 pm.
- **Reason for warfarin:** 'To thin the blood' and treat DVT, PE, AF, etc. (this should be tailored to the individual patient).
- **Risks and side effects**: Discuss the risk of bleeding, when to seek help (e.g. if you experience unexplained bruising) and the possible side effects that may be experienced.

Table 2.6 Indications for Starting Warfarin and Target INRs

CONDITION	TARGET INR	DURATION OF THERAPY
Isolated DVT in a nonsurgical patient with no risk factors	2.5	3 months
DVT in a postsurgical patient with no other risk factors	2.5	6 weeks
Recurrent DVT/PE when on warfarin	3.5	Long term (or until risk factors resolve)
Continuous or paroxysmal AF	2.5	Long term
AF to be electively cardioverted	2.5	3 weeks prior to procedure, and 4 weeks postprocedure
Mechanical mitral valve	3.5	Long term
Valvular disease with previous emboli or AF	2.5	Long term
Ischaemic stroke and AF	2.5	Long term
Peripheral arterial embolic disease and AF	2.5	Long term

AF, Atrial fibrillation; *DVT,* deep vein thrombosis; *INR,* international normalised ratio; *PE,* pulmonary embolism.

Table 2.7 Modified Fennerty Regimen (Age Adjusted) for Initiating Warfarin

		DOSE (MG) ACCORDING TO AGE			
DAY	INR	<50 YEARS	50–65 YEARS	66–80 YEARS	>80 YEARS
1	<1.4	10	9	7.5	6
2	<1.6	10	9	7.5	6
	<1.7	0.5	0.5	0.5	0.5
3	<1.8	10	9	7.5	6
	1.8–2.3	5	4.5	4	3
	2.4–2.7	4	3.5	3	2
	2.8–3.1	3	2.5	2	1
	3.2–3.3	2	2	1.5	1
	3.4	1.5	1.5	1	1
	3.5	1	1	1	0.5
	3.3–4.0	0.5	0.5	0.5	0.5
	>4	Withhold dose	Withhold dose	Withhold dose	Withhold dose
4	<1.6	10–15	9–14	7.5–11	6–9
	1.6	8	7	6	5
	1.7–1.8	7	6	5	4
	1.9	6	5	4.5	3.5
	2.0–2.6	5	4.5	4	3
	2.7–3.0	4	3.5	3	2.5
	3.1–3.5	3.5	3	2.5	2
	3.6–4.0	3	2.5	2	1.5
	4.1–4.5	Omit next dose, then 1–2	Omit next dose, then 0.5–1.5	Omit next dose, then 0.5–1.5	Omit next dose, then 0.5–1
	>4.5	Withhold dose	Withhold dose	Withhold dose	Withhold dose
Warfarin dose should be taken at 6 pm each day Blood for INR should be taken at between 9 and 11 am the next morning					

INR, International normalised ratio.

- **Supply:** Provide information regarding the tablets provided, the dose strength of each tablet and that the different colours of warfarin tablets correspond to particular strengths.
- **Monitoring**: Discuss the importance of regular INR checks and how/where this will be performed for the particular individual.
- **Missed doses:** Take warfarin as soon as you remember, but do not double up doses.
- **Changing the dose:** Explain how the dose will be altered according to INR.
- **Drug interactions:** Many drugs and herbal remedies have the potential to interact with warfarin. Patients should be advised to alert other practitioners

(doctors, dentists, pharmacists or herbalists) to the fact that they take warfarin when any new treatment is being considered.

- **Diet:** Avoid large quantities of food rich in vitamin K, e.g. liver, green vegetables. Avoid cranberry juice.
- **Alcohol:** Do not binge drink. Drink alcohol in moderation with a maximum of 2 units/day. If you are going to drink, try and drink the same amount every day. Acute 'binge' drinking can increase the INR while chronic alcohol consumption can reduce the INR.
- **Surgical and dental procedures:** Patients should discuss warfarin with their doctor or dentist prior to any procedure.
- **Injections:** Intramuscular (IM) injections should be avoided if possible. Intraarticular injections are contraindicated.
- **Pregnancy (if relevant):** Warfarin is teratogenic and should be avoided in pregnancy. Women may require treatment with heparin during this time.
- **Leisure:** Avoid activities that could increase risk of bleeding, e.g. rugby.

Some common drugs should be avoided (unless specifically advised) when taking warfarin because they *increase* the likelihood that warfarin anticoagulation will cause bleeding (pharmacodynamic interactions):

- Aspirin (including low dose)
- NSAIDs (ibuprofen, diclofenac, naproxen)
- Other antiplatelet drugs (clopidogrel)
- Other anticoagulants (heparins, DOACs)

Note that enteral feeds may contain vitamin K and decrease the effect of warfarin.

Some common drugs have an effect on the metabolism of warfarin via the cytochrome P450 system (pharmacokinetic interactions), which either reduces or increases the metabolism of warfarin. This leads to an increased or decreased anticoagulant effect of warfarin. Examples of these drugs are listed in the previous box about enzyme inhibitors and inducers that alter the effects of warfarin (check the BNF for a full list of interacting drugs).

Try to avoid starting drugs that will interact with warfarin. However, if this is unavoidable:

- If a short course of the new drug is needed, e.g. less than 7 days, then warfarin dose adjustments are generally not required.
- If a course of >7 days is required, then check INR 3 to 7 days after starting the new medication and adjust the dose accordingly. You then may need to monitor INR more frequently until stable.

Side Effects of Warfarin

- Bleeding (common, even if INR within target range)
- Alopecia
- Skin necrosis
- Urticaria
- Dermatitis
- Anorexia
- GI upset
- Hepatic dysfunction
- Pancreatitis

STARTING WARFARIN IN A HOSPITALISED PATIENT

Common indications for starting warfarin are shown in Table 2.6.

- Usually following an age-adjusted Fennerty regimen (see Table 2.7, if target INR is 2–3). Seek specialist advice if a different target INR is required.
- Prior to discharge, the INR must be stable and therapeutic, with plans for GP follow-up and community monitoring in place.

STARTING WARFARIN IN THE COMMUNITY

- For patients who do not require urgent anticoagulation (e.g. stroke prevention in patients with AF), warfarin can be started in the community with a more gentle loading regimen, reflecting the less regular monitoring and supervision in that setting (see example in Table 2.8).
- INR should be checked weekly for the first 6 weeks.

When the INR has been therapeutic on at least two consecutive measurements, then the frequency of INR monitoring can be reduced. The exact frequency will depend on your local policy, but an example would be to check INR twice per week for 2 weeks, then weekly for 2 weeks.

For long-term treatment the maximum monitoring intervals are:

- One INR result within therapeutic range: check in 2 weeks.
- Two INR results within therapeutic range at two weekly monitoring intervals: check in 4 weeks.
- Two INRs therapeutic at four weekly monitoring: check in 8 weeks.
- Two INRs therapeutic at eight weekly monitoring: check in 12 weeks.
- Patients with prosthetic valves: maximum period between INR checks is 6 weeks.

ADJUSTING MAINTENANCE WARFARIN DOSE

Minor fluctuations in INR around the target do not require a change of dose. For example, for a patient with a target INR of 2.5, an INR between 2 and 3 is acceptable. If the INR control changes then it is important to explore adherence to treatment, possible coadministration of new medicines, changes in food or drink intake and the emergence of new diseases.

Here is a *guide* to how to adjust warfarin dose (although this may need to be amended for individual patients).

For INR results <2.0 or >3.0 in a patient with a target INR of 2.5:

- **INR 1.1 to 1.4**: First, give a once-off dose of 20% of the weekly dose plus the usual daily dose Increase weekly total dose by 20%. Recheck INR in 1 week.
- **INR 1.5 to 1.9**: Increase weekly dose by 10%. Recheck INR in 1 week.
- **INR 3.1 to 3.9**: Reduce weekly dose by 10%. Recheck INR in 1 week.
- **INR 4.0 to 5.0**: Omit one dose. Reduce weekly dose by 10% to 20%. Recheck INR in 4 to 5 days.

Table 2.8 Prescribing Warfarin

Table 2.8A Loading Regimen	
Day 1	Start warfarin at 2 mg per day
Day 7	Check INR. If it is 3.0 or less then continue 2 mg/day; if it is >3.0, reduce the dose to 1 mg/day
Day 14	Check INR. Calculate predicted maintenance dose depending on the sex of the patient and their INR on day 14
Days 21, 28, 35 and 42	Check INR and adjust as necessary
Table 2.8B Predicting the Daily Maintenance Dose (Males)	
Males	
INR ON DAY 14	**PREDICTED DAILY MAINTENANCE DOSE**
1.0	6 mg
1.1–1.2	5 mg
1.3–1.5	4 mg
1.6–2.1	3 mg
2.2–3.0	2 mg
>3	1 mg
Table 2.8C Predicting the Daily Maintenance Dose (Females)	
Females	
INR ON DAY 14	**PREDICTED DAILY MAINTENANCE DOSE**
1.0–1.1	5 mg
1.2–1.3	4 mg
1.4–1.9	3 mg
2.0–3.0	2 mg
>3	1 mg

INR, International normalised ratio.

- **INR >5:** Manage as overcoagulation (see later).

For INR results <3.0 or >4.0 in a patient with a target INR of 3.5:

- **INR 1.1 to 1.4**: First, give a once-off dose of 20% of the weekly dose plus the usual daily dose. Then, increase weekly total dose by 20%. Recheck INR in 1 week.
- **INR 1.5 to 1.9**: Increase weekly dose by 20%. Recheck INR in 1 week.
- **INR 2.0 to 2.9**: Increase weekly dose by 10%. Recheck INR in 1 week.
- **INR 4.1 to 4.9**: Reduce weekly dose by 10%. Recheck INR in 1 week.
- **INR 5.0 to 6.0**: Omit 1 dose, reduce weekly dose by 10% to 20%. Recheck INR in 4 to 5 days.
- **INR >6.0**: Manage as overcoagulation.

It may take a few days after changing the dose of warfarin before you see a change in the INR. Therefore avoid over-frequent dosage adjustments.

MANAGEMENT OF OVERCOAGULATION

- Assess any patient with a high INR for evidence of bleeding.
- Look for a cause of the high INR, e.g. change in medication, alcohol binge.
- The most common cause of fatal bleeding in patients on warfarin is due to intracranial or intraspinal bleeding.
- Any patient on warfarin who presents with a headache, confusion, reduced GCS or head injury should be assessed for an urgent computed tomography (CT).

WHAT SHOULD YOU DO IF A PATIENT TAKING WARFARIN IS BLEEDING?

Major Bleeding (i.e. Requiring Hospitalisation and Blood Transfusion, Potentially Life-Threatening)

- Stop warfarin.
- Give phytomenadione (vitamin K_1) 5 mg by slow IV injection.
- Give dried prothrombin complex (or fresh frozen plasma).

Minor Bleeding With INR >8.0

- Stop warfarin (until INR <5.0).
- Give phytomenadione (vitamin K_1) 1 to 3 mg by slow IV injection (repeat if INR >5.0 after 24 hours.

Minor Bleeding With INR 5.0 to 8.0

- Stop warfarin (until INR <5.0).
- Give phytomenadione (vitamin K_1) 1 to 3 mg once by slow IV injection.

No Bleeding With INR >8.0

- Stop warfarin (until INR <5.0).

- Give phytomenadione (vitamin K_1) 1 to 5 mg by mouth using the IV preparation (repeat if INR >5.0 after 24 hours).

No Bleeding With INR 5.0 to 8.0

- Stop warfarin for 1 or 2 days before rechecking INR and recommencing at a lower maintenance dose.

ADDITIONAL EXAMPLE SCENARIOS

Example 2: Mrs Smith has been taking 6 mg of warfarin per day for AF (target INR 2.5) and has been stable on this regimen over the last 4 months in the community. However, over the last 2 weeks, she has cut down her daily alcohol intake and her latest INR has come back at 1.3. What do you do?

- Usual weekly dose: 42 mg (usual daily dose 6 mg).
- One-off additional dose: 20% of 42 mg = 8.4 mg (round this up to 8.5 mg). Give 8.5 mg plus usual 6 mg (i.e. 14.5 mg).
- New daily dose: weekly dose + 20% of weekly dose = 42 + 8.5 = 50.5. Divide this by 7 = 7.2.
- Therefore, new daily dose = 7 mg.
- Recheck INR in 1 week.

Example 3: Mrs Lawson is an 87-year-old woman who started warfarin 2 years ago after her GP diagnosed AF. Her INR has been stable and she is currently having it checked every 6 weeks. She is admitted to the A&E department with a nosebleed which is controlled in the department. Swallowing blood has led Mrs Lawson to feel nauseated and she has vomited once in the department. Her INR on admission is 8.1. Her daughter voices concern that she has been becoming more forgetful over the last 6 months, and she has had a few falls when getting up to go to the toilet during the night. On further questioning, Mrs Lawson admits she often forgets which tablets she has taken each day and will often take them again 'just in case'.

- Stop the warfarin.
- Assess for any further bleeding—has she had another fall recently? Could she have had an intracranial haemorrhage?
- Give vitamin K 2 mg IV. Vitamin K is necessary because of the bleeding (minor) and must be given IV because she is vomiting.
- Recheck INR after 4 to 6 hours.
- Consider overnight admission for observation. This is likely to be required in an elderly woman who lives alone.
- Recheck the INR daily over the next few days.
- Consider the risks versus the benefits of continuing to treat Mrs Lawson with warfarin.

You request a CT head given her history of falls and 'forgetfulness'. This shows generalised cerebral atrophy but no intracranial haemorrhage. Over the next few days, the INR goes down and Mrs Lawson has no further episodes of bleeding. She is noted to be unsteady on her feet and this is felt to be due to a combination of poor eyesight and osteoarthritis in both knees. Your consultant agrees that it is not appropriate to continue warfarin in this woman due to the risk of falls and cognitive impairment. Both she and her daughter are happy with this plan.

Stopping Warfarin

- There is no convincing evidence of clinically relevant rebound hypercoagulability occurring after stopping warfarin.
- Warfarin can therefore be stopped suddenly rather than tailed off.
- Further INR monitoring is not needed.

FURTHER READING

European Society of Cardiology, 2015. 2015 ESC Guidelines for the diagnosis and management of pericardial diseases. European Heart Journal 36, 2921–2964. https://doi.org/10.1093/eurheartj/ehv318 (Last accessed 24.12.23).

National Institute for Health and Care Excellence (NICE). Acute heart failure: diagnosis and management. Clinical guideline [CG187]. Last updated: 17 November 2021. https://www.nice.org.uk/guidance/cg187 (Last accessed 24.12.23).

National Institute for Health and Care Excellence (NICE). Acute coronary syndromes. Clinical guideline [NG185]. Last updated: 18 November 2020. https://www.nice.org.uk/guidance/ng185 (Last accessed 24.12.23).

British National Formulary. Arrhythmias. https://bnf.nice.org.uk/treatment-summaries/arrhythmias/ (Last accessed 24.12.23).

Kotadia, I.D., Williams, S.E., O'Neill, M., 2020. Supraventricular tachycardia: an overview of diagnosis and management. Clinical Medicine 20, 43–47. https://doi.org/10.7861/clinmed.cme.20.1.3 (Last accessed: 24.12.23).

National Institute for Health and Care Excellence (NICE). Clinical knowledge summaries. Scenario: warfarin. October 2023. https://cks.nice.org.uk/topics/anticoagulation-oral/management/warfarin/ (Last accessed 24.12.23).

Tideman, P.A., Tirimacco, R., St John, A., Roberts, G.W., 2015. How to manage warfarin therapy. Aust Prescr. 38, 44–48. https://australianprescriber.tg.org.au/articles/how-to-manage-warfarin-therapy.html (Last accessed 24.12.23).

Keeling, D., Baglin, T., Tait, C., Watson, H., Perry, D., Baglin, C., Kitchen, S., Makris, M., 2011. Guidelines on oral anticoagulation with warfarin – fourth edition. Br J Haematol 154, 311–324. https://doi.org/10.1111/j.1365-2141.2011.08753.x (Last accessed: 24.12.23).

PRESCRIPTION CHARTS

PRESCRIPTION AND ADMINISTRATION RECORD

Standard Chart

Hospital/Ward: RIE WARD 6	**Consultant:** DR CHANG	**Name of Patient:** JASON ANDERSON
Weight: 60kg	**Height:** 180cm	**Hospital Number:** 4495039943
If re-written, date:		**D.O.B.:** 22/03/95
DISCHARGE PRESCRIPTION **Date completed:-**	**Completed by:-**	

OTHER MEDICINE CHARTS IN USE		PREVIOUS ADVERSE REACTIONS This section must be completed before any medicine is given		Completed by (sign & print)	Date
Date	Type of Chart	None known ☒		E. Smith E. SMITH	19/10/24
		Medicine/Agent	Description of Reaction		

CODES FOR NON-ADMINISTRATION OF PRESCRIBED MEDICINE

If a dose is not administered as prescribed, initial and enter a code in the column with a circle drawn round the code according to the reason as shown below. **Inform the responsible doctor in the appropriate timescale.**

1. Patient refuses
2. Patient not present
3. Medicines not available – CHECK ORDERED
4. Asleep/drowsy
5. Administration route not available – CHECK FOR ALTERNATIVE
6. Vomiting/nausea
7. Time varied on doctor's instructions
8. Once only/as required medicine given
9. Dose withheld on doctor's instructions
10. Possible adverse reaction/side effect

ONCE-ONLY

Date	Time	Medicine (Approved Name)	Dose	Route	Prescriber – Sign + Print	Time Given	Given By
19/10//24	07.30	CO-CODAMOL (30/500)	2 tablets	ORAL	E. Smith E. SMITH	07.45	FN
19/10//24	07.30	IBUPROFEN	400mg	ORAL	E. Smith E. SMITH	07.45	FN

OXYGEN	Start Date	Start Time	Route Mask (%)	Route Prongs (L/min)	Prescriber – Sign + Print	Administered by	Stop Date	Stop Time

Fig. 2.1 Prescription and administration record prescription chart for Jason Anderson.

Name: JASON ANDERSON

Date of Birth: 22/03/95

REGULAR THERAPY

PRESCRIPTION		Date → / Time ↓	19/10/24	20/10/24										
Medicine (Approved Name): IBUPROFEN		6												
Dose: 400mg	Route: ORAL	(8)	X											
		12												
Notes	Start Date: 19/10/24	(14)	SD											
		18												
Prescriber – sign + print: K. Morris KATE MORRIS		(22)	SD											
Medicine (Approved Name): OMEPRAZOLE		6												
Dose: 20mg	Route: ORAL	(8)	SD											
		12												
Notes	Start Date: 19/10/24	14												
		18												
Prescriber – sign + print: K. Morris KATE MORRIS		22												
Medicine (Approved Name): CO-CODAMOL 30/500		6												
Dose: 2 tablets	Route: ORAL	(8)	X											
		(12)	SD											
Notes	Start Date: 19/10/24	14												
		(18)	SD											
Prescriber – sign + print: K. Morris KATE MORRIS		(22)	SD											
Medicine (Approved Name): TED STOCKINGS		(6)												
Dose: 1 pair	Route: TOP	(8)	SD											
		(12)												
Notes	Start Date: 19/10/24	(14)												
		(18)												
Prescriber – sign + print: K. Morris KATE MORRIS		(22)												
Medicine (Approved Name)		6												
Dose	Route	8												
		12												
Notes	Start Date	14												
		18												
Prescriber – sign + print		22												
Medicine (Approved Name)		6												
Dose	Route	8												
		12												
Notes	Start Date	14												
		18												
Prescriber – sign + print		22												

Fig. 2.2 Regular therapy prescription chart for Jason Anderson.

PRESCRIPTION AND ADMINISTRATION RECORD

Standard Chart

Hospital/Ward: LGH WARD 45 **Consultant:** DR ROSS

Weight: 58 kg **Height:** 150 cm

If re-written, date:

DISCHARGE PRESCRIPTION
Date completed:- **Completed by:-**

Name of Patient: MARGARET JENKINS

Hospital Number: 2008306547

D.O.B.: 20/08/1940

OTHER MEDICINE CHARTS IN USE

Date	Type of Chart

PREVIOUS ADVERSE REACTIONS
This section must be completed before any medicine is given

Medicine/Agent	Description of Reaction	Completed by (sign & print)	Date
None known ☐			
Medicine/Agent	Description of Reaction		
CLARITHROMYCIN	RASH	E. Smith E. SMITH	21/10/24

CODES FOR NON-ADMINISTRATION OF PRESCRIBED MEDICINE

If a dose is not administered as prescribed, initial and enter a code in the column with a circle drawn round the code according to the reason as shown below. **Inform the responsible doctor in the appropriate timescale.**

1. Patient refuses
2. Patient not present
3. Medicines not available – CHECK ORDERED
4. Asleep/drowsy
5. Administration route not available – CHECK FOR ALTERNATIVE
6. Vomiting/nausea
7. Time varied on doctor's instructions
8. Once only/as required medicine given
9. Dose withheld on doctor's instructions
10. Possible adverse reaction/side effect

ONCE-ONLY

Date	Time	Medicine (Approved Name)	Dose	Route	Prescriber – Sign + Print	Time Given	Given By
22/10/24	19.30	FUROSEMIDE	40 mg	IV	E. Smith E. SMITH	19.35	FN
22/10/24	19.30	MORPHINE (titrate to response)	1 to 10 mg	IV	E. Smith E. SMITH	19.35	FN (5 mg)
22/10/24	19.30	METOCLOPRAMIDE	10 mg	IV	E. Smith E. SMITH	19.40	FN
22/10/24	19.30	GLYCERYL TRINITRATE SPRAY	800 micrograms (2 sprays)	SL	E. Smith E. SMITH	19.40	FN

OXYGEN

Start Date	Start Time	Route Mask (%)	Route Prongs (L/min)	Prescriber – Sign + Print	Administered by	Stop Date	Stop Time
22/10/24	19.30	15L/min via NON-REBREATHER MASK		E. Smith E. SMITH	GH		

Fig. 2.3 Prescription and administration record prescription chart for Margaret Jenkins.

Name: MARGARET JENKINS

Date of Birth: 20/08/40

REGULAR THERAPY

PRESCRIPTION

Medicine (Approved Name): FUROSEMIDE
Dose: 60 mg | Route: IV
Notes: Give over at least 15 minutes (4 mg/min) | Start Date: 23/10/24
Prescriber – sign + print: E. Smith E. SMITH

Date → / Time ↓	22/10/24	23/10/24	24/10/24									
6												
(8)		AD	SD									
12												
14												
18												
22												

Medicine (Approved Name): FUROSEMIDE
Dose: 40 mg | Route: IV
Notes: | Start Date: 23/10/24
Prescriber – sign + print: E. Smith E. SMITH

Date → / Time ↓	22/10/24	23/10/24	24/10/24									
6												
8												
12												
(14)		AD	SD									
18												
22												

Medicine (Approved Name): RAMIPRIL
Dose: 1.25 mg | Route: ORAL
Notes: Titrate dose up. Monitor BP and renal function | Start Date: 24/10/24
Prescriber – sign + print: E. Smith E. SMITH

Date → / Time ↓	22/10/24	23/10/24	24/10/24									
6												
(8)			SD									
12												
14												
18												
22												

Medicine (Approved Name): BISOPROLOL
Dose: 1.25 mg | Route: ORAL
Notes: Titrate dose up. Monitor BP + HR | Start Date: 24/10/24
Prescriber – sign + print: E. Smith E. SMITH

Date → / Time ↓	22/10/24	23/10/24	24/10/24									
6												
(8)			SD									
12												
14												
18												
22												

Medicine (Approved Name): ENOXAPARIN
Dose: 40 mg | Route: SC
Notes: | Start Date: 22/10/24
Prescriber – sign + print: E. Smith E. SMITH

Date → / Time ↓	22/10/24	23/10/24	24/10/24									
6												
8												
12												
14												
(18)	DF	DF	SD									
22												

Medicine (Approved Name):
Dose: | Route:
Notes: | Start Date:
Prescriber – sign + print:

Date → / Time ↓	22/10/24	23/10/24	24/10/24									
6												
8												
12												
14												
18												
22												

Fig. 2.4 Regular therapy prescription chart for Margaret Jenkins.

FLUID PRESCRIPTION CHART

Hospital/Ward: LGH WARD 45	**Consultant:** DR ROSS	**Name of Patient:** MARGARET JENKINS **Hospital Number:** 2008306547
Weight: 58 kg	**Height:** 150cm	**D.O.B:** 20/08/1940

Date/ Time	FLUID / ADDED DRUGS	VOLUME / DOSE	ROUTE	RATE	PRESCRIBER – SIGN AND PRINT
22/10/24 18.00	SODIUM CHLORIDE 0.9%	500 mL	IV	125 mL/h	N. Black NATHAN BLACK Stopped due to acute LVF. 22/10/24 E. Smith EMMA SMITH
22/10/24 22.00	SODIUM CHLORIDE 0.9% POTASSIUM CHLORIDE	500 mL 20 mmol	IV	125 mL/h	N. Black NATHAN BLACK Stopped due to acute LVF. 22/10/24 E. Smith EMMA SMITH
23/10/24 02.00	SODIUM CHLORIDE 0.9% POTASSIUM CHLORIDE	500 mL 20 mmol	IV	125 mL/h	N. Black NATHAN BLACK Stopped due to acute LVF. 22/10/24 E. Smith EMMA SMITH

Fig. 2.5 Fluid Prescription chart for Margaret Jenkins.

PRESCRIPTION AND ADMINISTRATION RECORD

Standard Chart

Hospital/Ward: KGH WARD 26	**Consultant:** DR JAMES	**Name of Patient:** JOHN DRUMMOND
Weight: 72 kg	**Height:** 186 cm	**Hospital Number:** 1510421543
If re-written, date:		**D.O.B.:** 15/10/1952
DISCHARGE PRESCRIPTION Date completed:-	Completed by:-	

OTHER MEDICINE CHARTS IN USE		**PREVIOUS ADVERSE REACTIONS** This section must be completed before any medicine is given		Completed by (sign & print)	Date
Date	Type of Chart	None known ☒		E. Smith E. SMITH	8/10/24
		Medicine/Agent	Description of Reaction		

CODES FOR NON-ADMINISTRATION OF PRESCRIBED MEDICINE

If a dose is not administered as prescribed, initial and enter a code in the column with a circle drawn round the code according to the reason as shown below. **Inform the responsible doctor in the appropriate timescale.**

1. Patient refuses
2. Patient not present
3. Medicines not available – CHECK ORDERED
4. Asleep/drowsy
5. Administration route not available – CHECK FOR ALTERNATIVE
6. Vomiting/nausea
7. Time varied on doctor's instructions
8. Once only/as required medicine given
9. Dose withheld on doctor's instructions
10. Possible adverse reaction/side effect

ONCE-ONLY

Date	Time	Medicine (Approved Name)	Dose	Route	Prescriber – Sign + Print	Time Given	Given By
22/10/24	19.30	ASPIRIN	300 mg	ORAL	E. Smith E. SMITH	19.35	FV
22/10/24	19.30	MORPHINE (titrate to response)	1 to 10 mg	IV	E. Smith E. SMITH	19.35	FV (7 mg)
22/10/24	19.30	METOCLOPRAMIDE	10 mg	IV	E. Smith E. SMITH	19.40	FV
22/10/24	19.30	GLYCERYL TRINITRATE SPRAY	800 micrograms (2 sprays)	SL	E. Smith E. SMITH	19.40	FV
22/10/24	19.30	CLOPIDOGREL	300 mg	ORAL	E. Smith E. SMITH	19.45	FV
22/10/24	19.30	FONDAPARINUX	2.5 mg	SC	E. Smith E. SMITH	19.45	FV

OXYGEN	Start Date	Start Time	Route Mask (%)	Route Prongs (L/min)	Prescriber – Sign + Print	Administered by	Stop Date	Stop Time
	22/10/24	19.30	15L via NON-REBREATHER MASK		E. Smith E. SMITH	AP	22/10/24	20.15
	22/10/24	20.15		2L/min via NASAL CANNULAE	E. Smith E. SMITH	AP		

Fig. 2.6 Prescription and administration record prescription chart for John Drummond.

Name: *JOHN DRUMMOND*

Date of Birth: *15/10/52*

REGULAR THERAPY

PRESCRIPTION	Date → / Time ↓	22/10/24	23/10/24

Medicine (Approved Name)	Route	Time	22/10/24	23/10/24
ENOXAPARIN (crossed through)		6		
Dose: *40 mg*	*SC*	8		
Notes:	Start Date: *8/10/24*	12		
Prescriber – sign + print: *E. Smith E. SMITH*		14		
		(18)	*SD*	
		22		

Stopped due to acute coronary syndrome treatment being commenced
E. Smith E. SMITH 22/10/24

Medicine (Approved Name)	Route	Time	22/10/24	23/10/24
CLOPIDOGREL		6		
Dose: *75 mg*	*ORAL*	(8)		*SD*
Notes:	Start Date: *22/10/24*	12		
Prescriber – sign + print: *E. Smith E. SMITH*		14		
		18		
		22		

Medicine (Approved Name)	Route	Time	22/10/24	23/10/24
ASPIRIN		6		
Dose: *75 mg*	*ORAL*	(8)		*SD*
Notes:	Start Date: *22/10/24*	12		
Prescriber – sign + print: *E. Smith E. SMITH*		14		
		18		
		22		

Medicine (Approved Name)	Route	Time	22/10/24	23/10/24
FONDAPARINUX		6		
Dose: *2.5 mg*	*SC*	8		
Notes: *For eight days*	Start Date: *22/10/24*	12		
Prescriber – sign + print: *E. Smith E. SMITH*		14		
		(18)		*SD*
		22		

Medicine (Approved Name)	Route	Time	22/10/24	23/10/24
SIMVASTATIN		6		
Dose: *40 mg*	*ORAL*	8		
Notes:	Start Date: *22/10/24*	12		
Prescriber – sign + print: *E. Smith E. SMITH*		14		
		18		
		(22)	*SD*	

Medicine (Approved Name)	Route	Time	22/10/24	23/10/24
BISOPROLOL		6		
Dose: *1.25 mg*	*ORAL*	(8)		*SD*
Notes: *Monitor HR + BP*	Start Date: *22/10/24*	12		
Prescriber – sign + print: *E. Smith E. SMITH*		14		
		18		
		22		

Fig. 2.7 Regular therapy prescription chart for John Drummond.

Name: JOHN DRUMMOND

Date of Birth: 15/10/52

REGULAR THERAPY

PRESCRIPTION	
Medicine (Approved Name) RAMIPRIL	
Dose 2.5 mg	Route ORAL
Notes Monitor renal function and BP	Start Date 22/10/24
Prescriber – sign + print E. Smith E. SMITH	

Date → / Time ↓		22/10/24	23/10/24										
6													
(8)			SD										
12													
14													
18													
22													

Medicine (Approved Name)	
Dose	Route
Notes	Start Date
Prescriber – sign + print	

Time													
6													
8													
12													
14													
18													
22													

Medicine (Approved Name)	
Dose	Route
Notes	Start Date
Prescriber – sign + print	

Time													
6													
8													
12													
14													
18													
22													

Medicine (Approved Name)	
Dose	Route
Notes	Start Date
Prescriber – sign + print	

Time													
6													
8													
12													
14													
18													
22													

Medicine (Approved Name)	
Dose	Route
Notes	Start Date
Prescriber – sign + print	

Time													
6													
8													
12													
14													
18													
22													

Medicine (Approved Name)	
Dose	Route
Notes	Start Date
Prescriber – sign + print	

Time													
6													
8													
12													
14													
18													
22													

Fig. 2.7 cont'd

PRESCRIPTION AND ADMINISTRATION RECORD

Standard Chart

Hospital/Ward: JDH MEDICAL WARD	Consultant: DR JONES	Name of Patient: JACK LEWIS
Weight: 75kg	Height: 1.88 m	Hospital Number: 0308406874
If re-written, date:		D.O.B.: 03/08/1950
DISCHARGE PRESCRIPTION Date completed:-	Completed by:-	

OTHER MEDICINE CHARTS IN USE		PREVIOUS ADVERSE REACTIONS This section must be completed before any medicine is given		Completed by (sign & print)	Date
Date	Type of Chart	None known ☒		L. Manning LUCY MANNING	19/10/24
		Medicine/Agent	Description of Reaction		

CODES FOR NON-ADMINISTRATION OF PRESCRIBED MEDICINE

If a dose is not administered as prescribed, initial and enter a code in the column with a circle drawn round the code according to the reason as shown below. **Inform the responsible doctor in the appropriate timescale.**

1. Patient refuses
2. Patient not present
3. Medicines not available – CHECK ORDERED
4. Asleep/drowsy
5. Administration route not available – CHECK FOR ALTERNATIVE
6. Vomiting/nausea
7. Time varied on doctor's instructions
8. Once only/as required medicine given
9. Dose withheld on doctor's instructions
10. Possible adverse reaction/side effect

ONCE-ONLY

Date	Time	Medicine (Approved Name)	Dose	Route	Prescriber – Sign + Print	Time Given	Given By
19/10/24	09.30	ATROPINE	500 micrograms	IV	L. Manning LUCY MANNING	09.30	SF
19/10/24	09.35	ATROPINE	500 micrograms	IV	L. Manning LUCY MANNING	09.40	SF

OXYGEN	Start Date	Start Time	Route Mask (%)	Route Prongs (L/min)	Prescriber – Sign + Print	Administered by	Stop Date	Stop Time

Fig. 2.8 Prescription and administration record prescription chart for Jack Lewis.

PRESCRIPTION AND ADMINISTRATION RECORD

Standard Chart

Hospital/Ward: LDH MEDICAL WARD **Consultant:** DR JONES	**Name of Patient:** BENJAMIN GREEN
Weight: 82 kg **Height:** 1.92 m	**Hospital Number:** 3009573361
If re-written, date:	**D.O.B.:** 30/09/1967
DISCHARGE PRESCRIPTION **Date completed:-** **Completed by:-**	

OTHER MEDICINE CHARTS IN USE		PREVIOUS ADVERSE REACTIONS This section must be completed before any medicine is given		Completed by (sign & print)	Date
Date	Type of Chart	None known ☒		L. Manning LUCY MANNING	19/10/24
		Medicine/Agent	Description of Reaction		

CODES FOR NON-ADMINISTRATION OF PRESCRIBED MEDICINE

If a dose is not administered as prescribed, initial and enter a code in the column with a circle drawn round the code according to the reason as shown below. **Inform the responsible doctor in the appropriate timescale.**

1. Patient refuses
2. Patient not present
3. Medicines not available – CHECK ORDERED
4. Asleep/drowsy
5. Administration route not available – CHECK FOR ALTERNATIVE
6. Vomiting/nausea
7. Time varied on doctor's instructions
8. Once only/as required medicine given
9. Dose withheld on doctor's instructions
10. Possible adverse reaction/side effect

ONCE-ONLY

Date	Time	Medicine (Approved Name)	Dose	Route	Prescriber – Sign + Print	Time Given	Given By
19/10/24	12.30	ADENOSINE (over 2 secs)	6 mg	IV	L. Manning LUCY MANNING	12.30	LH

OXYGEN	Start Date	Start Time	Route Mask (%)	Route Prongs (L/min)	Prescriber – Sign + Print	Administered by	Stop Date	Stop Time

Fig. 2.9 Prescription and administration record prescription chart for Benjamin Green.

PRESCRIPTION AND ADMINISTRATION RECORD

Standard Chart

Hospital/Ward: HGH WARD 4 **Consultant:** DR JAMES	**Name of Patient:** JIM JACKSON
Weight: 60 kg **Height:** 1.7 m	**Hospital Number:** 0607471232
If re-written, date:	**D.O.B.:** 06/07/37
DISCHARGE PRESCRIPTION **Date completed:-** **Completed by:-**	

OTHER MEDICINE CHARTS IN USE		PREVIOUS ADVERSE REACTIONS This section must be completed before any medicine is given		Completed by (sign & print)	Date
Date	Type of Chart	None known ☒		L. Grey GREY	10/11/24
		Medicine/Agent	Description of Reaction		

INDICATION	Duration of treatment	Target INR	Completed by (sign & print)	Date
PE	6 MONTHS	2.5	L. Grey GREY	10/11/24

CODES FOR NON-ADMINISTRATION OF PRESCRIBED MEDICINE

If a dose is not administered as prescribed, initial and enter a code in the column with a circle drawn round the code according to the reason as shown below. **Inform the responsible doctor in the appropriate timescale.**

1. Patient refuses
2. Patient not present
3. Medicines not available – CHECK ORDERED
4. Asleep/drowsy
5. Administration route not available – CHECK FOR ALTERNATIVE
6. Vomiting/nausea
7. Time varied on doctor's instructions
8. Once only/as required medicine given
9. Dose withheld on doctor's instructions
10. Possible adverse reaction/side effect

ONCE-ONLY

Date	Time	INR	Dose of warfarin	Prescriber – Sign + Print	Time Given	Given By
10/11/24	18.00	1.0	10 mg	L. Grey GREY	18.00	PY
11/11/24	18.00	1.6	10 mg	L. Grey GREY	18.00	EM
12/11/24	18.00	2.1	5 mg	L. Grey GREY	18.00	EM
13/11/24	18.00	2.6	4.5 mg	L. Grey GREY	18.00	SW
14/11/24	18.00	–	4.5 mg	L. Grey GREY	18.00	PY
15/11/24	18.00	2.6	4.5 mg	L. Grey GREY	18.15	PY
16/11/24	18.00	–	4.5 mg	L. Grey GREY	18.00	PY
17/11/24	18.00	–	4.5 mg	L. Grey GREY	18.05	PY
18/11/24	18.00	2.5	4.5 mg	L. Grey GREY	18.00	PY
19/11/24	18.00	–	4.5 mg	L. Grey GREY	18.00	PY

Fig. 2.10 **Prescription and administration record prescription chart for Jim Jackson.** Note hospitals will usually have a special warfarin chart. The format may vary significantly from the above, so therefore consult local guidelines.

Respiratory Medicine

3

Simon R.J. Maxwell

Chapter Outline

Station 3.1: Acute Exacerbation of Asthma
Station 3.2: Exacerbation of COPD
Station 3.3: Community-Acquired Pneumonia (CAP)
Station 3.4: Hospital-Acquired Pneumonia
Station 3.5: Pulmonary Embolism (PE)

STATION 3.1: ACUTE EXACERBATION OF ASTHMA

You are the junior doctor working in the emergency department. You are asked urgently to review Mr Cannon, a 23-year-old man with asthma, who has presented with breathlessness and wheeze.

Patient Details

Name:	Russell Cannon
DOB:	21/03/01
Hospital number:	2103014532
Weight:	65 kg
Height:	1.6 m
Consultant:	Dr Roy
Hospital/Ward:	WGH Ward 4
Current medications:	Salbutamol (100 micrograms/ metered dose) 2 puffs INH PRN
Allergies:	None known
Admission date:	22/10/24

Initial Differential Diagnosis of Acute Dyspnoea

- Respiratory: Asthma, pneumothorax, pulmonary embolism (PE), pneumonia
- Cardiac: Myocardial infarction (MI), pulmonary oedema, cardiac tamponade, valvular pathology, e.g. aortic stenosis
- Anaphylaxis
- Inhaled foreign body
- Metabolic acidosis
- Sepsis

Complications of an Acute Exacerbation of Asthma

- Pneumothorax
- Respiratory failure/arrest
- Hypokalaemia (from salbutamol treatment)
- Right heart failure (chronic asthma)

INITIAL ASSESSMENT

AIRWAY

- Assess patency of the airway. Can you hear any added airway noises?

'The patient is maintaining their airway and no stridor is audible.'

No additional airway support is required at present but remember that the patient could deteriorate quickly.

BREATHING

- Check respiratory rate and oxygen saturations.
- Look at the work of breathing: nasal flaring, use of accessory muscles. Is the patient able to complete sentences? Often patients with respiratory distress fix their rib cage and shoulder girdle by supporting themselves on straight arms and grasping the sides of the bed.
- Perform a respiratory examination, particularly assessing for chest wall movement, air entry into the lungs and additional sounds (crackles or wheeze) on auscultation. Also look for signs of a pneumothorax such as hyperresonant percussion and unequal breath sounds. Tracheal deviation, displacement of the apex beat away from the side of the pneumothorax and haemodynamic instability are clinical findings indicating a pneumothorax is under tension. This is a medical emergency, requiring urgent needle decompression.

'RR 35/min, oxygen saturations are 89% on room air. The patient is using his accessory muscles and unable to speak in full sentences. On auscultation, there is symmetrical chest wall movement, lung fields are resonant throughout, with reduced air entry at the base of the lungs, and a widespread bilateral polyphonic wheeze.'

You start the patient on high-flow oxygen via a non-rebreather mask (to maintain saturations between 94%

and 98%). You prescribe 5 mg of salbutamol to be nebulised with oxygen.

Prescribe (Figs 3.1 and 3.2)

Bronchodilator:
- SALBUTAMOL 5 mg NEB (driven with oxygen) STAT

High-flow OXYGEN:
- OXYGEN 15 L/min via NONREBREATHER MASK

CIRCULATION

- Assess haemodynamic status by measuring pulse, blood pressure (BP) and capillary refill time (CRT). A tachycardia indicates worsening asthma, whereas a bradycardia can be a preterminal event.
- Perform a cardiovascular (CVS) examination, as breathlessness may be due to a cardiovascular cause such as aortic stenosis or left heart failure.
- Obtain intravenous (IV) access and take bloods.
- Consider commencing IV fluids, particularly if there is evidence of shock.

'The patient's heart rate is 134 bpm, with a BP of 145/95 mmHg and CRT of 2 seconds. There is no evidence of heart failure or valvular disease on cardiovascular examination.'

No cardiovascular support is required at present.

DISABILITY

- Assess the patient's Glasgow Coma Scale (GCS) or AVPU (is the patient Alert? If not, do they respond to Verbal or Painful stimuli? Or are they Unresponsive?) level—are they becoming exhausted? Check the blood glucose.

'The patient is GCS 15 (E4, M6, V5). His blood glucose is 4.8 mmol/L.'

When describing a GCS score to a senior, always divide it into the separate categories (e.g. E3, M4, V4)—this allows them to get a more accurate picture.

EXPOSURE

- Examine the abdomen, check the temperature and remember to check the legs for any sign of a deep vein thrombosis (DVT).

'The patient's abdomen is soft and nontender, and there is no evidence of DVT. He is apyrexial.'

INITIAL INVESTIGATIONS

Ask one of your colleagues, if available, to perform the arterial blood gas (ABG) or request the chest radiography (CXR) while you continue your assessment (see Table 3.1).

- **ABG**: Perform if (a) the SpO_2 is <92% or (b) there are any features of life-threatening asthma. Patients are likely to be hypoxic. The $PaCO_2$ is likely to be low (due to hyperventilation), causing a respiratory alkalosis (low H^+/high pH). However, if a patient becomes exhausted, their respiratory rate will reduce and the $PaCO_2$ will go from low to normal to high (indicating a near-fatal exacerbation).
- **Bloods**: Check Hb (for anaemia), urea and electrolytes (U&Es) (for dehydration and to monitor potassium when giving salbutamol), white cell count (WCC), C-reactive protein (CRP) ± blood cultures (for evidence of infection). Theophylline levels if on aminophylline (Table 3.2).
- **Peak flow**: This helps to measure the severity of an asthma attack (Table 3.1), as well as the response to treatment. It is most useful if measured as a percentage of a patient's previous best, but it can also be measured as a percentage of predicted (which is based on height, sex and age).
- **Electrocardiogram (ECG)**: Arrhythmias can be a sign of a life-threatening attack (or might suggest an alternative diagnosis as a cause of the breathlessness).
- **CXR** is indicated if:
  - There are any life-threatening features of asthma.
  - There is another diagnosis suspected, e.g. pneumothorax.
  - Bacterial infection is suspected.
  - Failure to respond to treatment.
  - Prior to continuous positive airway pressure (CPAP)/bilevel positive airway pressure (BiPAP)/intubation.

'The patient's peak flow is 40% of his usual best. ABG on air shows hypoxaemia and a respiratory alkalosis (PaO_2 7.0 kPa, $PaCO_2$ 3.1 kPA, H^+ 28 nmol/L (pH 7.55) and HCO_3^- 20 mmol/L). CXR shows hyperinflation. The lungs are clear, no pneumothorax. ECG shows sinus tachycardia. Bloods are normal.'

INITIAL MANAGEMENT

Asthma Initial Management Summary

- Resuscitate using an ABCDE approach
- Oxygen
- Bronchodilators
- Corticosteroids
- Regular assessment

- **Oxygen:** Should be given to all hypoxic patients. Aim for saturations of 94% to 98%.
- **Salbutamol:** 5 mg nebulised with oxygen should be given as soon as possible. These can then be given 'back-to-back', i.e. every 10 minutes if the initial response is poor. Only consider IV beta-2 agonists for those who are unable to undergo inhaled therapy. Nebulisers should be driven with oxygen (flow rate of 6 L/min usually needed) to avoid worsening hypoxia.

Table 3.1 Assessment of Severity of Asthma

MODERATE	ACUTE SEVERE	LIFE THREATENING
Increasing symptoms	Any one of:	Acute severe asthma + any one of:
Peak expiratory flow 50%–75% of best or predicted	Peak expiratory flow 33%–50% of best or predicted	Peak expiratory flow <33% of best or predicted
No features of acute severe asthma	Respiratory rate ≥25/min	Oxygen saturations <92%
	Heart rate ≥110/min	PaO_2 <8 kPa
	Unable to complete sentences in one breath	Normal $PaCO_2$ (4.6–6 kPa)
	Unable to perform peak flow	Silent chest
		Cyanosis
		Poor respiratory effort
		Arrhythmia
		Exhaustion, altered conscious level

Table 3.2 Mr Cannon's Blood and ABG Results

PARAMETER	VALUE	NORMAL RANGE (UNITS)
WCC	10.0 × 10^9/L	4.0–11.0 (×10^9/L)
Neutrophil	5.0 × 10^9/L	2.0–7.5 (×10^9/L)
Lymphocyte	2.1 × 10^9/L	1.4–4.0 (×10^9/L)
Platelet	250 × 10^9/L	150–400 (×10^9/L)
Haemoglobin	140 g/L	Men: 135–177 (g/L) Women: 115–155 (g/L)
CRP	2 mg/L	0–5 (mg/L)
Urea	5.3 mmol/L	2.5–6.7 (mmol/L)
Creatinine	90 µmol/L	79–118 (µmol/L)
Sodium	140 mmol/L	135–146 (mmol/L)
Potassium	4.2 mmol/L	3.5–5.0 (mmol/L)
eGFR	>60 mL/min	>60 (mL/min)
pH	**7.55**	**7.35–7.45**
H^+	**28 nmol/L**	**35–45 (nmol/L)**
PaO_2	**7.0 kPa on air**	**>10.0 on air (kPa)**
$PaCO_2$	**3.1 kPa**	**4.7–6.0 (kPa)**
HCO_3^-	**20 mmol/L**	**22–26 (mmol/L)**

Data in bold signifies results that are outside the normal laboratory range.
ABG, Arterial blood gas; *CRP*, C-reactive protein; *eGFR*, estimated glomerular filtration rate.

- **Ipratropium bromide:** 500 micrograms nebulised every 4 to 6 hours, if the attack is severe or life-threatening or if there is a poor response to nebulised salbutamol.
- **Corticosteroids:** Prednisolone 40 to 50 mg PO or hydrocortisone 100 mg IV if unable to swallow. Corticosteroids should be given in all cases of acute asthma. Oral corticosteroids are as effective as IV corticosteroids if the patient can swallow and absorb them. Continue for at least 5 days or until recovery.
- **Antibiotics:** Only required if there is any evidence of an infection (pyrexia, crackles on auscultation/consolidation on CXR or raised WCC/CRP).
- **Review medications:** May need to stop drugs such as beta-blockers and sedatives.

Prescribe (see Figs 3.1 and 3.2)

Corticosteroids:
- PREDNISOLONE 40 mg PO STAT

Bronchodilators:
- IPRATROPIUM BROMIDE 500 micrograms NEB (driven with oxygen) STAT and SALBUTAMOL 5 mg NEB (driven with oxygen) STAT

- Remember to involve your senior early. They may consider giving a single dose of magnesium sulfate 1.2–2 g IV in a life-threatening or near-fatal attack, or to patients who have not made a good response to nebulised salbutamol.
- Involve HDU/ITU early on. Patients with severe asthma may eventually require intubation.
- IV aminophylline is occasionally given by senior doctors. This may be considered in patients who have a severe or life-threatening attack and have responded poorly to initial treatment. Theophylline levels should be checked if the patient is already on theophylline or aminophylline, as it has a narrow therapeutic index.

REASSESSMENT

- Repeat the ABCDE process.
- Peak flow should be repeated at 15 and 30 minutes.
- ABGs should be repeated within 30 minutes if there is a poor response to treatment (Table 3.3).
- Titrate oxygen to the saturations and ABG results.

Table 3.3 Mr Cannon's Repeat ABG

PARAMETER	VALUE	NORMAL RANGE (UNITS)
pH	**7.52**	**7.35–7.45**
H^+	**30 nmol/L**	**35–45 (nmol/L)**
PaO_2	15.0 kPa on 2 L of nasal cannula oxygen	>10.0 (kPa) on air
$PaCO_2$	**3.8 kPa**	**4.7–6.0 (kPa)**
HCO_3^-	23 mmol/L	22–26 (mmol/L)

Data in bold signifies results that are outside the normal laboratory range.
ABG, Arterial blood gas.

'The patient is starting to improve. Airway is patent and RR is now 20/min. Oxygen saturations are now 95% on 2 L of nasal cannula oxygen. There is still expiratory wheeze; however, air entry has improved. HR is 118 bpm and BP is 120/80 mmHg. Peak flow is now 60% of predicted. Repeat ABG on 2 L oxygen shows PaO_2 15.0 kPa, $PaCO_2$ 3.8 kPA, H^+ 30 nmol/L (pH 7.52) and HCO_3^- 23 mmol/L.'

Side effects of salbutamol include tremor, tachycardia and hypokalaemia. Keep an eye on the U&Es and replace potassium with slow IV fluids if required.

FURTHER MANAGEMENT

- Ideally patients should be admitted under the care of a respiratory specialist rather than to a general ward.
- Aim to identify the trigger that precipitated the asthma attack.
- Continue regular nebulised therapy initially, e.g. salbutamol 5 mg every 4 hours ± ipratropium bromide 500 micrograms every 6 hours.
- After 24 hours, consider changing nebulised salbutamol to inhaled salbutamol, and adding in high-dose inhaled corticosteroid.
- Continue 40 mg of prednisolone for at least 5 days. The dose does not need to be tapered down, unless the patient is on maintenance corticosteroid treatment or has been on corticosteroid treatment for >3 weeks.
- Prescribe ongoing oxygen requirement, e.g. 2 L/min via nasal cannulae.
- Don't forget to prescribe DVT prophylaxis as long as there are no contraindications.
- Patients can be discharged when they are no longer requiring nebulised therapy and when the beta-2 agonist therapy can be extended to every 4 hours.
- Prior to discharge, the peak expiratory flow rate should be >75% of best/predicted, with <25% diurnal variation.
- Patients should be discharged with a personal self-management asthma plan and their inhaler technique should be assessed.
- After discharge, patients should be reviewed by an asthma specialist within 30 days.

Prescribe (see Figs 3.1 and 3.2)

START

Bronchodilators:

- SALBUTAMOL 5 mg NEB (driven with oxygen or air) 2 HOURLY
- IPRATROPIUM BROMIDE 500 micrograms NEB (driven with oxygen or air) 6 HOURLY

Corticosteroids:

- PREDNISOLONE 40 mg PO OD for 5 DAYS

Thromboprophylaxis:

- ENOXAPARIN 40 mg SC OD or FONDAPARINUX 2.5 mg SC OD

Oxygen:

- OXYGEN 2 L/min via NASAL CANNULAE

STOP

High-flow oxygen

HANDING OVER THE PATIENT

'Mr Cannon is a 23-year-old man who presented this evening with a life-threatening exacerbation of asthma. He was acutely breathless, with a RR 35/min, saturations of 89% on air, widespread wheeze in the lung field and poor basal lung entry. He has been treated with oxygen, 2 × 5 mg salbutamol nebulisers back-to-back, ipratropium bromide and prednisolone, and is responding well.

Current observations are RR 20/min, SpO_2 95% on 2 L of O_2. HR is 118/min and BP is 120/80 mmHg. Peak flow is 60% of predicted, and ABG shows a respiratory alkalosis. He has been reviewed by the HDU registrar who is happy with ward level management at present.

He is being transferred to the ward on 2-hourly salbutamol nebulisers and 6-hourly ipratropium. CXR shows hyperexpanded lungs, and bloods are normal. Please could you review him in one hour and check his peak flow again within 30 minutes.'

Features of a Near-Fatal Attack of Asthma

- Raised $PaCO_2$
- Patient requiring mechanical ventilation
- Bradycardia

STATION 3.2: EXACERBATION OF COPD

You are the junior doctor working in the medical assessment unit. Your next patient is Mrs Johnson, an acutely breathless 67-year-old woman with a history of chronic obstructive pulmonary disease (COPD). She normally controls this with inhalers alone and has no home nebulisers or long-term oxygen therapy. She says she is more breathless and wheezy but her sputum has not changed in colour.

Patient Details

Name:	Mary Johnson
DOB:	13/09/57
Hospital number:	1309576374
Weight:	78 kg
Height:	1.55 m
Consultant:	Dr Jones
Hospital/Ward:	WGH Ward 4
Current medications:	Salbutamol (100 micrograms/metered dose) 2 puffs INH PRN
Allergies:	None known
Admission date:	19/10/24

Initial Differential Diagnosis of Acute Breathlessness and Wheeze

- Respiratory: Exacerbation of COPD, exacerbation of asthma, acute viral or bacterial bronchitis
- Cardiac: Acute left ventricular failure
- Other: Anaphylaxis, inhaled foreign body

Long-term Complications of COPD

- Noninfective exacerbation of COPD
- Infective exacerbation of COPD
- Pneumothorax
- Weight loss
- Depression/anxiety
- Right heart failure
- Sleep disturbance

INITIAL ASSESSMENT

AIRWAY

- Assess patency of the airway.

  'The airway is patent.'

  No additional airway support is currently required.

BREATHING

- Assess respiratory rate, oxygen saturations, work of breathing and evidence of tiring. Percuss carefully, particularly to exclude pneumothoraces (increased risk in COPD, especially bullous emphysema). Auscultate for air entry, wheeze and crepitations.

  'RR 30/min, oxygen saturations are 82% on 2 L oxygen, with increased work of breathing. Resonant lung fields. There is good bilateral air entry with widespread inspiratory wheeze. No crepitations.'

You give oxygen via a Venturi mask and nebulised salbutamol and ipratropium. You also perform an ABG.

COPD Exacerbation Management

- Resuscitate using an ABCDE approach
- Oxygen with ABGs
- Bronchodilators
- Corticosteroids
- Antibiotics and fluids (if indicated)

Prescribe (Figs 3.3 and 3.4)

Bronchodilators:

- SALBUTAMOL 5 mg NEB (driven with oxygen) STAT
- IPRATROPIUM BROMIDE 500 micrograms NEB (driven with oxygen) STAT

Controlled OXYGEN:

- via a VENTURI MASK at a percentage determined by blood gas analysis

CIRCULATION

- Assess haemodynamic stability by measuring pulse, BP, CRT (centrally and peripherally).
- Perform a cardiovascular examination, looking at the jugular venous pressure (JVP) and listening to the lung bases for evidence of heart failure, and assessing the heart sounds for evidence of valvular disease, all of which can cause dyspnoea.

  'HR 84 bpm, BP 122/74 mmHg. Mrs Johnson has warm peripheries with a CRT <2 seconds. She has good volume peripheral pulses. CVS examination reveals normal HS, no murmurs, and no evidence of heart failure.'

  Secure IV access and take bloods.

DISABILITY

- Assess her conscious level, using AVPU (is the patient Alert? If not, do they respond to Verbal or Painful stimuli? Or are they Unresponsive?) or GCS. Check glucose levels.

  'She is alert but finding it difficult to speak in sentences. Her blood glucose is 9.5 mmol/L.'

EXPOSURE

- Check the patient's temperature. Expose the patient. Look for sources of infection, evidence of anaphylaxis (urticaria, erythema and oedema), and of a DVT.

  'Mrs Johnson's temperature is 36.9°C. The rest of the examination is normal.'

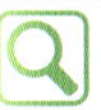

In contrast to asthma, peak flow is not useful in the management of acute COPD.

INITIAL INVESTIGATIONS

- **ABG:** One of the most important investigations in an exacerbation of COPD. It allows assessment of the degree of oxygenation (PaO_2) and ventilation ($PaCO_2$). Check within 20 minutes of starting or changing flow of oxygen. Aim for PaO_2 >6.6 kPa and H^+ <55 (pH >7.25). If this is achieved, increase the oxygen to achieve PaO_2 >7.5 kPa. Aim for oxygen saturations of 88% to 92%. If possible, compare to a baseline, e.g. clinic ABG result.
- **CXR:** To exclude other causes of dyspnoea, especially a pneumothorax. Look for areas of consolidation. This is a priority investigation and may need to be a portable CXR if the patient is not stable enough to go to the X-ray department.
- **ECG:** Look for evidence of an MI or arrhythmias.
- **Bloods:** Full blood count (FBC), U&Es, CRP. Look for evidence of infection, check for anaemia, assess renal function. Theophylline levels if on aminophylline (Table 3.4).
- **Blood culture:** If the patient is pyrexial.
- **Sputum culture:** If the patient has purulent sputum.

'ABG (on 2 L/min oxygen) PaO_2 6.0 kPa, $PaCO_2$ 3.1 kPa, H^+ 33 nmol/L (pH 7.48), HCO_3^- 26 mmol/L. WCC 8.6 × 10^9/L. CRP is 12 mg/L. Renal function is normal. CXR shows hyperinflated lungs with coarsening of the background markings in keeping with COPD. No consolidation or pneumothorax. ECG: sinus rhythm.'

Table 3.4 Mrs Johnson's Blood Test and ABG Results

PARAMETER	VALUE	NORMAL RANGE (UNITS)
WCC	8.6 × 10^9/L	4–11 (×10^9/L)
Neutrophil	5.8 × 10^9/L	2–7.5 (×10^9/L)
Lymphocyte	2.3 × 10^9/L	1.4–4.0 (×10^9/L)
Platelet	220 × 10^9/L	150–400 (×10^9/L)
Haemoglobin	150 g/L	Men: 135–177 (g/L) Women: 115–155 (g/L)
CRP	**12 mg/L**	**0–5 (mg/L)**
Urea	4.5 mmol/L	2.5–6.7 (mmol/L)
Creatinine	112 µmol/L	79–118 (µmol/L)
eGFR	>60 mL/min	>60 (mL/min)
Sodium	140 mmol/L	135–146 (mmol/L)
Potassium	4.5 mmol/L	3.5–5.0 (mmol/L)
pH	**7.48**	**7.35–7.45**
PaO_2	**6.0 kPa on air**	**>10.0 (kPa) on air**
$PaCO_2$	**3.1 kPa**	**4.7–6.0 (kPa)**
HCO_3^-	26 mmol/L	22–26 (mmol/L)
H^+	**33 nmol/L**	**35–45 (nmol/L)**

Data in bold signifies results that are outside the normal laboratory range.
ABG, Arterial blood gas; *CRP*, C-reactive protein; *eGFR*, estimated glomerular filtration rate; *WCC*, white cell count.

INITIAL MANAGEMENT

- This patient has a noninfective exacerbation of COPD.
- **Airway support:** Airway patent, no intervention required.
- **High-flow oxygen:** Best delivered by a Venturi mask, which allows controlled oxygen delivery regardless of the respiratory pattern or rate. Oxygen has to be used carefully in a certain cohort of COPD patients who rely on a hypoxic drive for respiration. However, in the acute setting the patient will die faster from hypoxia than hypercapnia. Titrate oxygen therapy using ABGs as indicated earlier.
- **Bronchodilators:** Nebulised salbutamol 5 mg and ipratropium bromide 500 micrograms immediately and then 4 to 6 hourly. Nebulisers can be driven with oxygen or air, depending on the result of ABGs. If the patient is not responding, salbutamol can be given more frequently and the respiratory registrar on call should be contacted.
- **Corticosteroids:** Prednisolone 30 mg PO OD (or hydrocortisone 200 mg IV if oral route unavailable) should be given for 5 days as standard but may require a longer course depending on the rate of recovery. Osteoporosis prophylaxis should be considered in patients having frequent courses of corticosteroids.
- **Antibiotics:** Used for patients with more purulent sputum or evidence of pneumonia clinically or radiologically. The choice depends on local policy. One option is amoxicillin 500 mg PO TDS or clarithromycin 250 to 500 mg BD if penicillin allergy. Adjust antibiotics according to sputum and blood culture results.
- **IV fluids:** If clinically dehydrated, or not tolerating oral fluids.
- **Venous thromboembolism prophylaxis.**

Remember oxygen saturation readings give no information about CO_2 or pH—ABGs are needed to assess these parameters.

Prescribe (see Figs 3.3 and 3.4)

Bronchodilator:
- SALBUTAMOL 5 mg NEB (driven with oxygen or air) 4 HOURLY
- IPRATROPIUM BROMIDE 500 micrograms NEB (driven with oxygen or air) 6 HOURLY

Corticosteroids:
- PREDNISOLONE 30 mg PO STAT then OD for 5 days

Thromboprophylaxis:
- ENOXAPARIN 40 mg SC OD or FONDAPARINUX 2.5 mg SC OD

REASSESSMENT

- After controlled oxygen, nebulisers and corticosteroids, the patient is reassessed (Table 3.5).

'Mrs Johnson does not look much better. Her airway is patent. RR 28/min, oxygen saturations are 96%, on 60% oxygen. Her chest is wheezy throughout. HR 88 bpm, BP 136/78 mmHg, CRT 2 seconds. Repeat ABG on 60% oxygen shows PaO_2 12.8 kPa, $PaCO_2$ 7.6 kPa, H^+ 53 nmol/L (pH 7.28), HCO_3^- 26 mmol/L.'

The patient is relatively hypoxic (given she is breathing 60% oxygen) and has developed a respiratory acidosis, probably secondary to the high concentration of inspired oxygen. You reduce the concentration of supplementary oxygen, since saturations are above 92%, and phone the respiratory registrar for review. After his review, he decides to commence the patient on a theophylline (aminophylline) infusion given the limited response to repeated bronchodilators.

Table 3.5 Mrs Johnson's Repeat ABG

PARAMETER	VALUE	NORMAL RANGE (UNITS)
pH	**7.28**	**7.35–7.45**
PaO_2	12.8 kPa on 60% oxygen	>10.0 (kPa) on air
$PaCO_2$	**7.6 kPa**	**4.7–6.0 (kPa)**
HCO_3^-	26 mmol/L	22–26 (mmol/L)
H^+	**53 nmol/L**	**35–45 (nmol/L)**

Data in bold signifies results that are outside the normal laboratory range.
ABG, Arterial blood gas.

Prescribe (see Figs 3.3 and 3.4)

AMINOPHYLLINE 250 mg IV (over 20 minutes)
Controlled OXYGEN:

- 35% via VENTURI MASK

STOP
60% OXYGEN via VENTURI MASK

FURTHER MANAGEMENT

- **Theophylline:** Should be considered as an adjunct if there is inadequate response to nebulised bronchodilators. Theophylline levels should be monitored within 24 hours of starting treatment.
- **Noninvasive ventilation:** Treatment of choice for persistent hypercapnic ventilation failure despite optimal medical treatment.
- **Invasive ventilation:** May be considered for patients not responding to noninvasive ventilation.
- **Chest physiotherapy**: Physiotherapy using positive expiratory pressure masks may be useful in certain COPD patients during an exacerbation to help clear sputum. Secretions may also be cleared using saline nebulisers and mucolytic agents such as carbocisteine.
- **Reassessment**: Regular reassessment of symptoms and functional capacity is required. Oxygen saturations can be used to monitor the recovery of patients with nonacidotic, nonhypercapnic respiratory failure. ABGs are needed for monitoring in patients with hypercapnic or acidotic respiratory failure.
- **Maintenance therapy**: Patients should be established on their optimal maintenance bronchodilator therapy prior to discharge. Withhold regular inhaler while on nebulisers.

HANDING OVER THE PATIENT

'Mrs Johnson is a 67-year-old woman with a noninfective exacerbation of COPD.

She usually has a good exercise tolerance and maintains an active life. She does not have home oxygen or nebulisers and has had one previous admission in the last 5 years, requiring nebulisers only.

She presented in respiratory distress with marked wheeze. Bloods were normal, and CXR showed no pneumothorax or consolidation. Initial ABG on air showed hypoxaemia and a respiratory alkalosis. She was treated for a noninfectious exacerbation of COPD but responded poorly to initial treatment with high-flow oxygen, nebulisers and corticosteroids. Repeat ABG showed a respiratory acidosis and relative hypoxaemia. She has been reviewed by the respiratory registrar who has commenced an aminophylline infusion.

The plan is to admit her to the respiratory ward, on 35% oxygen, 6-hourly ipratropium, 4-hourly salbutamol, aminophylline infusion, and prednisolone. She will require a repeat ABG in 30 minutes, and titration of her oxygen. She would be a candidate for escalation of her care if required and has been discussed with HDU already.'

STATION 3.3: COMMUNITY-ACQUIRED PNEUMONIA (CAP)

You are a junior doctor working in the medical assessment unit. Your next patient is Mr Taylor, an 84-year-old man with mild dementia, who presents with a cough and fever. His daughter tells you he has been coughing up green sputum for the last couple of days. She has also noticed he is more confused than normal.

Patient Details

Name:	William Taylor
DOB:	16/10/40
Hospital number:	1610401289
Weight:	72 kg
Height:	1.65 m
Consultant:	Dr Jones
Hospital/Ward:	WGH Ward 4
Current medications:	Nil
Allergies:	Trimethoprim (rash)
Admission date:	19/10/24

Initial Differential Diagnosis of Cough With Sputum

- Pneumonia
- Acute viral bronchitis
- COPD (including exacerbation)
- Lung abscess
- Tuberculosis
- Broncho-alveolar carcinoma
- Left ventricular failure

Acute Complications of Pneumonia

- Pleural effusion
- Empyema
- Lung abscess
- Septicaemia
- Respiratory failure (type 1 or type 2 if severe)
- Atrial fibrillation
- Confusion

CAP Management

- Resuscitate using an ABCDE approach
- Oxygen
- Antibiotics
- IV fluids

INITIAL ASSESSMENT

AIRWAY

- Is the airway patent?

'The airway is patent.'

No additional airway support is currently required.

BREATHING

- Assess respiratory rate, oxygen saturations, work of breathing. Percuss for evidence of consolidation and pleural effusions. Auscultate for air entry, wheeze and crepitations.

'RR 25/min, oxygen saturations are 88% on room air. Chest expansion is reduced on the right and the right lower zone is dull to percussion. Crepitations and increased vocal resonance in the right lower zone.'

Given these findings, you give high-flow oxygen.

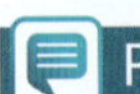

Prescribe (Figs 3.5–3.7)

High-flow OXYGEN:
- 15 L/min via NONREBREATHER MASK

CURB 65: CAP Severity Assessment

C—New-onset confusion
U—Urea >7 mmol/L
R—Respiratory rate ≥30/min
B—Systolic BP <90 mmHg, diastolic ≤60 mmHg
65—Age ≥65 years

SEVERITY

0: low risk (less than 1% mortality risk)
1 or 2: intermediate risk (1%–10% mortality risk)
3 or 4: high risk (more than 10% mortality risk).
Consider hospital assessment for people with a CURB 65 score of 2 or higher

CIRCULATION

- Assess haemodynamic stability by measuring pulse, BP, CRT (centrally and peripherally). Review urine output.
- Perform a cardiovascular examination, in particular looking for evidence of heart failure which can cause a productive cough.

'HR 110 bpm, BP 142/86 mmHg. His peripheries are warm with a CRT <2 seconds. He has good volume peripheral pulses. CVS examination reveals normal HS, with no murmurs. The JVP is not elevated.'

Secure IV access and take bloods.

DISABILITY

In patients with a background of dementia, it is important to assess for an acute change in confusion levels—compare current AMT with previous if available.

- Assess his conscious level, using AVPU (is the patient Alert? If not, do they respond to Verbal or Painful stimuli? Or are they Unresponsive?). Use the abbreviated mental test (AMT) to assess confusion. Check glucose levels.

'He is alert but confused with an AMT of 2/10. His AMT on the previous admission 4 months ago was 7/10. His blood glucose is 8.5 mmol/L.'

EXPOSURE

- Check the patient's temperature. Examine the patient, looking in particular for other sources of infection.

'Mr Taylor's temperature is 38.9°C. His mucous membranes are dry. His abdomen is soft, nontender and there is no sign of cellulitis. The rest of the examination is normal.'

Infection is one cause of acute confusion. Others include:
- Metabolic abnormalities (hypoglycaemia, hyponatraemia, hypercalcaemia, etc.)
- Drugs such as opioids, corticosteroids, benzodiazepines
- Alcohol withdrawal
- Surgery
- Intracranial pathology such as subdural haematoma

INITIAL INVESTIGATIONS

Remember infection can cause arrhythmias, such as atrial fibrillation.

- **Bloods:** FBC, U&E, CRP, liver function tests (LFTs), calcium. Look for evidence of infection, causes of confusion, assess renal function. Deranged LFTs may indicate biliary pathology or can occur with pneumonia. Mycoplasma blood test (Table 3.6).
- **Blood cultures:** Recommended for all patients with moderate to severe CAP. Ideally, send at least two sets before starting antibiotics.
- **Sputum culture:** Recommended for patients with moderate to severe CAP.
- **Urine:** Pneumococcal urine antigen test should be performed in moderate or severe CAP. Test urine for Legionella if the patient has severe CAP or there is clinical suspicion of Legionella pneumonia.
- **ABG:** Consider performing an ABG. This allows assessment of oxygenation (PaO_2), ventilation ($PaCO_2$) and acid–base status.
- **CXR:** Look for areas of consolidation and effusions.
- **ECG:** To assess the rate and rhythm.

'WCC 18.6 × 10⁹/L, neutrophils 15.8 × 10⁹/L. CRP is 163 mg/L. Urea 14.3 mmol/L, creatinine 170 µmol/L, eGFR 40 mL/min (baseline urea 7.3 mmol/L, creatinine 101 µmol/L, eGFR >60 mL/min), LFTs normal. One

Table 3.6 Mr Taylor's Blood Results

PARAMETER	VALUE	NORMAL RANGE (UNITS)
WCC	**18.6 × 10^9/L**	**4.0–11.0 (×10^9/L)**
Neutrophil	**15.8 × 10^9/L**	**2.0–7.5 (×10^9/L)**
Lymphocyte	2.2 × 10^9/L	1.4–4.0 (×10^9/L)
Platelet	200 × 10^9/L	150–400 (×10^9/L)
Haemoglobin	160 g/L	Men: 135–177 (g/L) Women: 115–155 (g/L)
CRP	**163 mg/L**	**0–5 (mg/L)**
Urea	**14.3 mmol/L**	**2.5–6.7 (mmol/L)**
Creatinine	**170 µmol/L**	**79–118 (µmol/L)**
eGFR	**40 mL/min**	**>60 (mL/min)**
Sodium	140 mmol/L	135–146 (mmol/L)
Potassium	4.5 mmol/L	3.5–5.0 (mmol/L)
pH	7.38	7.35–7.45
PaO_2	12.8 kPa on 15 L/min of oxygen	>10.0 (kPa) on air
$PaCO_2$	5.0 kPa	4.7–6.0 (kPa)
HCO_3^-	23 mmol/L	22–26 (mmol/L)

Data in bold signifies results that are outside the normal laboratory range. *CRP*, C-reactive protein; *eGFR*, estimated glomerular filtration rate; *WCC*, white cell count.

set of blood cultures are in progress. The nursing staff will obtain a sputum sample as soon as possible. ABG shows a PaO_2 12.8 kPa on 15 L/min of oxygen. CXR shows right lower lobe consolidation. ECG shows a sinus tachycardia.'

INITIAL MANAGEMENT

- This patient has sepsis from severe CAP (CURB 65 score = 3) and acute kidney injury.
- **High-flow oxygen:** To correct hypoxia. Aim for oxygen saturations 94% to 98%.
- **Antibiotics:** Should be tailored to the likely organism and severity of the pneumonia. Consult your local antibiotic guidelines. One option is amoxicillin 500 mg PO TDS for CURB 65 score 0 to 1 (alternatively doxycycline 200 mg on first day then 100 mg OD or clarithromycin 500 mg BD if penicillin allergy or atypical pathogens suspected). Co-amoxiclav 1.2 g IV TDS and clarithromycin 500 mg BD PO or IV for CURB 65 score 2 to 5. Adjust antibiotics according to sputum and blood culture results.
- **IV fluids:** To correct hypovolaemia, compensate for increased insensible losses when pyrexial, and reverse acute kidney injury (secondary to hypoperfusion of the kidneys from shock).
- **Antipyretic**: Paracetamol can be used to help reduce a raised temperature.
- **Venous thromboembolism prophylaxis:** It is important to consider venous thromboembolism prophylaxis.
- **Early senior review:** Patients with a CURB 65 score of ≥3 are at high risk of death and should be reviewed by a senior physician at the earliest opportunity.

The distinction between community- and hospital-acquired pneumonia is important because the likely causative organisms and empirical antibiotics differ.

Prescribe (see Figs 3.6–3.8)

Antibiotics:
- CO-AMOXICLAV (1000 mg/200 mg) 1.2 g IV STAT and then TDS
- CLARITHROMYCIN 500 mg PO STAT and then BD

Antipyretics:
- PARACETAMOL 1 g STAT and then QDS

Thromboprophylaxis:
- DALTEPARIN 5000 UNITS SC OD

Fluids:
- SODIUM CHLORIDE 0.9% 500 mL 250 mL/h and then SODIUM CHLORIDE 0.9% 500 mL 250 mL/h

OXYGEN:
- 4 L/min via NASAL CANNULAE

STOP

High-flow oxygen

Dosage of antibiotics and DVT prophylaxis may need to be adjusted in renal failure—consult appropriate prescribing guidance, e.g. the British National Formulary (BNF).

REASSESSMENT

- After supplementary oxygen, antibiotics and IV fluids, the patient is reassessed.

'Mr Taylor looks better. His airway is patient. RR 16/min, oxygen saturations are 95%, on 4 L of oxygen. He has crackles at the right base, the rest of his chest is clear. HR 86 bpm, BP 140/70 mmHg, CRT 2 seconds. Temperature 37.9°C. His mucous membranes remain dry.'

FURTHER MANAGEMENT

- **Antibiotics**: Adjust antibiotics according to culture results. Change IV to oral antibiotics as soon as clinical improvement occurs and the temperature has been normal for >24 hours. Duration of antibiotic therapy depends on clinical response. Five days is usually recommended for mild or moderate community-acquired pneumonia unless microbiological results suggest a longer course is needed or the patient is not clinically stable.
- **Fluid support**: Regular fluids reviews are needed as it is easy to put a patient into heart failure with overzealous fluid resuscitation, especially elderly patients.

- In many patients with pneumonia, a repeat chest X-ray should be performed in 6 weeks to ensure resolution and exclude an underlying malignancy.

HANDING OVER THE PATIENT

'Mr Taylor is an 84-year-old man with sepsis secondary to community-acquired pneumonia, and acute kidney injury.

He presented with a cough, fever and confusion and on admission had a CURB 65 score of 3 (for worsening confusion, raised urea and age). Bloods show raised inflammatory markers, and evidence of acute renal failure.

He has mild dementia, is on no regular medication and is otherwise well.

He has been treated with antibiotics, IV fluids and supplementary oxygen, and has shown signs of improvement. Current observations: oxygen saturations are 95% (on 4 L of oxygen), HR 86 bpm, BP 140/70 mmHg, temperature 37.9°C. He has been reviewed by the medical consultant on call, who feels he would be suitable for escalation above ward-based care should he deteriorate. I have spoken with his next of kin, who are in agreement.

The plan is to continue antibiotics, maintain saturations above 94% with oxygen, and repeat bloods in the morning. He will require a fluid review in the evening.'

STATION 3.4: HOSPITAL-ACQUIRED PNEUMONIA

You are a junior doctor working on an orthopaedic ward. You are asked to review Mrs Jackson, an 80-year-old woman who is 4 days post a left dynamic hip screw for a femoral neck fracture. She has a background of hypertension, and gastro-oesophageal reflux. The nurse tells you she has developed a temperature.

Patient Details

Name:	Patricia Jackson
DOB:	21/06/44
Hospital number:	2106442256
Weight:	64 kg
Height:	1.6 m
Consultant:	Mr Kaye
Hospital/Ward:	WGH Ortho Ward
Current medications:	Fondaparinux 2.5 mg SC OD (started this admission—thromboprophylaxis) Omeprazole 20 mg PO OD (for gastro-oesophageal reflux) Lisinopril 10 mg PO OD (for hypertension) Paracetamol 1 g PO QDS (for pain)
Allergies:	Nil
Admission date:	15/10/24

Initial Differential Diagnosis of Pyrexia in a Hospitalised Patient

- Respiratory: Hospital-acquired pneumonia, aspiration pneumonia
- Urology: Urinary tract infection
- Skin: Wound infection, cellulitis
- Other: Gastroenteritis, *Clostridium difficile* infection, surgical causes, e.g. perforation, cholecystitis

Acute Complications of Pneumonia

- Pleural effusion
- Empyema
- Lung abscess
- Septicaemia
- Respiratory failure (type 1 or type 2 if severe)
- Atrial fibrillation
- Confusion

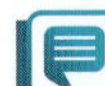

Hospital-Acquired Pneumonia Management

- Resuscitate using an ABCDE approach
- Oxygen
- IV fluids
- Consider chest physiotherapy
- Antibiotics

INITIAL ASSESSMENT

AIRWAY

- Assess patency of the airway.

  'The airway is patent.'

  No additional airway support is currently required.

BREATHING

- Assess respiratory rate, oxygen saturations and work of breathing. Percuss for evidence of a pleural effusion or pneumothorax. Auscultate for air entry and crepitations or wheeze.

  'RR 23/min, oxygen saturations are 90% on air. At the right base there is dullness, reduced air entry and crackles. The left lung is clear.'

You give supplementary oxygen to maintain oxygen saturations >94%.

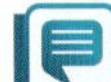

Prescribe (see Figs **3.8–3.10**)

OXYGEN:
- 4 L/min via NASAL CANNULAE

Fluid bolus:
- SODIUM CHLORIDE 0.9% 500 mL (over 15 minutes)

CIRCULATION

- Assess haemodynamic stability by measuring pulse, BP, CRT (centrally and peripherally). Review urine output.
- Perform a cardiovascular examination.

'HR 125 bpm, BP 102/78 mmHg. Mrs Jackson has warm peripheries with a CRT <2 seconds. She has good volume peripheral pulses, and good urine output. CVS examination shows normal HS, with no murmurs.'

Secure IV access and take bloods, including blood cultures. Give a fluid bolus. Supplementary IV fluids are likely to be required.

DISABILITY

- Assess her conscious level, using AVPU (is the patient Alert? If not, do they respond to Verbal or Painful stimuli? Or are they Unresponsive?). Check glucose levels.

'She is alert but disorientated to time and place. You note that on admission she was orientated, with an AMT score of 9/10. Her blood glucose is 8.2 mmol/L.'

Infection is one cause of acute confusion. Others include:

- Metabolic abnormalities (hypoglycaemia, hyponatraemia, etc.)
- Drugs such as opiates, corticosteroids, benzodiazepines
- Alcohol withdrawal
- Surgery
- Intracranial pathology such as subdural haematoma

EXPOSURE

- Check the patient's temperature. Expose the patient and look for other possible sources of infection—pay close attention to the skin (cellulitis or wound infection) and abdomen (cholecystitis). Assess for a neurological cause of confusion (subdural haematoma or stroke). Check lines such as urinary catheters and IV cannulae, which may be a source of infection.

'Mrs Jackson's temperature is 39.0°C. The abdomen is soft and nontender. The wound looks healthy. No evidence of cellulitis. The rest of the examination is normal.'

You may have to remove dressings from wounds to assess for surgical site infections.

INITIAL INVESTIGATIONS

- **Bloods:** FBC, U&Es, CRP, LFTs, calcium. Look for evidence of infection, assess renal function and look for causes of confusion. Deranged LFTs may indicate biliary pathology or can occur with pneumonia (Table 3.7).

Table 3.7 Mrs Jackson's Blood Results

PARAMETER	VALUE	NORMAL RANGE (UNITS)
WCC	**17.6 × 10^9/L**	**4.0–11.0 (×10^9/L)**
Neutrophil	**14.0 × 10^9/L**	**2.0–7.5 (×10^9/L)**
Lymphocyte	3.1 × 10^9/L	1.4–4.0 (×10^9/L)
Platelet	300 × 10^9/L	150–400 (×10^9/L)
Haemoglobin	140 g/L	Men: 135–177 (g/L) Women: 115–155 (g/L)
CRP	**125 mg/L**	**0–5 (mg/L)**
Urea	**15.3 mmol/L**	**2.5–6.7 (mmol/L)**
Creatinine	**120 μmol/L**	**79–118 (μmol/L)**
eGFR	**40 mL/min**	**>60 (mL/min)**
Sodium	137 mmol/L	135–146 (mmol/L)
Potassium	4.3 mmol/L	3.5–5.0 (mmol/L)
pH	7.38	7.35–7.45
PaO_2	**9.8 kPa on air**	**>10.0 (kPa) on air**
$PaCO_2$	4.9 kPa	4.7–6.0 (kPa)
HCO_3^-	24 mmol/L	22–26 (mmol/L)

Data in bold signifies results that are outside the normal laboratory range.
CRP, C-reactive protein; *eGFR*, estimated glomerular filtration rate; *WCC*, white cell count.

- **ABG:** Consider performing an ABG.
- **Blood culture:** Ideally, send at least two sets before starting antibiotics.
- **Sputum culture:** Ask the nursing staff to obtain a sputum sample and nasopharyngeal swab.
- **Urinalysis:** Dipstick test for leucocytes, nitrites and blood. Send for culture if positive.
- **Wound swab:** Send if the wound looks infected.
- **Stool culture:** Send if the patient has diarrhoea.
- **CXR:** To assess for pneumonia and pleural effusions.

Always remember to compare the results of investigations, such as renal function and chest X-rays, with previous results.

'WCC 17.6 × 10^9/L, neutrophils 14 × 10^9/L. CRP is 125 mg/L. Urea 15.3 mmol/L, creatinine 120 μmol/L, eGFR 40 mL/min (baseline—urea 8 mmol/L, creatinine 65 μmol/L, eGFR >60 mL/min). Electrolytes and LFTs are normal. Urinalysis shows no blood, leucocytes or nitrites. Blood cultures are in progress. Blood gas shows mild hypoxaemia, with a normal carbon dioxide and pH. The nurses will send sputum samples when possible. CXR shows right lower lobe consolidation with a small parapneumonic effusion, new compared with the admission CXR.'

INITIAL MANAGEMENT

- This patient has sepsis secondary to hospital-acquired pneumonia.
- **Airway support:** Airway patent in this case, with no intervention required.

- **Supplementary oxygen**: If oxygen saturations are <94%.
- **Antibiotics:** Choice of empirical antibiotics depends on local knowledge of the nature and susceptibility patterns of pathogens. For early onset infections (<5 days of admission) of lower severity with no recent antibiotics, then co-amoxiclav PO is usually appropriate (other oral options are doxycycline, cefalexin and co-trimoxazole). For more severe infections, IV therapy with piperacillin and tazobactam would be more appropriate. Consult local antibiotic guidelines or a microbiologist for late-onset infections (>5 days).
- **Fluid support**: Septic patients usually require IV fluids as they have a relative hypovolaemia secondary to vasodilatation. Furthermore, they have increased insensible losses. Regular reassessment of fluid status is needed, particularly in elderly patients.
- **Antipyretic**: Paracetamol can be used to help reduce a high temperature.
- **Review current medications**: Discontinue any medications that may worsen renal failure and consider any potential drug interactions. Ensure the patient is on appropriate thromboprophylaxis.

Hospital-acquired pneumonia is defined as a respiratory infection developing >48 hours after hospital admission.

Prescribe (see Figs 3.8–3.10)

Antibiotics:
- PIPERACILLIN WITH TAZOBACTAM (4 g/500 mg) 4.5 g IV STAT and then TDS

Fluids:
- SODIUM CHLORIDE 0.9% 125 mL/h

STOP
Lisinopril (until renal function has improved)

REASSESSMENT

- After IV antibiotics and fluids, paracetamol and supplemental oxygen, the patient is reassessed.

'Mrs Jackson looks better. Her airway is patent. RR 18/min, oxygen saturations are 96%, on 4 L of oxygen via nasal prongs. Crackles are heard at the right base. HR 88 bpm, BP 142/74 mmHg, CRT 2 seconds. She remains disorientated.'

FURTHER MANAGEMENT

- **Antibiotics**: Adjust antibiotics according to culture results. Duration of antibiotic therapy depends on clinical response, but should routinely be less than 8 days.
- **Fluid support**: Regular fluids reviews are needed as it is easy to put a patient into heart failure with overzealous fluid resuscitation, especially elderly patients.
- **Chest physiotherapy**: May be useful for some patients with hospital-acquired pneumonia, but there is currently no evidence it improves outcome.

HANDING OVER THE PATIENT

'Mrs Jackson is a 80-year-old woman, 4 days post left dynamic hip screw repair of a NOF fracture, with a hospital-acquired pneumonia.

She was noted today to have a temperature, and to be acutely confused. Clinical examination and CXR confirm a right lower lobe hospital-acquired pneumonia with a small parapneumonic effusion. Bloods show elevated inflammatory markers and acute kidney injury. Blood cultures have been sent, but we are waiting for a sputum sample.

IV piperacillin with tazobactam, supplementary oxygen and IV fluids have been started. Her nephrotoxic drugs have been withheld.

Current observations: oxygen saturations are 96% on 4 L/min of oxygen, HR 88 bpm, BP 142/72 mmHg. She is on 4-hourly observations. The plan is to continue antibiotics, chase blood/sputum cultures, and for a fluid review in a few hours. Prior to this admission she was fit and well. She would therefore be a candidate for escalation of care if she deteriorates.'

STATION 3.5: PULMONARY EMBOLISM (PE)

You are a junior doctor working in the Medical Admission Unit on the evening shift. Your next patient is a 69-year-old man who is visiting the UK. He arrived 4 days ago from Australia. Today he has become acutely breathless, with small volume haemoptysis, and left-sided pleuritic chest pain. Please assess the patient and start appropriate management.

Patient Details

Name:	Steven Peters
DOB:	02/10/55
Hospital number:	0210556647
Weight:	110 kg
Height:	1.78 m
Consultant:	Dr Jones
Hospital/Ward:	WGH MAU
Current medications:	Nil
Allergies:	Nil
Admission date:	18/10/24

Initial Differential Diagnosis of Acute Dyspnoea and Chest Pain

- Respiratory: Pulmonary embolus, pneumothorax, pneumonia
- Cardiac: Acute coronary syndrome, pericarditis
- Musculoskeletal: Musculoskeletal chest pain, rib fractures

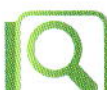

Complications of Pulmonary Embolism

- Haemoptysis
- Right heart failure
- Respiratory failure
- Atrial fibrillation/cardiac arrhythmia
- Pulmonary hypertension

INITIAL ASSESSMENT

AIRWAY

- Assess patency of the airway.

'The airway is patent.'

No additional airway support is required.

BREATHING

- Assess respiratory rate, oxygen saturations and work of breathing. Look for cyanosis.
- Palpate for chest wall tenderness.
- Percuss for hyperresonance (pneumothorax) or hyporesonance (pleural effusion).
- Auscultate for air entry, any additional sounds of wheeze and crepitations.

'RR 25/min, oxygen saturations are 90% on air. No increased work of breathing or chest wall tenderness. Percussion and breath sounds are normal throughout with no added sounds.'

You give supplementary oxygen (since saturations are below 94%).

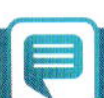

Prescribe (Fig. 3.11)

OXYGEN:
- 4 L/min via NASAL CANNULAE

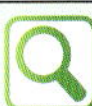

Don't forget that heart failure can be a consequence of PE, as well as a cause of breathlessness.

CIRCULATION

- Assess haemodynamic stability by measuring pulse, BP, CRT (centrally and peripherally).
- Perform a cardiovascular examination, looking at the JVP for evidence of right heart failure, which can occur with PE. Auscultate the heart looking for evidence of pericarditis (pericardial rub), or valvular heart disease (murmurs, thrills, heaves).

'HR 106 bpm regular, BP 158/90 mmHg, CRT 2 seconds. The JVP is not elevated. CVS examination shows normal HS, with no murmurs or pericardial rub.'

This patient will require IV access. Bloods should be sent at the same time.

DISABILITY

- Assess the patient's conscious level, using AVPU (is the patient Alert? If not, do they respond to Verbal or Painful stimuli? Or are they Unresponsive?) or GCS. Check glucose levels.

'The patient is alert, and has blood glucose of 6.9 mmol/L.'

EXPOSURE

- Expose the patient and perform a full examination, looking particularly for evidence of a deep vein thrombosis (swollen lower limb with tenderness along the distribution of the deep veins).

In patients with PE, there is often no clinical evidence of DVT—don't let this put you off the diagnosis of PE.

'Temperature is 37.5°C, and examination is otherwise normal, with no evidence of DVT.'

INITIAL INVESTIGATIONS

- **ABG:** The ABG can vary depending on the size of the PE:
  - With small or medium-sized PEs, there may not be a significant ventilation–perfusion mismatch (the ABG can be normal).
  - A medium or large PE may show a respiratory alkalosis, with a low $PaCO_2$, due to hyperventilation, and a low PaO_2. The PaO_2 will be lower the larger the PE. A massive PE will also cause a metabolic acidosis due to hypoxaemia and anaerobic metabolism. Usually, even in a massive PE, the $PaCO_2$ is low due to hyperventilation, although rarely it may become high if the patient has progressed to type 2 respiratory failure.
- **Bloods:** FBC, U&Es, CRP, prothrombin time (PT), activated partial thromboplastin time (APTT), D-dimer. Look for evidence of infection and assess renal function. D-dimer is sensitive but not specific for venous thromboembolism. It should be used to exclude venous thromboembolism in patients who are at low or intermediate risk of PE. Baseline coagulation screen is useful in patients with bleeding, and those commencing treatment with heparin or warfarin. Troponin should only be requested if the history, examination and ECG are suggestive of

ACS: it will be high with a big PE/right ventricular strain (Table 3.8).

- **CXR:** It will often be normal in PE, but may show atelectasis, pleural effusions, linear shadows or wedge-shaped peripheral opacities. Useful for excluding other differential diagnoses, such as pneumothorax, pneumonia or acute rib fractures.
- **ECG:** Usually nonspecific, with sinus tachycardia being the most common abnormality. There may be evidence of right ventricular strain (T-wave inversion in lead V1–V4) and right bundle branch block. The classic S1Q3T3 pattern (large S wave in lead I, large Q wave in lead III and T-wave inversion in lead III) is uncommon.
- **Computed tomographic pulmonary angiography (CTPA):** Gold standard investigation for PE. It is sensitive and specific for PE. Additionally, it allows identification of other pathologies contributing to the clinical findings.
- **Weight:** Important for calculating the dose of LMWH.

The CXR and ECG are often nonspecific in PE. Their value lies primarily in excluding differential diagnoses.

'ABG on air shows a PaO_2 7.0 kPa, $PaCO_2$ 3.8 kPa, H^+ 28 nmol/L (pH 7.55), HCO_3^- 25 mmol/L, BE 2.0 mmol/L. Hb is 185 g/L, WCC 11 × 10^9/L. Urea 6.2 mmol/L, creatinine 60 µmol/L. D-dimer is positive 1264 µg/L, clotting otherwise normal. CXR is normal. ECG shows sinus tachycardia. Weight is 110 kg.'

Table 3.8 Mr Peters' Blood and ABG Results

PARAMETER	VALUE	NORMAL RANGE (UNITS)
WCC	11.0 × 10^9/L	4.0–11.0 (×10^9/L)
Neutrophil	7.6 × 10^9/L	2.0–7.5 (×10^9/L)
Lymphocyte	2.5 × 10^9/L	1.4–4.0 (×10^9/L)
Platelet	200 × 10^9/L	150–400 (×10^9/L)
Haemoglobin	185 g/L	Men: 135–177 (g/L) Women: 115–155 (g/L)
CRP	3 mg/L	0–5 (mg/L)
Urea	6.2 mmol/L	2.5–6.7 (mmol/L)
Creatinine	60 µmol/L	79–118 (µmol/L)
Sodium	140 mmol/L	135–146 (mmol/L)
Potassium	4.3 mmol/L	3.5–5.0 (mmol/L)
eGFR	>60 mL/min	>60 (mL/min)
PT	12 seconds	11.5–13.5 seconds
APTT	30 seconds	26–37 seconds
D-dimer	**1264 µg/L**	**<500 (µg/L)**
pH	**7.55**	**7.35–7.45**
PaO_2	**7.0 kPa on air**	**>10.0 (kPa) on air**
$PaCO_2$	**3.8 kPa**	**4.7–6.0 (kPa)**
HCO_3^-	25 mmol/L	22–26 (mmol/L)
H^+	**28 nmol/L**	**35–45 (nmol/L)**
Base excess	2 mmol/L	±2 (mmol/L)

Data in bold signifies results that are outside the normal laboratory range. *ABG*, Arterial blood gas; *APTT*, activated partial thromboplastin time; *CRP*, C-reactive protein; *eGFR*, estimated glomerular filtration rate; *PT*, prothrombin time; *WCC*, white cell count.

Table 3.9 Revised Geneva Score

CRITERIA	SCORE
Age 65 years or over	1
Previous DVT or PE	3
Surgery or fracture in the last month	2
Active malignant condition	2
Unilateral lower limb pain	3
Haemoptysis	2
Heart rate 75–94 bpm	3
Heart rate >94 bpm	5
Pain on deep palpation of lower limb and unilateral oedema	4
0–3 = Low probability of PE (8%)	
4–10 = Intermediate probability (28%)	
>10 = High probability (74%)	

Data in bold signifies results that are outside the normal laboratory range. *DVT*, Deep vein thrombosis; *PE*, pulmonary embolism.

Clinical Decision Rules for Determining the Probability of PE

- Presentations with acute breathlessness *suspected* to be caused by a PE are common and so there is a need to have criteria for risk stratification (e.g. Geneva Score, Wells score) (Table 3.9).
- Patients with a high probability of PE should proceed to imaging to confirm or exclude PE.
- Patients with a low or intermediate probability should have a D-dimer checked:
  - If there is likely to be a delay before the D-dimer result can be obtained, then initial therapeutic anticoagulation should be given (e.g. LMWH or fondaparinux).
  - If the D-dimer is positive, they should undergo imaging to confirm or exclude PE.
  - If the D-dimer is negative, then PE is effectively ruled out.

INITIAL MANAGEMENT

Pulmonary Embolus Management

- Resuscitate using an ABCDE approach
- Breathing: Supplementary oxygen
- Circulation: low-molecular-weight heparin (LMWH) ± warfarin, may require IV fluids or inotropes

- **Airway support:** Airway patent in this case, with no intervention required.
- **Supplementary oxygen**: If oxygen saturations are <94%.
- **Heparin:** Patients with *suspected* PE should be treated with therapeutic doses of an anticoagulant such as

an LMWH (e.g. enoxaparin), fondaparinux or a factor Xa inhibitor (e.g. apixaban) without preliminary heparin, until the diagnosis has been deemed very unlikely. Unfractionated heparin may be preferred in severe renal impairment (creatinine clearance (CrCl) <15 mL/min) because its effects diminish rapidly on discontinuation and can be reversed (with protamine). These anticoagulants have an immediate effect, unlike warfarin, which requires time before a therapeutic level is reached. Care is needed if there is an increased bleeding risk—in such patients a CTPA may be needed to confirm the diagnosis before starting treatment. Note that the dosage of treatments such as LMWHs may need to be adjusted because of weight and renal function.

- **Analgesia:** Use the WHO pain ladder to prescribe adequate analgesia to reduce pleuritic chest pain.
- **Fluid support and inotropes**: These may be required in patients with large PEs who are haemodynamically unstable.
- **Thrombolysis (systemic)**: This should be considered in patients with large PEs with right ventricular dysfunction who are haemodynamically unstable.
- **Endovascular interventions**: In some specialist centres, patients with large PEs are occasionally managed with catheter-directed thrombolysis or percutaneous mechanical thrombectomy.

CTPAs are often not performed 'out of hours.' Patients with suspected PEs and no significant bleeding risk should still receive treatment dose heparin/LMWH while awaiting CTPA.

Haemodynamically Unstable Patients

- Require circulatory support
- May need thrombolysis
- Call for senior help early

Prescribe (see Fig. 3.11)

PE treatment:

- ENOXAPARIN 110 mg SC STAT or FONDAPARINUX 10 mg SC STAT

Analgesia:

- PARACETAMOL 1 g PO STAT

REASSESSMENT

- After commencing supplementary oxygen, the patient is reassessed.

'The airway is patient. RR 20/min, oxygen saturations are 96% on 4 L of nasal canula oxygen. HR 96 bpm, BP 138/78 mmHg. The lungs remain clear, the JVP is not raised and there are no murmurs.'

FURTHER MANAGEMENT

- **Heparin**: Once a PE is *confirmed*, the LMWH (or fondaparinux) can be switched to an oral anticoaugulant (such as apixaban) unless the intention is to continue longer-term anticoagulation with a vitamin K antagonist (e.g. warfarin sodium), in which case LMWH must continue until a therapeutic INR is established. This approach is much less common now unless the patient has active cancer (continued LMWH is also an option) or antiphospholipid syndrome.
- **Direct inhibitors of activated factor X (e.g. apixaban):** Direct oral anticoagulants are increasingly preferred over vitamin K antagonists for long-term anticoagulation because of their more rapid onset of action, convenience for patients and lack of requirement for regular monitoring. Anticoagulation will normally be given for at least 3 months, taking into account contraindications, comorbidities and the patient's preferences. After 3 months, an assessment of the benefits and risks of continuing, stopping or changing the anticoagulant should be made.
- **Mechanical interventions (e.g. inferior vena cava filter):** Such measures are occasionally considered if anticoagulation therapy is contraindicated or a pulmonary embolus has been confirmed in a patient who is already appropriately anticoagulated.

HANDING OVER THE PATIENT

'Mr Peters is a previously well 69-year-old man with a probable PE.

He presented with acute-onset dyspnoea and left-sided pleuritic chest pain following a long-haul flight. He was hypoxic on arrival with tachypnoea and mild tachycardia.

Initial investigations show ABG of PaO_2 7.0 kPa, $PaCO_2$ 3.8 kPa, H^+ 28 nmol/L (pH 7.55), HCO_3^- 25 mmol/L, BE 2.0 mmol/L on room air. Hb 185 g/L, WCC 11.0 × 10^9/L. Urea 9.3 mmol/L, creatinine 60 µmol/L, normal clotting. CXR is normal. ECG shows sinus tachycardia.

Revised Geneva Score is 8 (age, haemoptysis, heart rate) and his D-dimer was positive. He is awaiting CTPA, but this will not be performed until the morning. His current treatment is supplementary oxygen, simple analgesia and enoxaparin. He has not required any circulatory support.

The plan is to transfer to the ward, continue with enoxaparin and supplementary oxygen to maintain oxygen saturations >94%. If a PE is confirmed, he will be prescribed apixaban for three months. Please monitor for any deterioration as thrombolysis may be considered.'

Heparin/LMWH will not dissolve emboli—it is used to prevent emboli increasing in size and prevent further emboli forming. If the patient deteriorates, they may need thrombolysis.

FURTHER READING

CKS summary (May 2024). https://cks.nice.org.uk/topics/chronic-obstructive-pulmonary-disease/management/acute-exacerbation/.

National Institute for Health and Care Excellence (NICE). Asthma: diagnosis, monitoring and chronic asthma management. NICE guideline [NG80]. Published: 29 November 2017. Last updated: 22 March 2021. https://www.nice.org.uk/guidance/ng80 (Last accessed 28.12.23).

National Institute for Health and Care Excellence (NICE). Chronic obstructive pulmonary disease in over 16s: diagnosis and management. Clinical guideline [NG115]. Published: 5 December 2018. Updated: 26 July 2019. https://www.nice.org.uk/guidance/ng115 (Last accessed 28.12.23).

National Institute for Health and Care Excellence (NICE). Pneumonia in adults: diagnosis and management. Clinical guideline [CG191]. Published: 03 December 2014. Last updated: 31 October 2023. https://www.nice.org.uk/guidance/cg191 (Last accessed 28.12.23).

National Institute for Health and Care Excellence (NICE). Pneumonia (hospital-acquired): antimicrobial prescribing. NICE guideline [NG139]. Published: 16 September 2019. https://www.nice.org.uk/guidance/ng139 (Last accessed 28.12.23).

National Institute for Health and Care Excellence (NICE). Venous thromboembolic diseases: diagnosis, management and thrombophilia testing. NICE guideline [NG158]. Updated: 2 August 2023. https://www.nice.org.uk/guidance/ng158 (Last accessed 28.12.23).

National Institute for Health and Care Excellence (NICE). Asthma: Scenario: Acute exacerbation of asthma. Clinical guideline. Last revised: July 2024. https://cks.nice.org.uk/topics/asthma/management/acute-exacerbation-of-asthma/ (Last accessed 26.11.24).

PRESCRIPTION CHARTS

PRESCRIPTION AND ADMINISTRATION RECORD

Standard Chart

Hospital/Ward: WGH WARD 4 **Consultant:** DR ROY	**Name of Patient:** RUSSELL CANNON
Weight: 65 kg **Height:** 1.6 m	**Hospital Number:** 2103014532
If re-written, date:	**D.O.B.:** 21/03/01
DISCHARGE PRESCRIPTION **Date completed:-** **Completed by:-**	

OTHER MEDICINE CHARTS IN USE		PREVIOUS ADVERSE REACTIONS This section must be completed before any medicine is given		Completed by (sign & print)	Date
Date	Type of Chart	None known ☒		E. Smith E. SMITH	22/10/24
		Medicine/Agent	Description of Reaction		

CODES FOR NON-ADMINISTRATION OF PRESCRIBED MEDICINE

If a dose is not administered as prescribed, initial and enter a code in the column with a circle drawn round the code according to the reason as shown below. **Inform the responsible doctor in the appropriate timescale.**

1. Patient refuses
2. Patient not present
3. Medicines not available – CHECK ORDERED
4. Asleep/drowsy
5. Administration route not available – CHECK FOR ALTERNATIVE
6. Vomiting/nausea
7. Time varied on doctor's instructions
8. Once only/as required medicine given
9. Dose withheld on doctor's instructions
10. Possible adverse reaction/side effect

ONCE-ONLY

Date	Time	Medicine (Approved Name)	Dose	Route	Prescriber – Sign + Print	Time Given	Given By
22/10/24	17.00	SALBUTAMOL (driven with oxygen)	5 mg	NEB	E. Smith E. SMITH	17.10	YP
22/10/24	17.00	PREDNISOLONE	40 mg	ORAL	E. Smith E. SMITH	17.10	YP
22/10/24	17.10	IPRATROPIUM BROMIDE (driven with oxygen)	500 micrograms	NEB	E. Smith E. SMITH	17.20	YP
22/10/24	17.10	SALBUTAMOL (driven with oxygen)	5 mg	NEB	E. Smith E. SMITH	17.20	YP

OXYGEN	Start Date	Start Time	Route Mask (%)	Route Prongs (L/min)	Prescriber – Sign + Print	Administered by	Stop Date	Stop Time
	22/10/24	17.00	NON-REBREATHER MASK (15 L/min)		E. Smith E. SMITH	YP	22/10/24	20.10
	22/10/24	20.10		2 L/min via NASAL CANNULAE	E. Smith E. SMITH	YP		

Fig. 3.1 Prescription and administration record (standard chart) for Russell Cannon.

Name: RUSSELL CANNON
Date of Birth: 21/03/01

REGULAR THERAPY

PRESCRIPTION	Date → Time ↓		22/10/24	23/10/24										
Medicine (Approved Name) SALBUTAMOL	6													
Dose 5mg; **Route** NEB	8													
	12													
Notes Review at 01.00 23/10/24. Driven with oxygen or air.; **Start Date** 22/10/24	14	(19)	FG											
	18	(21)	FG											
Prescriber – sign + print E. Smith E. SMITH	22	(23)	FG											
Medicine (Approved Name) IPRATROPIUM BROMIDE	(6)													
Dose 500 micrograms; **Route** NEB	8													
	(12)													
Notes Driven with oxygen or air.; **Start Date** 22/10/24	14													
	(18)		x											
Prescriber – sign + print E. Smith E. SMITH	22	(24)	FG											
Medicine (Approved Name) PREDNISOLONE	6													
Dose 40mg; **Route** ORAL	(8)		x											
	12													
Notes For 5/7. Stop on 27/10/24; **Start Date** 22/10/24	14													
	18													
Prescriber – sign + print E. Smith E. SMITH	22													
Medicine (Approved Name) FONDAPARINUX	6													
Dose 2.5mg; **Route** SC	8													
	12													
Notes; **Start Date** 22/10/24	14													
	(18)		FG											
Prescriber – sign + print E. Smith E. SMITH	22													
Medicine (Approved Name)	6													
Dose; **Route**	8													
	12													
Notes; **Start Date**	14													
	18													
Prescriber – sign + print	22													
Medicine (Approved Name)	6													
Dose; **Route**	8													
	12													
Notes; **Start Date**	14													
	18													
Prescriber – sign + print	22													

Fig. 3.2 **Prescription and administration record (regular therapy) for Russell Cannon.**

PRESCRIPTION AND ADMINISTRATION RECORD

Standard Chart

Hospital/Ward: WGH WARD 4 **Consultant:** DR JONES	**Name of Patient:** MARY JOHNSON
Weight: 78 kg **Height:** 1.55 m	**Hospital Number:** 1309576374
If re-written, date:	**D.O.B.:** 13/09/1957
DISCHARGE PRESCRIPTION **Date completed:-** **Completed by:-**	

OTHER MEDICINE CHARTS IN USE		PREVIOUS ADVERSE REACTIONS This section must be completed before any medicine is given		Completed by (sign & print)	Date
Date	Type of Chart	None known ☒		L. Manning LUCY MANNING	19/10/24
		Medicine/Agent	Description of Reaction		

CODES FOR NON-ADMINISTRATION OF PRESCRIBED MEDICINE

If a dose is not administered as prescribed, initial and enter a code in the column with a circle drawn round the code according to the reason as shown below. **Inform the responsible doctor in the appropriate timescale.**

1. Patient refuses
2. Patient not present
3. Medicines not available – CHECK ORDERED
4. Asleep/drowsy
5. Administration route not available – CHECK FOR ALTERNATIVE
6. Vomiting/nausea
7. Time varied on doctor's instructions
8. Once only/as required medicine given
9. Dose withheld on doctor's instructions
10. Possible adverse reaction/side effect

ONCE-ONLY

Date	Time	Medicine (Approved Name)	Dose	Route	Prescriber – Sign + Print	Time Given	Given By
19/10/24	14.30	SALBUTAMOL (driven with oxygen)	5 mg	NEB	L. Manning LUCY MANNING	14.35	AD
19/10/24	14.30	IPRATROPIUM BROMIDE (driven with oxygen)	500 micrograms	NEB	L. Manning LUCY MANNING	14.35	AD
19/10/24	15.00	PREDNISOLONE	30 mg	ORAL	L. Manning LUCY MANNING	15.10	AD
19/10/24	15.25	AMINOPHYLLINE (over at least 20 minutes)	250 mg	IV	L. Manning LUCY MANNING	15.30	AD

OXYGEN	Start Date	Start Time	Route Mask (%)	Route Prongs (L/min)	Prescriber – Sign + Print	Administered by	Stop Date	Stop Time
	19/10/24	14.30	VENTURI (60%) Repeat blood gas at 15.00		L. Manning LUCY MANNING	AD	19/10/24	15.25
	19/10/24	15.25	VENTURI (35%) Repeat blood gas at 16.00		L. Manning LUCY MANNING			

Fig. 3.3 Prescription and administration record (standard chart) for Mary Johnson.

Name: MARY JOHNSON

Date of Birth: 13/09/57

REGULAR THERAPY

PRESCRIPTION	Date → / Time ↓		19/10/24	20/10/24										
Medicine (Approved Name) SALBUTAMOL	6	(2)		FD										
Dose 5mg — **Route** NEB	8	(6)		FD										
Notes Review at 10.00 20/10/24. Driven with oxygen or air.	12	(10)												
Start Date 19/10/24	(14)													
Prescriber – sign + print L. Manning LUCY MANNING	(18)		FD											
	(22)		FD											
Medicine (Approved Name) IPRATROPIUM BROMIDE	(6)			FD										
Dose 500 micrograms — **Route** NEB	8													
Notes Driven with oxygen or air.	(12)			FD										
Start Date 19/10/24	14													
Prescriber – sign + print L. Manning LUCY MANNING	(18)		FD											
	22	(24)	FD											
Medicine (Approved Name) PREDNISOLONE	6													
Dose 30mg — **Route** ORAL	(8)		X	FD										
Notes For 7 days. Stop on 26/10/24	12													
Start Date 19/10/24	14													
Prescriber – sign + print L. Manning LUCY MANNING	18													
	22													
Medicine (Approved Name) FONDAPARINUX	6													
Dose 2.5mg — **Route** SC	8													
Notes	12													
Start Date 19/10/24	14													
Prescriber – sign + print L. Manning LUCY MANNING	(18)		FD											
	22													
Medicine (Approved Name)	6													
Dose — **Route**	8													
Notes	12													
Start Date	14													
Prescriber – sign + print	18													
	22													
Medicine (Approved Name)	6													
Dose — **Route**	8													
Notes	12													
Start Date	14													
Prescriber – sign + print	18													
	22													

Fig. 3.4 Prescription and administration record (regular therapy) for Mary Johnson.

PRESCRIPTION AND ADMINISTRATION RECORD

Standard Chart

Hospital/Ward: WGH WARD 4	Consultant: DR JONES	Name of Patient: WILLIAM TAYLOR
Weight: 72 kg	Height: 1.65 m	Hospital Number: 1610401289
If re-written, date:		D.O.B.: 16/10/1940
DISCHARGE PRESCRIPTION Date completed:-	Completed by:-	

OTHER MEDICINE CHARTS IN USE		PREVIOUS ADVERSE REACTIONS This section must be completed before any medicine is given		Completed by (sign & print)	Date
Date	Type of Chart	None known ☐			
		Medicine/Agent	Description of Reaction		
		TRIMETHOPRIM	RASH	L. Manning LUCY MANNING	19/10/24

CODES FOR NON-ADMINISTRATION OF PRESCRIBED MEDICINE

If a dose is not administered as prescribed, initial and enter a code in the column with a circle drawn round the code according to the reason as shown below. **Inform the responsible doctor in the appropriate timescale.**

1. Patient refuses
2. Patient not present
3. Medicines not available – CHECK ORDERED
4. Asleep/drowsy
5. Administration route not available – CHECK FOR ALTERNATIVE
6. Vomiting/nausea
7. Time varied on doctor's instructions
8. Once only/as required medicine given
9. Dose withheld on doctor's instructions
10. Possible adverse reaction/side effect

ONCE-ONLY

Date	Time	Medicine (Approved Name)	Dose	Route	Prescriber – Sign + Print	Time Given	Given By
19/10/24	15.10	CO-AMOXICLAV (1000 mg/200 mg)	1.2 g	IV	L. Manning LUCY MANNING	15.14	FR
19/10/24	15.10	CLARITHROMYCIN	500 mg	ORAL	L. Manning LUCY MANNING	15.14	FR
19/10/24	15.10	PARACETAMOL	1 g	ORAL	L. Manning LUCY MANNING	15.14	FR

OXYGEN	Start Date	Start Time	Route: Mask (%)	Route: Prongs (L/min)	Prescriber – Sign + Print	Administered by	Stop Date	Stop Time
	19/10/24	15.00	15 L/min (VIA NON REBREATHER MASK)		L. Manning LUCY MANNING	FR	19/10/24	17.30
	19/10/24	17.30		4 L/min VIA NASAL CANNULAE	L. Manning LUCY MANNING	FR		

Fig. 3.5 Prescription and administration record (standard chart) for William Taylor.

Name: WILLIAM TAYLOR
Date of Birth: 16/10/40

REGULAR THERAPY

PRESCRIPTION	Date → / Time ↓	19/10/24											
Medicine (Approved Name): PARACETAMOL	6												
Dose: 1g; Route: ORAL	(8)												
Notes: ; Start Date: 19/10/24	12												
Prescriber – sign + print: L. Manning LUCY MANNING	(14)												
	(18)	X											
	(22)	DF											
Medicine (Approved Name): CO-AMOXICLAV (1000 mg/200 mg)	6												
Dose: 1.2g; Route: IV	(8)												
Notes: Community acquired pneumonia. Review after 48H; Start Date: 19/10/24	12												
Prescriber – sign + print: L. Manning LUCY MANNING	(14)												
	18												
	(22)	DF											
Medicine (Approved Name): CLARITHROMYCIN	6												
Dose: 500 mg; Route: ORAL	(8)												
Notes: Community acquired pneumonia. Review after 48H; Start Date: 19/10/24	12												
Prescriber – sign + print: L. Manning LUCY MANNING	14												
	18												
	(22)	DF											
Medicine (Approved Name): DALTEPARIN	6												
Dose: 5000 units; Route: SC	8												
Notes: ; Start Date: 19/10/24	12												
Prescriber – sign + print: M. Fisher MARTIN FISHER	14												
	(18)	DF											
	22												
Medicine (Approved Name):	6												
Dose: ; Route:	8												
Notes: ; Start Date:	12												
Prescriber – sign + print:	14												
	18												
	22												
Medicine (Approved Name):	6												
Dose: ; Route:	8												
Notes: ; Start Date:	12												
Prescriber – sign + print:	14												
	18												
	22												

Fig. 3.6 Prescription and administration record (regular therapy) for William Taylor.

FLUID PRESCRIPTION CHART

Hospital/Ward: WGH WARD 4 **Consultant:** DR JONES

Weight: 72 kg **Height:** 1.65 m

Name of Patient: WILLIAM TAYLOR

Hospital Number: 1610401289

D.O.B: 16/10/1940

Date/ Time	FLUID	VOLUME	ROUTE	RATE	PRESCRIBER – SIGN AND PRINT
	ADDED DRUGS	DOSE			
19/10/24	SODIUM CHLORIDE 0.9%	500 mL			
17.30			IV	250 mL/h	L. Manning LUCY MANNING
19/10/24	SODIUM CHLORIDE 0.9%	500 mL			
21.30			IV	250 mL/h	L. Manning LUCY MANNING

Fig. 3.7 Fluid prescription chart for William Taylor.

PRESCRIPTION AND ADMINISTRATION RECORD

Standard Chart

Hospital/Ward: WGH ORTHO WARD **Consultant:** MR KAYE	**Name of Patient:** PATRICIA JACKSON
Weight: 64 kg **Height:** 1.4 m	**Hospital Number:** 2106442256
If re-written, date:	**D.O.B.:** 21/6/1944
DISCHARGE PRESCRIPTION **Date completed:-** **Completed by:-**	

OTHER MEDICINE CHARTS IN USE		PREVIOUS ADVERSE REACTIONS This section must be completed before any medicine is given		Completed by (sign & print)	Date
Date	Type of Chart	None known ☒		M. Fisher MARTIN FISHER	15/10/24
		Medicine/Agent	Description of Reaction		

CODES FOR NON-ADMINISTRATION OF PRESCRIBED MEDICINE

If a dose is not administered as prescribed, initial and enter a code in the column with a circle drawn round the code according to the reason as shown below. **Inform the responsible doctor in the appropriate timescale.**

1. Patient refuses
2. Patient not present
3. Medicines not available – CHECK ORDERED
4. Asleep/drowsy
5. Administration route not available – CHECK FOR ALTERNATIVE
6. Vomiting/nausea
7. Time varied on doctor's instructions
8. Once only/as required medicine given
9. Dose withheld on doctor's instructions
10. Possible adverse reaction/side effect

ONCE-ONLY

Date	Time	Medicine (Approved Name)	Dose	Route	Prescriber – Sign + Print	Time Given	Given By
19/10/24	14.00	CO-AMOXICLAV (1000 mg/200 mg)	1.2 g	IV	M. Fisher MARTIN FISHER	14.00	EM

OXYGEN	Start Date	Start Time	Route Mask (%)	Route Prongs (L/min)	Prescriber – Sign + Print	Administered by	Stop Date	Stop Time
	19/10/24	13.45		4 L/min via NASAL CANNULAE	M. Fisher MARTIN FISHER	EM		

Fig. 3.8 Prescription and administration record (standard chart) for Patricia Jackson.

Name: PATRICIA JACKSON
Date of Birth: 21/6/44

REGULAR THERAPY

PRESCRIPTION

Medicine (Approved Name)	Dose	Route	Notes	Start Date	Prescriber – sign + print
PARACETAMOL	1g	ORAL		15/10/24	M. Fisher MARTIN FISHER

Time		15/10/24	16/10/24	17/10/24	18/10/24	19/10/24							
6													
(8)			AS	GR	GR	GR							
12													
(14)		AS	AS	GR	GR	GR							
(18)		AS	AS	AS	GR	GR							
(22)		PF	PF	PF	PF	PF							

Medicine (Approved Name)	Dose	Route	Notes	Start Date	Prescriber – sign + print
OMEPRAZOLE	20mg	ORAL		15/10/24	M. Fisher MARTIN FISHER

Time		15/10/24	16/10/24	17/10/24	18/10/24	19/10/24							
6													
(8)			AS	GR	GR	GR							
12													
14													
18													
22													

Medicine (Approved Name)	Dose	Route	Notes	Start Date	Prescriber – sign + print
LISINOPRIL	10mg	ORAL		15/10/24	M. Fisher MARTIN FISHER

Time		15/10/24	16/10/24	17/10/24	18/10/24	19/10/24							
6													
(8)			AS	GR	GR	GR							
12													
14													
18													
22													

Stopped due to acute kidney injury 19/10/24
M. Fisher MARTIN FISHER

Medicine (Approved Name)	Dose	Route	Notes	Start Date	Prescriber – sign + print
FONDAPARINUX	2.5mg	SC		15/10/24	M. Fisher MARTIN FISHER

Time		15/10/24	16/10/24	17/10/24	18/10/24	19/10/24							
6													
8													
12													
14													
(18)		AS	AS	AS	GR	GR							
22													

Medicine (Approved Name)	Dose	Route	Notes	Start Date	Prescriber – sign + print
CO AMOXICLAV (1000mg/200mg)	1.2g	IV	Hospital acquired pneumonia review after 48h	19/10/24	M. Fisher MARTIN FISHER

Time		15/10/24	16/10/24	17/10/24	18/10/24	19/10/24							
6													
(8)													
12													
(14)						X							
18													
(22)						GR							

Medicine (Approved Name)	Dose	Route	Notes	Start Date	Prescriber – sign + print

Time													
6													
8													
12													
14													
18													
22													

Fig. 3.9 Prescription and administration record (regular therapy) for Patricia Jackson.

FLUID PRESCRIPTION CHART

Hospital/Ward: WGH ORTHO WARD	**Consultant:** MR KAYE	**Name of Patient:** PATRICIA JACKSON **Hospital Number:** 2106442256
Weight: 64 kg	**Height:** 1.4 m	**D.O.B:** 21/06/1944

Date/ Time	FLUID / ADDED DRUGS	VOLUME / DOSE	ROUTE	RATE	PRESCRIBER – SIGN AND PRINT
19/10/24 14.00	SODIUM CHLORIDE 0.9%	500 mL	IV	Over 15 min	M. Fisher MARTIN FISHER
19/10/24 15.00	SODIUM CHLORIDE 0.9%	500 mL	IV	125 mL/h	M. Fisher MARTIN FISHER

Fig. 3.10 Fluid prescription chart for Patricia Jackson.

PRESCRIPTION AND ADMINISTRATION RECORD

Standard Chart

Hospital/Ward: WGH MAU	**Consultant:** DR JONES	**Name of Patient:** STEVEN PETERS
Weight: 110 kg	**Height:** 1.78 m	**Hospital Number:** 0210556647
If re-written, date:		**D.O.B.:** 2/10/1955
DISCHARGE PRESCRIPTION **Date completed:-**	**Completed by:-**	

OTHER MEDICINE CHARTS IN USE		**PREVIOUS ADVERSE REACTIONS** This section must be completed before any medicine is given		Completed by (sign & print)	Date
Date	Type of Chart	None known ☒		P. Gibson PETER GIBSON	18/10/24
		Medicine/Agent	Description of Reaction		

CODES FOR NON-ADMINISTRATION OF PRESCRIBED MEDICINE

If a dose is not administered as prescribed, initial and enter a code in the column with a circle drawn round the code according to the reason as shown below. **Inform the responsible doctor in the appropriate timescale.**

1. Patient refuses
2. Patient not present
3. Medicines not available – CHECK ORDERED
4. Asleep/drowsy
5. Administration route not available – CHECK FOR ALTERNATIVE
6. Vomiting/nausea
7. Time varied on doctor's instructions
8. Once only/as required medicine given
9. Dose withheld on doctor's instructions
10. Possible adverse reaction/side effect

ONCE-ONLY

Date	Time	Medicine (Approved Name)	Dose	Route	Prescriber – Sign + Print	Time Given	Given By
18/10/24	20.00	PARACETAMOL	1g	ORAL	P. Gibson PETER GIBSON	20.05	DF
18/10/24	20.45	FONDAPARINUX	10mg	SC	P. Gibson PETER GIBSON	20.50	DF

OXYGEN	Start		Route		Prescriber – Sign + Print	Administered by	Stop	
	Date	Time	Mask (%)	Prongs (L/min)			Date	Time
	18/10/24	20.00		4L/min via NASAL CANNULAE	P. Gibson PETER GIBSON	DF		

Fig. 3.11 Prescription and administration record (standard chart) for Steven Peters.

Gastroenterology

4

Ali B.A.K. Al-Hadithi

Chapter Outline

Station 4.1: Severe Ulcerative Colitis
Station 4.2: Spontaneous Bacterial Peritonitis
Station 4.3: Paracetamol Overdose
Station 4.4: Abdominal Sepsis
Station 4.5: Acute Upper GI Bleed

STATION 4.1: SEVERE ULCERATIVE COLITIS

You are the junior doctor covering the medical assessment unit overnight. You are to see a 27-year-old man (John Smith, 12/08/97) who has been admitted with a 48-hour history of bloody diarrhoea (>10 stools a day). You are told he has a previous diagnosis of ulcerative colitis (UC), normally well controlled with sulfasalazine.

Patient Details

Name:	John Smith
DOB:	12/08/97
Hospital number:	1208970076
Weight:	72 kg
Height:	1.7 m
Consultant:	Dr Cox
Hospital/Ward:	WGH Ward 3
Current medications:	Sulfasalazine 500 mg PO QDS
Allergies:	Penicillin (rash)
Admission date:	12/11/24

Initial Differential Diagnosis

- Flare up of UC
- Infective colitis (bacterial, viral, e.g. CMV)
- Ischaemic colitis
- Angiodysplasia, bleeding vessel

Complications of Severe Ulcerative Colitis

- Toxic megacolon
- Perforation
- Sepsis

INITIAL ASSESSMENT

AIRWAY

- Assess patency of the airway. The patient may have also been vomiting and is at risk of aspirating. A quick way to assess the airway is to see whether the patient can speak back to you.

'The patient is speaking back to you in full sentences. He denies any episodes of vomiting.'

You are satisfied that the airway is patent.

BREATHING

- Assess the respiratory rate and oxygen saturations. A dehydrated, shocked patient may have an increased respiratory rate while trying to compensate for a presumed metabolic acidosis.
- Perform a respiratory examination looking for evidence of aspiration.

'The patient is visibly tachypnoeic with a respiratory rate of 24/min. On examination, his chest is clear with vesicular breath sounds and good air entry bilaterally. Oxygen saturations are 98% on air, so supplementary oxygen is not required.'

You are satisfied that there is no evidence of an aspiration pneumonia. However, you will still order a chest radiography (CXR) (to rule out perforation), as well as performing an arterial blood gas (ABG), which has already been sent for processing. Oxygen saturations are 98% on air.

Acute Severe Colitis Is Best Defined by the Truelove and Witts' Criteria

- ≥6 stools/day
- HR >90 bpm
- T >37.5°C
- Hb <105 g/L
- ESR >30 mm/h

CIRCULATION

- Perform a cardiovascular (CVS) examination. Cool peripheries, delayed capillary refill time (CRT), tachycardia, a weak central pulse, dry mucous membranes and nonvisible jugular venous pressure (JVP) are all signs of hypovolaemia.

- Assess fluid balance by measuring pulse (rate, rhythm and character), BP, CRT, JVP and urine output (if being recorded). This patient is likely to be hypovolaemic given his history of diarrhoea. Tachycardia in a young patient is of concern despite a normal BP due to their ability to still maintain a normal BP in the initial stages of shock.

'On examination the patient is tachycardic with a raised CRT. He is cool peripherally and has a weak brachial pulse. JVP is not visible and his mucous membranes are dry. Heart rate is 108 bpm and BP is 108/76 mmHg. He denies any chest pain and, on ausculation, heart sounds are normal with no added sounds.'

Following this assessment, you establish intravenous (IV) access and send off urgent bloods. You also perform an ECG. You start a urine chart, measuring hourly urine output.

 Prescribe (Figs 4.1–4.3)

Fluid bolus:
- SODIUM CHLORIDE 0.9% 500 mL (over 15 minutes)

DISABILITY

- Assess the patient's conscious level, either using AVPU (is the patient Alert? If not, do they respond to Verbal or Painful stimuli? Or are they Unresponsive?) or Glasgow Coma Scale (GCS).
- Check blood glucose levels.

'Glucose level is 5.8 mmol/L and he is alert although visibly tired.'

EXPOSURE

- Expose the patient and look for further evidence of bloody diarrhoea. Examine the abdomen for any tenderness or masses. Listen for bowel sounds. Look at the calves and examine for tenderness (UC, alongside hypovolaemia are risk factors for a deep vein thrombosis (DVT)).

'There is no obvious bleeding and no calf tenderness. Abdomen is soft but generally tender, with hyperactive bowel sounds on auscultation. There is no organomegaly or signs of peritonism. Temperature is 37.9°C.'

INITIAL INVESTIGATIONS

- **ABG:** Important to assess patient acid–base status. Look out for evidence of a metabolic acidosis. A lactate of >2.5 suggests significant tissue hypoperfusion.
- **CXR:** To rule out possible aspiration. Ensure you look under the diaphragm for free air, a radiological sign of perforation.
- **Abdominal radiograph (AXR):** Urgent investigation to rule out the presence of toxic megacolon, which is a surgical emergency. Consider a need for daily AXR, especially if there are signs of colonic distension and/or there is significant deterioration in clinical condition/blood parameters.
- **Electrocardiogram (ECG):** Diarrhoea and vomiting may lead to dangerous electrolyte imbalances, which may in turn predispose the individual to potentially fatal arrhythmias.
- **Bloods:** Full blood count (FBC), clotting, urea and electrolytes (U&Es), liver function tests (LFTs), glucose, C-reactive protein (CRP), erythrocyte sedimentation rate (ESR), blood cultures, group and save. Look for evidence of infection, assess renal function and possible electrolyte abnormalities. Ensure blood cultures are taken. Group and save is vital as the patient may require early surgical intervention. Daily bloods are required in severe UC (Table 4.1).
- **Stool samples:** Stool culture and *Clostridium difficile* assay on at least three stool samples to detect 90% of cases. Cytomegalovirus (CMV) should be considered in severe or refractory colitis. Results should not delay the administration of corticosteroid treatment.
- **Flexible sigmoidoscopy:** Flexible sigmoidoscopy and biopsy should be requested and available within 72 hours (ideally 24 hours) and a histological diagnosis within 5 days to confirm diagnosis and exclude CMV.
- **Urine dipstick:** To look for possible evidence of a urinary tract infection (UTI) (with abdominal pain) and for evidence of bleeding elsewhere (in urine).

'Blood tests: Hb 110 g/L, WCC 14 × 10^9/L, CRP 120 mg/L with normal clotting, glucose, liver and renal function. ABG: PaO_2 14 kPa, $PaCO_2$ 3.2 kPa, HCO_3 19 mmol/L, lactate 2.7 mmol/L, pH 7.3 (metabolic acidosis with partial respiratory compensation). AXR: distal faecal loading, featureless descending colon consistent with colitis and no evidence of toxic megacolon. Urine dipstick: positive for ketones (+).'

INITIAL MANAGEMENT

 Management of Severe Ulcerative Colitis

- Resuscitate using an ABCDE approach
- Fluids
- Corticosteroids
- Early specialist input including consideration of need for surgery

- **Withdraw agents that may precipitate colonic dilatation:** Anticholinergics, antidiarrhoeal agents, non-steroidal antiinflammatory drugs (NSAIDs) and opioid drugs increase the risk of precipitating colonic dilatation.
- **IV fluids:** IV fluid and electrolyte replacement to correct and prevent dehydration or electrolyte imbalance.
- **Isolation:** Keep patient isolated until it is clear that the diarrhoea is noninfective in nature.

Table 4.1 Mr Smith's Blood Results

PARAMETER	VALUE	NORMAL RANGE (UNITS)
WCC	**14 × 10^9/L**	**4–11 (×10^9/L)**
Neutrophil	6 × 10^9/L	2–7.5 (×10^9/L)
Lymphocyte	3 × 10^9/L	1.4–4 (×10^9/L)
Platelet	220 × 10^9/L	150–400 (×10^9/L)
Haemoglobin	**110 g/L**	**Men: 135–180 (g/L) Women: 115–160 (g/L)**
CRP	**120 mg/L**	**0–5 (mg/L)**
Urea	6.4 mmol/L	2.5–6.7 (mmol/L)
Creatinine	90 μmol/L	79–118 (μmol/L)
eGFR	>60 mL/min	>60 (mL/min)
Sodium	138 mmol/L	135–146 (mmol/L)
Potassium	3.8 mmol/L	3.5–5.0 (mmol/L)
Lactate	**2.7 mmol/L**	**0.6–2.4 (mmol/L)**
Bilirubin	8 μmol/L	<17 (μmol/L)
ALT	20 IU/L	<40 (IU/L)
ALP	55 IU/L	39–117 (IU/L)
Albumin	40 g/L	35–50 (g/L)
Glucose	5 mmol/L	4.5–5.6 (mmol/L) (fasting)
PT	12 seconds	11.5–13.5 seconds
APTT	30 seconds	26–37 seconds
pH	**7.3**	**7.35–7.45**
PaO_2	14 kPa	10.6–13.3 (kPa) on air
$PaCO_2$	**3.2 kPa**	**4.8–6.1 (kPa)**
HCO_3	**19 mmol/L**	**22–26 (mmol/L)**

Data in bold signifies results that are outside the normal laboratory range.
ALP, Alkaline phosphatase; *ALT,* alanine transaminase; *APTT,* activated partial thromboplastin time; *CRP,* C-reactive protein; *eGFR,* estimated glomerular filtration rate; *PT,* prothrombin time; *WCC,* white cell count.

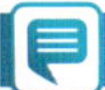

Prescribe (see Figs 4.1–4.3)

Further fluids (depending on response):
- 0.9% SODIUM CHLORIDE 500 mL (over 15 minutes)

REASSESSMENT

'Following IV fluid resuscitation, the patient is maintaining his airway and talking comfortably in full sentences. He is apyrexial, his respiratory rate is 18/min, heart rate 95 bpm and BP 130/74 mmHg. The patient looks more comfortable and settled.'

FURTHER MANAGEMENT

- **IV corticosteroids:** Either hydrocortisone 100 mg four times a day or methylprednisolone 60 mg/day. IV corticosteroids are generally given for up to 5 days. Consider giving a proton pump inhibitor (PPI) for gastric protection.
- **IV antibiotics:** Only if infection is considered or immediately prior to surgery.
- **Subcutaneous LMWH:** To reduce the risk of thromboembolism.
- **Bone protection:** Current guidelines recommend the use of calcium and vitamin D (e.g. Adcal D3 one tablet BD or Calcichew D3 Forte one tablet BD) during chronic corticosteroid use.
- **Stool chart:** To record number and character of bowel movements, including the presence or absence of blood and liquid versus solid stool.
- **Toxic megacolon:** If there is evidence of toxic megacolon (diameter >5.5 cm or caecum >9 cm), organise an urgent surgical review.
- **Surgical input:** A stool frequency of >8/day or CRP >45 mg/L at 3 days appears to predict the need for surgery in 85% of cases. Surgical review and input from specialist colorectal nurse or stoma therapist are appropriate at this stage.
- **Early specialist input:** Patients admitted with known or suspected inflammatory bowel disease (IBD) should be discussed with (and normally transferred to the care of) a consultant gastroenterologist or colorectal surgeon within 24 hours of admission. Joint surgical and medical management is appropriate.
- **Disease modifying agents:** Consider use of disease-modifying agents such as infliximab or cyclosporin in severe cases that fail to respond to treatment with systemic corticosteroids.

Prescribe (see Figs 4.1–4.3)

Corticosteroids:
- HYDROCORTISONE 100 mg IV STAT then 100 mg IV QDS

Thromboprophylaxis:
- DALTEPARIN 5000 units SC OD

Bone protection:
- ADCAL D3 1 tablet PO BD

Patient's regular aminosalicylate prescription:
- SULFASALAZINE 500 mg PO QDS

HANDING OVER THE PATIENT

'This is a 27-year-old patient presenting with a severe exacerbation of ulcerative colitis.

He presented with a 2-day history of bloody diarrhoea on a background of a known diagnosis of ulcerative colitis, normally well controlled with aminosalicylate treatment.

On initial assessment, the patient was significantly dehydrated with a HR 108 bpm and BP 108/76 mmHg. The abdomen was soft with generalised tenderness but no peritonism. An abdominal film shows no evidence of toxic megacolon. Routine bloods demonstrate raised inflammatory markers and a slight reduced Hb at 110 g/L, probably partly related to chronic disease and partly due to acute bleeding.

The patient showed good response to IV fluid resuscitation. The current plan is commencing maintenance IV fluids, IV corticosteroid treatment, daily blood tests, sending four stool samples to exclude infective colitis and urgent referral to gastroenterology.'

STATION 4.2: SPONTANEOUS BACTERIAL PERITONITIS

You are the junior doctor covering the medical assessment unit. You are called to see a 72-year-old man (Andrew Reddy, 12/08/52) with known alcoholic liver cirrhosis who presents with mild abdominal pain and confusion. You recognise him immediately as you also work on the gastroenterology ward where this patient attends every few weeks for therapeutic paracentesis.

Patient Details

Name:	Andrew Reddy
DOB:	12/08/52
Hospital number:	1208520060
Weight:	70 kg
Height:	1.76 m
Consultant:	Dr Bing
Hospital/Ward:	WGH Ward 4
Current medications:	Thiamine 100 mg PO TDS (for malnutrition), furosemide 40 mg PO OD and spironolactone 100 mg PO OD (for ascites)
Allergies:	No known drug allergies
Admission date:	12/11/24

Initial Differential Diagnosis

- Infection (SBP, lower respiratory tract infection, UTI)
- Constipation
- Hepatocellular carcinoma
- Wernicke's encephalopathy
- Alcohol intoxication
- Alcoholic hepatitis
- Upper gastrointestinal bleed

Complications of Chronic Liver Disease

Portal hypertension:
- Ascites
- Hypersplenism
- Varices

Synthetic dysfunction:
- Hypoalbuminaemia
- Coagulopathy

Hepatopulmonary syndrome
Hepatorenal syndrome
Encephalopathy
Hepatocellular carcinoma

Management of Chronic Liver Disease

- Resuscitate using an ABCDE approach
- Diagnostic paracentesis
- Albumin infusion
- IV antibiotics

INITIAL ASSESSMENT

AIRWAY

- Assess patency of the airway.

'The patient is drowsy but speaks in full sentences and rousable.'

Secure the airway if necessary. Encephalopathic patients are often drowsy, confused, and risk of aspiration is very high. You are satisfied that the airway is safe and proceed to assess breathing.

BREATHING

- Assess the respiratory rate and oxygen saturations.
- Give supplementary oxygen to maintain oxygen saturations >94%.
- Perform a respiratory examination, listening for basal crepitations which may suggest a lower respiratory tract infection. This patient is at risk of community-acquired pneumonia, hospital-acquired pneumonia (recurrent admissions) and aspiration pneumonia.
- Request a CXR.

'Saturations are 92% on 1 L/min supplemental oxygen with a respiratory rate of 22/min. Percussion reveals dull bases, and on auscultation, there is reduced air entry bilaterally. Portable CXR confirms small bilateral pleural effusions.'

Bilateral pleural effusions may be secondary to hypoalbuminaemia or congestive heart failure. No obvious consolidation is visible. You administer 2 L/min of oxygen to maintain saturations >94% and proceed to assess circulation.

CIRCULATION

- Assess haemodynamic stability by feeling the pulse, measuring capillary refill, looking at the JVP and measuring BP and urine output.
- Perform a full CVS examination.
- Obtain IV access and take bloods.
- Perform ABG if unwell to assess both oxygenation and his metabolic status.
- Perform an ECG.

'The patient is slightly tachycardic (95 bpm), with a normal BP (120/75 mmHg). ECG shows sinus tachycardia. His JVP is not visible. However, on examination, he has obvious abdominal distension and bilateral pitting oedema to the knees.'

This patient appears to be fluid overloaded but mildly intravascularly depleted. You prescribe IV fluids (human albumin solution or gelofusine) and go on to assess disability.

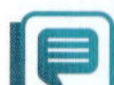

Prescribe (Figs **4.4–4.6**)

Oxygen:
- 2 L/min via NASAL CANNULAE

Fluids:
- HUMAN ALBUMIN SOLUTION 20% 500 mL IV 83 mL/h

DISABILITY

- Assess the patient's conscious level, either using AVPU (is the patient Alert? If not, do they respond to Verbal or Painful stimuli? Or are they Unresponsive?) or GCS. Check blood glucose.

'The patient is rousable on voice. Blood glucose is 5.8 mmol/L.'

EXPOSURE

- Expose the patient and perform a full examination focusing on signs of chronic liver disease (spider naevi, Dupuytren's contracture, loss of secondary hair, gynaecomastia) and any obvious precipitating factors of decompensated disease (haemorrhage, sepsis). Assess for evidence of decompensated liver disease (ascites, jaundice, encephalopathy, hepatic flap). Look for evidence of an upper gastrointestinal (GI)/variceal bleed (digital rectal examination). Examine the abdomen looking for obvious ascites (shifting dullness) or signs suggestive of peritonism (tender, rigid abdomen, guarding).

'There are >10 spider naevi in the SVC distribution with loss of secondary hair and gynaecomastia. The patient is jaundiced. The patient is holding his abdomen in some distress but there are no signs of peritonism. Abdominal distension with positive shifting dullness is in keeping with ascites.'

You request the nurse to prepare a trolley for an urgent ascitic tap to rule out spontaneous bacterial peritonitis (SBP) while you attempt to find an ultrasound machine.

INITIAL INVESTIGATIONS

A diagnostic paracentesis should be performed in all cirrhotic patients with ascites, in those who have signs and symptoms of peritoneal infection, including the development of encephalopathy, renal impairment or peripheral leucocytosis without a precipitating factor.

- **Bloods:** FBC, U&Es, LFT, clotting screen, CRP, lactate. Patients with alcoholic liver disease are almost invariably thrombocytopaenic; however, ensure that the platelet count is stable and at least in double figures. Haemoglobin may be low due to anaemia of chronic disease. Liver failure and renal failure are both associated with a low sodium(Table 4.2).
- **ABG:** Allows assessment of the patient's metabolic state as well as ventilation/oxygenation. You may find a metabolic acidosis secondary to sepsis.
- **CXR:** Look for evidence of a lower respiratory tract infection precipitating the patient's decompensated liver disease. Evidence of an aspiration pneumonia secondary to encephalopathy may also exist.

Table 4.2 Mr Reddy's Blood Results

PARAMETER	VALUE	NORMAL RANGE (UNITS)
Hb	**104 g/L**	**Men: 135–180 (g/L) Women: 115–160 (g/L)**
WCC	**16 × 10^9/L**	**4–11 (×10^9/L)**
Neutrophil	**12 × 10^9/L**	**2–7.5 (×10^9/L)**
Lymphocyte	2.7 × 10^9/L	1.4–4 (×10^9/L)
Platelet	**95 × 10^9/L**	**150–400 (×10^9/L)**
CRP	**170 mg/L**	**0–5 (mg/L)**
Urea	6.4 mmol/L	2.5–6.7 (mmol/L)
Creatinine	90 μmol/L	79–118 (μmol/L)
eGFR	>60 mL/min	>60 (mL/min)
Sodium	**128 mmol/L**	**135–146 (mmol/L)**
Potassium	3.6 mmol/L	3.5–5.0 (mmol/L)
Lactate	**2.7 mmol/L**	**0.6–2.4 (mmol/L)**
Bilirubin	**60 μmol/L**	**<17 (μmol/L)**
ALT	**140 IU/L**	**<40 (IU/L)**
ALP	**180 IU/L**	**39–117 (IU/L)**
PT	12 seconds	11.5–13.5 seconds
APTT	30 seconds	26–37 seconds
pH	**7.3**	**7.35–7.45**
PaO_2	13 kPa	10.6–13.3 (kPa) on air
$PaCO_2$	5 kPa	4.8–6.1 (kPa)
HCO_3	**19 mmol/L**	**22–26 (mmol/L)**

Data in bold signifies results that are outside the normal laboratory range. *ALP*, Alkaline phosphatase; *ALT*, alanine transaminase; *APTT*, activated partial thromboplastin time; *CRP*, C-reactive protein; *eGFR*, estimated glomerular filtration rate; *PT*, prothrombin time; *WCC*, white cell count.

- **ECG:** Look for evidence of myocardial ischaemia or arrhythmias from electrolyte imbalances or an acute bleed.
- **Urine dipstick and culture:** Performed as part of septic screen.
- **Diagnostic paracentesis:** Mandatory in all patients with cirrhosis requiring hospital admission as part of a general septic screen. It should further be performed in all cirrhotic patients with ascites who have signs and symptoms of peritoneal infection, including the development of encephalopathy, renal impairment or peripheral leucocytosis without a precipitating factor. Ascitic fluid should be inoculated into blood culture bottles at the bedside. If the neutrophil count is >250 cells/mm^3, treat for SBP.

'Hb 104 g/L, WCC 16 × 10^9/L, platelets 95 × 10^9/L, bilirubin 60 μmol/L, ALT 140 IU/L, ALP 180 IU/L, Na 128 mmol/L, K 3.6 mmol/L, urea 6.4 mmol/L, creatinine 90 μmol/L, CRP 170 mg/L and lactate 2.7 mmol/L. Clotting is normal. Blood gas shows a metabolic acidosis with a pH 7.3, a bicarbonate of 19 mmol/L and $PaCO_2$ of 5 kPa. You are bleeped from the microbiology lab with the ascitic fluid results: neutrophil count >250 cells/mm^3.'

INITIAL MANAGEMENT

- **Oxygen:** Maintain saturations >94%.
- **IV access:** Large-bore cannulae preferred in patients with chronic liver disease and evidence of portal hypertension as they are at increased risk of having a life-threatening upper GI bleed.
- **IV antibiotics:** When the neutrophil count is >250 cells/mm^3 in ascitic fluid, patients should be treated for SBP as per local microbiology guidelines. Third-generation cephalosporins such as cefotaxime have been most extensively studied in the treatment of SBP and have been shown to be effective. Five days of treatment with cefotaxime is as effective as 10 days of therapy. Recently, tazobactam/piperacillin has also been used for the treatment of SBP. Resolution of infection in SBP is associated with an improvement in symptoms and signs. A reduction in ascitic fluid neutrophil count of less than 25% of the pretreatment value after 2 days of antibiotic treatment suggests failure to respond to therapy, and should raise the suspicion of 'secondary peritonitis' (secondary to perforation or inflammation of intraabdominal organs). An erect CXR and abdominal computed tomography (CT) scan are the most useful in practice.
- **Pabrinex IV High Potency Injection:** Urgent vitamin replacement (vitamins B_1, B_2, B_3, B_6, C) should be provided in suspected malnutrition and Wernicke's encephalopathy.
- **Lactulose:** May reduce risk of hepatic encephalopathy by reducing ammonia production in the gut as well as improving concomitant constipation.
- **Albumin infusion:** 30% of patients with SBP develop renal impairment. Consider giving an infusion of 1.5 g albumin/kg (equates to 1.5 × 70 = 105 g. 500 mL of Human albumin solution 20% contains 100 g of albumin) in the first 6 hours, followed by 1 g/kg on day 3, although this is a contentious area.
- **Thromboprophylaxis:** Important to consider this in all medical admissions: check renal function and clotting first.

Prescribe (see Figs **4.4–4.6**)

Antibiotics:

- TAZOBACTAM/PIPERACILLIN 4.5 G IV (over 30 minutes) STAT then TDS

Vitamin replacement:

- PABRINEX (HIGH POTENCY) Ampoules 1 and 2 IV (over 30 minutes) STAT then TDS

Thromboprophylaxis:

- DALTEPARIN 5000 units SC OD

Lactulose:

- 30 mL (20 mg) PO TDS

WITHHOLD

Furosemide and spironolactone

Thiamine (since vitamin replacement being given intravenously)

REASSESSMENT

'The patient has responded to antibiotics and is now apyrexial. Heart rate is 90 bpm and BP is still normal. Patient is more rousable and now opening eyes spontaneously.'

HANDING OVER THE PATIENT

'This is a 72-year-old patient with a background of chronic liver disease presenting with decompensated disease secondary to SBP.

He presented with a 3-day history of confusion, abdominal distension and fevers. On examination, he was jaundiced, had a coarse flapping tremor and was clinically dehydrated (tachycardic, weak pulse, dry mucous membranes, JVP not visible). However, he also had evidence of fluid overload in his extravascular space (ascites, pleural effusions, pitting oedema). Abdominal examination demonstrated ascites, and generalised tenderness but no signs of peritonism.

Observations were as follows: HR 90 bpm, BP 120/80 mmHg, RR 22/min, saturations 95% on 2 L, temperature 37.8°C. Bloods showed a CRP of 110 mg/L, lactate of 2.7 mmol/L, deranged LFTs (as previously known) but preserved renal function. He has anaemia, likely anaemia of chronic disease and no evidence of bleeding at present. There was a metabolic acidosis on the gas. Microbiology has just informed us that his ascitic tap had a neutrophil count in excess of 250 × 10^9/L. Urine dipstick was negative.

He has been started on tazobactam/piperacillin and cautious intravenous fluid replacement with 20% human albumin. He will require a fluid review tonight and repeat bloods in the morning. Blood cultures have been collected and sensitivities from the ascitic fluid will be back tomorrow.'

STATION 4.3: PARACETAMOL OVERDOSE

You are an emergency department junior doctor working on a night shift. A 37-year-old woman (Miss Joanne Macphee, 19/02/87), normally fit and well, accompanied by her friend, presents to the emergency department with an overdose of paracetamol following an argument with her parents. She did not coingest any alcohol or other drugs. Please assess her and instigate appropriate management.

Patient Details

Name:	Joanne Macphee
DOB:	19/02/87
Hospital number:	1902870900
Weight:	65 kg
Height:	1.68 m
Consultant:	Dr Jacobs
Hospital/Ward:	RIE CAA6
Current medications:	Nil
Allergies:	No known drug allergies
Admission date:	12/11/24

Management Summary

- Establish amount and timing of overdose.
- Paracetamol level 4 hours postingestion (please note exceptions in text).
- Identify high-risk group patients.
- Protect the liver—start NAC if needed.

Complications of Paracetamol Overdose

- Acute liver failure
- Hypoglycaemia
- Coagulopathy
- Hypotension
- Encephalopathy
- Acute tubular necrosis
- Pancreatitis

INITIAL ASSESSMENT

AIRWAY

- Assess patency of the airway.
- In patients who have taken an overdose, the airway may also be obstructed as a result of (a) vomiting or (b) reduced GCS due to coingestion of other drugs, e.g. central nervous system (CNS) depressants—alcohol, benzodiazepines.

'She tells you that she had intentionally ingested 15 × 500 mg paracetamol tablets 4 hours ago to upset her parents. Since then, she felt nauseous and had vomited twice.'

As she is speaking comfortably, there is no acute airway compromise. She now feels tearful and remorseful.

BREATHING

- Assess respiratory rate, breathing effort and pattern and oxygen saturation.
- Auscultate the chest.

'Her breathing rate is 20/min and oxygen saturations are 98% on room air. Chest auscultation is clear.'

In this case, she would not require a CXR. Bear in mind that patients who have taken an overdose may require a CXR to rule out aspiration, especially if there is airway compromise.

CIRCULATION

- Assess haemodynamic stability by measuring pulse, BP, CRT and JVP. Perform a CVS examination and ECG. Nausea and vomiting could be early features of poisoning or due to the effect of paracetamol upsetting the GI system.

'She is well hydrated. HR 70/min, BP 136/88 mmHg, CRT <2 seconds peripherally and CVS examination was normal.'

She requires IV access (with bloods sent simultaneously). No fluid resuscitation is currently required.

DISABILITY

- Assess the patient's consciousness level by using either AVPU (is the patient Alert? If not, do they respond to Verbal or Painful stimuli? Or are they Unresponsive?) or GCS score.
- Check blood glucose.
- Reduced consciousness level could indicate coingestion of other drugs (e.g. alcohol) or encephalopathy from liver failure. Low glucose raises suspicion of paracetamol-induced acute liver failure.

'She is alert with a blood glucose of 5 mmol/L.'

EXPOSURE

- Check temperature. Expose the patient and perform a full examination, focusing on the abdominal examination.
- Look for signs of decompensated liver disease, malnutrition, evidence of attempted/previous self-harm and IV drug use.

'Her temperature is 36.5°C. Abdominal examination is normal with no evidence of liver disease.'

INITIAL INVESTIGATIONS

- **Calculate timing and amount of overdose:** Take an accurate history of (1) amount ingested (you may need to work out the amount from the emptied packaging supplied by patients/family members/paramedics), (2) timing from ingestion, (3) time period over which it was ingested and (4) calculate mg/kg paracetamol ingested.
- **Serum paracetamol concentration:** In an acute single overdose, measure paracetamol concentration at least 4 hours after time of ingestion. If uncertain of time of ingestion or if there was a staggered overdose, check at time of presentation.
- **Bloods:** Check clotting screen, U&E, LFT, glucose and FBC to assess severity of hepatotoxicity. Include amylase in cases of abdominal pain as pancreatitis is a recognised complication of paracetamol overdose (Table 4.3).
- **ABG:** Allows assessment of acid–base status; it may show decreased pH and elevated lactate level. It is useful in assessing the severity of liver failure, if present.
- **ECG:** Paracetamol does not usually result in direct ECG changes; however, the patient may potentially coingest other medications that could cause changes, e.g. prolonged QT interval with antidepressants overdose.

'Serum paracetamol concentration comes back at 120 mg/L'.

Table 4.3 Miss Macphee's Blood Results

PARAMETER	VALUE	NORMAL RANGE (UNITS)
Hb	140 g/L	Men: 135–180 (g/L) Women: 115–160 (g/L)
WCC	11 × 10^9/L	4–11 (×10^9/L)
Neutrophil	5 × 10^9/L	2–7.5 (×10^9/L)
Lymphocyte	3 × 10^9/L	1.4–4 (×10^9/L)
Platelet	200 × 10^9/L	150–400 (×10^9/L)
Urea	5 mmol/L	2.5–6.7 (mmol/L)
Creatinine	90 μmol/L	79–118 (μmol/L)
eGFR	>60 mL/min	>60 (mL/min)
Sodium	140 mmol/L	135–146 (mmol/L)
Potassium	3.6 mmol/L	3.5–5.0 (mmol/L)
Lactate	2 mmol/L	0.6–2.4 (mmol/L)
Bilirubin	6 μmol/L	<17 (μmol/L)
ALT	14 IU/L	<40 (IU/L)
ALP	40 IU/L	39–117 (IU/L)
PT	12 seconds	11.5–13.5 seconds
APTT	30 seconds	26–37 seconds
Glucose	5 mmol/L	4.5–5.6 (mmol/L) (fasting)
Paracetamol concentration	**120 mg/L**	**Undetectable**
pH	7.4	7.35–7.45
PaO_2	13 kPa	10.6–13.3 (kPa) on air
$PaCO_2$	5 kPa	4.8–6.1 (kPa)
HCO_3	24 mmol/L	22–26 (mmol/L)

ALP, Alkaline phosphatase; *ALT,* alanine transaminase; *APTT,* activated partial thromboplastin time; *eGFR,* estimated glomerular filtration rate; *PT,* prothrombin time; *WCC,* white cell count.

INITIAL MANAGEMENT

- Calculate amount of paracetamol ingested.

  'Miss MacPhee took 15 × 500 mg tablets and her weight is 65 kg; the amount of paracetamol ingested is 115 mg/kg (=15 × 500/65).'

- If ingestion occurred in the last hour and a toxic quantity has been ingested (>150 mg/kg), consider activated charcoal 50 g orally with IV antiemetic. If >75 mg/kg is ingested (as in this case), IMMEDIATE NAC is indicated.

N-ACETYLCYSTEINE (NAC) ADMINISTRATION

- *N*-Acetylcysteine (NAC) is usually started when the serum paracetamol concentration is above the treatment line (based on Fig. 4.7). However, be mindful that NAC should be considered as an IMMEDIATE treatment in the following situations:
  - Patients with significant overdose (>75 mg/kg), staggered ingestion or uncertainty with the timing of the overdose.
  - Serum paracetamol level will not be available at 8 hours postingestion.
  - The patient presents in a coma.
  - Ingestion more than 36 hours ago with presentations of jaundice or liver tenderness.
- In the previous cases, NAC can always be stopped depending on the paracetamol levels when they come back. For those that present before 4 hours or at 4 to 8 hours postingestion, NAC commencement is guided by paracetamol levels taken at least 4 hours postingestion.
- Maximal liver protection is achieved if NAC is given within 8 hours postingestion.
- Following a Commission on Human Medicines (CHM) review, a single treatment line normogram regardless of risk factors of hepatotoxicity is now used.

'The patient required NAC immediately due to the overdose being >75 mg/kg. Her serum paracetamol level 4 hours postingestion returns as 120 mg/L and this is plotted on the treatment nomogram. The serum paracetamol concentration plots above the treatment line (Fig. 4.7). The paracetamol level has confirmed the need for NAC.'

High-risk groups:
- Chronic liver failure
- Malnutrition or not eaten for a few days (clue: may be reflected in raised urea)
- On drugs that induce liver enzymes, e.g. antiepileptics, carbamazepine, phenobarbitone, phenytoin, rifampicin, regular alcohol excess
- HIV
- Cystic fibrosis

- **Prescribing NAC:** NAC doses are normally given according to patient's weight in three infusions of different dose, volume and rate over 21 hours. If the weight of the patient is above 110 kg, use a weight of 110 kg for the purpose of the calculation (Table 4.4). A newer simpler 12-hour NAC regimen ('SNAP'), based on only two infusions, is gaining popularity because of a reduced incidence of adverse effects and shorter treatment time.

Prescribe (Fig. 4.8)
- ACETYLCYSTEINE 9750 mg IV in 200 mL GLUCOSE 5%, over 1 hour (200 mL/h)
- ACETYLCYSTEINE 3250 mg IV in 500 mL GLUCOSE 5%, over 4 hours (125 mL/h)
- ACETYLCYSTEINE 6500 mg IV in 1000 mL GLUCOSE 5%, over 16 hours (62.5 mL/h)

Table 4.4 NAC Dosage Calculation Based on Body Weight

	NAC DOSES	DILUENT	DURATION
First infusion	150 mg/kg	200 mL glucose 5%	1 hour
Second infusion	50 mg/kg	500 mL glucose 5%	4 hours
Third infusion	100 mg/kg	1000 mL glucose 5%	16 hours

NAC, N-acetyl cysteine.

MONITORING FOR LIVER FAILURE

- If there is clinical or biochemical evidence of liver failure, NAC should be given continuously and discussion with a Liver Unit is essential (for assessment of suitability for liver transplant).
- This is usually based on the King's College criteria. Transplant should be considered if either:
  - Arterial pH <7.3 OR
  - If all three of the following occur in a 24-hour period: creatinine >300 µmol/L, PT >100 seconds (INR >6.5) AND Grade III/IV encephalopathy
- Involve ITU early if there is significant liver failure.

REASSESSMENT

'Four hours later with her NAC running, she is now comfortably asleep with no further nausea and vomiting. Observations: RR 18/min, 98% RA, HR 80 bpm, BP 130/70 mmHg. Temp 36.0°C. Glucose 6.5 mmol/L. Her renal and liver functions are normal.'

- Recheck bloods after NAC therapy has been completed (LFTs, coagulation, U&E, ABG, with lactate). Further treatment with NAC is indicated if there are deranged LFTs or an elevated INR (>1.3). A minimal rise (an INR <1.3) is often seen purely due to NAC treatment and requires no action.
- Refer to psychiatry if overdose was in the context of a suicide attempt (Table 4.5).

HANDING OVER THE PATIENT

'Miss MacPhee is a 37-year-old lady who is usually fit and well. She presented with a single overdose of 15 x 500-mg paracetamol tablets following an argument with her boyfriend. She ingested 115 mg/kg of paracetamol and therefore NAC was immediately commenced. Levels came back above the treatment line at 120 mg/L. She is currently asymptomatic and has no clinical or laboratory evidence of acute liver injury. Bloods and gas were both normal.

Table 4.5 Common Overdoses

DRUGS	BE AWARE OF	SPECIFIC MANAGEMENT
Benzodiazepines	Respiratory and CNS depression	Supportive care Consider flumazenil (although increases risk of seizures and arrhythmias)
Salicylates	Confusion, metabolic acidosis, seizures, pulmonary oedema, coma, hypokalaemia	Consider bicarbonate
Antidepressants: Tricyclics, SSRIs, SNRIs, mirtazapine	Arrhythmias, GI upset, serotonin syndrome, acidosis, seizures	Supportive management
Opioids	CNS and respiratory depression	Naloxone

CNS, Central nervous system; *GI*, gastrointestinal; *SNRI*, serotonin norepinephrine reuptake inhibitor; *SSRI*, selective-serotonin reuptake inhibitor.

The plan is to repeat her bloods at the end of the infusion. She requires review by the liaison psychiatry team with regard to her suicide risk and safe discharge.'

STATION 4.4: ABDOMINAL SEPSIS

You are the junior doctor working on a general surgical admissions unit. Your next patient is a 47-year-old woman (Jennifer Williams, 12/05/77) who has presented with a 3-day history of worsening left iliac fossa pain and vomiting. She has had some loose stools over the last couple of days and has a background of diverticular disease. She is clearly in pain.

Patient Details

Name:	Jennifer Williams
DOB:	12/05/77
Hospital number:	1205772015
Weight:	72 kg
Height:	1.7 m
Consultant:	Mr Mann
Hospital/Ward:	WGH Ward 5
Current medications:	Nil
Allergies:	Erythromycin (rash)
Admission date:	12/11/24

Initial Differential Diagnosis

- Diverticulosis/diverticulitis
- Neoplasia
- Infective colitis
- UC
- Mesenteric adenitis
- Ectopic pregnancy
- Gynaecological malignancy
- Kidney stone

Common Complications of Diverticulitis

- Sepsis
- Perforation
- Obstruction
- Collection

INITIAL ASSESSMENT

AIRWAY

- Assess patency of the airway.

'She is able to speak in full sentences and is alert and orientated.'

You are satisfied that the airway is safe and proceed to assess breathing.

BREATHING

- Assess the respiratory rate and oxygen saturations.
- Perform a respiratory examination, particularly looking for signs of pneumonia.
- Request an erect CXR.

'Respiratory rate is 24/min, saturations 98% on air. On auscultation, there are vesicular breath sounds throughout. CXR confirms clear lung fields and no evidence of a pneumoperitoneum.'

You proceed to assess circulation.

CIRCULATION

- Assess haemodynamic stability by examining and measuring pulse, BP, CRT and JVP. Review urine output.
- Obtain two sites of IV access and take bloods.
- Perform an ABG and an ECG.
- Commence IV fluids.

'The patient is tachycardic at a rate of 110 bpm with a weak brachial pulse. JVP is not visible and heart sounds are unremarkable. BP is 90/63 mmHg, CRT = 3 seconds. ECG shows sinus tachycardia. She is pyrexial (38°C).'

You give a fluid bolus and monitor observations looking for a good response. A second bolus is given due to poor response. Consider catheterisation if the patient is unstable to help assess fluid balance.

Prescribe (Figs **4.9–4.11**)

Fluids, e.g. SODIUM CHLORIDE 0.9% 500 mL (over 15 minutes) followed by SODIUM CHLORIDE 0.9% 500 mL (over 15 min)

DISABILITY

- Assess the patient's conscious level, either using AVPU (is the patient Alert? If not, do they respond to Verbal or Painful stimuli? Or are they Unresponsive?) or GCS.

'The patient is alert and orientated in time, person and place.'

EXPOSURE

- Expose the patient and perform a full examination, particularly focusing on the abdomen.
- Examine the entire patient looking for sources of infection.

'Abdominal examination demonstrates left iliac fossa tenderness and involuntary guarding.'

You keep the patient nil by mouth, administer IV antibiotics to cover for possible intraabdominal sepsis as per local hospital guidelines (one option is tazobactam/piperacillin) and consider organising urgent imaging to rule out perforation/abscess formation (CT abdomen/pelvis scan).

Systemic inflammatory response syndrome (SIRS) is defined by two or more of the following:

- Pulse greater than 90 bpm
- Respiratory rate greater than 20/min or $PaCO_2$ less than 4.3 kPa
- WCC greater than 12 × 10^9/L or less than 4 × 10^9/L
- Temperature greater than 38°C or less than 36°C

SEPSIS = SIRS + suspected or confirmed source of infection.

INITIAL INVESTIGATIONS

- **Bloods:** Check FBC, U&E, LFT, amylase, lactate, CRP, glucose, group and save, and send off blood cultures (Table 4.6).
- **Urinalysis:** Look for evidence of a UTI as a source of sepsis. Offer a pregnancy test in women of childbearing age.
- **ABG:** Allows assessment of the metabolic status of the patient as well as the ventilation/oxygenation.
- **Erect CXR:** Look for free air under the diaphragm suggestive of a perforation. There may be evidence

of consolidation if the source of the sepsis is pneumonia. This will need to be a portable CXR if the patient is not stable enough to go to the X-ray department.

- **AXR:** To assess for obstruction (dilated bowel loops) and perforation.
- **ECG:** To assess the rhythm and look for evidence of a myocardial infarction.
- **CT scan:** Consider an urgent CT scan of the abdomen to rule out a perforation or collection.

'Blood tests: Hb 140 g/L, WCC 18.9 × 10⁹/L (neutrophils 13 × 10⁹/L), platelets 532 × 10⁹/L, urea 6.4 mmol/L, creatinine 109 µmol/L, Na 135 mmol/L, K 4 mmol/L, bilirubin 8 µmol/L, ALT 20 IU/L, ALP 100 IU/L, CRP 286 mg/L, lactate 4.3 mmol/L, amylase normal and pregnancy test negative. CT scan demonstrated complex diverticulitis and abscess formation.'

INITIAL MANAGEMENT

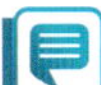

Management of Abdominal Sepsis

- Nil by mouth
- Antibiotics
- IV fluids
- Analgesia

- This patient is probably septic. (Note: Sepsis is an objective term: Sepsis = systemic inflammatory response syndrome (SIRS) plus confirmed or suspected source of infection.) Sepsis is a serious condition with a high mortality rate.
- Given the clear CXR, negative urinalysis and normal pregnancy test, the clinical picture of left iliac fossa pain and diarrhoea fits with diverticulitis.
- **Nil by mouth:** This patient may require surgical intervention. She should be nil by mouth until the senior review.
- **Antibiotics:** Recent case control studies have not found a significant benefit to prescribing antibiotics for mild diverticulitis. A randomised clinical trial that compared an oral versus an IV antibiotic regimen could not establish differences in outcome between the groups. The time between onset of sepsis and delivery of antibiotics is important for prognosis. In this scenario, however, we are dealing with severe diverticulitis and possible abscess formation. Antibiotic choice will be dependent on local antibiotic policies. One option is 4.5 g of piperacillin and tazobactam IV TDS.
- **IV fluids:** Septic patients require IV fluids as they are relatively hypovolaemic due to peripheral vasodilatation. In addition, they have increased insensible losses due to their raised respiratory rate and pyrexia. Furthermore, they may be nil by mouth. Patients with septic shock who are unresponsive to fluid resuscitation should be discussed with the high-dependency unit and considered for inotropic support (e.g. noradrenaline).
- **Catheter:** A urethral catheter should be considered to help assess fluid balance.
- **Analgesia:** This patient is clearly in pain. An appropriate regimen would be regular paracetamol 1 g IV and as required morphine IV/IM/SC 10 mg hourly.
- **Antiemetic:** Cyclizine 50 mg IV/IM/SC 8 hourly is one potential choice.
- Ensure the patient is on appropriate thromboprophylaxis as per local protocol. Liaise with seniors before prescribing anticoagulants in emergency surgical patients.

Table 4.6 Miss William's Blood Test Results

PARAMETER	VALUE	NORMAL RANGE (UNITS)
WCC	**18.9 × 10⁹/L**	**4–11 (×10⁹/L)**
Neutrophils	**13 × 10⁹/L**	**2–7.5 (×10⁹/L)**
Lymphocytes	4 × 10⁹/L	1.4–4 (×10⁹/L)
Platelets	**532 × 10⁹/L**	**150–400 (×10⁹/L)**
Haemoglobin	140 g/L	Men: 135–180 (g/L) Women: 115–160 (g/L)
CRP	**286 mg/L**	**0–5 (mg/L)**
Urea	6.4 mmol/L	2.5–6.7 (mmol/L)
Creatinine	109 µmol/L	79–118 (µmol/L)
Sodium	135 mmol/L	135–146 (mmol/L)
Potassium	4 mmol/L	3.5–5.0 (mmol/L)
eGFR	>60 mL/min	>60 (mL/min)
Lactate	**4.3 mmol/L**	**0.6–2.4 (mmol/L)**
Bilirubin	8 µmol/L	<17 (µmol/L)
ALT	20 IU/L	<40 (IU/L)
ALP	100 IU/L	39–117 (IU/L)
Amylase	95 IU/L	25–125 (IU/L)
Glucose	5 mmol/L	4.5–5.6 (mmol/L) (fasting)

Data in bold signifies results that are outside the normal laboratory range.
ALP, Alkaline phosphatase; *ALT*, alanine transaminase; *CRP*, C-reactive protein; *eGFR*, estimated glomerular filtration rate; *WCC*, white cell count.

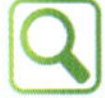

- Mild diverticulitis is a self-limiting process.
- CT is the imaging modality of choice.
- In complicated diverticulitis, clinicians now favour antibiotics and percutaneous drainage compared to surgical intervention.

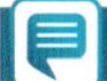

Prescribe (see Figs 4.9–4.11)

Antibiotics:

- PIPERACILLIN/TAZOBACTAM 4.5 g IV STAT (over 30 minutes) then TDS

Analgesia:
- PARACETAMOL 1 g IV STAT (over 15 minutes) then QDS, and MORPHINE 5 to 10 mg (titrate to response) IV STAT

Antiemetics:
- CYCLIZINE 50 mg IV STAT

Thromboprophylaxis:
- DALTEPARIN 5000 units SC OD

Maintenance fluids:
- SODIUM CHLORIDE 0.9% 500 mL IV 125 mL/h

REASSESSMENT

'Miss Williams looks significantly better. Work of breathing is reduced, RR 18/min and oxygen saturations 98% on air. After fluid boluses, the patient is now haemodynamically stable with HR 84 bpm, BP 128/60 mmHg, CRT <2 seconds and good urine output. There is still a low-grade pyrexia 37.6°C.'

FURTHER MANAGEMENT

- This patient needs early senior review to decide on possible percutaneous drainage or even a surgical procedure if perforation or obstruction is suspected.

HANDING OVER THE PATIENT

'This 47-year-old lady with a background of diverticulosis is being admitted with a diverticular abscess.

She presented with a 3-day history of vomiting and severe left iliac fossa pain. On examination, she was dehydrated and demonstrated left iliac fossa tenderness with guarding. She was pyrexial and hypotensive on admission. Inflammatory markers were raised. CT scan confirmed a diagnosis of diverticulitis with abscess formation.

Initial management included IV antibiotics, IV fluid resuscitation and catheterisation for closer fluid balance monitoring. Her observations quickly responded and she now has a satisfactory urine output (100 mL/h).

The plan is to admit, keep nil by mouth, continue IV maintenance fluids and IV antibiotics. She needs to be discussed with the surgical SpR on call as she may require percutaneous drainage of the collection.'

STATION 4.5: ACUTE UPPER GI BLEED

You are the junior doctor cross-covering GI medicine one evening. You are paged: a patient on the ward is having haematemesis (Steve Smith, 01/03/65). He was admitted directly from the medical outpatient clinic yesterday as he 'was yellow' and had a scan of his abdomen yesterday showing liver cirrhosis and portal hypertension. He is currently on Pabrinex and lactulose. He has never vomited blood before and he does not get indigestion. On arriving at the ward, you are shown into a side room where a dishevelled man is vomiting frank blood into a sick bowl. He is alert but is slurring his speech. He has blood on his hospital gown and there is blood on the floor around him. He tells you that he was sitting in bed when he vomited 30 minutes ago. He has vomited repeatedly since then.

Patient Details

Name:	Steve Smith
DOB:	01/03/65
Hospital number:	0103651252
Weight:	72 kg
Height:	1.7 m
Consultant:	Dr Khan
Hospital/Ward:	WGH Ward 2
Current medications:	Lactulose 30 mL (20 mg) PO TDS (started on admission—for liver failure) Pabrinex IV High Potency Injection (ampoules 1 and 2) IV TDS (started on admission—for liver failure) Enoxaparin 40 mg SC OD (started on admission—thromboprophylaxis)
Allergies:	None
Admission date:	11/11/24

Initial Differential Diagnosis

- Variceal bleed
- Gastric ulcer
- Mallory–Weiss tear
- Oesophagitis
- Vascular malformation
- Gastritis

Complications

- Aspiration
- Sepsis
- Encephalopathy
- Coagulopathy

Management of Massive Upper GI Bleed

- Major haemorrhage protocol (or equivalent at your hospital)
- Cross-match blood
- Oxygen
- IV fluids

INITIAL ASSESSMENT

AIRWAY

- Assess patency of the airway.

'The patient is drowsy and at high risk of aspirating. However, he can speak in full sentences.'

No action is currently required but continually reassess his airway.

BREATHING

- Assess the respiratory rate and oxygen saturations.
- Perform a respiratory examination, particularly listening for crepitations which may suggest aspiration pneumonia.
- Request an erect CXR.

'RR is 25/min, saturations 96% on room air. Chest is clear on auscultation with good bilateral air entry. CXR is clear, with no evidence of a pneumoperitoneum.'

You are satisfied with breathing at this point and continue by assessing circulation.

CIRCULATION

- Assess haemodynamic stability by measuring pulse, BP, CRT and JVP. Review urine output.
- Obtain two sites of IV access and take bloods.
- Perform an ABG and ECG.
- Commence IV fluids.

'On examination, the patient is tachycardic, with a heart rate of 110 bpm and sinus tachycardia on ECG. BP is 115/70 mmHg and CRT 3 seconds. He is covered in crusted and fresh blood.'

You send off blood tests to cross-match blood in preparation for transfusion. You administer fast IV fluids while waiting for cross-matched units to arrive.

DISABILITY

- Assess the patient's conscious level, either using AVPU (is the patient Alert? If not, do they respond to Verbal or Painful stimuli? Or are they Unresponsive?) or GCS. Check blood glucose.

'Patient is alert but is slurring his speech. Blood glucose is 5.4 mmol/L.'

Prescribe (Figs **4.12–4.14**)

Fluids:
- GELOFUSINE 500 mL (over 15 minutes) and then GELOFUSINE 500 mL (over 15 minutes) again

Blood:
- RED CELL CONCENTRATE 1 unit (over 15 minutes) and then again RED CELL CONCENTRATE 1 unit (over 15 minutes)

EXPOSURE

- Expose the patient and perform a full examination, particularly focusing on the abdomen. Is there evidence of perforation (e.g. peritonism)?
- Examine the entire patient looking for sources of bleeding.

'Abdomen is soft and nontender. He is unkempt and smells of alcohol. Bowel sounds are present. PR examination—no obvious masses or blood.'

Since the patient has signs of chronic liver disease, presenting with frank haematemesis in the absence of abdominal pain, variceal bleeding is likely.

INITIAL INVESTIGATIONS

- **Bloods:** Cross-match 6 units, FBC, U&E, LFT, clotting screen, amylase, lactate, CRP and glucose. Take venous blood cultures if the patient is pyrexial. Look for evidence of anaemia, infection, electrolyte derangement (raised urea suggestive of upper GI bleed), coagulation disorders and renal impairment (Table 4.10).
- **ABG:** This gives an immediate haemoglobin. It also allows assessment of the metabolic status of the patient as well as the ventilation/oxygenation.
- **Erect CXR:** Look for free air under the diaphragm suggestive of a perforation, for example from a GI ulcer. There may be evidence of consolidation (aspiration pneumonia). This will need to be a portable CXR if the patient is not stable enough to go to the X-ray department.
- **ECG:** Cardiac ischaemia may develop secondary to blood loss. This is something that should particularly be considered in the elderly or if there is massive blood loss or a history of cardiac disease.
- **Calculate Blatchford or Rockall score:** Blatchford score greater than 6 is associated with a high risk of needing intervention, while there is linear association between Rockall score and mortality. (Tables 4.7–4.9)

'Blood tests show Hb 67 g/L, WCC 17 × 10^9/L, platelets 200 × 10^9/L, urea 18 mmol/L, creatinine 115 μmol/L, SBR 250 μmol/L, ALT 600 IU/L, ALP 500 IU/L, normal clotting, lactate 2.7 mmol/L and CRP 20 mg/L. ECG demonstrates sinus tachycardia with possible ST depression in the lateral leads. CXR is clear with no evidence of a pneumoperitoneum. Blatchford score is 13 (urea 4 points, haemoglobin 6 points, pulse 1 point, hepatic disease 2 points), indicating high risk of needing intervention.'

INITIAL MANAGEMENT

- This patient shows features of a severe bleed (tachypnoea, tachycardia >100 bpm, reduced conscious level and likely variceal bleed).
- **The following risk assessment scores for all patients with acute upper GI bleeding should be done:** The Blatchford score at first assessment followed by an initial Rockall score before endoscopy (age, shock, comorbidity) and the full Rockall score after endoscopy. The importance of Rockall score before endoscopy is that it can give an initial measure of risk of death so that the patient is transferred to critical care (high dependency unit (HDU)/intensive care unit (ICU) if preendoscopy Rockall score is 3 or higher) for further management including endoscopy.

Table 4.7 The Blatchford Score

RISK MARKER	POINTS
Blood Urea (mmol/L)	
6.5–<8	2
≥8–<10	3
≥10–<25	4
≥25	6
Haemoglobin (g/L) (Men)	
≥12–13	1
≥10–<12	3
<10.0	6
Haemoglobin (g/L) (Women)	
≥10–12	1
<10.0	6
Blood Pressure (mmHg) (Sys)	
100–109	1
90–99	2
<90	3
Other Markers	
Pulse ≥100 bpm	1
Presentation with melaena	1
Presentation with syncope	2
Hepatic disease	2
Cardiac failure	2

- **Activate major haemorrhage protocol (or equivalent) if there is evidence of massive blood loss.**
- **Nil by mouth:** This patient may require surgical intervention. He should be nil by mouth until the senior review. Note any previous history of peptic ulcer, use of NSAIDs or anticoagulants, liver disease or dyspeptic symptoms. Look for evidence of chronic liver disease such as jaundice or spider naevi. If present, refer to the GI registrar and continue to stabilise the patient.
- **Oxygen:** Maintain oxygen saturations >94%.
- **Secure IV access:** Two large-bore cannulae (16 G or bigger).
- **IV fluids:** Rapid IV fluid resuscitation is required since the patient is hypovolaemic. Gelofusin or sodium chloride 0.9% can be used in the first instance until blood is available. If features of circulatory compromise persist after initial bolus of fluids, commence blood transfusion. If available, use type specific or cross-matched blood. If not, use O-negative blood. Coagulopathy should be corrected using appropriate blood products, such as fresh frozen plasma or vitamin K after consultation with haematology.
- **Continuous monitoring:** Cardiac rate and rhythm, BP and oxygen saturation. A urethral catheter should be considered to monitor urine output and help assess fluid balance.
- **PPIs:** Do not offer IV infusion of acid suppression drugs before endoscopy to patients with suspected nonvariceal upper GI bleeding.
- **Antibiotics:** Administer IV antibiotics (prophylaxis since there is a risk of developing bacterial infection in patients with liver cirrhosis presenting with haematemesis and sepsis is considered a risk factor for further bleeds). Antibiotic choice will depend on local antibiotic policies. One option is 4.5 g of piperacillin and tazobactam IV TDS.
- Do not give LMWH due to active bleeding but apply thromboembolic deterrent stockings.

Table 4.8 Calculating Rockall Score

VARIABLE	0 POINTS	1 POINT	2 POINTS	3 POINTS
Age	<60	60–79	≥80	
Shock	No shock	Pulse >100 bpm Systolic BP >100 mmHg	Systolic BP <100 mmHg	
Comorbidity	Nil major		Chronic heart failure, ischaemic heart disease, major morbidity	Renal failure, liver failure, metastatic cancer
Diagnosis	Mallory–Weiss	All other diagnoses	Gastrointestinal malignancy	
Evidence of bleeding	None		Blood, adherent clot, spurting vessel	

BP, Blood pressure.

Table 4.9 Mortality Risk According to Rockall Score

Rockall score	0	1	2	3	4	5	6	7	8+
Mortality (percentage)	0	0	0.2	2.9	5.3	10.8	17.3	27.0	41.1

Table 4.10 Mr Smith's Blood Test Results

PARAMETER	VALUE	NORMAL RANGE (UNITS)
WCC	**17 × 10^9/L**	**4–11 (×10^9/L)**
Neutrophils	**10 × 10^9/L**	**2–7.5 (×10^9/L)**
Lymphocytes	**5 × 10^9/L**	**1.4–4 (×10^9/L)**
Platelets	200 × 10^9/L	150–400 (×10^9/L)
Haemoglobin	**67 g/L**	**Men: 135–180 (g/L) Women: 115–160 (g/L)**
Urea	**18 mmol/L**	**2.5–6.7 (mmol/L)**
Creatinine	115 µmol/L	79–118 (µmol/L)
Sodium	138 mmol/L	135–146 (mmol/L)
Potassium	3.8 mmol/L	3.5–5.0 (mmol/L)
eGFR	>60 mL/min	>60 (mL/min)
Lactate	**2.7 mmol/L**	**0.6–2.4 (mmol/L)**
PT	12 seconds	11.5–13.5 seconds
APTT	30 seconds	26–37 seconds
Bilirubin	**250 µmol/L**	**<17 (µmol/L)**
ALT	**600 IU/L**	**<40 (IU/L)**
ALP	**500 IU/L**	**39–17 (IU/L)**
Amylase	50 IU/L	25–125 (IU/L)
Glucose	5.5 mmol/L	4.5–5.6 (mmol/L) (fasting)
CRP	**20 mg/L**	**0–5 (mg/L)**

Data in bold signifies results that are outside the normal laboratory range.
ALP, Alkaline phosphatase; *ALT,* alanine transaminase; *APTT,* activated partial thromboplastin time; *CRP,* C-reactive protein; *eGFR,* estimated glomerular filtration rate; *PT,* prothrombin time; *WCC,* white cell count.

- Consider continuing lactulose. It may reduce risk of hepatic encephalopathy by reducing ammonia production in the gut. However, at present, oral therapy will not be tolerated and putting an NG tube down would be high risk given active bleeding.

Prescribe (see Figs 4.12–4.14)

Antibiotic prophylaxis:
- PIPERACILLIN/TAZOBACTAM 4.5 g IV STAT (over 30 minutes), then TDS

Mechanical thromboprophylaxis:
- TED STOCKING TOP CONTINUOUS

STOP
Lactulose therapy
Enoxaparin therapy

REASSESSMENT

'Following aggressive fluid resuscitation with IV fluids and 2 units of red cell concentrate, the patient has been stabilised. RR is now 18/min and saturations 98% on air. HR is now 95 bpm and BP has come up to 100/60 mmHg with warm peripheries, and a CRT of 2 seconds. There is still ongoing bleeding but the patient is now stable enough for endoscopy and the on-call gastroenterologist is on his way to open up the endoscopy suite.'

FURTHER MANAGEMENT

- **Contact:** GI Registrar immediately and critical care areas. Endoscopy should be offered to unstable patients with severe acute upper GI bleed immediately after resuscitation. All other patients should have an endoscopy within 24 hours. Use band ligation in patients with upper GI bleeding from oesophageal varices. Offer endoscopic injection of N-butyl-2-cyanoacrylate to patients with GI bleeding from gastric varices.
- **Terlipressin:** 2 mg IV then 1 to 2 mg IV every 6 hours. Stop after definitive haemostasis has been achieved, or after 5 days, unless there is another indication for its use. Caution in ischaemic heart disease, peripheral vascular disease and unresuscitated patients.
- **Further interventions:** For example transjugular intrahepatic portosystemic shunt (TIPSS) may be considered if bleeding from oesophageal varices is not controlled by band ligation. Sengstaken–Blakemore tubes are used acutely in dire situations, where bleeding cannot be controlled: this is a temporary measure, using a balloon to apply pressure in the oesophagus directly to stop bleeding.
- **Calculate Rockall score:** Good marker of prognosis postbleed. A score of <3 suggests a good prognosis, while a score above 8 suggests poor prognosis.
  Score in this case: 1 point (age), 1 points (shock), 3 points (comorbidity), 1 point (diagnosis), 2 points (evidence of bleeding) = 8 points.

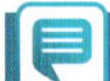
Prescribe (see Figs 4.12–4.14)

TERLIPRESSIN 2 mg IV STAT
Ongoing fluids:
- 500 mL GELOFUSINE 500 mL 500 mL/h

HANDING OVER THE PATIENT

'Mr Smith, a 59-year-old man with newly diagnosed liver cirrhosis and portal hypertension, presented with haematemesis likely from an oesophageal variceal bleed.

He had three episodes of haematemesis today. He was treated with aggressive IV fluid resuscitation. Admission haemoglobin was 67 g/L with normal platelets and clotting. Urea was elevated at 18 mmol/L with a normal creatinine. His Blatchford score was 13 (high risk). Following intravenous fluid resuscitation and 2 units of blood transfused, he was taken straight away for an urgent endoscopy.

Currently, he is on prophylactic antibiotics and continues Pabrinex. He has had one dose of terlipressin. There is currently no active bleeding. Please review and repeat his blood tests postendoscopy and perform a fluid review as ongoing fluids need to be prescribed.'

FURTHER READING

Aithal, G.P., Palaniyappan, N., China, L., et al., 2020. Guidelines to the management of ascites in cirrhosis. Gut 70 (1), 9–29.

Blatchford, O., Murray, W.R., Blatchford, M., 2000. A risk score to predict need for treatment for upper-gastrointestinal haemorrhage. Lancet 356 (9238), 1318–1321.

BMJ Best Practice. Paracetamol overdose in adults. https://bestpractice.bmj.com/topics/en-gb/3000110/management-recommendations. (Last accessed 22.09.23).

Joint Formulary Committee, 2023. British National Formulary 86. Pharmaceutical Press.

Lamb, C.A., Kennedy, N.A., Raine, T., et al., 2019. British Society of Gastroenterology consensus guidelines on the management of inflammatory bowel disease in adults. Gut 68 (Suppl 3), s1–106.

Patient.co.uk, 2019. Paracetamol poisoning. https://patient.info/doctor/paracetamol-poisoning [Last accessed 22.09.23].

Rockall, T.A., Logan, R.F., Devlin, H.B., 1996. Risk assessment after acute upper gastrointestinal haemorrhage. Gut 38 (3), 316–321.

PRESCRIPTION CHARTS

PRESCRIPTION AND ADMINISTRATION RECORD

Standard Chart

Hospital/Ward: WGH WARD 3 **Consultant:** DR COX	**Name of Patient:** JOHN SMITH
Weight: 72 kg **Height:** 1.70 m	**Hospital Number:** 1208970076
If re-written, date:	**D.O.B.:** 12/8/1997
DISCHARGE PRESCRIPTION **Date completed:-** **Completed by:-**	

OTHER MEDICINE CHARTS IN USE		**PREVIOUS ADVERSE REACTIONS** This section must be completed before any medicine is given		Completed by (sign & print)	Date
Date	Type of Chart	None known ☐			
		Medicine/Agent	Description of Reaction		
		PENICILLIN	RASH	MS (MI SMIG)	12/11/24

CODES FOR NON-ADMINISTRATION OF PRESCRIBED MEDICINE

If a dose is not administered as prescribed, initial and enter a code in the column with a circle drawn round the code according to the reason as shown below. **Inform the responsible doctor in the appropriate timescale.**

1. Patient refuses
2. Patient not present
3. Medicines not available – CHECK ORDERED
4. Asleep/drowsy
5. Administration route not available – CHECK FOR ALTERNATIVE
6. Vomiting/nausea
7. Time varied on doctor's instructions
8. Once only/as required medicine given
9. Dose withheld on doctor's instructions
10. Possible adverse reaction/side effect

ONCE-ONLY

Date	Time	Medicine (Approved Name)	Dose	Route	Prescriber – Sign + Print	Time Given	Given By
12/11/24	23.00	HYDROCORTISONE	100 mg	IV	MS (MI SMIG)	23.05	GH

OXYGEN	Start Date	Start Time	Route Mask (%)	Route Prongs (L/min)	Prescriber – Sign + Print	Administered by	Stop Date	Stop Time

Fig. 4.1 Prescription and administration record (standard chart) for John Smith.

Name: *JOHN SMITH*

Date of Birth: *12/8/1997*

REGULAR THERAPY

PRESCRIPTION

Medicine (Approved Name)		Time		12/11/24	13/11/24										
HYDROCORTISONE		(6)			FD										
Dose: *100 mg*	Route: *IV*	8													
Notes:	Start Date: *12/11/24*	(12)			FD										
Prescriber – sign + print: *MS (MI SMIG)*		14													
		(18)			FD										
		(22)			FD										

Medicine (Approved Name)		Time		12/11/24	13/11/24										
DALTEPARIN		6													
Dose: *5000 units*	Route: *SC*	8													
Notes:	Start Date: *12/11/24*	12													
Prescriber – sign + print: *MS (MI SMIG)*		14													
		(18)			FD										
		22													

Medicine (Approved Name)		Time		12/11/24	13/11/24										
ADCAL D3		6													
Dose: *1 tablet*	Route: *ORAL*	(8)			FD										
Notes: *While on steroids*	Start Date: *12/11/24*	12													
Prescriber – sign + print: *MS (MI SMIG)*		14													
		(18)			FD										
		22													

Medicine (Approved Name)		Time		12/11/24	13/11/24										
SULFASALAZINE		(6)			FD										
Dose: *500 mg*	Route: *ORAL*	8													
Notes:	Start Date: *12/11/24*	(12)			FD										
Prescriber – sign + print: *MS (MI SMIG)*		14													
		(18)			FD										
		(22)			FD										

Medicine (Approved Name)		Time													
		6													
Dose:	Route:	8													
Notes:	Start Date:	12													
Prescriber – sign + print:		14													
		18													
		22													

Medicine (Approved Name)		Time													
		6													
Dose:	Route:	8													
Notes:	Start Date:	12													
Prescriber – sign + print:		14													
		18													
		22													

Fig. 4.2 Prescription and administration record (regular therapy) for John Smith.

FLUID PRESCRIPTION CHART

Hospital/Ward: WGH WARD 3	**Consultant:** DR COX
Weight: 72 kg	**Height:** 1.70 m

Name of Patient: JOHN SMITH

Hospital Number: 1208970076

D.O.B: 12/8/97

Date/ Time	FLUID / ADDED DRUGS	VOLUME / DOSE	ROUTE	RATE	PRESCRIBER – SIGN AND PRINT
12/11/24 23.00	SODIUM CHLORIDE 0.9%	500 mL	IV	Over 15 min	MS (MI SMIG)
12/11/24 23.30	SODIUM CHLORIDE 0.9%	500 mL	IV	Over 15 min	MS (MI SMIG)

Fig. 4.3 Fluid prescription chart for John Smith.

PRESCRIPTION AND ADMINISTRATION RECORD

Standard Chart

Hospital/Ward: WGH WARD 4	Consultant: DR BING	Name of Patient: ANDREW REDDY
Weight: 70 kg	Height: 1.76 m	Hospital Number: 1208520060
If re-written, date:		D.O.B.: 12/8/1952
DISCHARGE PRESCRIPTION Date completed:-	Completed by:-	

OTHER MEDICINE CHARTS IN USE		PREVIOUS ADVERSE REACTIONS This section must be completed before any medicine is given		Completed by (sign & print)	Date
Date	Type of Chart	None known ☒		MS (MI SMIG)	12/11/24
		Medicine/Agent	Description of Reaction		

CODES FOR NON-ADMINISTRATION OF PRESCRIBED MEDICINE

If a dose is not administered as prescribed, initial and enter a code in the column with a circle drawn round the code according to the reason as shown below. **Inform the responsible doctor in the appropriate timescale.**

1. Patient refuses
2. Patient not present
3. Medicines not available – CHECK ORDERED
4. Asleep/drowsy
5. Administration route not available – CHECK FOR ALTERNATIVE
6. Vomiting/nausea
7. Time varied on doctor's instructions
8. Once only/as required medicine given
9. Dose withheld on doctor's instructions
10. Possible adverse reaction/side effect

ONCE-ONLY

Date	Time	Medicine (Approved Name)	Dose	Route	Prescriber – Sign + Print	Time Given	Given By
12/11/24	21.00	PIPERACILLIN/TAZOBACTAM (over 30 min)	4.5 g	IV	MS (MI SMIG)	21.05	CV
12/11/24	21.40	PABRINEX (HIGH POTENCY) (over 30 min)	Ampoules 1 and 2	IV	MS (MI SMIG)	21.45	CV

OXYGEN	Start Date	Start Time	Route Mask (%)	Route Prongs (L/min)	Prescriber – Sign + Print	Administered by	Stop Date	Stop Time
	12/11/24	21.00		2L/min via NASAL CANNULAE	MS (MI SMIG)	SB		

Fig. 4.4 Prescription and administration record (standard chart) for Andrew Reddy.

Name: ANDREW REDDY

Date of Birth: 12/8/1952

REGULAR THERAPY

PRESCRIPTION

Prescription	Time	12/11/24	13/11/24										
Medicine (Approved Name): PIPERACILLIN/TAZOBACTAM	6												
Dose: 4.5g	(8)		DW										
Route: IV	12												
Notes: for spontaneous bacterial peritonitis. Review in 48h. Given over 30mins	(14)		DW										
Start Date: 12/11/24	18												
Prescriber – sign + print: MS (MI SMIG)	(22)	x	DW										

Prescription	Time	12/11/24	13/11/24										
Medicine (Approved Name): LACTULOSE	6												
Dose: 30mL (20 mg)	(8)		DW										
Route: ORAL	12												
Notes:	(14)		DW										
Start Date: 12/11/24	18												
Prescriber – sign + print: MS (MI SMIG)	(22)	DW	DW										

Prescription	Time	12/11/24	13/11/24										
Medicine (Approved Name): PABRINEX (HIGH POTENCY)	6												
Dose: Ampoules 1 and 2	(8)		DW										
Route: IV	12												
Notes: For 3 days. Given over 30mins.	(14)		DW										
Start Date: 12/11/24	18												
Prescriber – sign + print: MS (MI SMIG)	(22)	x	DW										

Prescription	Time	12/11/24	13/11/24										
Medicine (Approved Name): DALTEPARIN	6												
Dose: 5000 units	8												
Route: SC	12												
Notes:	14												
Start Date: 12/11/24	(18)		DW										
Prescriber – sign + print: MS (MI SMIG)	22												

Prescription	Time												
Medicine (Approved Name):	6												
Dose:	8												
Route:	12												
Notes:	14												
Start Date:	18												
Prescriber – sign + print:	22												

Prescription	Time												
Medicine (Approved Name):	6												
Dose:	8												
Route:	12												
Notes:	14												
Start Date:	18												
Prescriber – sign + print:	22												

Fig. 4.5 Prescription and administration record (regular therapy) for Andrew Reddy.

FLUID PRESCRIPTION CHART

Hospital/Ward: WGH WARD 4	**Consultant:** DR BING	**Name of Patient:** ANDREW REDDY **Hospital Number:** 1208520060
Weight: 70 kg	**Height:** 1.76 m	**D.O.B:** 12/8/1952

Date/ Time	FLUID / ADDED DRUGS	VOLUME / DOSE	ROUTE	RATE	PRESCRIBER – SIGN AND PRINT
12/11/24 22.00	HUMAN ALBUMIN SOLUTION 20%	500 mL	IV	83 mL/h	MS (MI SMIG)

Fig. 4.6 **Fluid prescription chart for Andrew Reddy.** Note that human albumin solution prescriptions are often done on a separate chart.

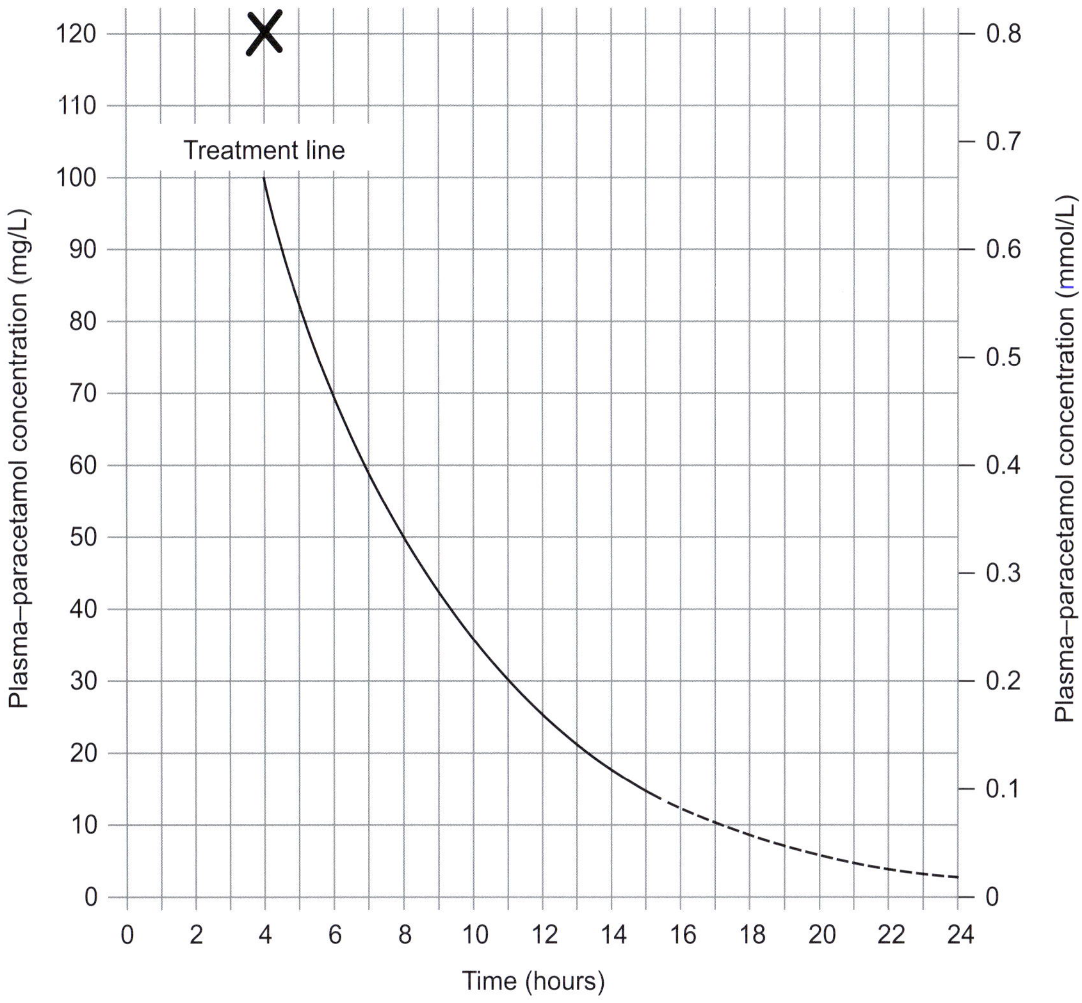

Fig. 4.7 Paracetamol overdose, treatment nomogram.

FLUID PRESCRIPTION CHART

Hospital/Ward: RIE CAA6	**Consultant:** DR JACOBS
Weight: 65 kg	**Height:** 1.68 m

Name of Patient: JOANNE MACPHEE

Hospital Number: 1902870900

D.O.B: 19/2/87

Date/ Time	FLUID / ADDED DRUGS	VOLUME / DOSE	ROUTE	RATE	PRESCRIBER – SIGN AND PRINT
12/11/24 22.15	GLUCOSE 5%	200 mL	IV	200 mL/h	MS (MI SMIG)
	ACETYLCYSTEINE	9750 mg			
12/11/24 23.15	GLUCOSE 5%	500 mL	IV	125 mL/h	MS (MI SMIG)
	ACETYLCYSTEINE	3250 mg			
13/11/24 03.15	GLUCOSE 5%	1000 mL	IV	62.5 mL/h	MS (MI SMIG)
	ACETYLCYSTEINE	6500 mg			

Fig. 4.8 Fluid prescription chart for Joanne MacPhee.

PRESCRIPTION AND ADMINISTRATION RECORD

Standard Chart

Hospital/Ward: WGH WARD 5 **Consultant:** MR MANN

Weight: 72 kg **Height:** 1.70 m

If re-written, date:

DISCHARGE PRESCRIPTION
Date completed:- **Completed by:-**

Name of Patient: JENNIFER WILLIAMS

Hospital Number: 1205772015

D.O.B.: 12/5/77

OTHER MEDICINE CHARTS IN USE	
Date	Type of Chart

PREVIOUS ADVERSE REACTIONS This section must be completed before any medicine is given		Completed by (sign & print)	Date
None known ☐			
Medicine/Agent	Description of Reaction		
ERYTHROMYCIN	RASH	MS (MI SMIG)	12/11/24

CODES FOR NON-ADMINISTRATION OF PRESCRIBED MEDICINE

If a dose is not administered as prescribed, initial and enter a code in the column with a circle drawn round the code according to the reason as shown below. **Inform the responsible doctor in the appropriate timescale.**

1. Patient refuses
2. Patient not present
3. Medicines not available – CHECK ORDERED
4. Asleep/drowsy
5. Administration route not available – CHECK FOR ALTERNATIVE
6. Vomiting/nausea
7. Time varied on doctor's instructions
8. Once only/as required medicine given
9. Dose withheld on doctor's instructions
10. Possible adverse reaction/side effect

ONCE-ONLY

Date	Time	Medicine (Approved Name)	Dose	Route	Prescriber – Sign + Print	Time Given	Given By
12/11/24	23.00	PIPERACILLIN/TAZOBACTAM (over 30 mins)	4.5g	IV	MS (MI SMIG)	23.00	AS
12/11/24	23.00	MORPHINE (titrate to response)	5 to 10 mg	IV	MS (MI SMIG)	23.05	AS (10 mg)
12/11/24	23.00	CYCLIZINE	50 mg	IV	MS (MI SMIG)	23.05	AS
12/11/24	23.00	PARACETAMOL (over 15 mins)	1g	IV	MS (MI SMIG)	23.10	AS

OXYGEN	Start Date	Start Time	Route Mask (%)	Route Prongs (L/min)	Prescriber – Sign + Print	Administered by	Stop Date	Stop Time

Fig. 4.9 Prescription and administration record (standard chart) for Jennifer Williams.

Name: JENNIFER WILLIAMS

Date of Birth: 12/5/1977

REGULAR THERAPY

PRESCRIPTION	Date → / Time ↓	12/11/24	13/11/24									
Medicine (Approved Name): PIPERACILLIN/TAZOBACTAM	6											
Dose: 4.5g; Route: IV	(8)		VB									
	12											
Notes: Abdominal sepsis. Review in 48 h. Given over 30 mins; Start Date: 12/11/24	(14)		VB									
	18											
Prescriber – sign + print: MS (MI SMIG)	(22)		VB									
Medicine (Approved Name): DALTEPARIN	6											
	8											
Dose: 5000 units; Route: SC	12											
Notes; Start Date: 12/11/24	14											
	(18)		VB									
Prescriber – sign + print: MS (MI SMIG)	22											
Medicine (Approved Name): PARACETAMOL	(6)		VB									
	8											
Dose: 1g; Route: IV	(12)		VB									
Notes: Given over 15 minutes; Start Date: 12/11/24	14											
	(18)		VB									
Prescriber – sign + print: MS (MI SMIG)	(22)		VB									
Medicine (Approved Name)	6											
	8											
Dose; Route	12											
Notes; Start Date	14											
	18											
Prescriber – sign + print	22											
Medicine (Approved Name)	6											
	8											
Dose; Route	12											
Notes; Start Date	14											
	18											
Prescriber – sign + print	22											
Medicine (Approved Name)	6											
	8											
Dose; Route	12											
Notes; Start Date	14											
	18											
Prescriber – sign + print	22											

Fig. 4.10 Prescription and administration record (regular therapy) for Jennifer Williams.

FLUID PRESCRIPTION CHART

Hospital/Ward: WGH WARD 5 **Consultant:** MR MANN	**Name of Patient:** JENNIFER WILLIAMS
	Hospital Number: 1205772015
Weight: 72 kg **Height:** 1.70 m	**D.O.B:** 12/5/77

Date/ Time	FLUID / ADDED DRUGS	VOLUME / DOSE	ROUTE	RATE	PRESCRIBER – SIGN AND PRINT
12/11/24 23.00	SODIUM CHLORIDE 0.9%	500 mL	IV	Over 15 min	MS (MI SMIG)
12/11/24 23.15	SODIUM CHLORIDE 0.9%	500 mL	IV	Over 15 min	MS (MI SMIG)
13/11/24 00.15	SODIUM CHLORIDE 0.9%	500 mL	IV	125 mL/h	MS (MI SMIG)

Fig. 4.11 Fluid prescription chart for Jennifer Williams.

PRESCRIPTION AND ADMINISTRATION RECORD

Standard Chart

Hospital/Ward: WGH WARD 2 **Consultant:** DR KHAN	**Name of Patient:** STEVE SMITH
Weight: 72 kg **Height:** 1.70 m	**Hospital Number:** 0103651252
If re-written, date:	**D.O.B.:** 1/3/65
DISCHARGE PRESCRIPTION **Date completed:-** **Completed by:-**	

OTHER MEDICINE CHARTS IN USE		PREVIOUS ADVERSE REACTIONS This section must be completed before any medicine is given		Completed by (sign & print)	Date
Date	Type of Chart	None known ☒		M. Jones (MJ JONES)	11/11/24
		Medicine/Agent	Description of Reaction		

CODES FOR NON-ADMINISTRATION OF PRESCRIBED MEDICINE

If a dose is not administered as prescribed, initial and enter a code in the column with a circle drawn round the code according to the reason as shown below. **Inform the responsible doctor in the appropriate timescale.**

1. Patient refuses
2. Patient not present
3. Medicines not available – CHECK ORDERED
4. Asleep/drowsy
5. Administration route not available – CHECK FOR ALTERNATIVE
6. Vomiting/nausea
7. Time varied on doctor's instructions
8. Once only/as required medicine given
9. Dose withheld on doctor's instructions
10. Possible adverse reaction/side effect

ONCE-ONLY

Date	Time	Medicine (Approved Name)	Dose	Route	Prescriber – Sign + Print	Time Given	Given By
12/11/24	21.00	PIPERACILLIN/TAZOBACTAM (over 30 mins)	4.5g	IV	M. Jones (MJ JONES)	21.05	KB
12/11/24	21.40	TERLIPRESSIN	2 mg	IV	M. Jones (MJ JONES)	21.45	KB

OXYGEN	Start Date	Start Time	Route Mask (%)	Route Prongs (L/min)	Prescriber – Sign + Print	Administered by	Stop Date	Stop Time

Fig. 4.12 Prescription and administration record (standard chart) for Steve Smith.

Name: STEVE SMITH
Date of Birth: 1/3/65

REGULAR THERAPY

PRESCRIPTION	Time \ Date	11/11/24	12/11/24	13/11/24
Medicine (Approved Name): PIPERACILLIN/TAZOBACTAM	6			
Dose: 4.5g; Route: IV	(8)			FD
Notes: Prophylaxis for 7 days due to upper GI bleed. Given over 30 mins	12			
Start Date: 12/11/24	(14)			FD
Prescriber – sign + print: M. Jones (MJ JONES)	18			
	(22)		x	

PRESCRIPTION	Time \ Date	11/11/24	12/11/24	13/11/24
Medicine (Approved Name): LACTULOSE	6			
Dose: 30 ml (20 mg); Route: ORAL	(8)	DF		
Notes:	12			
Start Date: 11/11/24	(14)	DF		
Prescriber – sign + print: M. Jones (MJ JONES)	18			
	(22)			

Stopped due to not tolerating oral medications 12/11/24 M. Jones (MJ JONES)

PRESCRIPTION	Time \ Date	11/11/24	12/11/24	13/11/24
Medicine (Approved Name): PABRINEX (HIGH POTENCY)	6			
Dose: Ampoules 1 and 2; Route: IV	(8)	DF		
Notes: Prescribed for 3 days. Given over 30 mins.	12			
Start Date: 11/11/24	(14)	DF		
Prescriber – sign + print: M. Jones (MJ JONES)	18			
	(22)	DF		

PRESCRIPTION	Time \ Date	11/11/24	12/11/24	13/11/24
Medicine (Approved Name): ENOXAPARIN	6			
Dose: 40mg; Route: TOP	8			
Notes:	12			
Start Date: 11/11/24	14			
Prescriber – sign + print: M. Jones (MJ JONES)	(18)	DF		
	22			

Stopped due to active bleeding 12/11/24 M. Jones (MJ JONES)

PRESCRIPTION	Time \ Date	11/11/24	12/11/24	13/11/24
Medicine (Approved Name): TED STOCKINGS	6		FG	
Dose: 1 pair; Route: TOP	8			
Notes:	12			
Start Date: 12/11/24	14			
Prescriber – sign + print: M. Jones (MJ JONES)	18			
	22			

PRESCRIPTION	Time \ Date			
Medicine (Approved Name):	6			
Dose: ; Route:	8			
Notes:	12			
Start Date:	14			
Prescriber – sign + print:	18			
	22			

Fig. 4.13 Prescription and administration record (regular therapy) for Steve Smith.

FLUID PRESCRIPTION CHART

Hospital/Ward: WGH WARD 2	**Consultant:** DR QURESHI	**Name of Patient:** STEVE SMITH
		Hospital Number: 0103651252
Weight: 72 kg	**Height:** 1.70 m	**D.O.B:** 1/3/65

Date/ Time	FLUID / ADDED DRUGS	VOLUME / DOSE	ROUTE	RATE	PRESCRIBER – SIGN AND PRINT
12/11/24 21.00	GELOFUSINE	500 mL	IV	Over 15 min	M. Jones (MJ JONES)
12/11/24 21.00	GELOFUSINE	500 mL	IV	Over 15 min	M. Jones (MJ JONES)
12/11/24 21.15	RED CELL CONCENTRATE	1 unit	IV	Over 15 min	M. Jones (MJ JONES)
12/11/24 21.15	RED CELL CONCENTRATE	1 unit	IV	Over 15 min	M. Jones (MJ JONES)
12/11/24 21.30	GELOFUSINE	500 mL	IV	500 mL/h	M. Jones (MJ JONES)

Fig. 4.14 **Fluid prescription chart for Steve Smith.** Note blood prescriptions are often done on a separate prescription chart.

Neurology

5

Ali B.A.K. Al-Hadithi

Chapter Outline

Station 5.1: Meningitis
Station 5.2: Seizures
Station 5.3: Subarachnoid Haemorrhage
Station 5.4: Ischaemic Stroke
Station 5.5: Myasthenia Gravis

STATION 5.1: MENINGITIS

You are the junior doctor working in the emergency department when a 22-year-old student, Simon Peters (01/07/02), is brought in by ambulance with a headache, vomiting and neck stiffness. He looks unwell and is shielding his eyes from the light. The ambulance crew report that he seems confused and his temperature is elevated at 38.5°C. Please assess him and instigate appropriate management.

Patient Details

Name:	Simon Peters
DOB:	01/07/02
Hospital number:	F2083912
Weight:	75 kg
Height:	1.8 m
Consultant:	Dr Epp
Hospital/Ward:	SGH Neurology
Current medications:	Nil
Allergies:	Nil
Admission date:	12/10/24

Differential Diagnosis of Headache With a Fever

- Meningitis/encephalitis
- Intracranial abscess
- Intracranial bleed
- Sinusitis

Complications of Meningitis

- Immediate: septic shock, disseminated intravascular coagulation (DIC), coma, seizures, raised intracranial pressure, adrenal haemorrhage, syndrome of inappropriate antidiuretic hormone (SIADH), multiorgan failure
- Long term: learning disability, memory impairment, hearing/visual loss, focal paralysis, hydrocephalus, subdural effusion, ataxia

INITIAL ASSESSMENT

AIRWAY

- Assess patency of the airway. Is there any stridor or noisy breathing? Is there any vomit that could be obstructing the airway? Is the patient conscious enough to maintain a safe airway?

'The airway is patent with no obstruction. The patient is maintaining a safe airway.'

No additional airway support is required.

BREATHING

- Assess respiratory rate, oxygen saturations and accessory muscle use. Auscultate for air entry, and additional sounds of wheeze or crepitations.

'The respiratory rate is 22/min and oxygen saturations are 99%. There are no signs of respiratory distress. The lung fields are clear.'

The oxygen saturations are normal and therefore supplementary oxygen is not required. The respiratory rate is mildly raised and this likely reflects a systemic inflammatory response.

In a case of suspected meningitis you must alert your senior immediately, assess the patient promptly and do not delay antibiotic treatment. Following an initial ABCDE assessment, obtain intravenous (IV) access and take blood cultures. Ideally, patients should have brain imaging prior to lumbar puncture (LP) (if computed tomography (CT) scanning is readily available and LP is not contraindicated) but antibiotic therapy should not be delayed beyond 3 hours after presentation.

CIRCULATION

- Assess circulatory status by measuring pulse, blood pressure (BP) and capillary refill time (CRT). Is the pulse bounding (seen early in sepsis) or weak (associated with hypotension)? Are the peripheries warm (vasodilatation secondary to sepsis) or cold (is the patient peripherally shut down)?

- The patient has been vomiting and it is therefore particularly important to assess fluid status. As well as BP and pulse, also examine skin turgor, mucous membranes and look for sunken eyes. None of these signs are particularly specific on their own, so an overall assessment should be made.
- Perform a cardiovascular (CVS) examination. Assess the jugular venous pressure (JVP) and central pulse. Auscultate for heart sounds and any additional murmurs. Examine for evidence of peripheral oedema.

'The HR is 110 bpm and BP 125/60 mmHg, CRT is 1 second peripherally. The pulse is bounding and the peripheries are warm. Mucous membranes are dry but skin turgor is normal. On cardiovascular examination the JVP is not visible. Heart sounds are normal with no murmurs. There is no evidence of peripheral oedema.'

- The patient is maintaining an adequate BP but is tachycardic and vasodilated. There are also some signs of dehydration which are likely to be secondary to vomiting.
- Obtain IV access, take bloods and start IV maintenance fluids at 125 mL/h (see initial management).
- Consider the need to insert a urinary catheter to measure urine output hourly and start a fluid balance chart. Urinary catheterisation should be performed in all patients with severe sepsis.

DISABILITY

- Assess the patient's conscious level using the Glasgow Coma Scale (GCS). Ask the nursing staff to start the patient on neurological observations. Check pupil sizes and reactions. Check bedside glucose levels.

'The patient is rousable to voice and confused with a GCS of 13 (E 3, V 4, M 6). The pupils are equal and reactive to light and the blood glucose is 4.5 mmol/L.'

- A full neurological examination is required to assess for any focal neurological deficit; however, initial antibiotic treatment should not be delayed while a lengthy examination is performed.
- Examine the cranial nerves (including fundoscopy), upper and lower limbs. If there is any focal neurological deficit, this could suggest raised intracranial pressure which would be a contraindication to LP. If there is a pressure difference between the supratentorial and infratentorial compartments, LP may increase this pressure difference and cause brain herniation. In such cases, LP should not be performed and antibiotics given immediately. Other signs that could suggest raised intracranial pressure include a reduced or fluctuating GCS and papilloedema.
- In a case of meningitis with signs of raised intracranial pressure, the nearest neurosurgical centre should be contacted and the patient should be cared for on an intensive care unit.

'Full neurological examination is limited due to patient confusion; however, there do not appear to be any focal neurological signs. Specifically, there is no evidence of papilloedema on fundoscopy; power, reflexes and tone are normal in all four limbs and there is no facial asymmetry or obvious cranial nerve deficit.'

Signs Suggestive of Raised Intracranial Pressure

- Reduced or fluctuating GCS
- Focal neurological deficit
- Unequal or abnormal pupils
- Papilloedema

EXPOSURE

- Expose the patient and in particular look for any evidence of rash. The presence of a nonblanching petechial rash indicates septicaemia and the patient should be reviewed by critical care for intensive care admission.
- Measure the temperature. Examine for neck stiffness and assess Kernig's sign (flex the patient's hip and when the knee is extended, there is pain and resistance). Palpate for any lymphadenopathy and examine the abdomen to exclude any pathology.

'The temperature is elevated at 38.1°C and there is no obvious rash. There is neck stiffness and Kernig's sign is positive.'

INITIAL INVESTIGATIONS

- **Bloods:** Full blood count (FBC), urea and electrolytes (U&Es), liver function tests (LFTs), glucose, C-reactive protein (CRP), clotting, meningococcal and viral PCR (polymerase chain reaction) (Table 5.1). Look for evidence of infection and check platelet count and clotting before performing LP. In severe meningitis, disseminated intravascular coagulation can occur, causing deranged clotting and low platelets, both of which would be a contraindication to LP.
- **Blood cultures:** Ensure aseptic technique when taking blood and that at least 10 mL of blood is collected in each blood culture bottle to give the highest chance of culturing an organism.
- **Venous blood gas:** This is useful to assess the patient's acid–base status and their lactate. A raised lactate may suggest reduced tissue perfusion which

Table 5.1 Mr Peters' Blood Test Results

PARAMETER	VALUE	NORMAL RANGE (UNITS)
WCC	**25 × 10⁹/L**	**4–11 (×10⁹/L)**
Neutrophil	**21 × 10⁹/L**	**2–7.5 (×10⁹/L)**
Lymphocyte	2 × 10⁹/L	1.4–4 (×10⁹/L)
Platelet	230 × 10⁹/L	150–400 (×10⁹/L)
Haemoglobin	150 g/L	Men: 135–177 (g/L) Women: 115–155 (g/L)
PT	11.8 seconds	11.5–13.5 seconds
APTT	30 seconds	26–37 seconds
CRP	**80 mg/L**	**0–5 (mg/L)**
Urea	6 mmol/L	2.5–6.7 (mmol/L)
Creatinine	100 µmol/L	79–118 (µmol/L)
Sodium	140 mmol/L	135–146 (mmol/L)
Potassium	4 mmol/L	3.5–5.0 (mmol/L)
eGFR	>60 mL/min	>60 (mL/min)
Bilirubin	10 µmol/L	<17 (µmol/L)
ALT	20 IU/L	<40 (IU/L)
ALP	40 IU/L	39–117 (IU/L)
Lactate	1.5 mmol/L	0.6–2.4 (mmol/L)
Bicarbonate	24 mmol/L	22–26 (mmol/L)
pH	7.4	7.3–7.45
$PaCO_2$	5 kPa	4.8–6.1 (kPa)

Data in bold signifies results that are outside the normal laboratory range.
ALP, Alkaline phosphatase; *ALT,* alanine transaminase; *APTT,* activated partial thromboplastin time; *CRP,* C-reactive protein; *eGFR,* estimated glomerular filtration rate; *PT,* prothrombin time; *WCC,* white cell count.

is a poor prognostic sign and an indicator of severe sepsis.

- **CT head:** If CT scanning is readily available and will not lead to significant delays, a CT head should be performed prior to LP in all cases. If CT scanning is not readily available, LP can be performed if deemed safe by a neurologist. If a neurologist is not available, then the European Federation of Neurological Societies (EFNS) guidelines state antibiotics should be given while awaiting imaging. The CT protocol may vary between individual hospitals.
- **LP:** This is the key investigation in this case which will give the most diagnostic information. However, as already described, there are a number of contraindications to performing an LP—these are reduced or fluctuating GCS, raised intracranial pressure, suspected intracranial mass, focal neurology, septicaemia, shock, respiratory failure, trauma and middle ear pathology. If there are no contraindications, proceed as described in the following:
  - Ensure that the platelets, clotting and CT scan are normal prior to LP and obtain the patient's consent if they are able to.
  - Measure the opening pressure using a manometer (normal <25 cmH_2O).
  - Send the first and third bottles for microscopy, culture and sensitivity.
  - Send the second bottle for biochemistry (protein and glucose) and send a paired serum glucose.
  - Send the fourth bottle for meningococcal PCR and viral PCR (if encephalitis suspected).
  - If subarachnoid haemorrhage is suspected, a CT head should be performed prior to LP. If this is clear, a fifth bottle can be sent for xanthochromia (taken at least 12 hours following the time of the suspected subarachnoid haemorrhage).
  - Send the samples urgently to the lab and contact the microbiologist on call to alert them of the patient (urgent microscopy will be required) and for advice on antibiotic choice.
- **Electroencephalography (EEG) and magnetic resonance imaging (MRI) head:** If there is concern of encephalitis then EEG and MRI can be useful, both usually illustrating changes in the fronto-temporal lobes.
- **Throat swab:** Send throat swabs for bacterial and viral culture.
- **Septic screen:** In view of the temperature, a chest X-ray and midstream urine analysis should be performed to exclude any evidence of pneumonia or urinary tract infection. In view of the vomiting, aspiration pneumonia should also be suspected; however, clinical examination in this case does not suggest any evidence of pneumonia.

'Blood testing reveals WCC 25 × 10⁹/L, neutrophils 21 × 10⁹/L and CRP 80 mg/L. Platelets and clotting are normal. Venous gas shows normal acid–base balance and a lactate of 1.5 mmol/L. CXR is clear, blood cultures and MSU are sent. A CT head is arranged prior to lumbar puncture.'

Common Organisms Causing Bacterial Meningitis

- *Neisseria meningitidis*
- *Streptococcus pneumoniae*
- *Haemophilus influenzae*

INITIAL MANAGEMENT

Management Summary

- Resuscitate using an ABCDE approach
- CT head
- Blood cultures and lumbar puncture (if no contraindications)
- Broad-spectrum antibiotics
- IV corticosteroids
- Consider antiviral agents if there is a concern about encephalitis
- IV fluids

- **Airway support:** In this case, no intervention required. Consider intubation in any patient with a GCS <8.

- **Supplementary oxygen:** Give supplementary oxygen in any patient with saturations <94% or severe sepsis.
- **IV fluids:** IV fluids should be given to all patients with sepsis. In this case, the patient is given sodium chloride 0.9% at 125 mL/h. Reassess fluid status frequently and titrate fluid therapy as necessary. Once the U&Es are available, further fluids can be prescribed with supplementary potassium added as necessary. In a case of suspected meningitis, it is important to maintain neutral fluid balance—patients with sepsis should be given IV fluid therapy to maintain good tissue perfusion; however, overhydration can worsen raised intracranial pressure which occurs in meningitis.
- **Antibiotics:** The choice of antibiotics depends on the local antibiotic policy and early microbiological advice should be sought. Usually, a third-generation cephalosporin is given as first line, e.g. cefotaxime 2 g IV 6-hourly. Atypical organisms should be considered in certain cases and advice from the microbiologist will be important in determining the most effective choice of antibiotics. In the elderly, consider *Listeria* infection which is covered by the addition of amoxicillin. If the patient has recently been abroad, they may have infection with penicillin-resistant pneumococci and you should add high-dose vancomycin.
- **Corticosteroids:** In cases of community-acquired meningitis (particularly pneumococcal meningitis), there is evidence that high-dose corticosteroids may reduce neurological complications if given before or at the same time as the first dose of antibiotics. Following senior advice, consider starting dexamethasone 10 mg IV QDS. These should preferably be started before or with the first dose of antibiotics. High-dose corticosteroids should not be given in those with meningococcal septicaemia, septic shock, in the immunosuppressed and those who have undergone recent neurosurgery. If corticosteroids are to be given, a proton pump inhibitor (PPI) (such as omeprazole 40 mg IV OD) should be given in addition to prevent gastric ulceration.
- **Antiviral treatment:** In cases where encephalitis is suspected (headache, fever, seizures, altered personality, focal neurology), also give aciclovir 10 mg/kg IV TDS. It is reasonable to give it in Simon Peters' case because of the patient's confusion. Outcomes in encephalitis significantly worsen the longer treatment is delayed; therefore, if you ever suspect encephalitis, you should start treatment immediately—this can easily be stopped later when the viral PCR results are available.
- **Analgesia:** Start regular paracetamol for the patient's headache. Use opioids with considerable caution in a patient with a reduced GCS.
- **Deep vein thrombosis (DVT) prophylaxis treatment:** Pharmacological prophylaxis with low-molecular-weight heparin (LMWH) should initially be avoided. Intracerebral and adrenal haemorrhage can both occur in meningitis as well as clotting abnormalities and consumption of platelets due to sepsis and disseminated intravascular coagulation. In all cases, LMWH treatment should be delayed until at least 4 hours after LP. Following initial investigations and treatment, the appropriateness of LMWH prescription for DVT prophylaxis can be determined.
- **Notify public health authority:** Meningitis is a notifiable disease and close contacts should be treated with antibiotic prophylaxis—the choice of antibiotic depends on the causative organism and microbiology advice should be taken.
- As the GCS is 13, all medications are given intravenously.

Prescribe (Figs 5.1–5.3)

Corticosteroids:
- DEXAMETHASONE 10 mg IV STAT then QDS (for FOUR DAYS)

Antibiotics:
- CEFOTAXIME 2 g IV (over 20–60 mins) STAT then QDS

Antivirals:
- ACICLOVIR 750 mg IV (over 1 hour) STAT then TDS

PPI:
- OMEPRAZOLE 40 mg IV (over 20–30 mins) STAT then OD

Maintenance fluids:
- 1 L SODIUM CHLORIDE 0.9% IV at 125 mL/h

Analgesia:
- PARACETAMOL 1 g (over 15 mins) STAT then IV QDS

DVT prophylaxis:
- TED STOCKINGS CONTINUOUS TOP

REASSESSMENT AFTER INVESTIGATION RESULTS

- After initial assessment, a CT head is undertaken in view of the reduced GCS—this shows no evidence of intracranial mass or raised intracranial pressure. LP is therefore performed, the results of which are WBC 5000 cells/mm^3 (95% polymorphs), protein 1 g/L and glucose 1.5 mmol/L (plasma glucose 4.5 mmol/L).

INTERPRETING LUMBAR PUNCTURE RESULTS

The lumbar puncture results are consistent with bacterial meningitis (Table 5.2). Following discussion with the microbiology consultant, cefotaxime and dexamethasone are continued while awaiting CSF culture and sensitivities. Aciclovir is continued pending viral PCR results.

Table 5.2 Lumbar Puncture Results

	NORMAL	VIRAL	BACTERIAL	TUBERCULOUS
Appearance	Clear	Clear	Turbid/purulent	Turbid/viscous
Predominant cell type	Lymphocytes	Lymphocytes	Polymorphs	Mixed
WBC count (cells/mm^3)	0–5	5–1000	1000–10,000	25–500
Protein (g/L)	0.15–0.5	<1.0	>0.5	>0.5
Glucose (CSF/blood ratio)	0.6	>0.5	<0.3	<0.5

CSF, Cerebrospinal fluid; *WBC*, white blood cell.

HANDING OVER THE PATIENT (IN THIS CASE THIS WOULD LIKELY BE TO INTENSIVE CARE)

'Simon is a 22-year-old student with community-acquired bacterial meningitis that has been started on IV cefotaxime, aciclovir and dexamethasone.

He presented with headache, vomiting and neck stiffness. On examination, he is maintaining his own airway and is not in any respiratory distress. BP is 125/60 mmHg and pulse rate is 110 bpm. There are some signs of dehydration and he has been started on intravenous fluids. The GCS is 13/15: he is eye opening to voice and is confused but he obeys commands and there are no focal neurological signs. The temperature is elevated at 38.1°C and there is no evidence of a rash but he is Kernig's positive. He has initially been treated with cefotaxime 2 g, dexamethasone 10 mg and aciclovir 750 mg.

Cerebrospinal fluid examination reveals a significantly raised white cell count predominantly of polymorphs. The CSF protein is elevated and glucose level reduced.

The lumbar puncture results are typical of bacterial meningitis and, following microbiology advice, the plan is to continue current medications.

The patient is to be transferred to the intensive care unit for closer observation. The local public health authority has been informed and close contacts are being traced. Bloods are to be repeated in the morning and CSF/blood cultures need to be chased, as well as meningococcal and viral PCR results.'

STATION 5.2: SEIZURES

A 37-year-old woman, Lucy, is brought to the emergency department by ambulance following a collapse. She is currently having a generalised seizure while lying on a bed. The ambulance crew has just managed to place a cannula and ask if you want to give any medication. They report that Lucy has been seizing for about 10 minutes. She is not on any regular medications, and has never had a seizure before. Please assess her and instigate appropriate management.

Patient Details

Name:	Lucy Wall
DOB:	02/02/87
Hospital number:	C1261452
Weight:	50 kg
Height:	1.6 m
Consultant:	Dr Epp
Hospital/Ward:	SGH Neurology
Current medications:	Nil
Allergies:	Nil
Admission date:	12/10/24

Causes of Seizures

- Epilepsy
- Metabolic disturbance (low sodium, calcium, magnesium, glucose levels)
- Hypoxia
- Alcohol withdrawal
- Drug withdrawal or overdose
- Cerebral pathology (meningitis, encephalitis, abscess, tumour, trauma, subarachnoid haemorrhage)
- Eclampsia in pregnancy

Seizure Complications

- Status epilepticus (associated with significant cerebral, cardiovascular and metabolic/systemic deterioration, including multiorgan failure)
- Injury secondary to seizure
- Cognitive and behavioural deterioration

INITIAL ASSESSMENT

AIRWAY

- Assess patency of the airway. In the case of a generalised seizure, it is critically important that the airway is protected and the patient is protected from injury. Open the airway and ensure it is patent. Is there any stridor or noisy breathing? Is there any vomit that could be obstructing the airway?

'The patient is actively seizing and has therefore been placed in the recovery position. The airway is patent and unobstructed.'

- First roll the patient onto their left side and into the recovery position if possible: if the patient vomits, this will reduce the risk of aspiration. Ensure that the patient is not at risk of falling out of bed and call for a nurse to help assist you.
- If there is a history of trauma, use cervical spine precautions as necessary.
- Remove any loose-fitting teeth but do not place anything in the mouth.
- If there are excess secretions or vomit, use suction to clear the airway.
- Use head tilt, chin lift or jaw thrust manoeuvres as necessary to maintain the airway.
- Insert a nasopharyngeal airway with lubrication (unless there is a suspected basal skull fracture).
- Intubation should be considered early if necessary and the on-call anaesthetist informed.

BREATHING

- Assess respiratory rate, oxygen saturations and accessory muscle use. Auscultate for air entry and additional sounds of wheeze or crepitations.

'The respiratory rate is 25/min, oxygen saturations are 100% on high-flow oxygen. There is accessory intercostal muscle use. The lung fields are clear to auscultation.'

- Apply high-flow oxygen via a nonrebreather mask—make sure you inflate the reservoir bag with oxygen before placing it on the patient.
- High-flow oxygen therapy should be given to all patients who are having a generalised seizure unless there is a specific contraindication (e.g. known CO_2 retainer). The respiratory rate is usually raised in the setting of a seizure. If oxygen saturations are reduced, consider performing an arterial blood gas (ABG)—hypoxia can be a cause of seizures.

 **Prescribe (Figs 5.4–5.6)**

HIGH-FLOW OXYGEN:
- 15 L/min via a NON-REBREATHER MASK

CIRCULATION

- Assess circulatory status by measuring pulse, BP and CRT.
- Perform a focused CVS examination. Assess the central pulse and auscultate for heart sounds and any murmurs. Examine for evidence of peripheral oedema.

'The pulse is regular at 110 bpm, BP 155/90 mmHg and CRT is 1 second peripherally. Heart sounds are normal with no added murmurs. There is no evidence of peripheral oedema.'

The BP and pulse are slightly elevated (possibly due to seizure activity). Obtain IV access and take bloods.

DISABILITY

- Attempt to assess the patient's conscious level using either AVPU (is the patient Alert? If not, do they respond to Verbal or Painful stimuli? Or are they Unresponsive?) or the GCS. Check bedside glucose levels.

'The patient is actively seizing and it is therefore difficult to assess the GCS. The pupils are equal and reactive to light and the blood glucose is 5.1 mmol/L.'

- It is important not to miss hypoglycaemia as a cause of seizures as it is easily treatable. Beware in those with malnutrition or individuals with alcohol use disorder that IV glucose can precipitate Wernicke's encephalopathy in the presence of thiamine deficiency—therefore, give IV thiamine at the same time if this is suspected.
- Once the patient has stopped seizing, it will be important to perform a full neurological examination to look for any deficits. Be aware, however, that following a seizure, patients can have a Todd's paresis—transient focal arm or leg weakness that occurs after a seizure.
- Ask the nursing staff to start the patient on neurological observations. Check pupil sizes and reactions.

EXPOSURE

- Expose the patient and in particular look for any evidence of rash that may indicate the underlying cause, e.g. petechial rash in meningococcal septicaemia, shingles associated with viral encephalitis. Examine for any obvious signs of injury.
- Measure the temperature. Examine the abdomen if possible to exclude any pathology.

'The temperature is 37.6°C; examination is otherwise unremarkable.'

INITIAL INVESTIGATIONS

- **Bloods:** FBC, U&Es, LFTs, glucose, CRP, calcium, magnesium and clotting. Look for evidence of infection or electrolyte abnormality that could have precipitated the seizure (Table 5.3). Note that the white blood cell count will often go up secondary to a seizure in and of itself. Consider sending toxicology screen and measure drug levels if the patient is known to be taking antiepileptic medications. If the patient is a woman of child-bearing potential, send beta-human chorionic gonadotropin (β-hCG) levels or perform a urinary pregnancy test after the seizure has terminated. If pregnancy is strongly suspected, perform an emergency ultrasound or auscultate for a fetal heart: eclampsia usually does not occur until about 20 weeks of pregnancy so evidence of a baby should be present!
- **Blood cultures:** Infection can precipitate seizures in those with epilepsy or be the primary cause; therefore blood cultures should be taken. If the

temperature is elevated this may not always be due to infection as seizures themselves can lead to a rise in body temperature.

- **ABG:** Perform an ABG if possible; otherwise, a venous blood gas can be taken at the same time as cannulation. In particular, check for hypoxia and hyponatraemia and confirm normal glucose levels. Most blood gas machines will also analyse carboxyhaemoglobin levels, although carbon monoxide poisoning is a very rare cause of seizures (Table 5.3).
- **Respiratory and cardiac monitoring:** Arrange for continuous monitoring of BP, oxygen saturations and electrocardiogram (ECG) tracing (to exclude arrhythmia). It is important to monitor for hypoxia during a seizure as well as changes in the pulse and BP. Some of the medications given to terminate seizures (e.g. phenytoin) can lead to arrhythmias and therefore continuous cardiac monitoring is required if these are given.

'Bloods show a raised white cell count but are otherwise normal, including the arterial blood gas.'

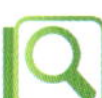

Status Epilepticus

A seizure lasting for more than 30 minutes or repeated seizures over 30 minutes with little or no recovery of consciousness between seizures

INITIAL MANAGEMENT

Management of Seizures

- Resuscitate using an ABCDE approach
- Oxygen
- Recovery position
- Consider reversible causes, e.g. hypoglycaemia
- Benzodiazepines

- **Airway support:** Place in the recovery position, perform airway manoeuvres as needed and insert a nasopharyngeal airway. Consider intubation if needed.
- **High-flow oxygen.**
- **Check blood glucose.**
- **Obtain IV access and perform ABG** (or venous gas if ABG not possible).
- **Terminating the seizure:** Many seizures self terminate without intervention; however, if the seizure is prolonged (i.e. greater than 5 minutes), treatment should be given to prevent hypoxic brain injury. In reality, if the patient hasn't stopped seizing by the time you have performed all of the previous steps, 5 minutes is likely to have passed and you should give medication to terminate the seizure:
  - The initial choice is a benzodiazepine, e.g. lorazepam 4 mg IV (as a slow injection over 2 minutes). Be aware that benzodiazepines can cause respiratory depression so have resuscitation equipment available in case it is needed. If it is not possible to obtain IV access then diazepam 10 mg can be given rectally or midazolam 10 mg buccally.
- **Consider reversible causes:**
  - The blood glucose should have already been checked and hypoglycaemia corrected.
  - In all individuals with alcohol use disorder and those who are malnourished, consider thiamine deficiency and give replacement with IV thiamine, e.g. Pabrinex IV High Potency Injection (ampoules 1 and 2) IV.
  - If the patient is pregnant, check the BP and consider eclampsia. Call for senior help immediately and contact the obstetric registrar on call. Following senior advice, treatment would consist of magnesium sulphate 4 g in 100 mL sodium chloride 0.9% given over 5 minutes with continuous respiratory and cardiac monitoring.
- **Prolonged seizures:**
  - If after 10 minutes the patient is still seizing, then repeat the same dose of benzodiazepine.
  - If despite two doses of benzodiazepines the patient continues to seize, load with phenytoin 20 mg/kg or levetiracetam 60 mg/kg (max dose 4500 mg) intravenously. Phenytoin should be given through a large-bore IV cannula followed by a flush of sodium chloride 0.9% as it can cause venous irritation. It is given at a maximum rate of 50 mg/min. It is diluted in sodium chloride 0.9% and the concentration should not exceed 10 mg/mL—therefore, usually doses of 1000 mg or less are made up in 100 mL, and doses above 1000 mg in 250 mL of 0.9% saline. Continuous monitoring of observations and ECG is necessary during phenytoin infusion and the infusion should be slowed or stopped if there is a fall in BP or arrhythmias develop.

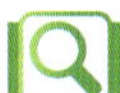

Example Prescription of Phenytoin

Patient weight = 50 kg
Dose of phenytoin is 20 mg/kg 20 × 50 = 1000 mg as phenytoin dose

Calculate how much sodium chloride 0.9% to put the 1000 mg phenytoin in:
Maximum safe concentration of phenytoin is 10 mg/mL
Therefore, to achieve this, divide the total dose of phenytoin (1000 mg) by 10
This gives 100 mL as volume of sodium chloride 0.9% diluent

Calculate the rate of the phenytoin infusion:
Maximum rate is 50 mg of phenytoin/min
Therefore, to achieve this, divide total dose of phenytoin (1000 mg) by 50
This gives 20 minutes as the minimum duration of infusion
This needs to be converted to mL/min:
If you are giving the total dose (1000 mg) over 20 minutes, this is equivalent to giving 100 mL of the infusion over 20 minutes. Therefore, the rate of infusion in mL/min is 100/20 = 5 mL/min.

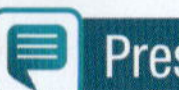

Prescribe (see Figs 5.4–5.6)

Benzodiazepine:

- LORAZEPAM 4 mg IV STAT. (Prescribe a second dose if the seizure has not terminated.)

If the patient continues to seize despite two doses of benzodiazepine:

- PHENYTOIN SODIUM 1000 mg in 100 mL SODIUM CHLORIDE 0.9%, at a rate of 5 mL/min (50 mg/min PHENYTOIN/MIN)

If the patient still continues to seize, senior help should already be present and expert advice is required. The patient should be transferred to intensive care for general anaesthesia. Agents used include propofol, midazolam or thiopental.

STOP

Oxygen prescription

REASSESSMENT ONCE THE SEIZURE HAS STOPPED

'The patient is given 4 mg lorazepam stat and a further 4 mg after 10 minutes but continues to seize. She is therefore loaded with phenytoin and subsequently stops seizing. Oxygen saturations are now 100% on air. A full history and examination can now be performed.'

- Usually, either spontaneously or after the measures described earlier, the patient will stop seizing. Your priorities now are to assess the patient post-seizure, investigate for an underlying cause and prevent further seizures.
- Assessment of a patient following a seizure serves three roles:
    - Assessment for harm during the seizure (e.g. injury, aspiration pneumonia)
    - Determination of the underlying cause of the seizure
    - Assessment of neurological recovery
- In the immediate period following a seizure, the patient may be confused and drowsy (particularly if given benzodiazepines) or have a focal neurological deficit (Todd's paresis). These should all improve with time—a persisting focal neurological deficit may suggest an underlying cause for the seizure (e.g. intracranial tumour).
- Perform a repeat ABCDE assessment, full neurological examination and repeat set of observations. Consider a chest radiography (CXR) if there is concern of aspiration pneumonia. When the patient is more alert, a full history should be taken.
- Further investigations to elucidate the cause of the seizure may include:
    - LP
    - CT head
    - EEG
- Ask the nursing staff to start the patient on a seizure chart and make sure the patient is located on the ward in an area that is clearly visible, e.g. next to the nurses' station. They will need regular neurological observations (pulse, BP, pupil diameter and reactivity, GCS, respiratory rate, temperature).
- Discuss the patient with your senior and decide if prophylaxis against further seizures is required.
- Assess the thromboprophylaxis risk: if there are any concerns regarding an intracranial bleed then avoid pharmacological intervention, but for the purpose of the drug charts here, we'll assume there are no concerns.

Table 5.3 Ms Wall's Blood and ABG Test Results

PARAMETER	VALUE	NORMAL RANGE (UNITS)
WCC	**15 × 10^9/L**	**4–11 (×10^9/L)**
Neutrophil	**8 × 10^9/L**	**2–7.5 (×10^9/L)**
Lymphocyte	**5 × 10^9/L**	**1.4–4 (×10^9/L)**
Platelet	200 × 10^9/L	150–400 (×10^9/L)
Haemoglobin	140 g/L	Men: 135–177 (g/L) Women: 115–155 (g/L)
PT	12 seconds	11.5–13.5 seconds
APTT	30 seconds	26–37 seconds
CRP	3 mg/L	0–5 (mg/L)
Urea	6 mmol/L	2.5–6.7 (mmol/L)
Creatinine	100 µmol/L	79–118 (µmol/L)
Sodium	140 mmol/L	135–146 (mmol/L)
Potassium	4 mmol/L	3.5–5.0 (mmol/L)
eGFR	>60 mL/min	>60 (mL/min)
Bilirubin	10 µmol/L	<17 (µmol/L)
ALT	14 IU/L	<40 (IU/L)
ALP	110 IU/L	39–117 (IU/L)
Glucose	5 mmol/L	4.5–5.6 (mmol/L) (fasting)
Calcium	2.23 mmol/L	2.20–2.67 (mmol/L)
Magnesium	1 mmol/L	0.7–1.1 (mmol/L)
pH	7.40	7.35–7.45
PaO_2	12.0 kPa on air	10.6–13.3 (kPa) on air
$PaCO_2$	5.0 kPa	4.8–6.1 (kPa)
HCO_3	24 mmol/L	22-26 (mmol/L)

Data in bold signifies results that are outside the normal laboratory range.
ABG, Arterial blood gas; *ALP*, alkaline phosphatase; *ALT*, alanine transaminase; *APTT*, activated partial thromboplastin time; *CRP*, C-reactive protein; *eGFR*, estimated glomerular filtration rate; *PT*, prothrombin time; *WCC*, white cell count.

PHENYTOIN THERAPY

- Following loading, a maintenance dose of phenytoin 100 mg TDS IV should be continued unless otherwise instructed. The first maintenance dose should be given 8 hours after the loading dose.
- There is no agreed consensus on when plasma-phenytoin concentration should be measured, and how the measurements should be interpreted.
- If a patient's seizure terminates after commencing phenytoin and they are exhibiting no signs of phenytoin toxicity, measuring phenytoin concentration has limited value.
- If the patient has further seizures after they have been loaded with phenytoin, then you should seek advice. Total plasma-phenytoin concentration is

usually checked at 24 hours after the loading dose and should be in the range of 10 to 20 mg/L. This can help guide whether a change of phenytoin dose is needed (if level is low) or if an alternative anticonvulsant will be required (if level is therapeutic).

- Remember to always interpret blood results in the clinical context (i.e. whether the patient is still having seizures and if there are any signs of toxicity). Be aware that small changes in the regular dose of phenytoin can cause large fluctuations in levels due to its zero-order pharmacokinetics. Cautious interpretation of total plasma-phenytoin concentration is also necessary in pregnancy, the elderly and certain disease states where protein binding may be reduced.
- Be aware that phenytoin exists mainly bound to albumin in plasma and therefore concentration will need to be adjusted depending on patient albumin levels. Phenytoin concentration can also be affected by significant renal impairment.
- Phenytoin levels can also be altered by many different medications and phenytoin itself is a CYP450 enzyme inducer and can therefore alter levels of other medications, e.g. warfarin.
- In view of the need for monitoring levels, various side effects and narrow therapeutic index, phenytoin is infrequently used in the long-term treatment of epilepsy but is an effective short-term treatment for prolonged seizures.
- Give advice to patients who drive that following a generalised seizure they should inform the Driver and Vehicle Licensing Agency (DVLA) and stop driving.

Prescribe (see Figs 5.4–5.6)

PHENYTOIN SODIUM 100 mg TDS IV Thromboprophylaxis:

- DALTEPARIN 5000 units SC OD

HANDING OVER THE PATIENT

'Lucy is a 37-year-old female who was admitted with a seizure.

She presented with a generalised tonic–clonic seizure which had been ongoing for 10 minutes. A nasopharyngeal airway was inserted and the airway was subsequently maintained. Initial treatment with lorazepam 4 mg IV given twice 10 minutes apart was not successful and she was therefore loaded with phenytoin 1 g intravenously.

Following phenytoin therapy, the seizure terminated and Lucy is now alert with a GCS of 15/15. There are no signs of injury and neurological examination is unremarkable.

At present, she remains on regular phenytoin therapy while awaiting review by the neurologist. A full set of bloods has been sent and are awaited but no further investigations are planned at present.'

STATION 5.3: SUBARACHNOID HAEMORRHAGE

William, a 67-year-old man, presents to the emergency department with a severe occipital headache. He reports that it came on suddenly an hour ago and is the worst headache he has ever had. While waiting to be assessed he has vomited twice. Please assess him and instigate appropriate management.

Patient Details

Name:	William Clark
DOB:	17/03/57
Hospital number:	H3742491
Weight:	80 kg
Height:	1.8 m
Consultant:	Dr Epp
Hospital/Ward:	SGH Neurology
Current medications:	Nil
Allergies:	Nil
Admission date:	12/10/24

Differential Diagnosis of Acute Headache

- Subarachnoid haemorrhage
- Meningitis
- Migraine
- Temporal arteritis
- Trigeminal neuralgia
- Cluster headache
- Tension headache
- Cerebral venous thrombosis

Complications of Subarachnoid Haemorrhage

- Rebleeding
- Vasospasm
- Hyponatraemia
- Hydrocephalus
- Epilepsy
- Cognitive and psychological impairment

INITIAL ASSESSMENT

AIRWAY

- Is the airway patent? Is there any vomit that could be obstructing the airway?

  'The patient is alert and talking, confirming that the airway is patent.'

The patient is able to talk to you, which confirms that the airway is patent and unobstructed. In cases of severe subarachnoid haemorrhage, patients can present with drowsiness or even coma. In such cases, assess the airway and use airway manoeuvres or adjuncts as necessary. If the GCS is less than 8, then intubation must be considered. Patients with subarachnoid haemorrhage can deteriorate rapidly, e.g. in the case of cerebral rebleeding, so always consider intubation early if the GCS begins to fall.

BREATHING

- Assess respiratory rate, oxygen saturations and any signs of respiratory distress, e.g. accessory muscle use. Auscultate for air entry and additional sounds of wheeze or crepitations.

'The respiratory rate is 18/min, oxygen saturations are 98% on air. The patient is breathing comfortably at rest and the lung fields are clear to auscultation.

There are no signs of respiratory distress and the oxygen saturations are normal; therefore, oxygen is not required. If the patient has been vomiting, make sure you exclude aspiration pneumonia, particularly if the GCS is reduced or if there have been seizures.

CIRCULATION

- Assess circulatory status by measuring pulse, BP and CRT.
- Perform a focused CVS examination. Assess the central pulse and JVP. Auscultate for heart sounds and any additional murmurs.
- Examine for evidence of peripheral oedema.

'The pulse is regular at 105 bpm, BP 135/90 mmHg and CRT is 2 seconds peripherally. The JVP is not elevated and heart sounds are normal with no murmurs. There is no evidence of peripheral oedema.'

Obtain IV access and take bloods. The BP is normal. Antihypertensive therapy may be considered if the BP is significantly elevated; however, this would only be on the advice of a specialist. A high BP may increase the risk of rebleeding but drops in BP can lead to a reduction in cerebral perfusion. If you are unsure, discuss the patient with your senior. If BP control is required, short-acting IV agents such labetalol are preferable.

DISABILITY

- Assess the patient's conscious level using the GCS. Ask the nursing staff to start the patient on neurological observations. Check pupil sizes and reaction. Check bedside glucose levels.

'The patient is alert with a GCS of 15/15 (E4, V5, M6). The pupils are equal and reactive to light and the blood glucose is 4.6 mmol/L.'

After initial assessment, a full neurological examination is required to assess for any focal signs. Fundoscopy should be performed to look for retinal haemorrhages (suggesting significant hypertension) or papilloedema suggesting raised intracranial pressure. The presence of focal neurology or reduced GCS is associated with a worse outcome in subarachnoid haemorrhage and the severity of subarachnoid haemorrhage can be graded using various different scoring systems, for example the Hunt and Hess scale (Box 5.1).

Box 5.1 Hunt and Hess Scale—A Predictor of Outcome in Subarachnoid Haemorrhage

Grade	Description
Grade 1	Mild headache, minimal neck stiffness
Grade 2	Neck stiffness, no neurological deficit except cranial nerve palsies
Grade 3	Drowsiness with mild focal neurological deficit
Grade 4	Drowsiness with significant neurological deficit, e.g. hemiplegia
Grade 5	Coma

EXPOSURE

- Expose the patient and examine for any rash (as the differential diagnosis of headache and vomiting must include meningitis). Examine for neck stiffness and Kernig's sign.
- Examine for any bleeding or bruising which may suggest underlying coagulopathy.
- Measure the temperature and examine the abdomen—patients with polycystic kidney disease have an increased risk of subarachnoid haemorrhage, so pay attention for bilaterally enlarged kidneys.

'The temperature is 37.0°C and there is neck stiffness. Examination is otherwise unremarkable.'

INITIAL INVESTIGATIONS

- **CT head:** This is the key initial investigation that should be performed urgently in all patients with a suspected diagnosis of subarachnoid haemorrhage. CT scanning within the first 12 hours has a sensitivity of 98% to 100%. The sensitivity declines, however, with delay from the initial event to imaging. CT imaging will also demonstrate if there are any contraindications to LP, e.g. intracranial mass, hydrocephalus or signs of mass effect.
- **Bloods:** FBC, U&Es, LFTs, CRP, clotting and group and save. Look for evidence of infection and ensure that the platelets and clotting are normal. Send a group and save as the patient may need to go for major surgery or be given blood products, e.g. platelets (Table 5.4).
- **Blood cultures and meningococcal PCR:** If the history is not definite for subarachnoid haemorrhage and you are considering meningitis.
- **LP:**
  - If the CT scan is normal, then an LP should be performed at least 12 hours after the onset of symptoms to exclude a subarachnoid haemorrhage.
  - Ensure that the platelets and clotting are normal prior to LP and consent the patient if they are able to.
  - Measure the opening pressure using a manometer (normal <25 cmH_2O).
  - Send the first and third bottles of cerebrospinal fluid (CSF) for microscopy, culture and

Table 5.4 Mr Clark's Blood Results

PARAMETER	VALUE	NORMAL RANGE (UNITS)
WCC	10 × 10^9/L	4–11 (×10^9/L)
Neutrophil	7 × 10^9/L	2–7.5 (×10^9/L)
Lymphocyte	4 × 10^9/L	1.4–4 (×10^9/L)
Platelet	200 × 10^9/L	150–400 (×10^9/L)
Haemoglobin	140 g/L	Men: 135–177 (g/L) Women: 115–155 (g/L)
PT	12 seconds	11.5–13.5 seconds
APTT	30 seconds	26–37 seconds
CRP	3 mg/L	0–5 (mg/L)
Urea	6 mmol/L	2.5–6.7 (mmol/L)
Creatinine	100 µmol/L	79–118 (µmol/L)
Sodium	140 mmol/L	135–146 (mmol/L)
Potassium	4 mmol/L	3.5–5.0 (mmol/L)
eGFR	>60 mL/min	>60 (mL/min)
Bilirubin	10 µmol/L	<17 (µmol/L)
ALT	20 IU/L	<40 (IU/L)
ALP	50 IU/L	39–117 (IU/L)

ALP, Alkaline phosphatase; *ALT,* alanine transaminase; *APTT,* activated partial thromboplastin time; *CRP,* C-reactive protein; *eGFR,* estimated glomerular filtration rate; *PT,* prothrombin time; *WCC,* white cell count.

sensitivity. Pay particular attention to the red cell count which, when elevated, may indicate the presence of blood in the CSF. Unfortunately, if the LP is traumatic, this will also cause the red cell count to be elevated. The first and third bottles can be compared, and if there are significantly less red cells in the third bottle, this suggests a traumatic tap. In reality, however, this technique is unreliable and unless there are no detectable red cells, you should base your diagnosis on the results of analysis for xanthochromia (see later).
- Send the second bottle for biochemistry (protein and glucose) and send a paired serum glucose.
- Most importantly, send the fourth bottle for examination for xanthochromia (CSF bilirubin) and send a paired serum sample for xanthochromia. When elevated, the presence of xanthochromia (or specifically bilirubin) indicates the breakdown of red blood cells in the CSF and is not affected by a traumatic tap. Note that if LP is performed before 12 hours, the red cells in the CSF may not have broken down and xanthochromia will not be present, giving a false-negative result—therefore, LP should be delayed until at least 12 hours after the onset of symptoms.

- **ECG:** An ECG should be performed on admission, which may show evidence of left ventricular hypertrophy suggesting longstanding hypertension (a risk factor for subarachnoid haemorrhage). Be aware that a significant number of patients with subarachnoid haemorrhage can have associated ECG abnormalities, such as T-wave inversion and ST changes. In such cases, it is useful to clarify if there has been any cardiac sounding chest pain and to compare old ECGs. Check cardiac enzymes and if there are any concerns you should discuss the patient with your senior or the cardiology registrar on call. The patient may need an echocardiogram to look for regional wall motion abnormalities or left ventricular systolic dysfunction. Do not give any antiplatelet or anticoagulant therapy as this will worsen cerebral bleeding.

'Initial bloods, CT head and ECG are normal.'

INITIAL MANAGEMENT

Management of Subarachnoid Haemorrhage

- Resuscitate using an ABCDE approach
- Treat any correctable coagulopathy
- CT head ± LP if CT negative
- Analgesia and antiemetics
- Nimodipine (to prevent vasospasm)
- IV fluids
- Neurosurgical intervention for aneurysms

- **Airway support:** Examine the airway and consider airway manoeuvres or adjuncts as necessary. Contact the on-call anaesthetist if intubation is required.
- **Obtain IV access and send bloods.**
- **Treat any correctable coagulopathy:** Contact your senior or the haematologist on call as soon as possible in any of the following:
  - If the platelet count is low
  - If the patient has been taking antiplatelet agents, e.g. aspirin, clopidogrel, prasugrel
  - If the clotting is deranged, e.g. raised international normalised ratio (INR) or activated partial thromboplastin time (APTT)
  - If there is a prior history of coagulopathy, e.g. haemophilia
- Caution may be required if the patient has a coronary artery stent, a metallic heart valve or a recent thrombosis. Expert advice from haematology is imperative to ensure optimal management.
- **Bed rest:** Keep the patient on bed rest to prevent fluctuations in BP and reduce the risk of rebleeding.
- **Analgesia:** Start with paracetamol (1 g PO QDS) and codeine phosphate (30–60 mg PO QDS). Do not give aspirin or non-steroidal antiinflammatory drugs such as ibuprofen (these will affect platelet function and may worsen bleeding). If the patient is still in pain, stronger opioids such as short-acting liquid morphine may be used with significant caution (due to the risks of causing additional confusion, vomiting and drowsiness).
- **Antiemetics:** Patients with subarachnoid haemorrhage may have significant nausea and vomiting which should be treated promptly to also avoid fluctuations in BP. Consider using metoclopramide 10 mg TDS (avoid in young people and those with Parkinson's

disease), cyclizine 50 mg TDS or ondansetron 4 mg TDS; all of these can be given orally or intravenously.

- **Venous thromboembolism (VTE) prophylaxis:** The patient cannot have LMWH so prescribe thromboembolic deterrent stockings.
- **Neurological observations:** Arrange hourly neurological observations to ensure that any deterioration in neurology is promptly identified as urgent neurosurgery may be required.
- **Neurosurgical advice:** If the patient has a reduced GCS or focal neurological deficit on admission, discuss the patient with your senior immediately and contact the local neurosurgical centre for advice.

Prescribe (Figs **5.7–5.9)**

Analgesia:
- PARACETAMOL 1 g PO STAT then QDS CODEINE PHOSPHATE 60 mg PO STAT then QDS

Antiemetic:
- METOCLOPROMIDE 10 mg PO STAT then TDS

Thromboprophylaxis:
- TED STOCKINGS TOP CONTINUOUS

FURTHER MANAGEMENT

'William is initially given analgesia and antiemetics and his headache improves. Blood testing is unremarkable with normal platelets and clotting. A CT head shows no evidence of cerebral haemorrhage. A lumbar puncture is subsequently performed at 12 hours which confirms an elevated CSF red cell count and the presence of xanthochromia.'

- The LP findings are consistent with subarachnoid haemorrhage. You should inform your senior and contact the local neurosurgical centre for advice and consideration of transfer for further investigation and treatment.
- The patient should be started on nimodipine 60 mg orally 4-hourly to reduce cerebral vasospasm, one of the complications of subarachnoid haemorrhage—it is usually given for 21 days in total.

Prescribe (see Figs **5.7–5.9)**

NIMODIPINE 60 mg PO STAT then 4 HOURLY

'The neurosurgical team is contacted and advises starting nimodipine 60 mg every 4 hours. Transfer is arranged to the nearest neurosurgical centre.'

- Cerebral aneurysms can be treated with either surgical clipping or endovascular coiling to prevent rebleeding.

MONITORING FOR COMPLICATIONS

- Following a subarachnoid haemorrhage, patients are usually cared for in a specialist neurosurgical centre. There are a number of potential complications that can occur following a subarachnoid haemorrhage.
- Cerebral rebleeding usually presents with rapid neurological deterioration with pupillary involvement (e.g. an unreactive, dilated pupil). The neurosurgical registrar should be contacted immediately as the patient may need urgent surgery or intubation and transfer to neurosurgical intensive care.
- Hydrocephalus can develop following subarachnoid haemorrhage due to interruption in the drainage of CSF. Patients usually deteriorate over hours with symptoms of headache, blurred vision and vomiting. The patient may require temporary or permanent diversion of CSF with a shunt or ventriculostomy.
- Cerebral vasospasm (or delayed cerebral ischaemia) can occur days after subarachnoid haemorrhage. It presents with focal neurological deficits, headache and reduced GCS. It is thought that the blood in subarachnoid haemorrhage irritates the walls of cerebral vessels leading to spasm and impairment of blood flow. The risk of vasospasm can be reduced by using nimodipine (as described earlier) and maintaining a good fluid intake.
- Patients with subarachnoid haemorrhage can develop abnormalities of sodium balance and subsequent hyponatraemia. Central salt wasting mediated by release of natriuretic factors can lead to excessive renal salt excretion and subsequent hypovolaemia and hyponatraemia. Because of this, sodium levels should be monitored daily in the period following subarachnoid haemorrhage and fluid balance documented.

FLUID PRESCRIBING IN PATIENTS WITH SUBARACHNOID HAEMORRHAGE

- To reduce the risk of cerebral vasospasm, patients with subarachnoid haemorrhage are often given IV fluids after their aneurysm is secured. Some centres advocate maintaining 3 L total volume intake, although evidence is lacking and others advise maintaining a state of euvolaemia. You should take advice from your local neurosurgical centre. Particular caution should be taken in the elderly and those with heart failure in whom excess IV fluids could precipitate pulmonary oedema.
- The IV fluid predominantly used is sodium chloride 0.9%. Other fluids such as glucose saline, glucose and Hartmann's solution are generally avoided because they are hypotonic and can therefore cause cerebral oedema due to their effects on serum osmolality.
- IV glucose should be avoided in any form of neurological injury as it can increase tissue acidosis in areas of ischaemia and increase neurological damage.

- U&E should be monitored daily in the immediate period following subarachnoid haemorrhage as well as fluid balance and the patient's weight to guide fluid prescription.

'Due to nausea, fluid intake is poor (approximately 1000 mL per day) and the patient is therefore prescribed 2 L of sodium chloride 0.9% over 24 hours to make a total input of 3 L per day; 60 mmol of KCl is added to fluids to meet daily requirements. U&Es are to be checked daily.'

Prescribe (see Figs 5.7–5.9)

SODIUM CHLORIDE 0.9% 1 L with 20 mmol KCl IV at 83 mL/h
SODIUM CHLORIDE 0.9% 1 L with 40 mmol KCl IV at 83 mL/h

HANDING OVER THE PATIENT

'William is a 67-year-old male with subarachnoid haemorrhage.

He initially presented with a severe sudden onset headache and vomiting. Neurological examination revealed a GCS of 15/15 and no focal neurological deficit. Initial CT head scan did not reveal any evidence of cerebral haemorrhage; however, lumbar puncture showed an elevated red cell count and the presence of xanthochromia, confirming the diagnosis. His headache has responded to analgesia and neurologically he has remained stable with a GCS of 15 and no focal deficits. He has been started on IV oral maintenance fluids because of poor oral fluid intake because of nausea.

Following discussion with the neurosurgeons he has been started on oral nimodipine and is due for transfer to the regional neurosurgical centre for further investigation and intervention.'

Under the care of the neurosurgical team, William undergoes CT cerebral angiography which confirms the presence of an aneurysm. He is taken to theatre and the aneurysm is successfully clipped.

STATION 5.4: ISCHAEMIC STROKE

You are on call in the emergency department when a 62-year-old man, Bernard, is brought in by ambulance with right-sided weakness, facial droop and difficulty getting his words out. His wife, who accompanies him, reports that he was completely normal the night before but awoke this morning with abnormal speech and right-sided weakness. Please assess him and instigate appropriate management.

Patient Details

Name:	Bernard White
DOB:	22/04/62
Hospital number:	W39203751
Weight:	78 kg
Height:	1.7 m
Consultant:	Dr Epp
Hospital/Ward:	SGH Neurology
Current medications:	Nil
Allergies:	Nil
Admission date:	12/10/24

Causes of Stroke

- Embolic stroke (often thrombi but may be fat or septic emboli)
- Thrombotic stroke (usually related to atherosclerosis)
- Haemorrhagic stroke (often related cerebral aneurysms, uncontrolled hypertension or arteriovenous malformations)
- Venous thrombosis (e.g. cerebral venous sinus thrombosis)
- Cerebral hypoperfusion (e.g. secondary to sepsis or heart failure)

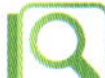
Complications of Stroke

- Muscle weakness/numbness
- Incontinence
- Speech/visual/hearing deficit
- Apraxia
- Poor swallow/aspiration pneumonia
- Psychological disturbance including depression
- Dementia
- Seizures

INITIAL ASSESSMENT

AIRWAY

- Assess patency of the airway. Is there any stridor or noisy breathing? Is there excess saliva or drooling to suggest swallowing difficulty? Is the patient conscious enough to maintain a safe airway?

'The airway is patent with no obstruction. The patient is alert and is maintaining his airway.'

You should consider dysphasia in all patients with suspected stroke and the risks of aspiration pneumonia. If there any concerns over safety of swallowing, place the patient nil by mouth until a swallowing assessment has been performed by either a trained nurse or the speech and language team.

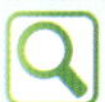
Up to 50% of acute stroke patients have some degree of dysphagia in the initial 72 hours following a stroke.

BREATHING

- Assess respiratory rate, oxygen saturations and accessory muscle use. Auscultate for air entry and additional sounds of wheeze or crepitations.

'The respiratory rate is 20/min and oxygen saturations are 98%. There are no signs of respiratory distress. The lung fields are clear.'

The patient is comfortable with normal oxygen saturations—supplementary oxygen is therefore not required. Pay attention for any signs of an aspiration pneumonia if the patient has dysphagia or respiratory signs and order a chest X-ray.

CIRCULATION

- Assess circulatory status by measuring pulse, BP and CRT.
- Perform a CVS examination. Assess the JVP and central pulse. Auscultate for heart sounds, additional murmurs and carotid bruits. Examine for evidence of peripheral oedema.
- Pay particular attention to the patient's pulse—is it regular or irregular? Remember that atrial fibrillation can predispose to stroke and future management will differ if the patient is in atrial fibrillation. Also listen carefully to the heart sounds for evidence of a metallic heart valve, a potential source of emboli.
- If the BP is significantly elevated in an acute stroke, antihypertensive treatment may need to be given (e.g. prior to thrombolysis); however, this would be a senior decision.

'The pulse is regular at 80 bpm, BP 125/70 mmHg and CRT is 1.5 seconds peripherally. The JVP is not visible and heart sounds are normal with no murmurs. There is no evidence of peripheral oedema.'

- The patient's observations are stable with a normal CVS examination.
- Obtain IV access and take bloods. If you have placed the patient nil by mouth, start them on maintenance IV fluids.

DISABILITY

- Assess the patient's conscious level using the GCS. Ask the nursing staff to start the patient on hourly neurological observations. Check pupil sizes and reactions. Check bedside glucose levels.
- Significant hypoglycaemia (and rarely hyperglycaemia) can cause symptoms mimicking a stroke. Therefore, ensure that a blood glucose level is checked in all patients with suspected stroke and correct abnormalities as necessary.
- A full neurological examination is required to assess for any focal neurological deficit. Examine the cranial nerves, upper and lower limbs. When checking cranial nerves, do not forget to examine for visual inattention, the visual fields and speech as well as for cerebellar signs.
- The stroke territory can be identified using the Oxford Stroke Classification (Box 5.2). This classification is also useful in predicting prognosis following a stroke.

'The patient is alert with a GCS of 14/15 (E 4, V 4, M 6). The pupils are equal and reactive to light and the blood glucose is 5.2 mmol/L. Cranial nerve examination reveals mixed (expressive and receptive) dysphasia, right homonymous hemianopia and right-sided upper motor neuron facial nerve palsy. In the limbs, there is right-sided hemiparesis and right-sided sensory loss. These findings are consistent with a left total anterior circulation infarct.'

Box 5.2 Oxford Stroke Classification (Also Known as Bamford Classification)

TOTAL ANTERIOR CIRCULATION INFARCT

Significant infarction in the territory of the middle and anterior cerebral arteries. Characterised by all of the following:

- Unilateral weakness and/or sensory deficit of at least two of the following: face, arm and leg
- Homonymous hemianopia
- Higher cortical dysfunction (e.g. dysphasia, dyscalculia, sensory neglect)

PARTIAL ANTERIOR CIRCULATION INFARCT

Infarction affecting part of the middle and anterior cerebral artery territory. Characterised by only two of the three criteria for total anterior circulation infarct, higher cerebral dysfunction alone or with a limited motor/sensory deficit (e.g. confined to one limb, or face and hand but not whole arm)

POSTERIOR CIRCULATION INFARCT

Infarction of the territory supplied by the posterior cerebral artery and vertebrobasilar arterial system causing any of the following:

- Cerebellar signs (without ipsilateral long tract deficit)
- Bilateral motor and/or sensory deficits
- Ipsilateral cranial nerve palsy with contralateral motor and/or sensory deficit
- Disorders of conjugate eye movement
- Isolated homonymous hemianopia

LACUNAR INFARCT

Subcortical infarction in the territory of deep penetrating arteries characterised by one of the following:

- Pure motor deficit
- Pure sensory deficit
- Sensorimotor deficit
- Ataxic hemiparesis
- Dysarthria/clumsy hand

EXPOSURE

- Expose the patient and examine for rashes or other abnormality. Measure the temperature and examine the abdomen to exclude any pathology.

'Temperature is 37.5°C and examination is otherwise normal.'

INITIAL INVESTIGATIONS

- **Bloods:** FBC, U&Es, LFTs, glucose, clotting, CRP, erythrocyte sedimentation rate (ESR), lipids. Pay attention to the FBC for any evidence of polycythaemia or thrombocythaemia which may predispose to stroke. Thrombocytopaenia or clotting abnormalities are important not to miss in the case of cerebral haemorrhage. Check U&Es to guide fluid management. Check lipids (risk factor for stroke) and LFTs in anticipation of starting statin therapy. Check CRP for evidence of infection, and if the ESR is raised, consider a vasculitis such as temporal arteritis (Table 5.5).
- **ECG:** Atrial fibrillation is a risk factor for stroke and therefore an ECG should be performed in all patients presenting with an acute stroke.
- **CXR:** A chest X-ray should also be performed in all patients with acute stroke. This may show evidence of aspiration pneumonia in those with dysphagia. Lung cancer may be seen on CXR associated with cerebral metastases. Otherwise, it is useful to have a baseline chest X-ray to compare to in the future.
- **CT head:** This should be done to confirm the diagnosis in all cases. It is important to exclude a haemorrhagic stroke if considering aspirin therapy. If thrombectomy might be indicated, perform CT contrast angiography (or CT/magnetic resonance (MR) perfusion imaging if beyond 6 hours of symptom onset) after the initial nonenhanced CT. Urgent CT scanning should be performed in any of the following situations:
  - The patient is suitable for thrombolysis or thrombectomy.
  - The patient is on anticoagulation.
  - There is a known bleeding tendency.
  - The patient's GCS is <13.
  - The patient has unexplained progressive or fluctuating symptoms.
  - The patient has papilloedema, neck stiffness or fever.
  - The patient experienced severe headache at onset of stroke symptoms.

'Bernard presents with symptoms and signs of a total anterior circulation infarct. The time of onset of symptoms is not known and the patient is therefore not suitable for thrombolysis. The patient is placed nil by mouth and maintenance intravenous fluids are started.'

'CT head scanning shows infarction in the territory of the left middle cerebral artery. There is no evidence of haemorrhage on the scan. The CT perfusion scan subsequently showed a large infarct core volume, so he was not eligible for thrombectomy. The time of onset of symptoms is not known and may extend to the previous night, so he is not eligible for thrombolysis. The patient is transferred to the acute stroke unit and started on aspirin 300 mg OD. A swallowing assessment reveals evidence of dysphagia and an NG tube is therefore inserted for feeding.'

Table 5.5 Mr White's Blood Results

PARAMETER	VALUE	NORMAL RANGE (UNITS)
WCC	10 × 10^9/L	4–11 (×10^9/L)
Neutrophil	7 × 10^9/L	2–7.5 (×10^9/L)
Lymphocyte	3 × 10^9/L	1.4–4 (×10^9/L)
Platelet	200 × 10^9/L	150–400 (×10^9/L)
Haemoglobin	140 g/L	Men: 135–177 (g/L) Women: 115–155 (g/L)
ESR	10 mm/h	<15 (mm/h)
PT	12 seconds	11.5–13.5 seconds
APTT	30 seconds	26–37 seconds
CRP	3 mg/L	0–5 (mg/L)
Urea	4 mmol/L	2.5–6.7 (mmol/L)
Creatinine	110 µmol/L	79–118 (µmol/L)
Sodium	140 mmol/L	135–146 (mmol/L)
Potassium	4.5 mmol/L	3.5–5.0 (mmol/L)
eGFR	>60 mL/min	>60 (mL/min)
Bilirubin	10 µmol/L	<17 (µmol/L)
ALT	20 IU/L	<40 (IU/L)
ALP	53 IU/L	39–117 (IU/L)
Total cholesterol	5 mmol/L	3.5–6.5 (mmol/L)
HDL cholesterol	1.2 mmol/L	Men: 0.8–1.8 (mmol/L) Women: 1.0–2.3 (mmol/L)
LDL cholesterol	2 mmol/L	<4.0 (mmol/L)
Glucose	5 mmol/L	4.5–5.6 (mmol/L) (fasting)

ALP, Alkaline phosphatase; *ALT,* alanine transaminase; *APTT,* activated partial thromboplastin time; *CRP,* C-reactive protein; *eGFR,* estimated glomerular filtration rate; *ESR,* erythrocyte sedimentation rate; *HDL,* high-density lipoprotein; *LDL,* low-density lipoprotein; *PT,* prothrombin time; *WCC,* white cell count.

INITIAL MANAGEMENT

Management of Stroke

- Resuscitate patient using an ABCDE approach
- Consider thrombolysis and mechanical thrombectomy
- CT head
- Cautious BP control
- Place patient NBM and assess swallow
- Aspirin if no evidence of bleeding
- Initiate secondary rehabilitation and secondary prevention

In patients with suspected stroke, when the time of onset is (a) *known* and (b) *within 4.5 hours*, thrombolysis should be considered. Each hospital usually has a stroke thrombolysis protocol which, when activated, results in a call being put out to either the stroke or medical registrar to attend the patient. In such a situation, the patient will need rapid assessment and urgent CT scanning before consideration of thrombolysis. More recently, mechanical thrombectomy for strokes has been more routinely used in select groups of patients depending on timing of presentation and the location and degree of infarction.

- **Airway support:** Support the airway using manoeuvres and adjuncts as necessary.
- **Supplementary oxygen:** Aim to maintain oxygen saturations above 94%.
- **Check blood glucose and correct hypoglycaemia.**
- **Place the patient nil by mouth:** A swallowing assessment should be performed by a trained healthcare professional in all patients with acute stroke. While awaiting this, start the patient on maintenance IV fluids. The daily fluid requirement for an adult is approximately 25–30 mL/kg per day. The patient's weight is 78 kg, so the daily fluid requirement using 30 ml/kg would be 2340 mL. Therefore, prescribe fluid at a rate of 100 mL/h and add potassium to meet the daily requirement of 60 mmol. Sodium chloride 0.9% is preferred initially to glucose 5%, which has the potential to worsen cerebral oedema and acute brain injury. Once a nasogastric (NG) tube is inserted, fluid boluses can be given down the tube and IV fluids stopped.
- **BP control:** In acute stroke, BP should only be controlled if the patient is to be thrombolysed or there is a hypertensive emergency with one or more of the following:
  - Hypertensive encephalopathy
  - Hypertensive nephropathy
  - Hypertensive cardiac failure/myocardial infarction
  - Aortic dissection
  - Preeclampsia/eclampsia
- **Consider thrombolysis:** In all patients presenting within 4.5 hours of acute stroke, thrombolysis should be considered. If this situation arises, contact your senior immediately for advice. Before thrombolysis can be delivered it must be ensured that there are no contraindications (Box 5.3). Patients should be consented if they are able to do so, otherwise a decision should be made in their best interests. Each hospital usually has a stroke thrombolysis protocol that should be followed. Once a CT has excluded any evidence of intracranial haemorrhage, thrombolysis can be administered. Alteplase (recombinant tissue plasminogen activator) is used at a dose of 900 micrograms/kg with a maximum dose of 90 mg. The initial 10% is administered as an IV bolus and the remaining 90% over 1 hour with close monitoring.
- **Consider thrombectomy:** In patients with acute ischaemic stroke presenting within 6 hours of symptoms onset, offer thrombectomy if there is occlusion of the proximal anterior circulation confirmed on CT angiography. In ischaemic stroke, patients presenting between 6 hours and 24 hours of symptom onset, offer thrombectomy if there is occlusion of the proximal anterior circulation with potential to salvage brain tissue (as evaluated by CT perfusion imaging). Consider thrombectomy up to 24 hours of symptom onset in those with proximal posterior circulation occlusion if there is potential to salvage brain tissue.
- **Thromboprophylaxis:** Avoid pharmacological treatment (due to risk of haemorrhagic transformation of the ischaemic territory) and compression stockings (due to risk of pressure ulcers). Instead, encourage early mobilisation and good hydration. Patients with immobility should be offered intermittent pneumatic compression devices.
- **Aspirin:** Once the CT has excluded any evidence of cerebral haemorrhage, the patient should be started on aspirin 300 mg OD. If the patient is nil by mouth, aspirin can be given via an NG tube (if already inserted because of dysphagia) or rectally.
- **Antiplatelet therapy:** Aspirin should continue at 300 mg for 2 weeks, after which decisions regarding long-term antiplatelet or anticoagulation can be made depending on what the patient was taking previously and if the patient has atrial fibrillation.

Prescribe (Figs 5.10–5.12)

Maintenance IV fluids:

- SODIUM CHLORIDE 0.9% 1 L with 20 mmol KCL IV at 100 mL/h then GLUCOSE 5% 1 L with 40 mmol KCL IV at 100 mL/h
- ASPIRIN 300 mg NG STAT then OD

FURTHER MANAGEMENT FOLLOWING AN ACUTE STROKE

- **Stroke unit:** Evidence has shown that patients cared for on a specialised stroke unit have a better outcome; therefore, all patients with an acute stroke should be cared for on a stroke unit where facilities such as physiotherapy, speech and language therapy and occupational therapy are provided.
- **Glycaemic control:** Aim to maintain blood glucose readings between 4 and 11 mmol/L. In patients with

Box 5.3 Potential Contraindications to Thrombolysis (Each Case Should Be Considered Individually)

- Intracranial haemorrhage (current or previous)
- Cerebral tumour, arteriovenous malformation (AVM), aneurysm or other abnormality on CT head
- Previous cerebral or spinal surgery
- Suspected subarachnoid haemorrhage (even if CT scan normal)
- Seizure at onset of symptoms
- Rapidly improving or minor neurological symptoms (risks outweigh benefits)
- Major trauma, cardiopulmonary resuscitation or surgery within 14 days
- Active internal bleeding
- Uncontrolled hypertension (BP >185/110 mmHg)
- Known bleeding disorder, abnormal clotting (INR >1.7) or low platelets (<100 × 10^9/L)
- Stroke, transient ischaemic attack (TIA) or serious head injury within 3 months
- Pregnancy
- Gastrointestinal or urinary tract haemorrhage in past 3 weeks
- Puncture of a noncompressible artery within the last 7 days
- Pericarditis or endocarditis
- Significant hypo- or hyperglycaemia (glucose <2.7 or >22 mmol/L)

diabetes, a sliding scale insulin and glucose infusion may be required to achieve normoglycaemia.

- **Statin therapy:** Statin therapy should be started at least 48 hours after an acute stroke as secondary prevention (unless there are contraindications, e.g. previous allergic reaction).
- **Nutrition:** All patients with dysphagia should have an NG tube placed for feeding and hydration. Patients who are able to swallow should have an assessment to estimate their risk of malnutrition (e.g. Malnutrition Universal Screening Tool) and receive nutritional support as necessary. Patients may need dietician assessment to ensure adequate nutritional intake if they are at risk of malnutrition.
- **Secondary prevention of future stroke:** Once a patient has recovered from a stroke, the emphasis should be on prevention of future stroke. Management includes antiplatelet and statin therapy in all patients and anticoagulation in patients with atrial fibrillation (after 2 weeks and provided the benefits outweigh the risks). Aim for optimum control of BP (current optimal systolic BP targets is <130 mmHg), diabetes and lipids (consider additional treatment if statin therapy alone is not sufficient). Discuss lifestyle modification with the patient regarding diet, exercise and smoking cessation as necessary.
- **Carotid endarterectomy:** This should be considered in all those with nondisabling stroke and significant symptomatic carotid artery stenosis (50%–99% by the North American Symptomatic Carotid Endarterectomy (NASCET) criteria or 70%–99% by European Carotid Surgery Trial (ECST) criteria) to prevent future stroke. Patients should be referred within 1 week of acute stroke and undergo surgery within a maximum of 2 weeks following the onset of symptoms.

HANDING OVER THE PATIENT

'Bernard is a 62-year-old man with a left total anterior circulation infarct. He presented with right-sided weakness and sensory loss with associated speech difficulties. Neurological examination confirmed right-sided hemiparesis and hemisensory loss with dysphasia and homonymous hemianopia.

CT head scanning confirms infarction in the territory of the left middle cerebral artery with a large infarct core with no evidence of haemorrhage. He has been started on aspirin 300 mg OD for 2 weeks. Simvastatin will be started at 48 hours after stroke and carotid Dopplers are requested to investigate for carotid artery disease. Swallowing assessment has revealed evidence of dysphagia and an NG tube has therefore been placed for feeding.

Currently he is alert but unable to communicate due to dysphasia. The current plan is to start rehabilitation with the assistance of the speech and language team and physiotherapists.'

STATION 5.5: MYASTHENIA GRAVIS

A 42-year-old woman, Sheila, is referred to hospital by her GP with progressive weakness, double vision and difficulty swallowing. She has a known history of myasthenia gravis for which she takes pyridostigmine and azathioprine. She reports that she takes her medications regularly and has only ever missed the occasional dose. Please assess her and instigate appropriate management.

Patient Details

Name:	Sheila Brown
DOB:	20/05/82
Hospital number:	K32904738
Weight:	66 kg
Height:	1.6 m
Consultant:	Dr Epp
Hospital/Ward:	SGH Neurology
Current medications:	Pyridostigmine 60 mg PO QDS and azathiopine 120 mg PO OD (for myasthenia gravis)
Allergies:	Nil
Admission date:	12/10/24

Causes of Relapse of Myasthenia Gravis

- Spontaneous
- Infection
- Surgery
- Nonadherence or reduction in medication
- Medications that interfere with neuromuscular junction

Complications of Myasthenia Gravis

- Myasthenic crisis
- Respiratory failure
- Dysphagia
- Aspiration pneumonia

INITIAL ASSESSMENT

AIRWAY

- Assess the patency of the airway. Is there any stridor or noisy breathing? Is there any evidence of poor swallow, e.g. excess saliva or dribbling?
- If there are signs of airway compromise use manoeuvres and adjuncts as necessary but have a low threshold for contacting the anaesthetist on call to arrange intubation.
- Myasthenia gravis can affect the swallowing muscles and patients can be at risk of aspiration pneumonia. If there is any history of swallowing difficulties or you have concerns, place the patient nil by mouth and start maintenance fluids until a swallowing assessment has been performed by a trained professional.

'The airway is patent with no obstruction. The patient is alert and maintaining a safe airway.'

The patient should be made nil by mouth in view of swallowing difficulties.

BREATHING

- Assess respiratory rate, oxygen saturations and accessory muscle use. Auscultate for air entry and additional sounds of wheeze or crepitations.
- Pay particular attention for any signs of pneumonia as infection is a common cause for deterioration in patients with myasthenia.

'The respiratory rate is 16/min and oxygen saturations are 96% on air. There is no evidence of respiratory distress and the chest is clear to auscultation.'

Perform an ABG to assess oxygenation and carbon dioxide levels. If there is severe respiratory muscle weakness, the patient will hypoventilate causing a raised CO_2. Arrange for bedside spirometry equipment to measure the patient's forced vital capacity (FVC) and negative inspiratory pressure.

CIRCULATION

- Assess circulatory status by measuring pulse, BP and CRT.
- Perform a CVS examination. Assess the JVP and central pulse. Auscultate for heart sounds and any additional murmurs. Examine for evidence of peripheral oedema.

'The HR is 90 bpm, BP 135/90 mmHg and CRT is 1 second peripherally. The pulse is regular and the JVP is not visible. Heart sounds are normal with no murmurs. There is no evidence of peripheral oedema.'

The observations are normal and examination is unremarkable. In view of the swallowing difficulties, the patient should be placed nil by mouth and maintenance fluids started (see initial management).

DISABILITY

- Assess the patient's conscious level using the GCS. Check pupil sizes and reactions. Check bedside glucose levels.

Features of a Relapse of Myasthenia Gravis

- Ptosis
- Ophthalmoplegia
- Diplopia
- Nasal speech
- Dysphagia
- Absent gag reflex
- Reduced cough
- Proximal limb weakness
- Respiratory muscle weakness

'The patient is alert with a GCS of 15/15 (E 4, V 5, M 6). The pupils are equal and reactive to light and the blood glucose is 4.3 mmol/L.'

- A full neurological examination is required to assess for any focal neurological deficit. Assess the cranial nerves, upper and lower limbs. Pay attention for specific features of myasthenia gravis remembering to assess eye movements, speech, swallowing and proximal muscle power.

'Neurological examination reveals ophthalmoplegia and diplopia. The patient is still able to swallow saliva but reports some difficulties drinking water. There is evidence of proximal muscle weakness in the arms and legs.'

EXPOSURE

- Expose the patient and examine for any rashes or other abnormality.
- Measure the temperature. Palpate for any lymphadenopathy and examine the abdomen.

'The temperature is 36.2°C. Examination is otherwise unremarkable.'

Table 5.6 Ms Brown's Blood Results

PARAMETER	VALUE	NORMAL RANGE (UNITS)
WCC	10 × 10^9/L	4–11 (×10^9/L)
Neutrophil	7 × 10^9/L	2–7.5 (×10^9/L)
Lymphocyte	3 × 10^9/L	1.4–4 (×10^9/L)
Platelet	300 × 10^9/L	150–400 (×10^9/L)
Haemoglobin	140 g/L	Men: 135–177 (g/L) Women: 115–155 (g/L)
Urea	6 mmol/L	2.5–6.7 (mmol/L)
Creatinine	90 µmol/L	79–118 (µmol/L)
Sodium	140 mmol/L	135–146 (mmol/L)
Potassium	4 mmol/L	3.5–5.0 (mmol/L)
eGFR	>60 mL/min	>60 (mL/min)
Bilirubin	10 µmol/L	<17 (µmol/L)
ALT	20 IU/L	<40 (IU/L)
ALP	100 IU/L	39–117 (IU/L)
pH	7.38	7.35–7.45
PaO_2	11.7 kPa	10.6–13.3 (kPa) on air
$PaCO_2$	4.9 kPa	4.8–6.1 (kPa)
HCO_3	24 mmol/L	22–26 (mmol/L)

ALP, Alkaline phosphatase; *ALT*, alanine transaminase; *eGFR*, estimated glomerular filtration rate; *WCC*, white cell count.

INITIAL INVESTIGATIONS

- **Bloods:** FBC, U&Es, LFTs, CRP. Look for evidence of infection paying particular attention to the white cell count and CRP. Measure U&Es to guide fluid therapy. Check LFTs prior to starting immunosuppressive agents such as azathioprine (Table 5.6).
- **Blood cultures:** Take blood cultures if the patient is febrile and before starting any antibiotic therapy.
- **ABG:** Assess the patient's gas transfer and acid–base status. Treat hypoxia with supplementary oxygen but consider the underlying cause. Note that a raised carbon dioxide level is a late sign of decompensation indicating that the patient requires urgent ventilation. Spirometry is a more sensitive marker of respiratory decline.
- **Bedside spirometry:** In patients with myasthenia gravis, respiratory muscle weakness can lead to hypoventilation and respiratory failure. The most useful measure of respiratory function is the FVC. If the FVC is less than 15 mL/kg (approximately 1 L in the average person), arrange for intensive care review and consideration of elective intubation and ventilation. Serial spirometry should be performed to detect clinical decompensation early so that ventilation can be undertaken on an elective basis before the patient becomes compromised. If negative inspiratory force (NIF) is available to be measured, this can also be useful in the assessment of respiratory function. NIF measures the negative pressure generated during inhalation: the greater the negative pressure, the better the respiratory function. Also consider ventilation if NIF is less than 20 cmH_2O.
- **CXR:** Perform a chest X-ray to exclude any evidence of community acquired or aspiration pneumonia.

'Blood testing reveals normal WCC and CRP. Arterial blood gas shows pH 7.38, $PaCO_2$ 4.9 kPa and PaO_2 11.7 kPa on room air. Bedside spirometry shows an FVC of 2.8 L (normal). The CXR is unremarkable.'

'The clinical picture suggests a relapse of myasthenia gravis. There is no clear evidence of infection. Arterial blood gas testing and spirometry are reassuring and ventilation is not required at present.'

INITIAL MANAGEMENT

Management of MG

- Resuscitate the patient using an ABCDE approach.
- Manage reversible causes, e.g. withdrawing offending medication.
- Monitor respiratory function.
- Optimise current myasthenia medication and consider corticosteroids, immunosuppressive therapy, immunoglobulin and plasma exchange.

- **Airway support:** Open the airway using manoeuvres and adjuncts as necessary. Use suction to clear any excess secretions. Contact the on-call anaesthetist early if you are not happy with the patient's airway or if the ABG or spirometry is abnormal.
- **Supplementary oxygen:** Give supplementary oxygen to maintain saturations of 94% and above. Consider why the patient is hypoxic—if there is no obvious explanation (e.g. pneumonia), consider respiratory muscle weakness and the need for ventilation.
- **Identify and treat infection:** If there is any evidence of infection or the patient is febrile, perform a septic screen and start antibiotics. Take care to avoid antibiotics that can worsen myasthenia gravis (see Box 5.4).
- **Stop any offending medications:** Stop any medications that could have precipitated the current deterioration in myasthenia (see Box 5.4).
- **Review myasthenia therapy:** Before making any changes to the patient's medications, you should discuss the patient with your senior or the on-call neurologist. Consider stopping immunosuppressive agents if there is severe infection. Very rarely, if a patient takes high doses of anticholinesterases, they can present in a cholinergic crisis, characterised by sweating, confusion, wheeze, abdominal pain, miosis, bradycardia, fasciculations, hypersalivation, diarrhoea and incontinence. In such cases, the anticholinesterase should be withheld and atropine may need to be given.
- **Anticholinesterase therapy:** Anticholinesterases reduce breakdown of acetylcholine in the neuromuscular junction, thus improving neuromuscular transmission. They are of symptomatic benefit but do not treat the underlying process. The main anticholinesterase that is used therapeutically is pyridostigmine.

Box 5.4 Medications That Can Worsen Myasthenia Gravis

- Antibiotics: aminoglycosides (e.g. gentamicin, neomycin, streptomycin), macrolides (erythromycin, clarithromycin), fluoroquinolones (ciprofloxacin, norfloxacin), tetracyclines (doxycycline, minocycline), clindamycin
- Antimalarials: quinine, hydroxychloroquine
- Cardiac medications: beta-blockers, calcium channel blockers, quinidine, procainamide, lidocaine
- Anticonvulsants: phenytoin, carbamazepine
- Antipsychotics: chlorpromazine, sulpiride
- Muscle relaxants: curare, suxamethonium
- D-penicillamine
- Interferon alpha
- Botulinum toxin
- Iodinated radiocontrast agents

Patients are started on a low dose such as 30 mg TDS and then the dose is escalated as tolerated until it is effective, usually up to 60 mg every 4 hours. Doses above 360 mg per day are usually avoided as they can be associated with significant side effects but also acetylcholine receptor downregulation. The main side effects of anticholinesterases are nausea, vomiting, increased salivation, abdominal cramps, diarrhoea and fasciculations. If side effects occur, the dose can be reduced or you can try adding glycopyrrolate (an antimuscarinic agent) 1 mg BD.

- **High-dose corticosteroids:** In addition to anticholinesterase treatment, high-dose corticosteroids can be used for their immunosuppressive effect in patients with significant symptoms. Paradoxically, when patients are started on corticosteroids, their myasthenia symptoms can initially worsen before they improve. Because of this, prednisolone is started at a lower dose such as 10 mg every other day and titrated up to a dose of 60 mg/kg, so the dosing on subsequent days would be 0 mg, 20 mg, 0 mg, 30 mg, 0 mg, 40 mg, 0 mg, 50 mg, 0 mg, 60 mg and then maintained at 60 mg every other day. You should only initiate such treatments under the guidance of a neurologist and the patient should be monitored for any deterioration after starting corticosteroid therapy. Be sure to prescribe a PPI at the same time for gastric protection. In addition, if patients are expected to be on long-term corticosteroids, consider adding calcium and vitamin D supplementation.
- **Immunosuppressive agents:** Azathioprine can also be started at the same time as corticosteroids to provide long-term control of myasthenia and allow tapering of corticosteroid therapy. It is usually started at a low dose and titrated up to a dose of 2 to 2.5 mg/kg. At such levels, you will usually see a raised MCV and low lymphocyte count. Thiopurine methyltransferase (TPMT) activity should also be measured when starting patients on azathioprine. It can often take months for azathioprine to act but it can reduce the need for prolonged corticosteroid therapy and its associated side effects. Other immunosuppressive agents that are used include methotrexate and ciclosporin.
- **IV immunoglobulins:** In severe myasthenia gravis or a myasthenic crisis (where ventilation is required), IV immunoglobulins can be given. The usual dose is 2 g/kg given over 5 days (0.4 g/day). Its advantages are that it is available in most hospitals and can be given in patients who have concurrent sepsis. Common side effects include headaches and flu-like symptoms. Less commonly, it can cause rashes, VTE and renal failure. It is contraindicated in those with known IgA deficiency as it can cause anaphylaxis.
- **Plasma exchange:** An alternative to IV immunoglobulins is plasma exchange, which may be more effective, particularly in a myasthenic crisis. It works by removing circulating antibodies to the acetylcholine receptor. Unfortunately, it is only available in certain hospitals and its use is contraindicated in sepsis, heart failure, hypotension and pregnancy.
- **IV fluids:** If there are concerns regarding an unsafe swallow, place the patient nil by mouth and start IV fluids, e.g. sodium chloride 0.9% at 85 mL/h (Weight = 66 kg, at 30 mL/kg/day = 85 mL/h), followed by one glucose 5% bag. Adding 40 mmol of potassium to one bag, and then 20 mmol to the next one gives approximately the right amount.
- **NG tube placement:** Swallowing assessment should be performed in any patient with dysphagia and, if present, an NG tube inserted for feeding and delivery of medication.
- **VTE prophylaxis:** Patients with myasthenia gravis are often bed bound due to muscular weakness and are therefore at high risk of developing DVTs. Follow your hospital protocol for VTE prevention, e.g. enoxaparin SC 40 mg OD.

Prescribe (Figs 5.13–5.15)

High-dose corticosteroids:
- PREDNISOLONE 10 mg PO/NG STAT then ALTERNATE DAYS titrated up

Anticholinesterase therapy:
- PYRIDOSTIGMINE BROMIDE 60 mg PO/NG STAT then QDS

Immunosuppressive agents:
- AZATHIOPRINE 120 mg PO/NG OD

Thromboprophylaxis:
- ENOXAPARIN 40 mg SC OD

Gastric protection:
- OMEPRAZOLE 20 mg PO/NG STAT then OD

Maintenance IV fluids:
- SODIUM CHLORIDE 0.9% 1 L IV with 40 mmol KCL IV 85 mL/h
- GLUCOSE 5% 1 L with 20 mmol KCL IV at 85 mL/h

HANDING OVER THE PATIENT

'Sheila is a 42 year old woman who has presented with a relapse of myasthenia gravis. There is no obvious infective precipitant.

Blood testing is unremarkable and chest X-ray is clear. Arterial blood gas testing and spirometry are reassuring. Swallowing assessment reveals dysphagia and she is therefore placed nil by mouth. Intravenous fluids have been commenced and an NG tube is to be inserted.

She is to continue her pyridostigmine (60 mg QDS) and azathioprine (120 mg OD) and has been prescribed 10 mg of prednisolone to be titrated up to 60 mg/kg. At present, the neurologist on call does not feel she requires intravenous immunoglobulin or plasma exchange. She is having regular spirometry monitoring and is written up for VTE prophylaxis.'

FURTHER READING

Bamford, J., Sandercock, P., Dennis, M., 1991. Classification and natural history of clinically identifiable subtypes of cerebral infarction. Lancet 337, 1521–1526.

Epilepsies in children, young people and adults. NICE guideline [NG217]Published: 27 April 2022. Available at https://www.nice.org.uk/guidance/ng217 (last accessed 30th August 2024).

European Federation of Neurological Societies, 2010. Guidelines for treatment of autoimmune neuromuscular transmission disorders. Eur J Neurol 17, 893–902.

Hunt, W.E., Hess, R.M., 1968. Surgical risk as related to time of intervention in the repair of intracranial aneurysms. J Neurosurg 28 (1), 14–20.

McGill, F., Heyderman, R., Michael, B., 2016. The UK joint specialist societies guideline on the diagnosis and management of acute meningitis and meningococcal sepsis in immunocompetent adults. J Infect 72, 768–769.

Meierkord, H., Boon, P., Engelsen, B., 2010. EFNS guideline on the management of status epilepticus in adults. Eur J Neurol 17, 348–355.

Meningitis (bacterial) and meningococcal disease: recognition, diagnosis and management. NICE guideline [NG240] Published: 19 March 2024. Available at https://www.nice.org.uk/guidance/ng240 (last accessed 30th August 2024)

National Institute for Health and Clinical Excellence. Stroke and transient ischaemic attack in over 16s: diagnosis and initial management (NICE clinical guideline 128). Issued May 2019 (updated April 2022).

National Institute for Health and Clinical Excellence. Hypertension in pregnancy (Clinical Guideline 133). Issued June 2019 (updated April 2023).

Nyström, P.O., 1998. The systemic inflammatory response syndrome: definitions and aetiology. J Antimicrob Chemother 41 (Suppl. 1), 1–7.

Ryu, T., 2021. Fluid management in patients undergoing neurosurgery. Anesth Pain Med (Seoul) 16 (3), 215–224.

Stroke and transient ischaemic attack in over 16s: diagnosis and initial management. NICE guideline [NG128] Published: 01 May 2019. Last updated: 13 April 2022. Available at https://www.nice.org.uk/guidance/ng128 (last accessed 30th August 2024).

Subarachnoid haemorrhage caused by a ruptured aneurysm: diagnosis and management NICE guideline [NG228] Published: 23 November 2022. Available at https://www.nice.org.uk/guidance/ng228 (last accessed 30th August 2024).

PRESCRIPTION CHARTS

PRESCRIPTION AND ADMINISTRATION RECORD

Standard Chart

Hospital/Ward: SGH/NEUROLOGY **Consultant:** DR EPP	**Name of Patient:** SIMON PETERS
Weight: 75kg **Height:** 180cm	**Hospital Number:** F2083912
If re-written, date:	**D.O.B.:** 01/07/2002
DISCHARGE PRESCRIPTION **Date completed:-** **Completed by:-**	

OTHER MEDICINE CHARTS IN USE		PREVIOUS ADVERSE REACTIONS This section must be completed before any medicine is given		Completed by (sign & print)	Date
Date	Type of Chart	None known ☒		P. Smith PAUL SMITH	12/10/24
		Medicine/Agent	Description of Reaction		

CODES FOR NON-ADMINISTRATION OF PRESCRIBED MEDICINE

If a dose is not administered as prescribed, initial and enter a code in the column with a circle drawn round the code according to the reason as shown below. **Inform the responsible doctor in the appropriate timescale.**

1. Patient refuses
2. Patient not present
3. Medicines not available – CHECK ORDERED
4. Asleep/drowsy
5. Administration route not available – CHECK FOR ALTERNATIVE
6. Vomiting/nausea
7. Time varied on doctor's instructions
8. Once only/as required medicine given
9. Dose withheld on doctor's instructions
10. Possible adverse reaction/side effect

ONCE-ONLY

Date	Time	Medicine (Approved Name)	Dose	Route	Prescriber – Sign + Print	Time Given	Given By
12/10/24	12.00	DEXAMETHASONE	10mg	IV	P. Smith PAUL SMITH	12.05	DF
12/10/24	12.00	CEFOTAXIME (over 20-60mins)	2g	IV	P. Smith PAUL SMITH	12.10	DF
12/10/24	12.00	ACICLOVIR (over 1hour)	750mg	IV	P. Smith PAUL SMITH	12.10	DF
12/10/24	12.00	OMEPRAZOLE (over 20-30mins)	40mg	IV	P. Smith PAUL SMITH	12.20	DF
12/10/24	12.00	PARACETAMOL (over 15mins)	1g	IV	P. Smith PAUL SMITH	12.30	DF

OXYGEN	Start Date Time	Route Mask (%)	Prongs (L/min)	Prescriber – Sign + Print	Administered by	Stop Date Time

Fig. 5.1 Prescription and administration record (standard chart) for Simon Peters.

Name: SIMON PETERS
Date of Birth: 01/07/2002

REGULAR THERAPY

PRESCRIPTION

Medicine (Approved Name): CEFOTAXIME
Dose: 2g | Route: IV
Notes: Bacterial meningitis. Review at 7 days. Given over 20–60 mins | Start Date: 12/10/24
Prescriber – sign + print: P. Smith PAUL SMITH

Date → / Time ↓		12/10/24	13/10/24										
(6)			DF										
8													
(12)		X	DF										
14													
(18)		FD	DF										
(22)		FD	DF										

Medicine (Approved Name): DEXAMETHASONE
Dose: 10mg | Route: IV
Notes: Bacterial meningitis 4 day course | Start Date: 12/10/24
Prescriber – sign + print: P. Smith PAUL SMITH

Time		12/10/24	13/10/24										
(6)			DF										
8													
(12)		X	DF										
14													
(18)		FD	DF										
(22)		FD	DF										

Medicine (Approved Name): ACICLOVIR
Dose: 750mg | Route: IV
Notes: To cover encephalitis. Review once PCR available. Give over 1h. | Start Date: 12/10/24
Prescriber – sign + print: P. Smith PAUL SMITH

Time		12/10/24	13/10/24										
(6)			DF										
8													
12													
(14)		X	DF										
18													
(22)		FD	DF										

Medicine (Approved Name): OMEPRAZOLE
Dose: 40mg | Route: IV
Notes: Give over 20–30mins | Start Date: 12/10/24
Prescriber – sign + print: P. Smith PAUL SMITH

Time		12/10/24	13/10/24										
(6)		X	DF										
8													
12													
14													
18													
22													

Medicine (Approved Name): PARACETAMOL
Dose: 1g | Route: IV
Notes: Analgesia. Give over 15 minutes. | Start Date: 12/10/24
Prescriber – sign + print: P. Smith PAUL SMITH

Time		12/10/24	13/10/24										
(6)			DF										
8													
(12)		X	DF										
14													
(18)		FD	DF										
(22)		FD	DF										

Medicine (Approved Name): TED STOCKINGS
Dose: One pair | Route: TOP
Notes: | Start Date: 12/10/24
Prescriber – sign + print: P. Smith PAUL SMITH

Time		12/10/24	13/10/24										
6													
8													
12		FD	DF										
14													
18													
22													

Fig. 5.2 Prescription and administration record (regular therapy) for Simon Peter.

FLUID PRESCRIPTION CHART

Hospital/Ward: SGH/NEUROLOGY WARD **Consultant:** DR EPP

Weight: 75kg **Height:** 180cm

Name of Patient: SIMON PETERS

Hospital Number: F2083912

D.O.B: 01/07/2002

Date/ Time	FLUID / ADDED DRUGS	VOLUME / DOSE	ROUTE	RATE	PRESCRIBER – SIGN AND PRINT
12/10/24 15.00	SODIUM CHLORIDE 0.9%	1L	IV	125mL/h	P. Smith PAUL SMITH

Fig. 5.3 Fluid prescription chart for Simon Peters.

PRESCRIPTION AND ADMINISTRATION RECORD

Standard Chart

Hospital/Ward: SGH/NEUROLOGY WARD **Consultant:** DR EPP	**Name of Patient:** LUCY WALL
Weight: 50 kg **Height:** 160 cm	**Hospital Number:** C1261452
If re-written, date:	**D.O.B.:** 02/02/1987
DISCHARGE PRESCRIPTION **Date completed:-** **Completed by:-**	

OTHER MEDICINE CHARTS IN USE		PREVIOUS ADVERSE REACTIONS This section must be completed before any medicine is given		Completed by (sign & print)	Date
Date	Type of Chart	None known ☒		P. Smith PAUL SMITH	12/10/24
		Medicine/Agent	Description of Reaction		

CODES FOR NON-ADMINISTRATION OF PRESCRIBED MEDICINE

If a dose is not administered as prescribed, initial and enter a code in the column with a circle drawn round the code according to the reason as shown below. **Inform the responsible doctor in the appropriate timescale.**

1. Patient refuses
2. Patient not present
3. Medicines not available – CHECK ORDERED
4. Asleep/drowsy
5. Administration route not available – CHECK FOR ALTERNATIVE
6. Vomiting/nausea
7. Time varied on doctor's instructions
8. Once only/as required medicine given
9. Dose withheld on doctor's instructions
10. Possible adverse reaction/side effect

ONCE-ONLY

Date	Time	Medicine (Approved Name)	Dose	Route	Prescriber – Sign + Print	Time Given	Given By
12/10/24	13.00	LORAZEPAM	4 mg	IV	P. Smith PAUL SMITH	13.05	SA
12/10/24	13.10	LORAZEPAM	4 mg	IV	P. Smith PAUL SMITH	13.15	SA

OXYGEN	Start Date	Start Time	Route Mask (%)	Route Prongs (L/min)	Prescriber – Sign + Print	Administered by	Stop Date	Stop Time
	12/10/24	13.00	15L/min (via NON – REBREATHER MASK)		P. Smith PAUL SMITH	SA	12/10/24	18.00

Fig. 5.4 Prescription and administration record (standard chart) for Lucy Wall.

Name: LUCY WALL

Date of Birth: 02/02/1987

REGULAR THERAPY

PRESCRIPTION	Date → / Time ↓	12/10/24	13/10/24									

Medicine (Approved Name): PHENYTOIN SODIUM	
Dose: 100 mg	Route: IV
Notes: Give over at least two minutes. Administration should be preceded and followed by an injection of sodium chloride 0.9%.	Start Date: 12/10/24
Prescriber – sign + print: P. Smith PAUL SMITH	

Time	12/10/24	13/10/24										
(6)		SD										
8												
12												
(14)		SD										
18												
(22)	SD	SD										

Medicine (Approved Name): DALTEPARIN	
Dose: 5000 units	Route: SC
Notes	Start Date: 12/10/24
Prescriber – sign + print: P. Smith PAUL SMITH	

Time	12/10/24	13/10/24										
6												
8												
12												
14												
(18)	SD	SD										
22												

Medicine (Approved Name)	
Dose	Route
Notes	Start Date
Prescriber – sign + print	

Time												
6												
8												
12												
14												
18												
22												

Medicine (Approved Name)	
Dose	Route
Notes	Start Date
Prescriber – sign + print	

Time												
6												
8												
12												
14												
18												
22												

Medicine (Approved Name)	
Dose	Route
Notes	Start Date
Prescriber – sign + print	

Time												
6												
8												
12												
14												
18												
22												

Medicine (Approved Name)	
Dose	Route
Notes	Start Date
Prescriber – sign + print	

Time												
6												
8												
12												
14												
18												
22												

Fig. 5.5 Prescription and administration record (regular therapy) for Lucy Wall.

FLUID PRESCRIPTION CHART

Hospital/Ward: SGH NEUROLOGY WARD **Consultant:** DR EPP **Weight:** 50kg **Height:** 160cm	**Name of Patient:** LUCY WALL **Hospital Number:** C1261452 **D.O.B:** 02/02/1987

Date/ Time	FLUID / ADDED DRUGS	VOLUME / DOSE	ROUTE	RATE	PRESCRIBER – SIGN AND PRINT
12/10/24 13.20	SODIUM CHLORIDE 0.9%	100 ml	IV	5 mL/min (50 mg/min)	P. Smith PAUL SMITH
	PHENYTOIN SODIUM	1000 mg			

Fig. 5.6 Fluid prescription chart for Lucy Wall.

PRESCRIPTION AND ADMINISTRATION RECORD

Standard Chart

Hospital/Ward: SGH/NEUROLOGY WARD **Consultant:** DR EPP	**Name of Patient:** WILLIAM CLARK
Weight: 80kg **Height:** 180cm	**Hospital Number:** H3742491
If re-written, date:	**D.O.B.:** 17/03/1957
DISCHARGE PRESCRIPTION **Date completed:-** **Completed by:-**	

OTHER MEDICINE CHARTS IN USE		**PREVIOUS ADVERSE REACTIONS** This section must be completed before any medicine is given		Completed by (sign & print)	Date
Date	Type of Chart	None known ☒		P. Smith PAUL SMITH	12/10/24
		Medicine/Agent	Description of Reaction		

CODES FOR NON-ADMINISTRATION OF PRESCRIBED MEDICINE

If a dose is not administered as prescribed, initial and enter a code in the column with a circle drawn round the code according to the reason as shown below. **Inform the responsible doctor in the appropriate timescale.**

1. Patient refuses
2. Patient not present
3. Medicines not available – CHECK ORDERED
4. Asleep/drowsy
5. Administration route not available – CHECK FOR ALTERNATIVE
6. Vomiting/nausea
7. Time varied on doctor's instructions
8. Once only/as required medicine given
9. Dose withheld on doctor's instructions
10. Possible adverse reaction/side effect

ONCE-ONLY

Date	Time	Medicine (Approved Name)	Dose	Route	Prescriber – Sign + Print	Time Given	Given By
12/10/24	12.00	PARACETAMOL	1g	ORAL	P. Smith PAUL SMITH	12.00	CF
12/10/24	12.00	CODEINE PHOSPHATE	60mg	ORAL	P. Smith PAUL SMITH	12.00	CF
12/10/24	12.00	METOCLOPRAMIDE	10mg	ORAL	P. Smith PAUL SMITH	12.00	CF
12/10/24	15.00	NIMODIPINE	60mg	ORAL	P. Smith PAUL SMITH	15.00	CF

OXYGEN	Start Date	Start Time	Route Mask (%)	Route Prongs (L/min)	Prescriber – Sign + Print	Administered by	Stop Date	Stop Time

Fig. 5.7 Prescription and administration record (standard chart) for William Clark.

Name: WILLIAM CLARK

Date of Birth: 17/03/1957

REGULAR THERAPY

PRESCRIPTION

Medicine (Approved Name): TED STOCKINGS
Dose: 1 pair | Route: TOP
Notes: | Start Date: 12/10/24
Prescriber – sign + print: P. Smith PAUL SMITH

Time		12/10/24	13/10/24										
6													
8													
12		DS	DS										
14													
18													
22													

Medicine (Approved Name): PARACETAMOL
Dose: 1g | Route: ORAL
Notes: | Start Date: 12/10/24
Prescriber – sign + print: P. Smith PAUL SMITH

Time		12/10/24	13/10/24										
(6)			DS										
8													
(12)		X	DS										
14													
(18)		DS	DS										
22	(24)	DS	DS										

Medicine (Approved Name): CODEINE PHOSPHATE
Dose: 60mg | Route: ORAL
Notes: | Start Date: 12/10/24
Prescriber – sign + print: P. Smith PAUL SMITH

Time		12/10/24	13/10/24										
(6)			DS										
8													
(12)		X	DS										
14													
(18)		DS	DS										
22	(24)	DS	DS										

Medicine (Approved Name): MAGNESIUM HYDROXIDE (8% solution)
Dose: 10mL | Route: ORAL
Notes: | Start Date: 12/10/24
Prescriber – sign + print: P. Smith PAUL SMITH

Time		12/10/24	13/10/24										
6													
(8)			DS										
12													
(14)		DS	DS										
18													
22													

Medicine (Approved Name): METOCLOPRAMIDE
Dose: 10mg | Route: ORAL
Notes: | Start Date: 12/10/24
Prescriber – sign + print: P. Smith PAUL SMITH

Time		12/10/24	13/10/24										
6													
(8)			DS										
12													
14	(16)	X	DS										
18													
22	(24)	DS	DS										

Medicine (Approved Name): NIMODIPINE
Dose: 60mg | Route: ORAL
Notes: Prevention of vasospasm. 21 days total | Start Date: 12/10/24
Prescriber – sign + print: P. Smith PAUL SMITH

Time		12/10/24	13/10/24										
6	(0)		DS										
8	(4)		DS										
12	(8)		DS										
14	(12)		DS										
18	(16)	X	DS										
22	(20)	DS	DS										

Fig. 5.8 Prescription and administration record (regular therapy) for William Clark.

FLUID PRESCRIPTION CHART

Hospital/Ward: SGH/NEUROLOGY WARD **Consultant:** DR EPP

Weight: 80kg **Height:** 180cm

Name of Patient: WILLIAM CLARK

Hospital Number: H3742491

D.O.B: 17/03/1957

Date/ Time	FLUID / ADDED DRUGS	VOLUME / DOSE	ROUTE	RATE	PRESCRIBER – SIGN AND PRINT
12/10/24 13.00	SODIUM CHLORIDE 0.9%	1L	IV	83mL/h	P. Smith PAUL SMITH
	POTASSIUM CHLORIDE	20mmol			
12/10/24 13.00	SODIUM CHLORIDE 0.9%	1L	IV	83mL/h	P. Smith PAUL SMITH
	POTASSIUM CHLORIDE	40mmol			

Fig. 5.9 Fluid prescription chart for William Clark.

PRESCRIPTION AND ADMINISTRATION RECORD

Standard Chart

Hospital/Ward: SGH NEUROLOGY WARD **Consultant:** DR EPP	**Name of Patient:** BERNARD WHITE
Weight: 78 kg **Height:** 170 cm	**Hospital Number:** W39203751
If re-written, date:	**D.O.B:** 22/04/1962
DISCHARGE PRESCRIPTION **Date completed:-** **Completed by:-**	

OTHER MEDICINE CHARTS IN USE		**PREVIOUS ADVERSE REACTIONS** This section must be completed before any medicine is given		Completed by (sign & print)	Date
Date	Type of Chart	None known ☒		P. Smith PAUL SMITH	12/10/24
		Medicine/Agent	Description of Reaction		

CODES FOR NON-ADMINISTRATION OF PRESCRIBED MEDICINE

If a dose is not administered as prescribed, initial and enter a code in the column with a circle drawn round the code according to the reason as shown below. **Inform the responsible doctor in the appropriate timescale.**

1. Patient refuses
2. Patient not present
3. Medicines not available – CHECK ORDERED
4. Asleep/drowsy
5. Administration route not available – CHECK FOR ALTERNATIVE
6. Vomiting/nausea
7. Time varied on doctor's instructions
8. Once only/as required medicine given
9. Dose withheld on doctor's instructions
10. Possible adverse reaction/side effect

ONCE-ONLY

Date	Time	Medicine (Approved Name)	Dose	Route	Prescriber – Sign + Print	Time Given	Given By
12/10/24	12.00	ASPIRIN	300 mg	NG	P. Smith PAUL SMITH	12.10	FG

OXYGEN	Start Date	Start Time	Route Mask (%)	Route Prongs (L/min)	Prescriber – Sign + Print	Administered by	Stop Date	Stop Time

Fig. 5.10 Prescription and administration record (standard chart) for Bernard White.

Name: BERNARD WHITE

Date of Birth: 22/04/1962

REGULAR THERAPY

PRESCRIPTION

Medicine (Approved Name): ASPIRIN

Dose: 300 mg | Route: NG

Notes: Acute stroke, review at 2 weeks | Start Date: 12/10/24

Prescriber – sign + print: P. Smith PAUL SMITH

Date → / Time ↓	12/10/24	13/10/24										
6												
(8)	X	DS										
12												
14												
18												
22												

Medicine (Approved Name)

Dose | Route

Notes | Start Date

Prescriber – sign + print

Time												
6												
8												
12												
14												
18												
22												

Medicine (Approved Name)

Dose | Route

Notes | Start Date

Prescriber – sign + print

Time												
6												
8												
12												
14												
18												
22												

Medicine (Approved Name)

Dose | Route

Notes | Start Date

Prescriber – sign + print

Time												
6												
8												
12												
14												
18												
22												

Medicine (Approved Name)

Dose | Route

Notes | Start Date

Prescriber – sign + print

Time												
6												
8												
12												
14												
18												
22												

Medicine (Approved Name)

Dose | Route

Notes | Start Date

Prescriber – sign + print

Time												
6												
8												
12												
14												
18												
22												

Fig. 5.11 Prescription and administration record (regular therapy) for Bernard White.

FLUID PRESCRIPTION CHART

Hospital/Ward: SGH NEUROLOGY WARD **Consultant:** DR EPP	**Name of Patient:** BERNARD WHITE
	Hospital Number: W39203751
Weight: 78 kg **Height:** 170 cm	**D.O.B:** 22/04/1962

Date/ Time	FLUID / ADDED DRUGS	VOLUME / DOSE	ROUTE	RATE	PRESCRIBER – SIGN AND PRINT
12/10/24	SODIUM CHLORIDE 0.9%	1 L			
14.00	POTASSIUM CHLORIDE	20 mmol	IV	100 mL/h	P. Smith PAUL SMITH
13/10/24	GLUCOSE 5%	1 L			
00.00	POTASSIUM CHLORIDE	40 mmol	IV	100 mL/h	P. Smith PAUL SMITH

Fig. 5.12 Fluid prescription chart for Bernard White.

PRESCRIPTION AND ADMINISTRATION RECORD

Standard Chart

Hospital/Ward: SGH NEUROLOGY WARD	**Consultant:** DR EPP	**Name of Patient:** SHEILA BROWN
Weight: 66 kg	**Height:** 160 cm	**Hospital Number:** K32904738
If re-written, date:		**D.O.B.:** 20/05/1982
DISCHARGE PRESCRIPTION **Date completed:-**	**Completed by:-**	

OTHER MEDICINE CHARTS IN USE		PREVIOUS ADVERSE REACTIONS This section must be completed before any medicine is given		Completed by (sign & print)	Date
Date	Type of Chart	None known ☒		P. Smith PAUL SMITH	12/10/24
		Medicine/Agent	Description of Reaction		

CODES FOR NON-ADMINISTRATION OF PRESCRIBED MEDICINE

If a dose is not administered as prescribed, initial and enter a code in the column with a circle drawn round the code according to the reason as shown below. **Inform the responsible doctor in the appropriate timescale.**

1. Patient refuses
2. Patient not present
3. Medicines not available – CHECK ORDERED
4. Asleep/drowsy
5. Administration route not available – CHECK FOR ALTERNATIVE
6. Vomiting/nausea
7. Time varied on doctor's instructions
8. Once only/as required medicine given
9. Dose withheld on doctor's instructions
10. Possible adverse reaction/side effect

ONCE-ONLY

Date	Time	Medicine (Approved Name)	Dose	Route	Prescriber – Sign + Print	Time Given	Given By
12/10/24	12.00	PREDNISOLONE	10 mg	NG	P. Smith PAUL SMITH	12.05	FD
12/10/24	12.00	OMEPRAZOLE	20 mg	NG	P. Smith PAUL SMITH	12.05	FD
12/10/24	12.00	PYRIDOSTIGMINE BROMIDE	60 mg	NG	P. Smith PAUL SMITH	12.20	FD
14/10/24	06.00	PREDNISOLONE	20 mg	NG	P. Smith PAUL SMITH		
16/10/24	06.00	PREDNISOLONE	30 mg	NG	P. Smith PAUL SMITH		
18/10/24	06.00	PREDNISOLONE	40 mg	NG	P. Smith PAUL SMITH		

OXYGEN	Start Date	Start Time	Route Mask (%)	Route Prongs (L/min)	Prescriber – Sign + Print	Administered by	Stop Date	Stop Time

Fig. 5.13 Prescription and administration record (standard chart) for Sheila Brown.

Name: SHEILA BROWN
Date of Birth: 20/05/1982

REGULAR THERAPY

PRESCRIPTION	Date → / Time ↓		12/10/24	13/10/24										
Medicine (Approved Name): ENOXAPARIN	6													
Dose: 40 mg	8													
Route: SC	12													
Notes:	14													
Start Date: 12/10/24	(18)		FD	FD										
Prescriber – sign + print: P. Smith PAUL SMITH	22													

PRESCRIPTION	Date → / Time ↓		12/10/24	13/10/24										
Medicine (Approved Name): PYRIDOSTIGMINE BROMIDE	(6)			FD										
Dose: 60 mg	8													
Route: NG	(12)		X	FD										
Notes:	14													
Start Date: 12/10/24	(18)		FD	FD										
Prescriber – sign + print: P. Smith PAUL SMITH	22	(24)	FD	FD										

PRESCRIPTION	Date → / Time ↓		12/10/24	13/10/24										
Medicine (Approved Name): AZATHIOPRINE	(6)			FD										
Dose: 120 mg	8													
Route: NG	12													
Notes:	14													
Start Date: 13/10/24	18													
Prescriber – sign + print: P. Smith PAUL SMITH	22													

PRESCRIPTION	Date → / Time ↓		12/10/24	13/10/24										
Medicine (Approved Name): OMEPRAZOLE	(6)			FD										
Dose: 20 mg	8													
Route: NG	12													
Notes: Gastric protection whilst on corticosteroids	14													
Start Date: 12/10/24	18													
Prescriber – sign + print: P. Smith PAUL SMITH	22													

PRESCRIPTION	Date → / Time ↓		12/10/24	13/10/24										
Medicine (Approved Name):	6													
Dose:	8													
Route:	12													
Notes:	14													
Start Date:	18													
Prescriber – sign + print:	22													

PRESCRIPTION	Date → / Time ↓		12/10/24	13/10/24										
Medicine (Approved Name):	6													
Dose:	8													
Route:	12													
Notes:	14													
Start Date:	18													
Prescriber – sign + print:	22													

Fig. 5.14 Prescription and administration record (regular therapy) for Sheila Brown.

FLUID PRESCRIPTION CHART

Hospital/Ward: NEUROLOGY WARD	Consultant: DR EPP	Name of Patient: SHEILA BROWN
		Hospital Number: K32904738
Weight: 66 kg	Height: 160 cm	D.O.B: 20/05/1982

Date/ Time	FLUID / ADDED DRUGS	VOLUME / DOSE	ROUTE	RATE	PRESCRIBER – SIGN AND PRINT
12/10/24 13.00	SODIUM CHLORIDE 0.9%	1L	IV	85 mL/h	P. Smith PAUL SMITH
	POTASSIUM CHLORIDE	40 mmol			
13/10/24 01.00	GLUCOSE 5%	1L	IV	85 mL/h	P. Smith PAUL SMITH
	POTASSIUM CHLORIDE	20 mmol			

Fig. 5.15 Fluid prescription chart for Sheila Brown.

Endocrinology

6

Ali B.A.K. Al-Hadithi

Chapter Outline

Station 6.1: Diabetic Ketoacidosis (DKA)
Station 6.2: Hyperosmolar Hyperglycaemic State (HHS)
Station 6.3: Hypoglycaemia
Station 6.4: Insulin Prescribing
Station 6.5: Hyperkalaemia
Station 6.6: Hypercalcaemia
Station 6.7: Hyponatraemia
Station 6.8: Addisonian Crisis
Station 6.9: Hyperthyroid Crisis (Thyroid Storm)
Station 6.10: Hypothyroidism

STATION 6.1: DIABETIC KETOACIDOSIS (DKA)

You are the junior doctor on the medical admission unit and are seeing a 21-year-old woman, Ms Brown, who has come in with shortness of breath (SOB), abdominal pain and vomiting. She is too confused to give you much history, but her mother tells you she has recently been mildly unwell with painful micturition and had been told by her GP that she had a urinary tract infection. She has been drinking a lot of water and using the bathroom frequently over the past week. She has no past medical history.

Patient Details

Name:	Sarah Brown
DOB:	11/11/02
Hospital number:	204684560
Weight:	70 kg (estimated)
Height:	172 cm (estimated)
Consultant:	Dr Brown
Hospital/Ward:	WGH 2B
Current medications:	Nil
Allergies:	Nil
Admission date:	02/02/24

Triggers of DKA

- New diagnosis of diabetes mellitus
- Insulin omission
- Inadequate insulin dosing
- Infection
- Myocardial infarction

Complications of Diabetes

- Microvascular: retinopathy, neuropathy, nephropathy
- Macrovascular: ischaemic heart disease, peripheral arterial disease, cerebrovascular accidents/transient ischaemic attacks (TIAs)
- Infection

INITIAL ASSESSMENT

AIRWAY

- Assess patency of the airway.

'Airway is patent and there is no snoring or other noises. Her breath smells strongly of nail polish remover.'

No action is currently required.

BREATHING

- Assess respiratory rate (RR), oxygen saturations and work of breathing. Look for Kussmaul breathing. Listen for evidence of lower respiratory tract infection.

'RR is 40/min. Oxygen saturations are 99% on air with good bilateral air entry and no additional breath sounds. The patient's breaths are deep and sighing.'

No action is currently required.

CIRCULATION

- Assess pulse, blood pressure (BP), capillary refill time (CRT) and signs of dehydration. In DKA, shock may occur due to osmotic diuresis, diarrhoea and/or precipitating infection.

'The patient is warm to touch. Her radial pulse feels bounding and regular at 128 bpm. CRT is 3 seconds. BP is 104/68 mmHg.'

The patient is shocked: obtain large-bore intravenous (IV) access, send off bloods and prescribe a fluid bolus. Ask the nursing staff to put the patient on continuous electrocardiogram (ECG) monitoring and pulse oximetry. Catheterisation may be required to allow accurate fluid balance.

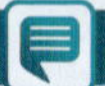

Prescribe (Figs 6.1–6.3)

Fluid challenge:

- 500 mL SODIUM CHLORIDE 0.9% IV (over 15 mins)

Antipyretics:

- PARACETAMOL 1 g PO STAT

Antibiotics:

- CO-AMOXICLAV (1000 mg/200 mg) 1.2 g IV STAT, GENTAMICIN 350 mg IV (over 1 H) STAT (5 mg/kg, estimating patient weight as 70 kg). In this case it is unlikely the gentamicin will need to be continued as a regular prescription unless an MCS result demonstrates resistance to penicillins.

DISABILITY

- Assess Glasgow Coma Scale (GCS) and blood glucose. Ketosis and/or current infection may make the patient obtunded.

'GCS is 14/15. Capillary blood glucose is 33.2 mmol/L.'

You suspect now that this is a case of DKA and start insulin therapy (see initial management).

EXPOSURE

- Look for evidence of possible triggers for DKA, particularly infection. In this case, there is a specific concern about a urinary tract infection (UTI), so look for evidence of pyelonephritis. Measure temperature.

'There is marked renal angle tenderness on the right side. Temperature is 39.1°C.'

There is strong clinical evidence the patient has pyelonephritis. There is a need for broad-spectrum antibiotic cover. One possible option would be a penicillin plus an aminoglycoside. Paracetamol should be given as an antipyretic.

INITIAL INVESTIGATIONS

- **Venous blood gas (VBG):** Assess for metabolic acidaemia (due to ketosis).
- **Capillary or urinary ketone measurement:** Capillary is preferred if available. Capillary ketones are a measure of 3-hydroxybutyrate. Urinary ketones measurement includes 3-hydroxybutyrate and acetoacetone but is less precise and subject to interreader variability.
- **Full blood count (FBC), urea and electrolytes (U&Es), chloride, bicarbonate, plasma glucose, C-reactive protein (CRP) and blood cultures:** Looking for evidence of infection or renal failure and to confirm the glucose level. In the context of a metabolic acidaemia, bicarbonate and chloride are useful to calculate the anion gap (Table 6.1).
- **Troponin:** Indicated in patients with chest pain/high risk of ischaemic heart disease—not in this case.
- **Chest radiography (CXR):** Part of a septic screen.
- **Urine dipstick:** Look for leucocytes and/or nitrites, which would be consistent with infection. Send urine cultures if the results are suggestive of an infection.
- **Pregnancy test:** If detected, current pregnancy would impact upon the investigation and management of this patient. Her abdominal pain could be related to a complication of pregnancy.
- **Renal ultrasound (USS):** To help assess for complications of pyelonephritis. If the diagnosis of pyelonephritis is uncertain, consider arranging a computed tomography (CT) of the kidneys, ureters and bladder.

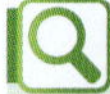

DKA definition

- Ketonaemia ≥3 mmol/L or ketonuria >2 mmol/L
- Blood glucose >11 mmol/L or known diabetes mellitus
- pH <7.3 and/or bicarbonate <15 mmol/L

'VBG: pH 7.11, PCO_2 3.8 kPa, HCO_3 5.8 mmol/L, BE –21.2 mmol/L. Capillary ketones are 6 mmol/L. Hb 125 g/L, WCC 17 × 10^9/L, neutrophil 15.6 × 10^9/L, platelet 198 × 10^9/L. CRP 250 mg/L. Urea 12.3 mmol/L, creatinine 134 μmol/L, Na 146 mmol/L, K 5.8 mmol/L, Cl 99 mmol/L. Glucose 31 mmol/L. Anion gap is 47 mmol/L [(Na + K) – (Cl + HCO_3) = (146 + 5.8) – (99 + 5.8) = 47 mmol/L]. CXR is normal. Urine dipstick shows +1 nitrites and +1 leucocytes.'

Blood Gases

ABGs are more painful than taking VBGs. Unless there is a specific reason to look at PO_2, the diagnosis and monitoring of the patient's acid–base status can be done with VBGs.

INITIAL MANAGEMENT

DKA Management Summary

- Fluid resuscitation
- Fixed rate insulin infusion
- Identifying cause of DKA

- **IV fluids:** First priority is to rehydrate. Maintain good fluid balance by measuring hourly urine volumes and consider a catheter; sodium chloride 0.9% is the rehydration fluid of choice, to replace not only water, but also correct sodium and chloride deficits.
- In DKA, typical water deficit is 100 mL/kg; therefore, for a 70-kg person, about 7 L of IV fluid may be needed in the first 24 hours. This should be given faster initially (i.e. 2–3 × 1 L bags over 1–2 hours), with regular titration of the rate depending on patient response (RR, heart rate (HR), BP, urine output).
- **Fixed rate IV insulin infusion:** This is *not* the same as a variable sliding scale (in which the rate of an

Table 6.1 Sarah Brown's Blood Results and VBG

PARAMETER	VALUE	NORMAL RANGE (UNITS)
Haemoglobin	125 g/L	Men: 135–177 (g/L) Women: 115–155 (g/L)
WCC	**17 × 10^9/L**	**4–11 (× 10^9/L)**
Neutrophil	**15.6 × 10^9/L**	**2.0–7.5 (× 10^9/L)**
Lymphocyte	2 × 10^9/L	1.5–4 (× 10^9/L)
Platelet	198 × 10^9/L	150–400 (× 10^9/L)
CRP	**250 mg/L**	**<5 (mg/L)**
Urea	**12.3 mmol/L**	**2.5–6.7 (mmol/L)**
Creatinine	**134** μmol/L	**79–118** (μmol/L)
Sodium	146 mmol/L	135–146 (mmol/L)
Potassium	**5.8 mmol/L**	**3.5–5.0 (mmol/L)**
eGFR	>60 mL/min	>60 (mL/min)
Chloride	99 mmol/L	98–106 (mmol/L)
Plasma glucose	**31 mmol/L**	**4.5–5.6 (mmol/L)**
pH	**7.11**	**7.35–7.45**
PCO_2	**3.8 kPa**	**4.8–6.1 (kPa)**
Bicarbonate	**5.8 mmol/L**	**22–26 (mmol/L)**
BE	**−21.2 mmol/L**	**±2 mmol/L**

Data in bold signifies results that are outside the normal laboratory range.
BE, Base excess; *CRP*, C-reactive protein; *eGFR*, estimated glomerular filtration rate; *VBG*, venous blood gas; *WCC*, white cell count.

insulin infusion is titrated against the blood glucose). The role of soluble insulin in DKA is to bring down the serum glucose but, more importantly, to suppress ketone production. Insulin should not be stopped until acidaemia has resolved and there is no remaining evidence of ketones. Insulin (Actrapid or similar) should be commenced at 0.1 units/kg per hour (70 kg × 0.1 is 7 units/h in this case).

- **Continue or commence long-acting insulin analogues.** This is to avoid rebound hyperglycaemia after discontinuation of IV insulin infusion. A typical starting dose is 6 units of insulin glargine (Lantus), although this can be altered depending on weight (discuss with diabetes team).
- **Potassium replacement:** Plasma potassium is often high on admission but falls rapidly as IV insulin and fluid replacement are commenced. For this reason, it is important to monitor potassium regularly and add potassium to ongoing maintenance fluids after initial resuscitation.
- **Thromboprophylaxis:** Sick medical patients are at risk of venous thromboembolism.
- **Continue treatment of trigger:** Regular co-amoxiclav should be given to treat the pyelonephritis (gentamicin here is given as a one-off dose to broaden initial antibiotic cover). Give further paracetamol if temperature persists or for any pain.

Prescribe (see Figs 6.1–6.3)

INSULIN (ACTRAPID) 50 units in 50 mL of SODIUM CHLORIDE 0.9% (concentration 1 unit/mL) infusing at a rate of 7 mL/h (use fluid chart)

Antibiotics:
- CO-AMOXICLAV (1000 mg/200 mg) 1.2 g TDS IV

Thromboprophylaxis:
- DALTEPARIN 5000 units OD SC

Long-acting insulin:
- INSULIN GLARGINE (LANTUS) 6 units OD at 18.00 h SC

REASSESSMENT

- You reevaluate Ms Brown 1 hour after the insulin infusion is commenced. U&Es and VBG are repeated (Table 6.2).

'RR has fallen to 36/min, HR is now 118 bpm and BP is 112/67 mmHg. She still seems a little confused. VBG shows pH 7.13, PCO_2 3.9 kPa, HCO_3 7 mmol/L, BE −15 mmol/L. Glucose is 27 mmol/L. K is 5.5 mmol/L, and renal function is slightly improved.'

The patient's HR and BP have responded to IV fluid, but she is still very fluid depleted.

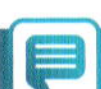

Prescribe (see Figs 6.1–6.3)

Further fluids:
- SODIUM CHLORIDE 0.9% at 1000 mL/h

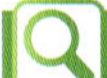

Cerebral Oedema

Although the mechanism has not clearly been elucidated, cerebral oedema can complicate DKA and lead to death. It is more common in children and adolescents; therefore, in this group, cautious fluid replacement is made over 48 hours. In adults, guidelines suggest cautious fluid replacement in nonshocked, small, young adults.

Table 6.2 Sarah Brown's Repeat Blood Results and VBG

PARAMETER	VALUE	NORMAL RANGE (UNITS)
Urea	**10 mmol/L**	**2.5–6.7 (mmol/L)**
Creatinine	**130 μmol/L**	**79–118 (μmol/L)**
eGFR	>60 mL/min	>60 (mL/min)
Sodium	145 mmol/L	135–146 (mmol/L)
Potassium	**5.5 mmol/L**	**3.5–5.0 (mmol/L)**
Chloride	99 mmol/L	98–106 (mmol/L)
Plasma glucose	**27 mmol/L**	**4.5–5.6 (mmol/L)**
pH	**7.13**	**7.35–7.45**
PCO_2	**3.9 kPa**	**4.8–6.1 (kPa)**
HCO_3	**7 mmol/L**	**22–26 (mmol/L)**
BE	**−15 mmol/L**	**±2 (mmol/L)**

Data in bold signifies results that are outside the normal laboratory range.
BE, Base excess; *eGFR*, estimated glomerular filtration rate; *VBG*, venous blood gas.

FURTHER MANAGEMENT

Ongoing management of this patient should involve the inpatient specialist diabetes team, senior medical doctors and high dependency unit (HDU) or intensive therapy unit (ITU) staff depending on the clinical condition. The aim should be to resolve the ketonaemia and acidosis within 24 hours.

- **Ongoing IV fluids:** If the patient has clinically responded to initial fast fluids (i.e. good urine output, falling HR, increasing BP), then the remaining fluid deficit can be replaced more slowly, e.g. sodium chloride 0.9% every 4 hours, based on regular clinical assessment, including a review of fluid balance, checking for clinical evidence of overload (i.e. increasing RR, wet crepitations in chest and peripheral oedema) and GCS.
- **Ketone monitoring and insulin infusion:** Blood ketones should be measured hourly. The target is a fall of ≥0.5 mmol/L per hour. If measurement of blood ketones is not available, then rate of glucose fall and bicarbonate increase can be used as proxies (see later). If the ketone target is not met, increase the insulin infusion at 1 unit/h until this is achieved. The insulin infusion can be stopped when the ketones are less than 0.3 mmol/L and the venous pH >7.3.
- **Glucose monitoring and glucose 10% solution:** Blood glucose should be measured hourly. A reduction of 3 mmol/L per hour or greater is the target. If the glucose falls below 14 mmol/L while the insulin infusion is still required, start glucose 10% at 125 mL/h. This is *in addition to*, not a replacement for, the sodium chloride 0.9% infusion, as the latter is more effective for replacement of circulatory volume.
- **VBG monitoring:** This is for the measurement of pH, bicarbonate and K^+. Repeat at 1 hour after initial assessment then every 2 hours for the first 6 hours. Frequency of measurement thereafter depends on the progress of the patient. The target increase in bicarbonate is >3 mmol/L per hour.
- With the introduction of insulin and IV rehydration, the potassium will start to fall. If K^+ is between 3.5 and 5.5 mmol/L, replace 40 mmol of potassium chloride with every 1 L of fluid given (but do not give more than 10 mmol/h of potassium). If <3.5 mmol/L, then more concentrated potassium solutions are likely to be needed: this may well require HDU.
- **Follow-on care:** Once ketonaemia and acidosis have resolved, the patient should be encouraged to eat and drink. A subcutaneous insulin regimen, often basal-bolus, will be needed for newly diagnosed patients. Known diabetic patients should be restarted on their SC insulin regimen, although this may need to be adjusted. The inpatient diabetes team should be involved and would include patient (re-)education.

HANDING OVER THE PATIENT

'Ms Brown is a 21-year-old patient presenting with diabetic ketoacidosis and sepsis secondary to pyelonephritis. This is a new diagnosis of type 1 diabetes.

I've started her on IV sodium chloride 0.9%. She's now on her 2nd litre over 1 hour. The insulin infusion has been commenced at a rate of 7 units/hour. She's had co-amoxiclav and gentamicin to cover for urinary sepsis. Initial blood tests show a WCC of 17 × 10^9/L and a CRP of 250 mg/L. The most recent K is 5.5 mmol/L and venous gases are improving, with the most recent one showing pH 7.13, PCO_2 3.9 kPa, HCO_3 7 mmol/L. Glucose is 27 mmol/L. Capillary ketones are 5.6 mmol/L, which is getting better. Urine and blood cultures have been sent.

Please repeat a VBG, capillary ketones, U&Es and evaluate hydration status in one hour and prescribe further sodium chloride 0.9% ± potassium chloride and, if needed, adjust the insulin infusion. She's still in MAU at the moment. Given the level of nursing support she will require for at least the next 12 hours, I think we should ask medical HDU whether they will take her with a plan to step down to the ward the next day.'

STATION 6.2: HYPEROSMOLAR HYPERGLYCAEMIC STATE (HHS)

You are the junior doctor on nights in the Medical Assessment Unit. You are called to attend a 69-year-old woman, Mrs Jones. The nurses tell you she is a frequent attender and is known to have type 2 diabetes. She appears drowsy and is unaccompanied.

Patient Details

Name:	Helen Jones
DOB:	14/09/54
Hospital number:	6481785610
Weight:	93 kg
Height:	151 cm
Consultant:	Dr Norris
Hospital/Ward:	WGH MAU
Current medications:	Nil
Allergies:	Nil
Admission date:	02/02/24

Differential Diagnosis of Presenting Complaint

- Infection: chest, urine, gastroenteritis
- Cardiovascular: MI, stroke
- Nonadherence with oral diabetic medication or insulin

Complications of HHS

- Coma
- Pressure sores
- Cerebral oedema
- Central pontine myelinolysis
- Arterial or venous thrombosis
- Death

INITIAL ASSESSMENT

AIRWAY

- Assess patency of the airway.

  'Airway is patent and there are no snoring or other noises.'

  No action is currently required.

BREATHING

- What is the RR, oxygen saturations and work of breathing? Look for Kussmaul breathing. Listen for evidence of lower respiratory tract infection.

  'RR is 24/min with oxygen saturations of 85% on air. There are moist crackles audible at the right base.'

High-flow oxygen is needed with the aim of maintaining saturations of 94% to 98%.

Request a CXR.

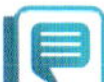

Prescribe (Figs 6.4–6.6)

HIGH-FLOW OXYGEN:
- 15 L/min via a NONREBREATHER MASK

Fluid bolus:
- SODIUM CHLORIDE 0.9% 500 ml IV (over 15 minutes)

CIRCULATION

- Assess pulse, BP, CRT and look for signs of dehydration.

  'CRT is 4 seconds. HR is 122 bpm and BP 103/59 mmHg. Her brow and hands feel warm to the touch.'

The patient is shocked: obtain large-bore IV access, send blood tests and prescribe a fluid challenge. Ask the nursing staff to put the patient on continuous ECG monitoring and pulse oximetry. Catheterisation may be required to allow accurate fluid balance.

DISABILITY

- Assess GCS and blood glucose. Ketosis and/or current infection may make the patient obtunded.

  'GCS is 14/15 as the patient is disorientated. The capillary blood glucose is 37.6 mmol/L and there are no urinary or blood ketones.'

This suggests a diagnosis of HHS, and aggressive fluid resuscitation should be continued.

EXPOSURE

- Measure temperature and look for potential reasons that might explain the patient's decompensation, particularly infection. Examine the skin carefully for evidence of cellulitis or infected ulcers, particularly on the heels. Also examine for abdominal tenderness or gastrointestinal upset, e.g. diarrhoea.

  'Temperature is 38.1°C. There is no evidence of sores including on pressure areas. The patient is obese with a soft and nontender abdomen.'

HHS: Definition

There are no strict criteria, but these are characteristic features:
- Hypovolaemia
- Hyperglycaemia (≥30 mmol/L) without significant ketonaemia (<3 mmol/L) or acidosis (pH >7.3, bicarbonate >15 mmol/L)
- Osmolality ≥320 mOsmol/kg

Alterations to mental state are common in HHS secondary to raised osmolality. This is a spectrum from mild confusion through to coma.

Remember that HHS and DKA are not mutually exclusive and may coexist.

- Given the patient is pyrexial with crepitations in her chest, she should be treated for pneumonia. Prescribe co-amoxiclav as a once-off dose since renal function is not yet known. While the nurses are preparing this ensure blood cultures are taken.
- Prescribe antipyretics.

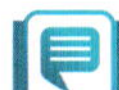

Prescribe (see Figs 6.4–6.6)

Antibiotics:
- CO-AMOXICLAV (1000 mg/200 mg) 1.2 g IV STAT

Antipyretics:
- PARACETAMOL 1 g PO STAT

INITIAL INVESTIGATIONS

- **VBG:** Perform for confirmatory blood glucose, rapid Na result and to assess acid–base status. Acidaemia could occur secondary to ketosis or sepsis (raised lactate).
- **Bloods:** FBC, U&Es, liver function tests (LFTs), CRP, glucose, blood cultures. Electrolytes can be deranged due to HHS and with subsequent fluid infusions. If available, (lab measured) osmolality should be requested. If this is not available, then calculate this using the formula $2 \times Na^+ + glucose + urea$ (estimated osmolality) (Table 6.3).
- **Capillary ketones:** Arrange if available, otherwise look at urine ketones. This is important for determining whether insulin should be started earlier and in determining whether this is DKA rather than HHS in situations where there is diagnostic doubt. If ketones are raised, they should be monitored.
- **Urine dipstick:** For markers of infection and for ketones.
- **CXR:** Look for consolidation.
- **ECG:** Look for evidence of cardiovascular precipitants of HHS, including myocardial infarction (MI).

'Bloods show Hb 134 g/L, WCC 16.7 × 10^9/L, platelets 198 × 10^9/L, urea 22 mmol/L, creatinine 170 µmol/L, K 3.7 mmol/L, Na 159 mmol/L. LFTs are normal. CRP is 123 mg/L. Glucose is 39 mmol/L. You calculate osmolality as 379 mOsmol/kg (range 278–305). Capillary ketones are 0.3 mmol/L. Venous blood gas shows a metabolic acidosis with partial respiratory compensation. CXR shows consolidation

Table 6.3 Helen Jones's Blood Results Including VBG

PARAMETER	VALUE	NORMAL RANGE (UNITS)
Haemoglobin	134 g/L	Men: 135–177 (g/L) Women: 115–155 (g/L)
WCC	**16.7 × 10⁹/L**	**4–11 (× 10⁹/L)**
Neutrophil	**15.6 × 10⁹/L**	**2.0–7.5 (× 10⁹/L)**
Lymphocyte	2 × 10⁹/L	1.4–4 (× 10⁹/L)
Platelet	198 × 10⁹/L	150–400 (× 10⁹/L)
CRP	**123 mg/L**	**<5 (mg/L)**
Urea	**22 mmol/L**	**2.5–6.7 (mmol/L)**
Creatinine	**170 μmol/L**	**79–118 (μmol/L)**
eGFR	**40 mL/min**	**>60 (mL/min)**
Sodium	**159 mmol/L**	**135–145 (mmol/L)**
Potassium	3.7 mmol/L	3.5–5.0 (mmol/L)
Plasma glucose	**39 mmol/L**	**4.5–5.6 (mmol/L)**
ALT	27 IU/L	<40 (IU/L)
ALP	92 IU/L	39–117 (IU/L)
Bilirubin	14 μmol/L	<17 (μmol/L)
pH	**7.25**	**7.35–7.45**
$PaCO_2$	**3.8 kPa**	**4.8–6.1 (kPa)**
Bicarbonate	**12.1 mmol/L**	**22–26 (mmol/L)**
BE	**−13.5 mmol/L**	**±2 (mmol/L)**

Data in bold signifies results that are outside the normal laboratory range. *ALP*, Alkaline phosphatase; *ALT*, alanine transaminase; *BE*, base excess; *CRP*, C-reactive protein; *eGFR*, estimated glomerular filtration rate; *VBG*, venous blood gas; *WCC*, white cell count.

at the right base. The ECG shows sinus tachycardia rate 116 bpm with no ST segment or T wave abnormalities.'

INITIAL MANAGEMENT

 **HHS Management Summary**

- Fluid resuscitation
- Potassium replacement
- Insulin therapy (when indicated)
- Identification of precipitant
- Thromboprophylaxis

IV FLUIDS

- IV fluids are used for the normalisation of plasma osmolality, sodium and glucose and to restore the circulating volume by replacing the considerable water and electrolyte deficit.
- In HHS, the plasma osmolality is significantly raised. High glucose is the significant contributor to this raised osmolality, but plasma sodium and urea concentration are usually raised as well, further increasing the osmolality.
- There is a total body deficit of electrolytes (principally sodium, potassium and chloride) due to their renal loss secondary to an osmotic diuresis driven by glycosuria.
- The key to treating HHS is to avoid too rapid correction of osmolality as this can be associated with seizures, cerebral oedema and central pontine myelinolysis.
- Methods of avoiding rapid changes in osmolality include regular monitoring of clinical state, U&Es and plasma osmolality (see Further Management). Furthermore, the rate of fluid administration needs to be carefully titrated and the fluid used should not be too hypotonic relative to the patient's plasma. Therefore, sodium chloride 0.9% is the fluid of choice. In healthy patients, this is isotonic. In HHS patients, this is hypotonic. Therefore, sodium chloride 0.45% is too hypotonic and if used initially risks precipitating rapid osmotic shifts; sodium chloride 0.45% can be considered at a later stage in refractory cases when a more rapid osmotic shift is needed (see Further Management).
- In HHS, the extent of dehydration is typically more profound than in DKA, requiring up to 200 mL/kg of fluid replacement over 2 or more days.
- Hourly urine volumes should be measured. Therefore, consider a catheter, particularly if the patient is immobile, confused and/or incontinent. Given Mrs Jones's reduced GCS, she should be catheterised and started on a fluid balance chart.
- **Insulin is not initially required:** In the majority of cases, the plasma glucose should begin to correct with sodium chloride 0.9% alone. Remember there is no absolute insulin deficit. Indications for *starting insulin immediately* are blood ketones >1 or urine ketones >2; otherwise, this should be initially postponed.
- **Replace potassium:** This is required even if the potassium is within normal limits. Avoid giving potassium supplementation to those with K >5.5 mmol/L.
- **Prescribe VTE prophylaxis:** Patients with HHS are at high risk of VTE and should be prescribed low-molecular-weight heparin (LMWH). Mrs Jones's Cockcroft–Gault creatinine clearance is 40.4 mL/min [(140–69) × 93 × 1.04/170 = 40.4]. Anti-factor Xa level monitoring is only required in patients with an estimated glomerular filtration rate (GFR) <20 mL/min. Therefore, this may be required should her renal function worsen.
- **Treat precipitant:** In this case, this is likely to be a lower respiratory tract infection. She would qualify as severe community-acquired pneumonia (CURB 65 score = 3 as over 65, confused, with a raised urea) and, therefore, add in clarithromycin 500 mg PO BD. Continue standard dose co-amoxiclav (it does not need to be renally adjusted until estimated GFR <30 mL/min). Paracetamol can be continued for pyrexia and pain control.

 Prescribe (see Figs 6.4–6.6)

Further IV fluids:
- SODIUM CHLORIDE 0.9% 1 L with 20 mmol KCl at 500 mL/h

Antibiotics:
- CLARITHROMYCIN 500 mg STAT PO, and then BD, CO-AMOXICLAV (1000 mg/200 mg) 1.2 g IV TDS

Thromboprophylaxis:
- DALTEPARIN 5000 units SC OD

Analgesia/antipyretic:
- PARACETAMOL 1 g PO QDS

REASSESSMENT

- You reevaluate the patient 90 minutes after first presentation.

  'Mrs Jones has a patent airway. Her oxygen saturations are 100% on 15 L high-flow oxygen. Her RR is now down to 18 breaths/min. Her HR is 110 bpm and BP is 110/70 mmHg. Her temperature is now 37.0°C. She's making orientated conversation with the nurses. She's been catheterised and in the first half an hour she's passed 45 mL of dark yellow urine. She's on continuous ECG and oxygen saturations monitoring and is still in MAU. Bloods taken 1 hour after presentation show urea 21 mmol/L, creatinine 165 μmol/L, K 3.4 mmol/L, Na 158 mmol/L, glucose 34 mmol/L with osmolality now 371 ((2 × 158) + 34 + 21 = 371 mOsmol/kg).'

The patient does not require as much oxygen as when she arrived, so this can be reduced.

 Prescribe (see Figs 6.4–6.6)

Oxygen, e.g. 40% OXYGEN via a FACE MASK

STOP

Initial oxygen prescription

FURTHER MANAGEMENT

- Ongoing management of this patient should involve the inpatient specialist diabetes team, senior medical doctors and HDU or ITU staff depending on the severity of the clinical condition.
- **Frequent monitoring** of clinical hydration status, GCS and fluid balance every 1 to 2 hours is needed, particularly looking for overload (i.e. SOB, wet crackles in the chest, peripheral oedema) and cerebral oedema (suggested by reduced GCS).
- **Measure blood glucose, Na, K and calculate osmolality** every hour for the first 6 hours, then, if biochemistry is normalising, 2-hourly for 6 hours.
- Aim to gradually drop osmolality by 3 to 8 mOsmol/kg per hour and achieve a positive fluid balance of 2 to 3 L at 6 hours and 3 to 6 L at 12 hours. Guidelines also suggest reducing plasma sodium by no more than 10 mmol/L per day. Note that full biochemical normalisation is unlikely to be achieved within 24 hours.
- **Insulin** as a fixed rate IV insulin infusion at 0.05 units/kg per hour can be started once the blood glucose is falling at less than 5 mmol/L per hour with adequate fluid balance. Adjust at 1 unit/h to achieve a target glucose between 10 and 15 mmol/L in the presence of adequate positive fluid balance.
- **IV fluids against fluid balance:** Increase the rate of IV fluids if target for positive balance is not met. If the osmolality is no longer declining despite adequate fluid replacement with sodium chloride 0.9% AND an adequate rate of fall of plasma glucose is not being achieved, then sodium chloride 0.45% should be used instead of sodium chloride 0.9%.
- **Glucose replacement:** If blood glucose falls below 14 mmol/L, prescribe additional glucose 10% at 125 mL/h.
- **Continue to treat and monitor for resolution of precipitant:** In this case, the lobar pneumonia is being treated with antibiotics.
- **Protect and monitor feet:** There is a high risk of pressure ulceration. Apply heel protectors if patient is at high risk, e.g. obtunded with known peripheral neuropathy.
- **Follow-on care:** Once the patient is biochemically normal, eating and drinking, the insulin infusion can be discontinued (if started) and regular oral hypoglycaemics and/or SC insulin started. This should be in liaison with the diabetes team.

HANDING OVER THE PATIENT

'69-year-old Mrs Jones has hyperosmolar hyperglycaemic state with a background of type 2 diabetes that is normally diet controlled. She is hypovolaemic and septic secondary to a right lower lobe pneumonia.

Her oxygen saturations were 85% when she came in but went up to 100% on high-flow oxygen. I've now put her on 40% via a face mask. She responded well to a fluid bolus of sodium chloride 0.9% and is currently having 1 L IV sodium chloride 0.9% over 2 hours, which will finish in an hour. The first doses of co-amoxiclav and clarithromycin have been given.

She's currently on a monitored bed in MAU. Her admission FBC was Hb 134 g/L, WCC 16.7 × 10^9/L, platelets 198 × 10^9/L. Her U&Es and glucose were repeated an hour ago and they show urea 21 mmol/L, creatinine 165 μmol/L, K 3.4 mmol/L, Na 158 mmol/L, glucose 34 mmol/L with osmolality now 371 mOsmol/kg, which is down from 379 mOsmol/kg on admission. Capillary ketones were only 0.3 mmol/L on arrival, so the patient hasn't been treated as DKA.

Can you review her now to check her oxygen saturations are adequate and repeat a VBG, U&Es and blood glucose? If she continues to respond, well she's likely to be okay to go to the ward, but if she remains shocked or hypoxaemic, consider discussing her case with HDU.'

STATION 6.3: HYPOGLYCAEMIA

You are the junior doctor on shift in the emergency department resus with your registrar. A 16-year-old girl, Yasmin Grey, presents unconscious brought in by ambulance. Her accompanying friends tell you that they were at a party and 15 minutes before they found her she was 'pretty drunk' but seemed otherwise fine. An electronic discharge summary from 6 months ago states a new diagnosis of type 1 diabetes.

Patient Details

Name:	Yasmin Grey
DOB:	15/05/07
Hospital number:	459023211
Weight:	50 kg (last admission)
Height:	164 cm (last admission)
Consultant:	Dr Taylor
Hospital/Ward:	WGH Emergency department
Current medications:	Insulin aspart (NovoRapid) 9 units SC before breakfast/lunch/dinner, plus insulin glargine (Lantus) 26 units SC before dinner
Allergies:	Nil
Admission date:	02/02/24

Initial Differential Diagnosis for a Coma

DRUGS
- Overdose
- Recreational drugs
- Alcohol
- Poisoning

METABOLIC
- Hypoxaemia
- Hypercapnia
- Sepsis
- Acidosis
- Hepatic encephalopathy

ENDOCRINE
- Hypo- or hyperglycaemia
- Severe hypothyroidism
- Addisonian crisis

NEUROLOGICAL
- Trauma
- Infection
- Haemorrhage
- Malignancy inc. metastases
- Epilepsy/post-ictal state

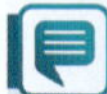

Complications of Hypoglycaemia

- Confusion
- Seizures
- Focal neurological signs
- Coma
- Death

Prescribe (Fig. 6.7)

Fluid challenge, e.g. SODIUM CHLORIDE 0.9% 500 mL IV (over 15 minutes)
IV glucose, e.g. GLUCOSE 20% 75 mL IV STAT

INITIAL ASSESSMENT

AIRWAY

- Assess patency of the airway.
- She is unconscious so at high risk of losing her airway. Vomiting is a particular risk given that she may have overdosed.

'There is no vomit or foreign material in the airway. There are obvious snoring noises audible.'

Your registrar asks you to apply a jaw thrust which relieves the airway noises. He asks the nurse to get an endotracheal tube ready but asks you to maintain the jaw thrust for the time being.

BREATHING

- Check RR, oxygen saturations, work of breathing and auscultate the chest. RR and oxygen saturations could be affected by alcohol or drugs. There is a risk of aspiration.

'RR is 15 breaths per minute. Saturations are 96% on air. The lung fields are clear to auscultation.'

No action required.

CIRCULATION

- Assess pulse, BP, CRT and look for other signs of dehydration or shock. Look particularly for hypertension and tachycardia, which could be caused by drugs.

'Yasmin is cool peripherally with a HR of 110 bpm, BP of 103/74 mmHg and CRT of 3 seconds.'

The patient is shocked and should be given a fluid challenge.

DISABILITY

- Assess GCS and blood glucose.

'The blood glucose is 1.1 mmol/L. Eyes open to voice stimuli (E3), there is moaning but no comprehensible words (V2), and arms flex to sternal pressure (M4): GCS 9/15.'

This patient is symptomatically hypoglycaemic and requires urgent treatment.

EXPOSURE

- Check temperature as this can be raised in overdoses of drugs such as ecstasy. Examine for evidence of self-harm. Look for evidence supporting other possible causes of reduced GCS, including infection. Check through possessions for other medications and recreational drugs.

'Temperature is 36.9°C. There is no evidence of previous or current self-harm.'

INITIAL INVESTIGATIONS

- **Bloods:** Including U&Es, LFTs, clotting (many drugs cause hepatic and renal impairment, including paracetamol, a common drug in overdose), paracetamol and salicylate levels (overdoses can include more than one drug).
- **VBG:** Confirmation of capillary blood glucose.
- **Urine drug screen:** This will look for amphetamines, benzodiazepines, cocaine, cannabis, ecstasy, opioids. This is particularly relevant if reduced consciousness persists or recurs despite treatment of hypoglycaemia.
- **Alcohol breathalyser.**
- **Arterial blood gas (ABG):** Many drugs can alter acid–base status, including paracetamol, alcohol and salicylates (Table 6.4).

'Initial bloods confirm hypoglycaemia with a blood glucose of 1.3 mmol/L. There is an associated CRP rise of 10 mmol/L with a lactate of 3 mmol/L. Blood gas shows a metabolic acidosis. Breathalyser shows low levels of alcohol in the bloodstream, urine toxicology is negative and paracetamol/salicylate levels are undetectable.'

Hypoglycaemia: When to Treat and Symptoms

A blood glucose ≤3 mmol/L requires urgent action.

≤3 = adrenergic symptoms:

- sweating
- flushing
- palpitations

≤2 = neuroglycopaenic symptoms:

- confusion
- tiredness
- focal neurological signs
- reduced consciousness

Causes of Hypoglycaemia in Type 1 Diabetes

- Alcohol ingestion
- Missed meal
- Exercise
- Chaotic lifestyle

INITIAL MANAGEMENT

Hypoglycaemia Management Summary

- Hypoglycaemia is an easily treatable medical emergency but, if unrecognised, can be fatal.
- First-line treatment is IV glucose and follow-up with longer acting oral carbohydrates.
- Monitor blood glucose.

- **Airway:** If consciousness level does not improve rapidly with treatment of hypoglycaemia, the patient will need a definitive airway.
- **Hypoglycaemia treatment:** In conscious patients, oral glucose or sweet drinks can be used. IV glucose is used for patients with reduced consciousness; 75 mL of glucose 20% or 150 mL of glucose 10% can be used; glucose 50% is not recommended due to the heightened risk of extravasation injury compared with less concentrated solutions. If given, it should be given into a large vein through a large-gauge needle.
- **1 mg of glucagon IM/SC/IV:** Is an alternative, particularly in out-of-hospital settings, or in hospital situations if there is difficult IV access. Glucagon is ineffective in those with low glycogen stores (e.g. malnourished patients) and can cause gastrointestinal side effects including nausea, vomiting and abdominal pain.

REASSESSMENT

'After about 5 minutes, Yasmin started to move around and groan and sat up on the trolley. Five minutes later, she was able to talk and could make orientated conversation. She says she drank a bottle of wine at the party and hasn't really drunk that much before. Also she injected herself with her normal dose of insulin at dinner time but ate very little.'

Hypoglycaemia in this case is likely multifactorial due to her insulin administration despite her missed meal and heavy alcohol consumption (alcohol inhibits gluconeogenesis).

FURTHER MANAGEMENT

- Regular ABCDE assessment, including capillary blood glucose needs to be continued, as there is a risk she will become hypoglycaemic again, particularly if she had injected a long-acting insulin.
- **Replenish glycogen stores:** The patient needs to eat a meal containing carbohydrate, e.g. two slices of toast.
- **Complete history:** This is now needed to determine the type of insulin injected, the dose injected and timing. Also check if any recreational drugs were taken.

Table 6.4 Yasmin's Blood Results and ABG

PARAMETER	VALUE	NORMAL RANGE (UNITS)
WCC	7 × 10^9/L	4–11 (× 10^9/L)
Neutrophil	4 × 10^9/L	2–7.5 (× 10^9/L)
Lymphocyte	2 × 10^9/L	1.4–4 (× 10^9/L)
Platelet	200 × 10^9/L	150–400 (× 10^9/L)
Haemoglobin	140 g/L	Men: 135–177 (g/L) Women: 115–155 (g/L)
PT	12 seconds	11.5–13.5 seconds
APTT	30 seconds	26–37 seconds
CRP	**10 mg/L**	**<5 (mg/L)**
Urea	6 mmol/L	2.5–6.7 (mmol/L)
Creatinine	80 µmol/L	79–118 (µmol/L)
Sodium	140 mmol/L	135–146 (mmol/L)
Potassium	4 mmol/L	3.5–5.0 (mmol/L)
eGFR	>60 mL/min	>60 (mL/min)
Bilirubin	7 µmol/L	<17 (µmol/L)
ALT	20 IU/L	<40 (IU/L)
ALP	100 IU/L	39–117 (IU/L)
Glucose	**1.3 mmol/L**	**4.5–5.6 (mmol/L) (fasting)**
Lactate	**3 mmol/L**	**0.6–2.4 (mmol/L)**
Paracetamol/ salicylate levels	Undetectable	Undetectable
pH	**7.30**	**7.35–7.45**
PaO_2	12 kPa	10.6–13.3 (kPa) on air
$PaCO_2$	5 kPa	4.8–6.1 (kPa)
HCO_3	**20 mmol/L**	**22–26 (mmol/L)**

Data in bold signifies results that are outside the normal laboratory range.
ABG, Arterial blood gas; *ALP*, alkaline phosphatase; *ALT*, alanine transaminase; *APTT*, activated partial thromboplastin time; *BE*, base excess; *CRP*, C-reactive protein; *eGFR*, estimated glomerular filtration rate; *PT*, prothrombin time; *WCC*, white cell count.

- **Counselling:** Before discharge about adherence with diabetic medications, the importance of adjusting insulin when meal size varies and trying to avoid binge-drinking.
- In cases of hypoglycaemia with **no obvious precipitant**, blood samples for insulin and c-peptide should be taken. If c-peptide levels are high this suggests increased endogenous insulin production, i.e. an insulinoma.

HANDING OVER THE PATIENT

'Yasmin Grey is a 16-year-old girl with type 1 diabetes who presented unconscious with a GCS of 9 on arrival and capillary blood glucose of 1.3 mmol/L. After giving IV glucose she regained full consciousness and is now back to her normal self and has eaten some toast.

Please repeat capillary blood glucose and neuro observations hourly overnight. If she's well in the morning she can be discharged. Can you please ensure she's referred to the inpatient diabetic nurse specialists for counselling and education before she goes?'

STATION 6.4: INSULIN PRESCRIBING

As a junior doctor working on the wards, you will often be called to prescribe insulin. This normally involves increasing or decreasing a dose and occasionally omitting a dose. You may be involved in the initiation of insulin for the first time, normally following discussion with the inpatient diabetes team. This section covers several common scenarios exposing you to the most frequently encountered insulin prescriptions in hospital. The prescriptions should be made on the separate insulin prescribing charts. The capillary blood glucose results relevant to the case (where applicable) are both in the text and on the prescription chart.

General Guide to Insulin Prescribing

- Target for capillary blood glucose (BM) readings is 4–7 mmol/L.
- Insulin dosing should be in the context of the last 48 hours BM readings (if available).
- Avoid knee-jerk reactive adjustments to or additions of insulin to treat hyperglycaemia: this can lead to hypoglycaemic episodes.
- Alter insulin dose by 10% when the BM is consistently out of range, e.g. increase breakfast insulin by 10% when prelunch glucose is repeatedly 8–10 mmol/L over the past few days. A larger proportional change of the insulin dose is sometimes needed if the BM is significantly out of range (discuss this with the diabetes team).
- Do not omit insulin due to mild hypoglycaemic episodes, e.g. if morning BM 2.9 mmol/L, give breakfast and normal morning insulin and consider dose adjustment of night-time long-acting insulin depending on recent trends.
- If already on insulin, take an accurate medication history—full name plus dose and timing of each insulin dose. For patients with insulin pumps, prescribe the type of insulin being infused and its dose—check these with the patient as they tend to be experts in their own management.
- Specify brand name as well as 'insulin' on prescriptions (e.g. 'insulin aspart (NovoRapid)'). Take great care as there are many sound-alike names (e.g. NovoRapid, Novomix).
- Prescribe as 'units' in full with a space after numbers (e.g. '8 units').
- Never abbreviate 'units' as 'u' to avoid the danger of 10-fold errors (i.e. 'u' can be mistaken for '0').
- If a specific insulin prescription chart is used, ensure its separate presence is made known on the main prescription chart (e.g. write 'Insulin', and then under dose write 'As Charted').
- There are different types of insulin (Table 6.5).

SCENARIO 1: STARTING A BASAL-BOLUS INSULIN

SCENARIO

You are called to see a 21-year-old girl with a new presentation of type 1 diabetes after presenting with DKA. Her name is Sarah Brown (DOB: 11/11/02, weight: 70 kg). It is now a day after presentation and

Table 6.5 Types of Insulin

INSULIN	EXAMPLE	APPROX ONSET OF ACTION	PEAK EFFECT	DURATION
Short-acting	Insulin aspart (NovoRapid)	10–20 minutes	1–3 hours	3–5 hours
Intermediate-acting	Insulin isophane (Humulin N)	1–2 hours	4–12 hours	14–24 hours
Long-acting	Insulin glargine (Lantus)	3–4 hours	No clear peak	22–24 hours

the patient is having a meal for the first time this evening. The nurses say the diabetes team have been to see her during the day and have written a plan in the notes for changing from IV to SC insulin 1 hour after her dinner.

EXPLANATION

New type 1 diabetic patients are put on a 'basal-bolus' insulin regimen. A rapid-acting humulin insulin analogue, such as insulin aspart (NovoRapid), is given three times a day before each meal. With the evening meal, a long-acting insulin, such as insulin glargine (Lantus), is given.

ACTION

You read what the diabetic team have written:

> *'If Sarah manages her evening meal tonight, stop IV insulin infusion and start SC regimen. Start with a total daily insulin dose in units of 0.75 × body weight. Give 50% of the total daily dose before the evening meal as insulin glargine (Lantus). Divide the other 50% up equally into three doses of insulin aspart (NovoRapid) which are given pre-breakfast, pre-lunch and pre-evening meal.'*

- Based on the patient's weight of 70 kg, prescribe evening and morning doses of insulin aspart (NovoRapid) and tonight's night-time dose of insulin glargine (Lantus) on the insulin prescribing chart.

TOTAL DAILY DOSE = 70 × 0.75 = 52.5 units
50% of this is 26.25 units, round to 26 units

For the insulin aspart (NovoRapid), a third of the remaining 50% is 8.75 units, round to 9 units.

Scenario 1: Prescribe (Fig. 6.8)

INSULIN GLARGINE (LANTUS) 26 units SC before evening meal today
INSULIN ASPART (NOVORAPID) 9 units SC before evening meal today
INSULIN ASPART (NOVORAPID) 9 units SC before breakfast tomorrow

SCENARIO 2: ADJUSTING SHORT-ACTING INSULIN

SCENARIO

You are called to see a 30-year-old man (Alex Smith, DOB: 1/7/93) with type 1 diabetes. Due to his diabetes, he has been admitted 1 day prior to his operation. He is going to have an anterior cruciate ligament repair.

The nurses tell you his pre-lunchtime BM is 10.3 mmol/L and they want you to prescribe his lunchtime insulin.

He is on a basal-bolus regimen and normally uses 35 units of insulin glargine (Lantus) at night and 12 units of insulin aspart (NovoRapid) with every meal.

His BM diary for the last 2 days shows prelunch readings of 9.7 mmol/L and 11.2 mmol/L and predinner readings of 13.1 mmol/L and 12.7 mmol/L.

EXPLANATION

Both his breakfast insulin dose (reflected in his lunchtime BM) and lunchtime insulin dose (reflected in his evening BM) are too low based on both today's readings and his own records.

ACTION

- His lunchtime dose today should be increased by 10%, i.e. 12 + (12 × 0.1) = 13.2, round to 13 units. Given he is due for an operation tonight, he is likely to be fasted from midnight and put on a variable sliding scale. He should be advised that after his operation he should increase his morning insulin dose to 13 units (based on the same principle).

Scenario 2: Prescribe (Fig. 6.9)

INSULIN ASPART (NOVORAPID) 13 units SC lunchtime on the insulin prescription chart

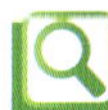

Causes of Derangements of Blood Glucose on Insulin Therapy

HYPOGLYCAEMIA

- Insulin overdose (accidental or intentional)
- Reducing insulin requirements (e.g. loss of weight, reduced dietary intake) but no insulin dose adjustment

HYPERGLYCAEMIA

- Omission of insulin (accidental or intentional, e.g. due to symptomatic hypos)
- Increasing insulin resistance, i.e. in worsening type 2 diabetes
- Increased insulin requirements, e.g. weight gain
- Increased insulin antagonism:
  - corticosteroid use
  - stress
  - intercurrent infection

SCENARIO 3: BIPHASIC INSULIN

SCENARIO

You are called to see a 65-year-old man (Boris Jones, DOB: 6/3/58) who presented with left lobar pneumonia 3 days ago. The nurses are concerned that his 'BMs are too high'. He is a patient with type 2 diabetes who normally takes biphasic isophane insulin (Humulin M3) 24 units in the morning and 12 units in the evening. His BMs before breakfast, lunch, dinner and bed were 12.1, 14.3, 13.6 and 10.2 mmol/L respectively, 2 days ago. They were 17.3, 13.2, 11.3 and 13.0 mmol/L, respectively, yesterday. Today the BM was 12.9 mmol/L before breakfast and 15.1 mmol/L before lunch.

EXPLANATION

Patients with type 2 diabetes are often on a twice-daily regimen of a biphasic isophane insulin (Humulin M3) which contains 30% fast-acting soluble insulin and 70% isophane intermediate-acting insulin. Typically, two-thirds of the daily dose is given in the morning and one-third is given with the evening meal.

In this case, capillary blood glucose is suboptimally controlled on average between 10.2 and 17.3 over a 3-day period (whereas the target should be 4.5–7.0) with no hypoglycaemic episodes. The patient's intercurrent pneumonia has increased the demand for insulin which is not currently being met.

ACTION

- Increase both doses of biphasic isophane insulin (Humulin M3) by 10% for the next 24 hours and prescribe on the chart. Based on the capillary blood glucose readings further incremental changes could be made the next day.

  New doses of insulin:

Morning: 24 + (24 × 0.1) = 26.4, round to 26 units
Evening: 12 + (12 × 0.1) = 13.2, round to 13 units.

 Scenario 3: Prescribe (Fig. 6.10)

BIPHASIC ISOPHANE INSULIN (HUMULIN M3) 13 units SC evening
BIPHASIC ISOPHANE INSULIN (HUMULIN M3) 26 units SC morning

SCENARIO 4: LONG-ACTING INSULIN

SCENARIO

You are called to see an 81-year-old man (Robert Appleby, DOB: 19/11/42) on the oncology ward. He weighs 60 kg. He is known to have bladder cancer and chronic kidney disease stage IV. He has type 2 diabetes and normally takes insulin detemir (Levemir) 34 units at night for glycaemic control. He says his appetite has been reasonably good but he has lost about 20 kg in the past 3 months. The nurses are concerned about his low blood glucose in the morning and ask you to adjust his insulin.

His blood glucose before breakfast, lunch, dinner and bed were 2.7, 6.9, 7.4 and 10.1 mmol/L respectively, 2 days ago. They were 3.1, 8.2, 5.7 and 9.9 mmol/L, respectively, yesterday. Today, the blood glucose was 3.0 mmol/L before breakfast and 7.4 mmol/L before lunch.

EXPLANATION

Long-acting insulins are used in patients with type 2 diabetes who need insulin but get significant recurrent hypoglycaemic episodes using a biphasic regimen and/or who need assistance with injecting insulin. Insulin is used in type 2 diabetes for patients who are suboptimally controlled on oral agents or where these are poorly tolerated or contraindicated (e.g. due to renal failure).

This patient's morning hypoglycaemic episodes are likely due to his insulin detemir (Levemir) dose being too high given he has reduced insulin requirements due to his lower body weight.

ACTION

- Reduce his dose of insulin detemir (Levemir) by 10%, i.e. 34 − (34 × 0.1) = 30.6, round to 31 units.

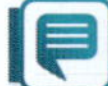 Scenario 4: Prescribe (Fig. 6.11)

INSULIN DETEMIR (LEVEMIR) 31 units SC before evening meal tonight

STATION 6.5: HYPERKALAEMIA

You are the junior doctor in the medical assessment unit. A frail 74-year-old patient, Mr White, has been admitted from emergency department with a 3-day history of vomiting and dehydration. He has a background of hypertension for which he is on ramipril. You are asked to chase his bloods and review him overnight. The nursing home say that they have continued to give him his antihypertensives until this evening when they omitted it because his BP was low.

Patient Details

Name:	Mark White
DOB:	14/04/49
Hospital number:	456488932
Weight:	50 kg (estimated)
Height:	164 cm (estimated)
Consultant:	Dr Olag
Hospital/Ward:	WGH MAU
Current medications:	Ramipril 2.5 mg PO OD
Allergies:	Nil
Admission date:	02/02/24

Causes of Hyperkalaemia

- Renal aetiology
  - Renal failure (acute and chronic)
  - Drugs, e.g. ACE inhibitors, NSAIDs
  - Type IV renal tubular acidosis
- Transcellular shift
  - Compensation for metabolic acidosis, e.g. in DKA
- Increased circulating potassium
  - Supplementation, e.g. excess Sando-K
  - Endogenous, e.g. rhabdomyolysis

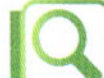

Complications of Renal Failure With Hyperkalaemia

- Arrhythmias: including ventricular tachycardia and fibrillation
- Pulmonary oedema
- Uraemic pericarditis
- Delirium
- Death: from pulmonary oedema or arrhythmia

INITIAL ASSESSMENT

AIRWAY

- Check patency as this may become compromised with vomiting.
- He is also at risk of delirium as he may be either septic or uraemic. This could reduce his level of consciousness and impair ability to maintain his airway.

'The airway is patent, there is no vomit within the oral cavity and there is no evidence of snoring or gurgling.'

No action is currently required.

BREATHING

- Measure RR. This will be increased if the patient is compensating for a metabolic acidosis secondary to sepsis or renal failure.
- Measure oxygen saturations. This could be low if the patient has developed pulmonary oedema as a complication of renal failure or if the patient has an aspiration pneumonia.
- Inspect. Deep, sighing breaths are consistent with Kussmaul breathing. Increased work of breathing may also be due to a chest infection or pulmonary oedema.
- Auscultate. Wet crepitations throughout the lung fields, particularly at the bases, would be consistent with pulmonary oedema.

'RR is 29/min, with oxygen saturations 97% on air. Auscultation reveals good bilateral air entry and there is no increased work of breathing.'

No action is currently required.

CIRCULATION

- Feel the peripheries, measure CRT and calculate the pulse rate. Cool peripheries with tachycardia would be consistent with dehydration, and would suggest prerenal renal failure.
- Measure the BP. Patients with uncontrolled chronic kidney failure are likely to be hypertensive, and patients in severe shock are likely to be hypotensive.
- Look at the urine in the catheter (if one is present), particularly checking whether the urine is dark and if any is being produced (are they anuric?).

'Peripheries are cool to the mid forearm with CRT of 5 seconds. HR is 125 bpm. The BP is 100/50 mmHg. There's evidence the patient has been incontinent: there is a small pool of dark yellow urine on the bed sheet that has a strong odour.'

The patient is clinically hypovolaemic. Prescribe a fluid challenge. You catheterise the patient as you will need an accurate fluid balance to assess response to aggressive IV fluid rehydration. A urine dipstick should be carried out on the initial catheter specimen.

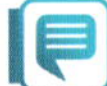

Prescribe (Figs 6.12–6.14)

Fluid challenge, e.g. SODIUM CHLORIDE 0.9% 500 mL IV (over 15 minutes)

'Urine dipstick from the catheter specimen urine reveals +2 leucocytes, +3 nitrites, trace protein and trace blood.'

DISABILITY

- Consciousness level may be impaired by delirium, as mentioned earlier.
- Check glucose. If the patient is diabetic and has been vomiting, he could be hypoglycaemic.

'There is localisation to sternal pressure, confused speech and eye opening to questioning (M5, V4, E3 = GCS 12/15). Glucose is 6.0 mmol/L.'

EXPOSURE

- Temperature.
- Look for burns or trauma. Both predispose to rhabdomyolysis, which can raise serum potassium.
- Arteriovenous (AV) fistulae or transplant scars would suggest the patient has chronic kidney failure and may be on a dialysis programme.
- Before catheter insertion, palpate and percuss suprapubically. A distended dull mass is most likely the bladder and would suggest urinary retention, often associated with postrenal renal failure.

'The thermometer reads 34.5°C and there is vomit staining the pillows. There is no palpable bladder but there is marked renal angle tenderness on the right side.'

- The patient needs urgent antibiotics for suspected pyelonephritis and additional blankets with regular assessment of temperature.

Initial Differential Diagnosis

Sepsis leading to hypovolaemia with likely prerenal failure. The most likely source of infection is pyelonephritis.

Prescribe (see Figs 6.12–6.14)

Antibiotics, e.g. CO-AMOXICLAV (1000 mg/200 mg) 1.2 g IV STAT, GENTAMICIN 125 mg IV (over 1 H) STAT (2.5 mg/kg of gentamicin, based on an estimated weight of 50 kg, the patient is unable to stand). In this case, it is unlikely the gentamicin will need to be continued as a regular prescription unless an MCS result demonstrates resistance to penicillins.

INITIAL INVESTIGATIONS

- **ABG:** The patient is clinically dehydrated and at risk of electrolyte disturbances, especially hyperkalaemia, given the angiotensin-converting enzyme (ACE) inhibitor and clinical signs that suggest prerenal failure. The patient is also likely to be acidotic secondary to renal failure and sepsis.
- **Bloods:** FBC and CRP looking for raised white cell count (WCC) and CRP suggestive of infection U&Es. Clinically, the patient has risk factors to be in renal failure and may have disturbances of electrolytes (Table 6.6).
- **ECG:** Important to evaluate the tachycardia and assess for changes that could be precipitated by hyperkalaemia. These features are T-wave tenting, P-wave flattening and PR interval prolongation. QRS widening, sine wave QRST segments and AV dissociation are late but very serious signs.
- **CXR:** Check for evidence of pulmonary oedema (given suspicion of renal failure) and consolidation (given septic presentation).
- **Renal USS:** Due to suspicion of pyelonephritis.

Hyperkalaemia: When to Treat?

- K^+ >6.5 mmol/L
- K^+ >5.5 mmol/L if:
  - Symptomatic (flaccid paralysis, weakness, palpitations, parasthesia) AND/OR
  - ECG changes are present.

Patients who have had a rapid rise in serum potassium are at the highest risk of developing cardiac conduction disturbances; chronic mild hyperkalaemia is well tolerated (e.g. in patients with chronic renal failure).

'The ABG shows pH 7.24, $PaCO_2$ 2.1 kPa, HCO_3 14 kPa, BE −8 mmol/L. K^+ is 7.2 mmol/L. CXR is normal. The ECG taken while you were at the gas analyser shows sinus rhythm, with tall, peaked T waves larger than the R waves in most complexes but is otherwise normal. Bloods come back showing: Hb 110 g/L, WCC 20 × 10^9/L, platelet 390 × 10^9/L, CRP 120 mg/L, Na 144 mmol/L, K 7.3 mmol/L, urea 24 mmol/L, creatinine 330 μmol/L.'

Table 6.6 Mr White's Blood Results and ABG

PARAMETER	VALUE	NORMAL RANGE (UNITS)
Haemoglobin	**110 g/L**	**Men: 135–177 (g/L)** **Women: 115–155 (g/L)**
WCC	**20 × 10^9/L**	**4–11 (× 10^9/L)**
Neutrophil	**15 × 10^9/L**	**2–7.5 (× 10^9/L)**
Lymphocyte	3 × 10^9/L	1.4–4 (× 10^9/L)
Platelet	390 × 10^9/L	120–400 (× 10^9/L)
CRP	**120 mg/L**	**<5 (mg/L)**
Urea	**24 mmol/L**	**2.5–6.7 (mmol/L)**
Creatinine	**330 μmol/L**	**79–118 (μmol/L)**
eGFR	**12 mL/min**	**>60 (mL/min)**
Sodium	144 mmol/L	135–146 (mmol/L)
Potassium	**7.3 mmol/L**	**3.5–5.0 (mmol/L)**
pH	**7.24**	**7.35–7.45**
$PaCO_2$	**2.1 kPa**	**4.8–6.1 (kPa)**
HCO_3	**14 mmol/L**	**22–26 (mmol/L)**
BE	**−8 mmol/L**	**±2 (mmol/L)**

Data in bold signifies results that are outside the normal laboratory range.
ABG, Arterial blood gas; *BE*, base excess; *CRP*, C-reactive protein; *eGFR*, estimated glomerular filtration rate; *WCC*, white cell count.

Blood Gases

ABGs or VBGs give useful initial results and can guide management before the lab results are ready.

INITIAL MANAGEMENT

Hyperkalaemia Management Summary

- Cardiac stabilisation (calcium gluconate and ECG monitoring)
- Reduce potassium (insulin, salbutamol)
- Treat underlying precipitant (e.g. IV fluids in prerenal renal failure)
- Regular reassessment

CARDIAC STABILISATION

- The ECG changes imply myocardial instability. If untreated, this could precipitate cardiac arrest.
- Urgent treatment is needed by giving IV 10% calcium chloride or calcium gluconate. The patient should be on continuous three-lead cardiac monitoring.
- If no continuous monitoring is available, slowly give the dose and repeat the ECG after 5 minutes: further doses will be needed if ECG changes have persisted. Prescribe this on the front of the drug chart and sign that you have given it; this drug is normally administered by a doctor.

LOWER SERUM POTASSIUM

These measures drive extracellular potassium into cells.

- **Salbutamol:** 10 mg nebulised. This can be prescribed and given quickly while you are waiting for other drugs to be prepared.
- **Insulin and glucose:** 10 units of insulin (Actrapid) in 250 mL of glucose 10% over 30 minutes. An alternative is 5 to 10 units of insulin (Actrapid) in 50 mL of glucose 50%, given IV over 5 to 15 minutes, which is more commonly recommended in guidelines; however, this is caustic and can cause skin damage if extravasated (if given, it should be given through a large vein). Ensure you ask the nurses to repeat the capillary blood glucose 30 minutes after starting insulin and glucose and hourly for 6 hours thereafter.
- The combination of salbutamol and insulin and glucose is more effective in lowering potassium than either alone. IV fluids will also help eliminate potassium by improving kidney perfusion and renal clearance of potassium.
- Review the prescription chart and stop any nephrotoxic drugs such as non-steroidal antiinflammatory drugs (NSAIDs) and ACE inhibitors.
- Thromboprophylaxis is required. Caution is required in patients with renal failure. Mr White's Cockcroft–Gault creatinine clearance is 12.3 mL/min [(140 – 74) × 50 × 1.23/330 = 12.3].

A standard dose of LMWH such as dalteparin can be prescribed but anti-factor Xa levels need to be monitored in patients with an estimated GFR less than 20 mL/min. The peak level is measured 4 hours postdose and trough level immediately predose. This should be done every 4 to 5 days while on LMWH. Peaks >0.6 and troughs >0.3 anti-Xa units/mL indicate a need for dose reduction.

Prescribe (see Figs 6.12–6.14)

Calcium gluconate, e.g. 30 mL of CALCIUM GLUCONATE 10%
Salbutamol, e.g. SALBUTAMOL 10 mg NEB (driven by air) STAT
Insulin and glucose, e.g. 10 units of INSULIN (ACTRAPID) in 250 mL of GLUCOSE 10% (over 30 minutes)
Thromboprophylaxis, e.g. DALTEPARIN 5000 units SC OD

REASSESSMENT

- You clinically reassess the patient after the fluid bolus, salbutamol, insulin and glucose, and calcium gluconate.

'RR is now 26/min with oxygen saturations still 97% on air. The peripheries feel a little warmer and temperature is now 36.0°C. The HR is down to 115 bpm but the BP is virtually unchanged (102/52 mmHg). A repeat ECG demonstrates resolution of the peaked T waves.'

The patient is still shocked and requires a further fluid bolus. There is no longer evidence of myocardial instability on the ECG.

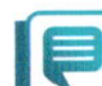

Prescribe (see Figs 6.12–6.14)

Further fluid challenge, e.g. SODIUM CHLORIDE 0.9% 500 mL IV (over 15 minutes)

FURTHER MANAGEMENT

- **Treatment of sepsis:** Dehydration and renal hypoperfusion related to sepsis are likely to be contributing to renal failure.
- **Eliminate potassium:** The patient should be assessed after the initial fluid challenge and ongoing IV fluids prescribed to aim for a urine output of at least 0.5 mL/kg per hour, but ideally 1 mL/kg per hour. You ask the nurses to start a fluid balance chart.
- **Further insulin and glucose:** Can be prescribed if potassium is still high despite initial treatment.
- **Increase faecal potassium excretion:** Sodium zirconium cyclosilicate (Lokelma) 10 g PO TDS can be used for up to 72 hours if Mr White stops vomiting. This acts by increasing potassium excretion through the gastrointestinal tract.
- **Withhold nephrotoxic drugs:** Ramipril needs to be withheld until the patient's renal function improves.
- **Monitor U&Es:** If the renal failure does not improve despite IV fluids, a renal USS is needed to ensure there is no evidence of obstruction (i.e. hydroureter and/or hydronephrosis). If there is obstruction. then a referral to urology is required. Intervention such as nephrostomy/ies may be needed.
- **Haemodialysis:** Is indicated if serum potassium remains >6.5 mmol/L and/or if ECG changes persist despite treatment.

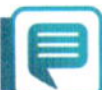

Prescribe (see Figs 6.12–6.14)

CO-AMOXICLAV (1000 mg/200 mg) 600 mg IV BD (reduced dose due to renal failure)

STOP

Ramipril for the next few days by putting crosses in the boxes on 03/02 and 04/02, and write r/v over the box on 05/02 so the appropriateness of restarting the drug can be considered by the medical staff before it is given, i.e. it would be reasonable to restart it if his renal function has improved.

HANDING OVER THE PATIENT

'Mr White, a 74-year-old male nursing home resident, has presented with hyperkalaemia secondary to prerenal failure in the context of likely urinary sepsis and ramipril prescription. Other than hypertension, there is no significant medical history.

On initial assessment, he was clinically hypovolaemic and shut down. The ECG showed peaked T waves consistent with an ABG K^+ of 7.2 mmol/L. I've given him an initial fluid challenge which he's responded to but he is still dry. A second fluid challenge is going through now. Salbutamol nebulisers and insulin and *glucose have been started, as well as 30 mL of calcium gluconate, after which the ECG changes have resolved.*

Please assess hydration status after the second fluid challenge is through and give further IV fluids as needed. An hour after the insulin and glucose have finished, please repeat another blood gas to see if the potassium is responding and give further insulin and glucose if the K^+ is greater than 6.5 mmol/L, or greater than 5.5 mmol/L with symptoms and/or ECG changes.'

STATION 6.6: HYPERCALCAEMIA

You are the junior doctor receiving patients while on an evening shift in oncology triage. A 77-year-old man, Mr Oldfield, with known prostate carcinoma is brought in by his family. A recent clinic letter states that he is known to have widespread bony metastases. He is also on bendroflumethiazide for hypertension, and on Adcal D3 supplements.

Mr Oldfield is groaning inexorably. His wife says that he has been wandering aimlessly for days, getting up at night and 'talking rubbish'. She is also concerned that he has not opened his bowels for over a week.

Patient Details

Name:	David Oldfield
DOB:	12/10/46
Hospital number:	432907155
Weight:	80 kg
Height:	176 cm
Consultant:	Dr Morris
Hospital/Ward:	WGH Oncology ward
Current medications:	Bendroflumethiazide 2.5 mg PO OD and Adcal D3 2 tablets PO OD
Allergies:	Nil
Admission date:	02/02/24

Differential Diagnosis

- Malignancy
- Hyperparathyroidism
- Multiple myeloma
- Hyperthyroidism

Complications of Hypercalcaemia

- Nausea, vomiting, constipation, abdominal pain
- Delirium
- Dehydration and renal failure
- Coma
- Cardiac arrest

INITIAL ASSESSMENT

AIRWAY

- Diminished consciousness level could impair maintenance of airway.

'Airway is patent.'

No action is currently required.

BREATHING

- Check RR and oxygen saturations. Auscultate lung fields.

'Saturations are 97% on room air with RR of 16/min. On auscultation the lung fields are clear.'

No action is currently required.

CIRCULATION

- The patient may well be dehydrated if oral intake has been limited while confused. Check for signs of shock, including increased CRT and HR, as well as hypotension.

'CRT is 3 seconds with slightly cool hands. HR is 90 bpm with a BP of 109/72 mmHg.'

- The patient is elderly and frail and clinically slightly dehydrated but not overtly shocked. He needs IV fluids at a rate faster than maintenance fluids (normally 8 hourly) but if given too rapidly could precipitate overload. Therefore, prescribe two consecutive bags of 1 L sodium chloride 0.9% over 6 hours IV. This can then be reviewed the following morning.

Prescribe (Figs 6.15 and 6.16)

Fluids, e.g. 1 L SODIUM CHLORIDE 0.9% IV at 166 mL/h and then 1 L SODIUM CHLORIDE 0.9% IV at 166 mL/h

DISABILITY

- There is a suspicion of confusion from the wife's history. This should be formally evaluated with the abbreviated mental test score (AMTS).

'AMTS was 5/10.'

EXPOSURE

- Make sure you do an abdominal examination. If the patient is severely constipated, he is at risk of bowel obstruction.

'Temperature is 36.9°C. The abdomen feels full and distended but not tympanic and bowel sounds are present.'

Calcium Adjustment

Remember that not all labs will provide a calcium adjusted according to serum albumin. In these cases, you will need to remember to request an albumin and manually adjust the calcium yourself.

Table 6.7 Mr Oldfield's Blood Results

PARAMETER	VALUE	NORMAL RANGE (UNITS)
Haemoglobin	**97 g/L**	**Men: 135–177 (g/L) Women: 115–155 (g/L)**
MCV	80 fL	80–96 (fL)
WCC	9 × 10^9/L	4–11 (× 10^9/L)
Neutrophil	6.0 × 10^9/L	2.0–7.5 (× 10^9/L)
Lymphocyte	3 × 10^9/L	1.5–4 (× 10^9/L)
Platelet	170 × 10^9/L	150–400 (× 10^9/L)
CRP	3 mg/L	<5 (mg/L)
Urea	**15.4 mmol/L**	**2.5–6.7 (mmol/L)**
Creatinine	**146 µmol/L**	**79–118 (µmol/L)**
eGFR	**42.5 mL/min**	**>60 (mL/min)**
Sodium	**133 mmol/L**	**135–146 (mmol/L)**
Potassium	4.2 mmol/L	3.5–5.0 (mmol/L)
Calcium	**3.23 mmol/L**	**2.20–2.67 (mmol/L)**
Albumin	**36 g/L**	**35–50 (g/L)**
Adjusted calcium	**3.31 mmol/L**	**2.20–2.67 (mmol/L)**
Phosphate	1.2 mmol/L	0.8–1.5 mmol/L
ALT	27 IU/L	<40 (IU/L)
ALP	**601 IU/L**	**39–117 (IU/L)**
Bilirubin	14 µmol/L	<17 (µmol/L)

Data in bold signifies results that are outside the normal laboratory range.
ALP, Alkaline phosphatase; *ALT,* alanine transaminase; *CRP,* C-reactive protein; *eGFR,* estimated glomerular filtration rate; *MCV,* mean cell volume; *WCC,* white cell count.

INITIAL INVESTIGATIONS

- **Bloods:** FBC, U&Es, LFTs, thyroid function tests (TFTs), CRP, calcium, albumin and phosphate. In particular, you are looking for causes of confusion, and possible renal failure. Raised calcium may have occurred due to malignancy. An elevated alkaline phosphatase (ALP) would be consistent with bony metastases as the source of raised calcium. Patients with carcinomatosis may have an anaemia of chronic disease (Table 6.7)
- **CXR and urine dipstick:** As part of a confusion screen to help exclude infection.

'Initial blood tests reveal some abnormalities: Hb 97 g/L, MCV 80 fL, urea 15.4 mmol/L, creatinine 146 µmol/L, Na 133 mmol/L, ALP 601 IU/L, adjusted Ca 3.31 mmol/L. TFT blood tests are in process. Urine dipstick is normal, as is the chest X-ray.'

INITIAL MANAGEMENT

Hypercalcaemia Management Summary

- IV fluids
- Bisphosphonates
- Stop medications increasing calcium levels
- Identify the underlying cause and, if possible, treat it

- **IV rehydration:** This is designed to both treat concomitant prerenal failure and reduce the serum calcium.
- **Stop contributing medications:** In particular thiazide diuretics, vitamin D and calcium supplements.
- **Bisphosphonate:** Disodium pamidronate is the most commonly used drug and it should be given by slow IV infusion (via a relatively large vein). This should be instigated after 24 hours of rehydration if the calcium remains high. If the repeat adjusted calcium is between 2.6 and 3.0 mmol/L then a dose of 30 to 60 mg is used. If >3.0 mmol/L, a dose of 90 mg is normally used, although there is local variation. Bisphosphonates have a long half-life and do not work immediately. Therefore, repeat bloods for calcium are normally rechecked 5 days following treatment. Disodium pamidronate can be diluted in glucose 5% or sodium chloride 0.9% after initial reconstitution with water for injection. Then it should be diluted with infusion fluid to a concentration of not more than 90 mg/250 mL, with the infusion being given at a rate not exceeding 1 mg/min.
- **Symptom control:** A stimulant laxative should be prescribed if there is constipation, e.g. senna 2 tablets oral nocte. If delirium and agitation worsen, then sedation with haloperidol (0.5 mg PO/IM PRN max 6-hourly) could be considered if he was a risk to himself or others.
- **Thromboprophylaxis:** LMWH should be given here, but caution is required in patients with renal failure. Mr Oldfield weighs 80 kg. Therefore, his Cockcroft–Gault creatinine clearance is 42.5 mL/min [(140 – 77) × 80 × 1.23/146 = 42.5 mL/min]. Anti-factor Xa level monitoring is only required in patients with an estimated GFR <20 mL/min; therefore, this may be required should his renal function worsen.

Based on these, discontinue the appropriate medications on the drug chart, prescribe the suggested laxative, dalteparin and continue IV fluids.

Bisphosphonates

Bisphosphonates, including pamidronate, are renally excreted. Therefore, it is important to calculate the patient's creatinine clearance before giving them. This requires the patient's weight in addition to serum creatinine.

Prescribe (see Figs 6.15 and 6.16)

Laxatives, e.g. SENNA 15 mg PO NOCTE
Thromboprophylaxis, e.g. DALTEPARIN 5000 units OD SC
Bisphosphonate, e.g. DISODIUM PAMIDRONATE 90 mg in 500 mL of SODIUM CHLORIDE 0.9% IV at 250 mL/h

WITHHOLD
Bendroflumethiazide and Adcal D3

REASSESSMENT

- You make a review with the consultant on the post-take ward round the next day.

'Patient reports feeling much better. He still thinks he is at home and does not know what day or month it is. He is now warm to touch and HR is 90 bpm with BP 127/86 mmHg. He has not yet opened his bowels. The repeat adjusted calcium is 3.21 mmol/L and creatinine is 122 μmol/L.'

In this case, a bisphosphonate is indicated. Based on the new creatinine result, his creatinine clearance is now 50.8 mL/min, so pamidronate is neither contraindicated nor does the dose or speed of infusion need to be reduced (this needs be considered when estimated GFR <30 mL/min).

HANDING OVER THE PATIENT

'Mr Oldfield is a 77-year-old man with known prostate carcinoma presenting with hypercalcaemia of 3.31 mmol/L corrected associated with renal failure.

He presented yesterday with confusion, constipation and dehydration. His bloods showed a persistent elevation in adjusted calcium despite 24 hours of IV fluid rehydration but his initial renal failure has improved. We have also stopped his Adcal D3 and thiazide diuretic as possible contributory factors to the hypercalcaemia. He may need ongoing IV fluids if he still has reduced oral intake on the ward.

I've started some senna but consider adding in another laxative if he hasn't opened his bowels by tomorrow. His calcium will need to be rechecked in 5 days.'

STATION 6.7: HYPONATRAEMIA

You are the haematology junior doctor on night ward cover. You are called to see 70-year-old Mr Shah on the ward who has just been admitted directly to the ward. He has a new diagnosis of non-Hodgkin's lymphoma and is due to start chemotherapy next week. The nurses say that he is confused and he has been trying to climb out of bed but he eats and drinks if supervised. Mr Shah normally lives with his son, who said that yesterday morning he was fully alert and orientated. On his drug chart, he is prescribed tramadol 50 mg PO QDS, bisoprolol 2.5 mg PO OD, bendroflumethiazide 2.5 mg PO OD and citalopram 10 mg PO OD.

Patient Details

Name:	Omar Shah
DOB:	02/02/1954
Hospital number:	549309293
Weight:	60 kg
Height:	169 cm
Consultant:	Dr Wilkins
Hospital/Ward:	WGH MAU
Current medications:	Tramadol 50 mg PO QDS, bisoprolol 2.5 mg PO OD, bendroflumethiazide 2.5 mg PO OD and citalopram 10 mg PO OD
Allergies:	Nil
Admission date:	02/02/24

Initial Differential Diagnosis for Delirium

This man has delirium, which has a very broad differential diagnosis, including:

- Cardiovascular: stroke, MI
- Hypoxaemia: due to respiratory or cardiac failure
- Electrolyte disturbances: hyponatraemia, hypercalcaemia
- Endocrine: hypothyroidism, hypoglycaemia
- Metabolic: renal or hepatic failure, anaemia
- Neurological: subdural haematoma, cerebral metastases, meningitis, encephalitis
- Nutritional: vitamin B_{12} deficiency
- Infection: UTI, pneumonia
- Medication side effects including opioids, sedatives

Causes of Hyponatra emia

Assessment of volume status and urine biochemistry are important in determining aetiology:

1. Dehydrated and urinary sodium >20 mmol/L
    - Addison's disease
    - Osmotic diuresis (e.g. diabetes mellitus)
2. Dehydrated and urinary sodium <20 mmol/L
    - Causes include diarrhoea, vomiting, small bowel obstruction
3. Oedematous
    - Cardiac, renal or hepatic failure
    - Nephrotic syndrome
4. Euvolaemic
    - Excessive water consumption
    - Hypothyroidism
    - Addison's disease
    - Syndrome of inappropriate of antidiuretic hormone (SIADH) (if plasma osmolality <260 mOsmol/kg, urine sodium >20 mmol/L, urine osmolality >500 mOsmol/kg)

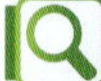

Complications of Hyponatraemia

- Seizures
- Delirium
- Coma
- Death

INITIAL ASSESSMENT

AIRWAY

- Check patency of airway. Diminished consciousness level could impair ability to maintain airway.

'Airway is patent.'

No action is currently required.

BREATHING

- What are the oxygen saturations, RR and work of breathing? RR may be elevated by acidaemia secondary to uraemia and/or sepsis. Examine for evidence of lower respiratory tract infection.

'RR is 16/min and oxygen saturations are 99% on air. Although it is difficult to examine the chest posteriorly (patient uncooperative), no obvious crepitations are audible.'

CIRCULATION

- Assess pulse, BP, CRT and for signs of dehydration. Shock could be associated with systemic infection, bleeding and acute coronary syndrome, all of which could make Mr Shah confused. Look for signs of organ failure such as raised JVP and pedal oedema.

'Mr Shah has moist mucous membranes, is warm to touch and has a CRT of 2 seconds. His HR is 54 bpm and BP 115/78 mmHg. The JVP is not raised and there is no pedal oedema.'

No action required.

DISABILITY

- Assess AMTS, measure capillary blood glucose and do a full neurological examination.

'AMTS is 5/10. Capillary blood glucose is 5.1 mmol/L. Unable to get the patient to cooperate with walking, testing of coordination and sensation, but otherwise the neurological examination is normal.'

EXPOSURE

- Pyrexia may indicate infection but could also be due to other causes, particularly if there is no infective focus, e.g. lymphoma.
- Look for precipitants of confusion, including smelling the breath for alcohol and looking for external signs of trauma as the patient may have had a seizure.

'Oral temperature is 36.6°C. There is evidence of bruising down the left arm but no bone or joint tenderness. There are no external signs of head trauma. He is not obviously in pain.'

The patient is confused and the unexplained external trauma could represent a fall out of bed or seizure prior to coming into hospital. You ask the nursing staff to put the bed sides up to avoid Mr Shah falling out of bed.

Management Summary of Hyponatraemia

- Identify and treat cause of hyponatraemia.
- Consider hypertonic sodium chloride if acute drop in sodium and/or symptomatic.
- Monitor sodium.
- Stop medications that might be contributing.

Drugs Which Cause Hyponatraemia

Diuretics, chlorpropramide, carbamazepine, selective serotonin reuptake inhibitor (SSRI) antidepressants, tricyclic antidepressants, lithium, MDMA/ecstasy, tramadol, haloperidol, vincristine, desmopressin, fluphenazine

INITIAL INVESTIGATIONS

- Screen for causes of delirium:
  - **Urine dipstick:** Check for the presence of nitrites and/or leucocytes (infection), protein and/or blood (renal failure).
  - **CXR:** Look for consolidation or pulmonary oedema.
  - **ECG:** Look for ischaemic changes, i.e. ST segment deflection, T-wave inversion.
  - **Bloods:** FBC, U&Es, calcium, LFTs, CRP, thyroid function tests (TFTs), glucose, troponin. Infection, anaemia, electrolyte disturbances, hypothyroidism and an MI are all possible causes of confusion (Table 6.8).
  - **CT head:** If no obvious cause for confusion identified.

'There are no abnormalities on the urine dipstick. The CXR shows bilateral hilar lymphadenopathy (as seen on previous X-ray). The ECG shows sinus bradycardia 54 bpm, with no evidence of heart-block. FBC, LFTs, renal function are normal. U&Es: Na 118 mmol/L, K 4.2 mmol/L.'

'Mr Shah has symptomatic hyponatraemia: confusion plus an injury that may be purely related to the confusion but a seizure is another possibility. The most likely explanation for this man's hyponatraemia is SIADH given that he is euvolaemic. This could be due to his lymphoma or be a side effect of his drugs, in

Table 6.8 Mr Shah's Blood Results

PARAMETER	VALUE	NORMAL RANGE (UNITS)
Haemoglobin	160 g/L	Men: 135–77 (g/L) Women: 115–155 (g/L)
WCC	8 × 10⁹/L	4–11 (× 10⁹/L)
Platelet	188 × 10⁹/L	150–400 (× 10⁹/L)
Urea	4.3 mmol/L	2.5–6.7 (mmol/L)
Creatinine	79 μmol/L	79–118 (μmol/L)
eGFR	>60 mL/min	>60 (mL/min)
Sodium	**118 mmol/L**	**135–146 (mmol/L)**
Potassium	4.2 mmol/L	3.5–5.0 (mmol/L)
Corrected calcium	2.40 mmol/L	2.20–2.67 (mmol/L)
ALT	24 IU/L	<40 (IU/L)
ALP	91 IU/L	39–117 (IU/L)
Bilirubin	11 μmol/L	<17 (μmol/L)

Data in bold signifies results that are outside the normal laboratory range. *ALP,* Alkaline phosphatase; *ALT,* alanine transaminase; *eGFR,* estimated glomerular filtration rate; *WCC,* white cell count.

particular citalopram or tramadol. His thiazide diuretic may also be contributing to renal sodium loss.'

INITIAL MANAGEMENT

- **Review recent bloods:** Look at recent U&Es (if available). This is an invaluable way of determining the acuity of the hyponatraemia.

  'Na was 135 mmol/L when check at an outpatient clinic 2 days ago.'

- **Measures to increase sodium:** The method chosen to do this should be based on the suspected speed of onset of hyponatraemia, the presence of symptoms and the fluid status of the patient:
  - Acute and/or symptomatic: sodium chloride 3% (hypertonic sodium chloride) should be used for Mr Shah following discussion with a senior clinician before commencement. Give at a rate of 1 mL/kg per hour until his symptoms have subsided or the serum sodium is greater than 120 mmol/L (whichever comes first). Given the patient is euvolaemic, fluid restriction should also be used (see later) and continued after the hypertonic sodium chloride has been stopped until the serum sodium is in, or close to, the reference range.
  - Chronic asymptomatic: If this was a less acute picture, then there would be less urgency in correcting the plasma sodium. If volume depleted, give IV sodium chloride 0.9%. If euvolaemic, then the patient's oral fluid intake should be restricted to 1.5 L per day.
- **Monitor plasma sodium carefully:** If this is corrected too quickly, it can lead to cerebral oedema or central pontine myelinolysis. The plasma sodium can be normalised more quickly in acute hyponatraemia, and correction is important to prevent complications of hyponatraemia itself. In acute and/or symptomatic hyponatraemia, plasma sodium should be corrected by no more than 1.5 to 2.0 mmol/L per hour. In chronic cases, the rate of correction should not exceed 12 mmol/L per day.
- If the sodium concentration does increase more quickly than these targets, then slow the rate of sodium chloride infusion. For patients who are being treated with fluid restriction, this should be temporarily postponed.
- Stop medications that could be contributing to hyponatraemia.
- Enhance orientation using nonpharmacological measures, e.g. nurse near to the nurses' station, put in a room with a clock, etc. If delirium and agitation worsen, then sedation with haloperidol (0.5 mg PO PRN maximum 6-hourly) could be considered if there is a risk of harm to self or others.
- **Thromboprophylaxis:** LMWH should be given here, as Mr Shah is an unwell, immobile medical patient. Standard dose can be given as he is not in renal failure.

Prescribe (Figs 6.17 and 6.18)

Hypertonic sodium chloride, i.e. 1 L SODIUM CHLORIDE 3% IV at 60 mL/h (patient's weight is 60 kg)
Thromboprophylaxis, e.g. DALTEPARIN 5000 units SC OD

STOP

Bendroflumethiazide, tramadol and citalopram

REASSESSMENT

- You go back to review the patient 4 hours later.

  'Mr Shah is easily roused from sleep. He now seems less confused and his repeat AMTS is 8/10. The repeat plasma sodium is 123 mmol/L (taken 5 hours after the initial dose—a rate of rise of 1 mmol/h).'

Mr Shah's sodium has increased to a safer level (greater than 120 mmol/L) and his symptoms have improved. Therefore, you discontinue the hypertonic sodium chloride.

STOP (see Figs 6.17 and 6.18)

Sodium chloride 3%

FURTHER MANAGEMENT

- The aim is to monitor for continued biochemical and clinical improvement after stopping his medications and start definitive treatment for any potential precipitants.
- Regular plasma sodium monitoring even once normalised. The sodium has started to normalise quickly in this case because the patient has been treated with hypertonic sodium chloride. Stopping some of his medications should help if they were the underlying cause. However, if it is SIADH due to lymphoma, then the sodium may start to fall again. It could also be multifactorial due to both drugs and lymphoma.
- Plasma osmolality and urine sodium and osmolality checks if the sodium does start to fall again. These results will be more accurate now that the diuretic has been stopped.
- Treat underlying cause. If lymphoma is leading to SIADH, then this will only improve with treatment of this. It may be pertinent to discuss with a senior the possibility of bringing forward Mr Shah's planned chemotherapy by a few days.
- Demeclocycline is another treatment option for hyponatraemia resulting from SIADH if fluid restriction alone is unsuccessful. Demeclocycline

acts by directly blocking the renal tubular effect of antidiuretic hormone. The starting dose is 0.9 to 1.2 g daily in divided doses, which is then reduced to 600 to 900 mg daily for maintenance.
- If delirium does not improve after correction of sodium, then investigate for other causes, e.g. doing a CT head to look for subdural haematoma.

HANDING OVER THE PATIENT

'Mr Shah is a 70-year-old diagnosed recently with non-Hodgkin's lymphoma who was admitted directly to the ward last night. He has acutely developed hyponatraemia over no more than the last 2 days: his sodium on admission was 118 mmol/L compared with 135 mmol/L 2 days ago. He is confused and has unexplained bruising down his left arm that could be due to an unwitnessed seizure.

We suspect that this is SIADH secondary to lymphoma but his regular bendroflumethiazide, tramadol and/or citalopram may be contributing so these have been stopped.

He initially received hypertonic sodium chloride 3% at 60 mL/h overnight and his sodium came up to 123 mmol/L at 01.30 and his confusion was better but not completely resolved. Therefore, the infusion was stopped at that point but I've maintained him on a fluid restriction of 1.5 L per day.

I've repeated his sodium at 06.00 this morning. Please can you follow up this result and then continue to monitor serum sodium regularly thereafter.'

STATION 6.8: ADDISONIAN CRISIS

You are the junior doctor on the surgical team. You are doing a routine postoperative review of a 40-year-old woman, Mrs Yu, post-laparoscopic cholecystectomy for recurrent episodes of biliary colic. The nurse tells you that she was about to bleep you because the patient is hypotensive despite having a recorded positive fluid balance of 4 L. She is known to have Addison's disease and is on regular steroid replacement (hydrocortisone 25 mg daily in divided doses (10 mg, 10 mg, 5 mg) PO, and fludrocortisone 100 micrograms PO OD). The patient postoperatively is on paracetamol 1 g PO QDS and as yet no thromboprophylaxis has been prescribed.

Patient Details

Name:	Abigael Yu
DOB:	30/08/83
Hospital number:	908236125
Weight:	52 kg
Height:	155 cm
Consultant:	Mr Smith
Hospital/Ward:	WGH General surgery
Current medications:	Hydrocortisone (10 mg PO BD, 5 mg PO OD) and fludrocortisone acetate (100 micrograms PO OD), paracetamol (1 g PO QDS started postoperatively)
Allergies:	Nil
Admission date:	01/02/24

Initial Differential Diagnosis of Presenting Complaint

- Addisonian crisis secondary to inadequate corticosteroid cover during the operation
- Bleeding
- Sepsis

Addisonian Crisis: Complications

- Shock
- Hyponatraemia
- Hyperkalaemia
- Arrhythmias secondary to hyperkalaemia
- Coma
- Death

INITIAL ASSESSMENT

AIRWAY

- Assess patency of the airway.

'Airway is patent.'

No action is currently required.

BREATHING

- Check RR and saturations, work of breathing and auscultate the chest.

'RR is 28/min with oxygen saturations of 95% on air (via ear lobe probe) and chest sounds clear.'

No action is currently required.

CIRCULATION

- Measure HR, BP and CRT. Assess for signs of shock.

'Mrs Yu feels shut down with cold hands and a thready radial pulse. Centrally, the HR is 140 bpm. The BP is 75/40 mmHg, and CRT is 3 seconds centrally.'

The patient is shocked: obtain large-bore IV access, send off bloods and run in a fluid challenge of sodium chloride 0.9%. You suspect that this is likely to be an Addisonian crisis so the patient needs urgent additional corticosteroids. Call for senior support.

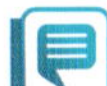

Prescribe (Figs 6.19–6.22)

Corticosteroids, e.g. HYDROCORTISONE 100 mg IV STAT
Fluid bolus, e.g. SODIUM CHLORIDE 0.9% 500 mL IV (over 15 minutes)

Route of Corticosteroid Injection

If IV access is a problem, hydrocortisone can be given by IM injection.

DISABILITY

- Assess GCS & capillary blood glucose. Note that an Addisonian crisis can lead to hypoglycaemia.

'The patient localises to sternal rub, is uttering confused speech and opens eyes to voice (GCS 12/15). Blood glucose is 4.1 mmol/L.'

EXPOSURE

- Check for signs of other causes of shock, such as postoperative bleeding and infection, by examining the abdomen and skin. Measure temperature.

'The laparoscopic port incisions are well apposed. The abdomen is soft, slightly tender in the right upper quadrant and bowel sounds are present but quiet. The patient's temperature is 36.1°C.'

INITIAL INVESTIGATIONS

- **ABG:** Given the clinical condition of the patient, there is a need to check acid–base status, electrolytes, glucose, lactate and Hb if available on the analyser.
- **Bloods:** Send for FBC, U&Es, CRP, glucose. Look for anaemia, prerenal failure and raised inflammatory markers. Characteristic electrolyte derangements of Addison's disease are hyponatraemia, hypoglycaemia and hyperkalaemia, but these are not present in all patients. Send blood cultures if an infectious aetiology is suspected (Table 6.9).
- **ECG:** Given the tachycardia, there is a need to check it is sinus rhythm and not an arrhythmia such as atrial flutter.
- **CXR/urine dipstick:** As part of a septic screen.

'The VBG shows pH 7.29, PO_2 11.5 kPa, PCO_2 2.3 kPa, bicarbonate 15 mmol/L, glucose 4.0 mmol/L, lactate 2.7 mmol/L, Hb 110 g/L, Na 125 mmol/L, K 5.9 mmol/L. Urea is 10 mmol/L, BE −6 mmol/L, with a creatine of 150 µmol/L. ECG shows sinus tachycardia with normal P and T waves. Urine dipstick is negative.'

INITIAL MANAGEMENT

Management Summary of Addisonian Crisis

- Resuscitate using an ABCDE approach
- Identify and treat precipitant for Addisonian crisis
- Corticosteroids

- **Aggressive IV fluid rehydration to normalise BP:** Use crystalloid IV fluids such as sodium chloride 0.9%. IV fluids should be titrated against HR, BP and urine output, aiming for at least 0.5 mL/kg per hour.
- **Continuing hydrocortisone:** This is given at a high dose parenterally to correct the glucocorticoid deficiency.
- **Thromboprophylaxis:** The patient needs mechanical prophylaxis (since she is postsurgery) and LMWH until she no longer has reduced mobility. This should have already been prescribed but always double check!

Table 6.9 Mrs Yu's Blood Results and ABG

PARAMETER	VALUE	NORMAL RANGE (UNITS)
Haemoglobin	**110 g/L**	**Men: 135–177 (g/L) Women: 115–155 (g/L)**
WCC	**15 × 10^9/L**	**4–11 (×10^9/L)**
Neutrophil	**10 × 10^9/L**	**2–7.5 (×10^9/L)**
Lymphocyte	4 × 10^9/L	1.4–4 (×10^9/L)
Platelet	188 × 10^9/L	150–400 (×10^9/L)
CRP	**10 mg/L**	**<5 (mg/L)**
Urea	**10 mmol/L**	**2.5–6.7 (mmol/L)**
Creatinine	**150 µmol/L**	**79–118 (µmol/L)**
eGFR	**36 mL/min**	**>60 (mL/min)**
Sodium	**125 mmol/L**	**135–146 (mmol/L)**
Potassium	**5.9 mmol/L**	**3.5–5.0 (mmol/L)**
Glucose	**4.0 mmol/L**	**4.5–5.6 (mmol/L)**
Lactate	**2.7 mmol/L**	**0.6–2.4 (mmol/L)**
pH	**7.29**	**7.35–7.45**
PCO_2	**2.3 kPa**	**4.8–6.1 (kPa)**
PO_2	11.5 kPa on air	10.6–13.3 (kPa) on air
HCO_3	**15 mmol/L**	**22–26 (mmol/L)**
BE	**−6 mmol/L**	**±2 (mmol/L)**

Data in bold signifies results that are outside the normal laboratory range.
ABG, Arterial blood gas; *BE*, base excess; *CRP*, C-reactive protein; *eGFR*, estimated glomerular filtration rate; *WCC*, white cell count.

Prescribe (see Figs 6.19–6.22)

Regular high-dose corticosteroids, e.g. HYDROCORTISONE 100 mg IV QDS

Thromboprophylaxis, e.g. DALTEPARIN 5000 units SC OD, TED STOCKINGS TOP CONTINUOUS

Further fluids, e.g. SODIUM CHLORIDE 0.9% 1 L IV at 1000 mL/h

STOP

Mrs Yu's previous regular dose of hydrocortisone on the drug chart

REASSESSMENT

- You review the patient again after 30 minutes (Table 6.10).

Table 6.10 Mrs Yu's Repeat Blood Results

PARAMETER	VALUE	NORMAL RANGE (UNITS)
Urea	**8.2 mmol/L**	**2.5–6.7 (mmol/L)**
Creatinine	80 µmol/L	79–118 (µmol/L)
eGFR	>60 mL/min	>60 (mL/min)
Sodium	**129 mmol/L**	**135–146 (mmol/L)**
Potassium	**5.6 mmol/L**	**3.5–5.0 (mmol/L)**
Glucose	**4.4 mmol/L**	**4.5–5.6 (mmol/L)**

Data in bold signifies results that are outside the normal laboratory range.
eGFR, Estimated glomerular filtration rate.

'Her HR is now 120 bpm, BP is 95/60 mmHg, she seems more alert and has passed 60 mL of urine over the past hour. Her repeat bloods show Na 129 mmol/L, K 5.6 mmol/L, urea 8.2 mmol/L, creatinine 80 µmol/L and glucose 4.4 mmol/L.'

- The patient is still fluid depleted and shocked but has responded to initial fluids. She needs subsequent fast IV fluids which can be further titrated against urine output.
- The team decision is for the patient to be transferred to HDU.

FURTHER MANAGEMENT

- HDU environment is appropriate until the patient has been stabilised (normalising HR, BP and improved urine output). This will facilitate continuous monitoring, hourly urine outputs and consideration of inotropic support if BP fails to respond to IV fluids and corticosteroids.
- **Glucose monitoring:** Initially, capillary blood glucose measurements should be measured hourly. If hypoglycaemia develops, commence IV glucose 10% solution in addition to sodium chloride 0.9%.
- **Ongoing hydrocortisone:** If the patient has clinically improved after 24 hours, the hydrocortisone can be converted to an oral dose. As long as there is continued clinical improvement, continue to reduce hydrocortisone daily aiming for the patient's maintenance dose within a few days.
- **Fludrocortisone:** Long term, hydrocortisone will not provide sufficient mineralocorticoid activity. This is why Mrs Yu's regular medication included fludrocortisone. Typical daily doses are 50 to 300 micrograms. Mrs Yu's regular prescription of fludrocortisone should be continued.
- **Contact endocrinology:** For inpatient input, particularly regarding ongoing corticosteroid replacement.

HANDING OVER THE PATIENT

'Mrs Yu is a 40-year-old with known Addison's disease who had an uncomplicated laparoscopic cholecystectomy earlier today and presented postoperatively in an Addisonian crisis.

I reviewed her postoperatively and found her severely shocked with an elevated urea of 10 mmol/L (8.2 mmol/L now). Her creatinine was 150 µmol/L (80 µmol/L now). Her abdomen was soft to examination with no evidence of peritonism. Given her endocrine history, the initial Na of 125 mmol/L, borderline hyperkalaemia of 5.9 mmol/L and blood glucose of 4 mmol/L, our working diagnosis is an Addisonian crisis. Her HR and BP have started to normalise with fast IV fluids and 100 mg of IV hydrocortisone.

Please continue hydrocortisone 6 hourly, continue IV fluids until she's fully rehydrated, monitor for hypoglycaemia and contact the endocrine team for review tonight.'

STATION 6.9: HYPERTHYROID CRISIS (THYROID STORM)

You are the junior doctor in emergency department majors. You attend a 77-year-old male patient, Mr Southern. His wife reports that he has been confused since this morning and has been saying that his heart is racing in his chest and it felt like his skin was 'burning up'. She said that he is known to have hyperthyroidism but has stopped taking his pills lately because he does not think he needs them. He has no other past medical history.

Patient Details

Name:	Matthew Southern
DOB:	02/02/47
Hospital number:	444829012
Weight:	75 kg
Height:	178 cm
Consultant:	Dr Rogers
Hospital/Ward:	WGH Emergency Department
Current medications:	Nil
Allergies:	Nil
Admission date:	27/10/24

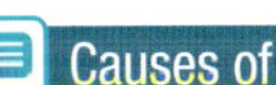

Causes of Atrial Fibrillation

CARDIAC
- Ischaemic heart disease
- Mitral valve disease
- Hypertension
- Cardiomyopathy

NONCARDIAC
- Acute infections, e.g. pneumonia
- Alcohol (acute and chronic use)
- Electrolyte disturbances
- Pulmonary embolism
- Thyrotoxicosis
- Following cardiac/chest surgery
- Lung cancer

Initial Differential Diagnosis

Hyperthyroid crisis has to be suspected given his medical history. It is most likely this has been precipitated by nonadherence with medication.

Other potential triggers include:

- MI
- surgery
- pulmonary embolism
- DKA
- severe infection

Complications of hyperthyroid storm

- Atrial fibrillation (10%–20%)
- Coma
- Death

INITIAL ASSESSMENT

AIRWAY

- Assess patency of the airway. There is a risk of coma and vomiting that might impair the airway.

  'Airway is patent.'

  No action required.

BREATHING

- What is the RR, oxygen saturations and work of breathing? Examine for evidence of pulmonary oedema.

  'You count the RR as 24/min and oxygen saturations are 85% on air. The patient cannot complete full sentences. Crepitations are audible at the lung bases bilaterally.'

- Prescribe high-flow oxygen in view of his low oxygen saturations (see later).

CIRCULATION

- Assess pulse, BP, CRT, look for signs of dehydration and carry out an ECG. Look for: tachycardia, hypotension and oedema. On the ECG look for atrial fibrillation (AF) and signs of ischaemia.

  'Mr Southern has strong bounding pulses, and you can see his heart beating in his praecordium. He is in atrial fibrillation at 144 bpm. There is no peripheral oedema and the JVP is not raised. The BP is 140/60 mmHg.'

- Given this patient is acutely unwell, you ask for him to be moved urgently to emergency department resus for stabilisation and ask for a senior colleague to assist you.
- The tachycardia is driven by the hyperthyroid crisis and AF. Prescribe a beta-blocker for rate control since the AF is most likely sympathetically driven. Given the suspicion of pulmonary oedema based on chest examination, IV fluids should not be currently considered.

DISABILITY

- Consciousness may be impaired by delirium or coma. Check blood glucose.

  'Although disorientated to time and place, Mr Southern answered all other questions appropriately. Blood glucose is 8 mmol/L.'

EXPOSURE

- Temperature: hyperpyrexia can occur in hyperthyroid crisis, although bear in mind other causes such as sepsis.
- Wounds or scars (over thyroid or nonthyroid area) would suggest a possible traumatic or surgical precipitant.

Prescribe (Figs 6.23 and 6.24)

High-flow OXYGEN e.g. 15 L/min via a NONREBREATHER MASK
Beta-blocker, e.g. PROPRANOLOL 80 mg PO STAT
Antipyretics, e.g. PARACETAMOL 1 g PO STAT
Loop diuretic, e.g. FUROSEMIDE 40 mg IV STAT

'Mr Southern is sweating profusely and the oral thermometer reads 40.5°C. There is no evidence of recent surgery.'

Antipyretics are required.

INTERPRETING TFTS

See Table 6.11 for an overview on how to interpret thyroid function tests.

INITIAL INVESTIGATIONS

- **Bloods:** FBC, U&Es, calcium, TFTs (including free T3, free T4 (FT4) and thyroid stimulating hormone (TSH)), CRP and blood cultures. Looking for possible infection, evidence of renal failure and acidosis and for confirmation of the diagnosis of hyperthyroidism. Calcium can be elevated with hyperthyroidism (Table 6.12).
- **Capillary blood glucose:** Looking for hypoglycaemia as a cause of confusion or hyperglycaemia (see Box 6.1).
- **CXR:** Looking for evidence of pulmonary oedema.
- **Urine dipstick:** As part of septic screen.

'FBC is within normal parameters. Urea 10.1 mmol/L, creatinine 120 µmol/L, normal electrolytes except elevated adjusted calcium of 2.74 mmol/L. CXR shows Kerley-B lines, perihilar shadowing and upper lobe diversion. Urine dipstick is normal. The lab phones you to say that thyroid function tests won't be ready for 3 hours. The capillary blood glucose is 10.1 mmol/L.'

Table 6.11 Interpreting Thyroid Function Tests

	PRIMARY HYPERTHYROID	PRIMARY HYPOTHYROID	SICK THYROID
TSH	↓	↑	→ or ↓
FT4	↑	↓	↓
FT3	↑	↓	↓

FT3, Free T3; *FT4*, free T4; *TSH*, thyroid stimulating hormone.

Table 6.12 Mr Southern's Blood Results

PARAMETER	VALUE	NORMAL RANGE (UNITS)
Haemoglobin	140 g/L	Men: 135–177 (g/L) Women: 115–155 (g/L)
WCC	8.5 × 10^9/L	4–11 (× 10^9/L)
Platelet	349 × 10^9/L	150–400 (× 10^9/L)
CRP	4 mg/L	<5 (mg/L)
Urea	**10.1 mmol/L**	**2.5–6.7 (mmol/L)**
Creatinine	**120 µmol/L**	**79–118 (µmol/L)**
eGFR	**48 mL/min**	**>60 (mL/min)**
Sodium	138 mmol/L	135–146 (mmol/L)
Potassium	4.2 mmol/L	3.5–5.0 (mmol/L)
Adjusted calcium	**2.74 mmol/L**	**2.20–2.67 (mmol/L)**
Blood glucose	**10.1 mmol/L**	**4.5–5.6 mmol/L**

Data in bold signifies results that are outside the normal laboratory range. *CRP*, C-reactive protein; *eGFR*, estimated glomerular filtration rate; *WCC*, white cell count.

Box 6.1 Glucose in Hyperthyroidism

Even in the absence of DKA, the blood glucose can be raised in a hyperthyroid crisis. This is due to the enhanced effect of catecholamines during a thyroid storm and the effect of thyroxine itself. These act antagonistically to insulin and increase the blood glucose concentration.

Mr Southern has evidence of pulmonary oedema. He needs a loop diuretic.

INITIAL MANAGEMENT

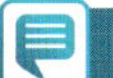

Hyperthyroidism Management Summary

Hyperthyroid crisis is essentially an extreme, life threatening version of thyrotoxicosis. The patient needs to be admitted. The management is twofold:

- **Supportive:** beta-blocker, diuretic if in heart failure, paracetamol, corticosteroids
- **Antithyroid drugs:** carbimazole or propylthiouracil followed by iodine solution after >1 hour

- **Beta-adrenergic blockade:** Propranolol 80 mg PO (or 1 mg IV doses if oral route not available) to reduce sympathetic drive from thyroxine, reduce the conversion of T4 to T3 and control AF (if present). Note that, as a general principle, beta-blockers should be avoided in acute heart failure; however, in this case they are appropriate. The patient does not have any past medical history except hyperthyroidism. Therefore, most likely the acute heart failure is genuinely acute (rather than acute-on-chronic) and the hyperthyroid crisis is driving his left ventricular failure and consequent pulmonary oedema, i.e. increased T4/T3 → propensity for AF → uncontrolled ventricular response → reduced cardiac output → heart failure. Giving beta-blockers in this circumstance will rate-control him and likely treat the underlying cause of the heart failure but close haemodynamic monitoring is required. A short-acting beta-blocker such as propranolol is preferred here since it will clear quickly if it does cause an unacceptable side effect, such as worsening heart failure.
- **Antipyretic:** Paracetamol, as prescribed. If this is not sufficient, external cooling can also be used.
- **Inhibit new thyroid hormone production:** Using carbimazole or propylthiouracil.
- **Nasogastric (NG) tube:** Should be considered for delivery of oral medications if the patient is vomiting or obtunded.
- **Thromboprophylaxis:** This is a sick medical patient at risk of venous thromboembolism. LMWH should be used. Mr Southern's weight is 75 kg. Cockcroft–Gault creatinine clearance is 48.4 mL/min [(140 − 77) × 75 × 1.23/120 = 48.4 mL/min]. This is above the eGFR threshold for factor Xa monitoring (20 mL/min).
- **Continuous monitoring:** To include three-lead ECG and oxygen saturations. Request regular (e.g. hourly) observations.
- **Fluid balance:** This is essential given that Mr Southern has received diuretics for his acute left ventricular failure. Urine volumes should be measured to confirm response to furosemide. Consider a catheter if the patient is struggling to get up to pass urine.
- **Corticosteroids:** Consider prescribing hydrocortisone 100 mg IV QDS in a thyrotoxic crisis because this acts to reduce the conversion of T4 to T3.

Prescribe (see Figs 6.23 and 6.24)

Short-acting beta-blocker, e.g. PROPRANOLOL 80 mg PO QDS
Antipyretic, e.g. PARACETAMOL 1 g PO QDS
Thyroid production inhibition, e.g. CARBIMAZOLE 20 mg PO STAT, then QDS
Thromboprophylaxis, e.g. DALTEPARIN 5000 units SC OD
HYDROCORTISONE 100 mg IV QDS STAT, then QDS

REASSESSMENT

- You make a full clinical assessment of the patient 1 hour after the initial treatments were given.

'Mr Southern's airway remains patent. His RR has fallen to 20/min with oxygen saturations of 99% on oxygen 15 L/min. His chest sounds much clearer to auscultation. His HR is now 90 bpm in sinus rhythm with a temperature of 38.1°C.'

The patient does not need as much as much oxygen currently, so this can be reduced.

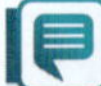

Prescribe (see Figs. 6.23 and 6.24)

OXYGEN, e.g. 40% via FACE MASK (reduced dose given oxygen saturations)

STOP
High-flow oxygen

FURTHER MANAGEMENT

- **Inhibit release of thyroid hormone:** With aqueous oral iodine solution (Lugol's iodine). This should be delayed at least 1 hour after carbimazole as it can paradoxically lead to massive thyroid hormone release.
- **Consider HDU/ITU**: Untreated or inadequately treated thyrotoxicosis is associated with high mortality. In scenarios such as this one, you should involve your seniors and the endocrine team early. ITU input will be required if there is ongoing evidence of haemodynamic compromise despite treatment or a need for ventilation. If available, medical HDU would be an appropriate place for initial management. Care should be under an endocrine team.
- **Education**: The patient needs to be counselled regarding the importance of taking his carbimazole.

Prescribe (see Figs 6.23 and 6.24)

Aqueous oral IODINE solution (iodine 5%, potassium iodide 10%) 0.3 mL STAT and then TDS PO (well diluted in water or milk)

HANDING OVER THE PATIENT

'Mr Southern is a 77-year-old man with known hyperthyroidism and poor recent adherence with medication who presented today in a hyperthyroid storm.

He presented with confusion, hyperpyrexia and atrial fibrillation with evidence of pulmonary oedema likely secondary to left ventricular failure. His FBC, Na and K are normal. Urea is 10.1 mmol/L, creatinine 120 µmol/L and adjusted calcium 2.74 mmol/L. CXR and urine dipstick are normal.

We have given the first doses of propranolol, carbimazole, hydrocortisone and paracetamol. He's also been given furosemide to reduce pulmonary oedema. Given his initial saturations on air were 85%, we started him initially on high-flow oxygen and he is now maintaining his saturations on 40% oxygen.

He has responded well to the above treatment and is stabilising. Please refer the patient to endocrinology for inpatient management and review regularly while still in the emergency department, particularly checking for further pyrexia and signs of heart failure as well as checking his fluid balance. He is due for a first dose of iodine solution in 30 minutes which is prescribed.

Please chase the outstanding thyroid function tests from the lab.

STATION 6.10: HYPOTHYROIDISM

You are the junior doctor working on the medical admissions unit (MAU). You see a 76-year-old woman, Mrs Phipps, who has been referred in by her GP. The daughter says that she is really worried her mother's memory has been deteriorating over the past month and she is more tired and sleepy during the day. She had a normal AMTS 1 year ago and she has no known medical problems.

Patient Details

Name:	Harriet Phipps
DOB:	12/02/47
Hospital number:	82948382
Weight:	60 kg
Height:	150 cm
Consultant:	Dr Horner
Hospital/Ward:	WGH 4B
Current medications:	Nil
Allergies:	Nil
Admission date:	02/02/24

Differential Diagnosis for Cognitive Impairment

SECONDARY (SOMETIMES REVERSIBLE) CAUSES, INCLUDING
- Hypothyroidism
- B_{12} and folate deficiency
- Subdural haematoma
- Depression
- HIV
- Normal pressure hydrocephalus

DEMENTIA
- Alzheimer's disease
- Vascular dementia
- Dementia with Lewy bodies
- Parkinson's disease dementia
- Frontotemporal lobe dementia

Hypothyroidism: Complications

- Skin: coarse features, puffy eye lids, dry skin
- Neck: goitre (in Hashimoto's thyroiditis)
- Hair: thinning
- Cardiovascular system: ischaemic heart disease, pericardial effusion
- Respiratory: pleural effusion
- Abdominal: obesity, ascites
- Neurological: neuropathy, somnolence, confusion, coma

INITIAL ASSESSMENT

AIRWAY, BREATHING, CIRCULATION

- Is the airway patent? What are the RR and oxygen saturations? Record HR and BP and look for signs of shock/dehydration.

'Airway is patent. RR is 14/min. Oxygen saturations 98% on room air. Pulse is 62 bpm and BP 138/79 mmHg. He is haemodynamically stable.'

No action is currently required.

DISABILITY

- Assess AMTS (see Abbreviated Mental Test Score (AMTS) box) and measure capillary blood glucose.

'AMTS is 6/10. Capillary blood glucose is 4.8 mmol/L.'

EXPOSURE

- Check temperature, examine the abdomen and do a neurological examination.

'Mrs Phipps feels cool to the touch. Her temperature is 35.8°C. She is obese but otherwise has a soft, nontender abdomen with no organomegaly. There is pitting oedema to her knees. Cranial nerves II–XII are normal. Peripheral neurological examination reveals slow-relaxing reflexes and reduced light touch sensation in a glove and stocking distribution.'

INITIAL INVESTIGATIONS

- **Urine dipstick:** In particular, look for the presence of leucocytes and/or nitrites, which would be consistent with infection.
- **CXR:** As part of a septic screen.
- **Bloods:** FBC, U&Es, LFTs, TFTs, B_{12} and folate. Hypothyroidism, electrolyte disturbances, B_{12} and folate deficiency are important reversible causes of cognitive impairment (Table 6.13).
- **Consider CT brain:** Assess for possible dementia or intracranial pathology leading to confusion, particularly if no cause is identified with the above investigations.

'Urine dipstick is negative and CXR is normal. Bloods show Hb 108 g/L, MCV 101 fL, WCC 7.4 × 10^9/L, platelet 155 × 10^9/L, urea 5.5 mmol/L, creatinine 89 μmol/L, Na 143 mmol/L, K 5.7 mmol/L, TSH 52 mU/L, free T4 (FT4) 6 pmol/L, B_{12} 209 pmol/L, folate 15 μg/L.'

The TSH is elevated and the FT4 is low. This is consistent with hypothyroidism.

Abbreviated Mental Test Score (AMTS)

- Give the patient an address to recall at the end
- Age
- Time (to nearest hour)
- What year is it?
- Recognise two people
- DOB
- Dates of Second World War
- Name of present monarch
- Name of hospital/institution
- Count backwards from 20 to 1

INITIAL MANAGEMENT

Hypothyroidism: Management Summary

- Replace thyroxine.
- Monitor TFTs monthly with levothyroxine dose adjustment.
- Monitor cholesterol.
- Screen for other autoimmune conditions if new symptoms develop.

- **Start levothyroxine:** At an initial dose of 25 micrograms daily. This is a more cautious dose than that used for younger people (typically 50–100 micrograms) to avoid precipitating AF or ischaemic heart disease.
- **Thyroid autoantibodies:** Check antithyroglobulin and antithyroid peroxidase antibodies. Primary hypothyroidism is most commonly an autoimmune disorder.

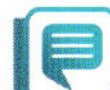

Prescribe (Fig. 6.25)

Thyroid replacement, e.g. LEVOTHYROXINE SODIUM 25 micrograms PO OD

REASSESSMENT

- After commencement on levothyroxine, Mrs Phipps is sent home from MAU with follow-up in medical outpatients in 4 weeks' time.

Table 6.13 Mrs Phipps' Blood Results

PARAMETER	VALUE	NORMAL RANGE (UNITS)
Haemoglobin	**108 g/L**	**Men: 135–177 (g/L) Women: 115–155 (g/L)**
Neutrophil	6.2 × 10^9/L	2.0–7.5 (× 10^9/L)
WCC	7.4 × 10^9/L	4–11 (× 10^9/L)
MCV	**101 fL**	**80–96 (fL)**
Platelet	155 × 10^9/L	150–400 (× 10^9/L)
B_{12}	209 pmol/L	150–675 (pmol/L)
Folate	15 μg/L	4–18 (μg/L)
Urea	5.5 mmol/L	2.5–6.7 (mmol/L)
Creatinine	89 μmol/L	79–118 (μmol/L)
[illegible]	44.[illegible] mL/min	[illegible] (mL/min)
Sodium	143 mmol/L	135–146 (mmol/L)
Potassium	**5.7 mmol/L**	**3.5–5.0 (mmol/L)**
ALT	17 IU/L	<40 (IU/L)
ALP	72 IU/L	39–117 (IU/L)
Bilirubin	10 μmol/L	<17 (μmol/L)
T3	1.2 pmol/L	0.9–2.4 (pmol/L)
T4	**6 pmol/L**	**9–21 (pmol/L)**
TSH	**52 mU/L**	**0.2–4.5 (mU/L)**

Data in bold signifies results that are outside the normal laboratory range. *ALP,* Alkaline phosphatase; *ALT,* alanine transaminase; *eGFR,* estimated glomerular filtration rate; *MCV,* mean cell volume; *TSH,* thyroid stimulating hormone; *WCC,* white cell count.

FURTHER MANAGEMENT

- **TFTs:** TFTs respond slowly to the initiation and adjustment of thyroxine supplementation. Therefore, these should be checked every 4 weeks until TSH and FT4 are in the normal range (keeping TSH >0.5). Then check TSH annually.
- **Adjust levothyroxine:** This should be increased in increments of 25 micrograms/day every 4 weeks until TFTs normalise.
- **Secondary prevention:** Hypothyroid patients are at risk of hyperlipidaemia. Measure baseline cholesterol and, if elevated, monitor and start a statin if cholesterol is persistently elevated despite rendering the patient euthyroid.
- **Other autoimmune conditions** occur more commonly in patients with autoimmune hypothyroidism and these include rheumatoid arthritis, pernicious anaemia, systemic lupus erythematosus, Addison's disease, coeliac disease and vitiligo. If patients develop new or nonspecific symptoms, then consider investigating for these other diseases.

REASSESSING THE PATIENT IN CLINIC

You see Mrs Phipps in clinic as planned.

'Mrs Phipps is much less confused with an AMTS of 10. Her peripheral oedema is now limited to her ankles and she says she feels less prone to cold. Her temperature is 36.9°C. The peripheral neuropathy persists. Her bloods show TSH 16.1 mU/L, FT4 8 pmol/L, triglycerides 1.5 mmol/L and total cholesterol 7.6 mmol/L.'

AFTERWARDS YOU WRITE A SHORT LETTER TO THE PATIENT'S GP

'Mrs Phipps presented to the medical take 4 weeks ago and was diagnosed with hypothyroidism leading to cognitive impairment, peripheral neuropathy, peripheral oedema and hypothermia. She was commenced on levothyroxine 25 micrograms daily for 4 weeks, which was increased in clinic today to 50 micrograms as her TFTs have improved but have not yet fully normalised. She has a high total cholesterol, please repeat this once the patient is euthyroid and treat with a statin if it remains elevated.

We discharge her back to your care. Please can you repeat her TFTs in 4 weeks and increase her levothyroxine to 75 micrograms daily if she is not yet euthyroid.'

FURTHER READING

BMJ Best Practice, 2022. Assessment of hyponatraemia. https://bestpractice.bmj.com/topics/en-gb/57 (Last accessed 22.09.23).

Joint British Diabetes Societies Inpatient Care Group, 2022. The management of the hypersomolar hyperglycaemic state (HHS) in adults. https://abcd.care/sites/default/files/site_uploads/JBDS_Guidelines_Current/JBDS_06_The_Management_of_Hyperosmolar_Hyperglycaemic_State_HHS_%20in_Adults_FINAL_0.pdf (Last accessed 22.09.23).

Joint British Diabetes Societies Inpatient Care Group, 2023. The management of diabetic ketoacidosis in adults. https://abcd.care/resource/current/jbds-02-management-diabetic-ketoacidosis-adults (Last accessed 22.09.23).

Joint British Diabetes Society, 2021. The hospital management of hypoglycaemia in adults with diabetes mellitus. https://abcd.care/sites/default/files/site_uploads/JBDS_Guidelines_Archive/JBDS_01_Hypo_Guideline_FINAL_23042021_Archive.pdf (Last accessed 22.09.23).

Joint Formulary Committee. British National Formulary (online). London: BMJ Group and Pharmaceutical Press. http://www.bnf.org (Last accessed 22.09.23).

Mahoney, B.A., Smith, W.A.D., Lo, D., 2005. Emergency interventions for hyperkalaemia. Cochrane Database Syst Rev (2).

National Collaborating Centre for Acute Care for NICE, 2018. Venous thromboembolism in over 16s: reducing the risk of hospital-acquired deep vein thrombosis or pulmonary embolism. https://www.nice.org.uk/guidance/ng89/resources/venous-thromboembolism-in-over-16s-reducing-the-risk-of-hospitalacquired-deep-vein-thrombosis-or-pulmonary-embolism-pdf-1837703092165 (Last accessed 22.09.23).

Nayak, B., Burman, K., 2006. Thyrotoxicosis and thyroid storm. Endocrinol Metab Clin N Am 35, 663–686.

NHS Tayside Diabetes MCN, 2021. Tayside diabetes MCN handbook insulin adjustment guidelines. http://www.diabetes-healthnet.ac.uk/Documents/Uploaded/HandbookInsulinadjustmentguidelines.pdf (Last accessed 22.09.23).

Patient.co.uk, 2020. Adrenal crisis. https://patient.info/doctor/adrenal-crisis (Last accessed 22.09.23).

Scottish Palliative Care Guidelines, 2021. Hypercalcaemia. https://www.palliativecareguidelines.scot.nhs.uk/guidelines/palliative-emergencies/hypercalcaemia.aspx (Last accessed 22.09.23).

The Renal Association, 2020. Clinical practice guidelines: treatment of acute hyperkalaemia in adults. https://ukkidney.org/sites/renal.org/files/RENAL%20ASSOCIATION%20HYPERKALAEMIA%20GUIDELINE%20-%20JULY%202022%20V2_0.pdf (Last accessed 22.09.23).

University Hospitals Sussex NHS Foundation Trust, 2015. Hypercalcaemia in malignancy guidelines. https://www.bsuh.nhs.uk/library/wp-content/uploads/sites/8/2019/03/HypercalcaemiaOfMaliganancy2015.pdf (Last accessed 22.09.23).

Wass, J.A.H., Arlt, W., 2012. How to avoid precipitating an acute adrenal crisis. BMJ 345, e6333.

Wilkinson, I.B., Raine, T., Wiles, K., et al., 2017. Oxford Handbook of Clinical Medicine, 10th edition. Oxford University Press, Oxford.

PRESCRIPTION CHARTS

PRESCRIPTION AND ADMINISTRATION RECORD

Standard Chart

Hospital/Ward: WGH 2B	**Consultant:** DR BROWN	**Name of Patient:** SARAH BROWN
Weight: 70 kg (ESTIMATED)	**Height:** 172 cm (ESTIMATED)	**Hospital Number:** 204684560
If re-written, date:		**D.O.B.:** 11/11/2002
DISCHARGE PRESCRIPTION **Date completed:-**	**Completed by:-**	

OTHER MEDICINE CHARTS IN USE		PREVIOUS ADVERSE REACTIONS This section must be completed before any medicine is given		Completed by (sign & print)	Date
Date	Type of Chart	None known ☒		P. Smith PAUL SMITH	02/02/24
		Medicine/Agent	Description of Reaction		

CODES FOR NON-ADMINISTRATION OF PRESCRIBED MEDICINE

If a dose is not administered as prescribed, initial and enter a code in the column with a circle drawn round the code according to the reason as shown below. **Inform the responsible doctor in the appropriate timescale.**

1. Patient refuses
2. Patient not present
3. Medicines not available – CHECK ORDERED
4. Asleep/drowsy
5. Administration route not available – CHECK FOR ALTERNATIVE
6. Vomiting/nausea
7. Time varied on doctor's instructions
8. Once only/as required medicine given
9. Dose withheld on doctor's instructions
10. Possible adverse reaction/side effect

ONCE-ONLY

Date	Time	Medicine (Approved Name)	Dose	Route	Prescriber – Sign + Print	Time Given	Given By
02/02/24	17.05	CO-AMOXICLAV (1000 mg/200 mg)	1.2 g	IV	P. Smith PAUL SMITH	17.10	AD
02/02/24	17.05	GENTAMICIN (over 1 H)	350 mg	IV	P. Smith PAUL SMITH	17.15	AD
02/02/24	17.05	PARACETAMOL	1 g	ORAL	P. Smith PAUL SMITH	17.15	AD

OXYGEN	Start Date	Start Time	Route Mask (%)	Route Prongs (L/min)	Prescriber – Sign + Print	Administered by	Stop Date	Stop Time

Fig. 6.1 Prescription and administration record (standard chart) for Sarah Brown.

Name: SARAH BROWN

Date of Birth: 11/11/2002

REGULAR THERAPY

PRESCRIPTION	Date → / Time ↓	02/02/24											
Medicine (Approved Name): CO-AMOXICLAV (1000 mg/200 mg)	6												
Dose: 1.2g — Route: IV	(8)												
Notes: pyelonephritis.14/7 r/v? switch to oral daily — Start Date: 02/02/24	12												
	(14)												
Prescriber – sign + print: P. Smith PAUL SMITH	18												
	(22)	FD											

PRESCRIPTION	Time	02/02/24											
Medicine (Approved Name): DALTEPARIN	6												
Dose: 5000 units — Route: SC	8												
Notes: — Start Date: 02/02/24	12												
	14												
Prescriber – sign + print: P. Smith PAUL SMITH	(18)	FD											
	22												

PRESCRIPTION	Time	02/02/24											
Medicine (Approved Name): INSULIN GLARGINE (LANTUS)	6												
Dose: 6 units — Route: SC	8												
Notes: — Start Date: 02/02/24	12												
	14												
Prescriber – sign + print: P. Smith PAUL SMITH	(18)	FD											
	22												

PRESCRIPTION	Time												
Medicine (Approved Name):	6												
Dose: — Route:	8												
Notes: — Start Date:	12												
	14												
Prescriber – sign + print:	18												
	22												

PRESCRIPTION	Time												
Medicine (Approved Name):	6												
Dose: — Route:	8												
Notes: — Start Date:	12												
	14												
Prescriber – sign + print:	18												
	22												

PRESCRIPTION	Time												
Medicine (Approved Name):	6												
Dose: — Route:	8												
Notes: — Start Date:	12												
	14												
Prescriber – sign + print:	18												
	22												

Fig. 6.2 Prescription and administration record (regular therapy) for Sarah Brown.

FLUID PRESCRIPTION CHART

Hospital/Ward: WGH 2B	**Consultant:** DR BROWN		**Name of Patient:** SARAH BROWN
Weight: 70kg (ESTIMATED)	**Height:** 172cm (ESTIMATED)		**Hospital Number:** 204684560
			D.O.B: 11/11/2002

Date/ Time	FLUID / ADDED DRUGS	VOLUME / DOSE	ROUTE	RATE	PRESCRIBER – SIGN AND PRINT
02/02/24 16.55	SODIUM CHLORIDE 0.9%	500mL	IV	Over 15min	P. Smith PAUL SMITH
02/02/24 17.00	SODIUM CHLORIDE 0.9%	50mL	IV	7mL/h	P. Smith PAUL SMITH
	INSULIN (ACTRAPID)	50 units			
02/02/24 18.00	SODIUM CHLORIDE 0.9%	1L	IV	1000mL/h	P. Smith PAUL SMITH

Fig. 6.3 Fluid prescription chart for Sarah Brown.

PRESCRIPTION AND ADMINISTRATION RECORD

Standard Chart

Hospital/Ward: WGH MAU	**Consultant:** DR NORRIS	**Name of Patient:** HELEN JONES
Weight: 93 kg	**Height:** 151 cm	**Hospital Number:** 3299206023
If re-written, date:		**D.O.B.:** 14/09/1954
DISCHARGE PRESCRIPTION **Date completed:-**	**Completed by:-**	

OTHER MEDICINE CHARTS IN USE		PREVIOUS ADVERSE REACTIONS This section must be completed before any medicine is given		Completed by (sign & print)	Date
Date	Type of Chart	None known ☒		P. Smith PAUL SMITH	02/02/24
		Medicine/Agent	Description of Reaction		

CODES FOR NON-ADMINISTRATION OF PRESCRIBED MEDICINE

If a dose is not administered as prescribed, initial and enter a code in the column with a circle drawn round the code according to the reason as shown below. **Inform the responsible doctor in the appropriate timescale.**

1. Patient refuses
2. Patient not present
3. Medicines not available – CHECK ORDERED
4. Asleep/drowsy
5. Administration route not available – CHECK FOR ALTERNATIVE
6. Vomiting/nausea
7. Time varied on doctor's instructions
8. Once only/as required medicine given
9. Dose withheld on doctor's instructions
10. Possible adverse reaction/side effect

ONCE-ONLY

Date	Time	Medicine (Approved Name)	Dose	Route	Prescriber – Sign + Print	Time Given	Given By
02/02/24	21.45	CO-AMOXICLAV (1000 mg/200 mg)	1.2g	IV	P. Smith PAUL SMITH	21.45	AS
02/02/24	21.45	PARACETAMOL	1g	ORAL	P. Smith PAUL SMITH	21.55	AS
02/02/24	22.00	CLARITHROMYCIN	500 mg	ORAL	P. Smith PAUL SMITH	22.15	AS

OXYGEN	Start Date	Start Time	Route Mask (%)	Route Prongs (L/min)	Prescriber – Sign + Print	Administered by	Stop Date	Stop Time
	02/02/24	21.30	15L/min via NON-REBREATHER MASK		P. Smith PAUL SMITH	BG 21:32	02/02/24	23.15
	02/02/24	23.15	40% via FACE MASK		P. Smith PAUL SMITH	BG 23:15		

Fig. 6.4 Prescription and administration record (standard chart) for Helen Jones.

Name: HELEN JONES
Date of Birth: 14/09/1954

REGULAR THERAPY

PRESCRIPTION		Date → / Time ↓		02/02/24	03/02/24										
Medicine (Approved Name): PARACETAMOL		6													
Dose: 1g	Route: ORAL	(8)			FD										
Notes:	Start Date: 02/02/24	(12)			FD										
Prescriber – sign + print: P. Smith PAUL SMITH		14													
		(18)			FD										
		(22)		X	FD										
Medicine (Approved Name): DALTEPARIN		6													
Dose: 5000 units	Route: SC	8													
Notes:	Start Date: 02/02/24	12													
Prescriber – sign + print: P. Smith PAUL SMITH		14													
		(18)			FD										
		22													
Medicine (Approved Name): CO-AMOXICLAV (1000 mg/200 mg)		6													
Dose: 1.2g	Route: IV	(8)			FD										
Notes: severe CAP 5/7 of treatment, r/v? switch to oral daily.	Start Date: 02/02/24	12													
Prescriber – sign + print: P. Smith PAUL SMITH		(14)			FD										
		18													
		(22)		X	FD										
Medicine (Approved Name): CLARITHROMYCIN		6													
Dose: 500 mg	Route: ORAL	(8)			FD										
Notes: severe CAP 5/7 of treatment	Start Date: 02/02/24	12													
Prescriber – sign + print: P. Smith PAUL SMITH		14													
		(18)			FD										
		22													
Medicine (Approved Name):		6													
Dose:	Route:	8													
Notes:	Start Date:	12													
Prescriber – sign + print:		14													
		18													
		22													
Medicine (Approved Name):		6													
Dose:	Route:	8													
Notes:	Start Date:	12													
Prescriber – sign + print:		14													
		18													
		22													

Fig. 6.5 Prescription and administration record (regular therapy) for Helen Jones.

FLUID PRESCRIPTION CHART

Hospital/Ward: WGH MAU	**Consultant:** DR NORRIS	**Name of Patient:** HELEN JONES
Weight: 93 kg	**Height:** 151 cm	**Hospital Number:** 6481785610
		D.O.B: 14/09/1954

Date/ Time	FLUID / ADDED DRUGS	VOLUME / DOSE	ROUTE	RATE	PRESCRIBER – SIGN AND PRINT
02/02/24 21.35	SODIUM CHLORIDE 0.9%	500 mL	IV	Over 15 mins	P. Smith PAUL SMITH
02/02/24 22.00	SODIUM CHLORIDE 0.9%	1 L	IV	500 mL/h	P. Smith PAUL SMITH
	POTASSIUM CHLORIDE	20 mmol			

Fig. 6.6 Fluid prescription chart for Helen Jones.

FLUID PRESCRIPTION CHART

Hospital/Ward: WGH A&E	Consultant: DR TAYLOR	Name of Patient: YASMIN GREY
Weight: 50 kg (LAST ADMISSION)	Height: 164 cm (LAST ADMISSION)	Hospital Number: 459023211
		D.O.B: 15/05/2007

Date/ Time	FLUID / ADDED DRUGS	VOLUME / DOSE	ROUTE	RATE	PRESCRIBER – SIGN AND PRINT
02/02/24 23.00	GLUCOSE 20%	50 mL	IV	STAT	P. Smith PAUL SMITH
02/02/24 23.05	SODIUM CHLORIDE 0.9%	500 mL	IV	Over 15 mins	P. Smith PAUL SMITH

Fig. 6.7 Fluid prescription chart for Yasmin Grey.

Name: SARAH BROWN
Date of Birth: 11/11/2002

SCENARIO 1: STARTING A BASAL-BOLUS

Blood glucose monitoring and subcutaneous insulin prescription chart

Date	BLOOD GLUCOSE (mmol/L)				INSULIN (units)							
	Before breakfast	Before lunch	Before dinner	Before bed	Before breakfast Type/units	Prescribed by / Given by	Before lunch Type/units	Prescribed by / Given by	Before evening meal Type/units	Prescribed by / Given by	Before bed Type/units	Prescribed by / Given by
03/02/24									INSULIN GLARGINE (LANTUS) 26 units INSULIN ASPART (NOVORAPID) 9 units	P. Smith PAUL SMITH		
04/02/24					INSULIN ASPART (NOVORAPID) 9 units	P. Smith PAUL SMITH						

Fig. 6.8 Blood glucose monitoring and subcutaneous insulin prescription chart for Sarah Brown.

Name: ALEX SMITH
Date of Birth: 01/07/1993

SCENARIO 2: ADJUSTING SHORT-ACTING INSULIN

Blood glucose monitoring and subcutaneous insulin prescription chart

Date	BLOOD GLUCOSE (mmol/L)				INSULIN (units)							
	Before breakfast	Before lunch	Before dinner	Before bed	Before breakfast Type/units	Prescribed by / Given by	Before lunch Type/units	Prescribed by / Given by	Before evening meal Type/units	Prescribed by / Given by	Before bed Type/units	Prescribed by / Given by
02/02/24		10.3					INSULIN ASPART (NOVORAPID) 13 units	P. Smith PAUL SMITH				

Fig. 6.9 Blood glucose monitoring and subcutaneous insulin prescription chart for Alex Smith.

Name: BORIS JONES

Date of Birth: 06/03/1958

SCENARIO 3: BIPHASIC INSULIN

Blood glucose monitoring and subcutaneous insulin prescription chart

Date	BLOOD GLUCOSE (mmol/L)				INSULIN (units)							
	Before breakfast	Before lunch	Before dinner	Before bed	Before breakfast Type/units	Prescribed by / Given by	Before lunch Type/units	Prescribed by / Given by	Before evening meal Type/units	Prescribed by / Given by	Before bed Type/units	Prescribed by / Given by
02/02/24	12.1	14.3	13.6	10.2	BIPHASIC ISOPHANE INSULIN (HUMULIN M3) 24 units	K. Jones KATE JONES / HM			BIPHASIC ISOPHANE INSULIN (HUMULIN M3) 12 units	K. Jones KATE JONES / HM		
03/02/24	17.3	13.2	11.3	13.0	BIPHASIC ISOPHANE INSULIN (HUMULIN M3) 24 units	K. Jones KATE JONES / HM			BIPHASIC ISOPHANE INSULIN (HUMULIN M3) 12 units	K. Jones KATE JONES / HM		
04/02/24	12.9	15.1			BIPHASIC ISOPHANE INSULIN (HUMULIN M3) 24 units	K. Jones KATE JONES / HM			BIPHASIC ISOPHANE INSULIN (HUMULIN M3) 13 units	P. Smith PAUL SMITH		
05/02/24					BIPHASIC ISOPHANE INSULIN (HUMULIN M3) 26 units	P. Smith PAUL SMITH						

Fig. 6.10 Blood glucose monitoring and subcutaneous insulin prescription chart for Boris Jones.

Name: ROBERT APPLEBY

Date of Birth: 19/11/1942

SCENARIO 4: LONG-ACTING INSULIN

Blood glucose monitoring and subcutaneous insulin prescription chart

Date	BLOOD GLUCOSE (mmol/L)				INSULIN (units)							
	Before breakfast	Before lunch	Before dinner	Before bed	Before breakfast Type/units	Prescribed by / Given by	Before lunch Type/units	Prescribed by / Given by	Before evening meal Type/units	Prescribed by / Given by	Before bed Type/units	Prescribed by / Given by
02/02/24	2.7	6.9	7.4	10.1					INSULIN DETEMIR (LEVEMIR) 34 units	K. Jones KATE JONES / HM		
03/02/24	3.1	8.2	5.7	9.9					INSULIN DETEMIR (LEVEMIR) 34 units	K. Jones KATE JONES / HM		
04/02/24	3.0	7.4							INSULIN DETEMIR (LEVEMIR) [illegible] units	P. Smith PAUL SMITH		
05/02/24												

Fig. 6.11 Blood glucose monitoring and subcutaneous insulin prescription chart for Robert Appelby.

PRESCRIPTION AND ADMINISTRATION RECORD

Standard Chart

Hospital/Ward: WGH MAU	**Consultant:** DR OLAG	**Name of Patient:** MARK WHITE
Weight: 50 kg (ESTIMATED)	**Height:** 164 cm (ESTIMATED)	**Hospital Number:** 456488932
If re-written, date:		**D.O.B.:** 14/04/1949
DISCHARGE PRESCRIPTION **Date completed:-**	**Completed by:-**	

IN USE		This section must be completed before any medicine is given		(sign & print)	Date
Date	Type of Chart	None known ☒		P. Smith PAUL SMITH	02/02/24
		Medicine/Agent	Description of Reaction		

CODES FOR NON-ADMINISTRATION OF PRESCRIBED MEDICINE

If a dose is not administered as prescribed, initial and enter a code in the column with a circle drawn round the code according to the reason as shown below. **Inform the responsible doctor in the appropriate timescale.**

1. Patient refuses
2. Patient not present
3. Medicines not available – CHECK ORDERED
4. Asleep/drowsy
5. Administration route not available – CHECK FOR ALTERNATIVE
6. Vomiting/nausea
7. Time varied on doctor's instructions
8. Once only/as required medicine given
9. Dose withheld on doctor's instructions
10. Possible adverse reaction/side effect

ONCE-ONLY

Date	Time	Medicine (Approved Name)	Dose	Route	Prescriber – Sign + Print	Time Given	Given By
02/02/24	19.05	CO-AMOXICLAV (1000 mg/200 mg)	1.2 g	IV	P. Smith PAUL SMITH	19.05	FD
02/02/24	19.05	GENTAMICIN (over 1 H)	250 mg	IV	P. Smith PAUL SMITH	19.10	FD
02/02/24	19.20	10% CALCIUM GLUCONATE (titrate in 1 mL aliquots to ECG changes)	10 mL	IV	P. Smith PAUL SMITH	19.20	PS (10 mL)
02/02/24	19.25	SALBUTAMOL (driven by air)	10 mg	NEB	P. Smith PAUL SMITH	19.30	FD

OXYGEN	Start Date	Start Time	Route Mask (%)	Route Prongs (L/min)	Prescriber – Sign + Print	Administered by	Stop Date	Stop Time

Fig. 6.12 Prescription and administration record (standard chart) for Mark White.

Name: MARK WHITE

Date of Birth: 14/04/1949

REGULAR THERAPY

PRESCRIPTION

Medicine (Approved Name)		Date → / Time ↓	02/02/24	03/02/24	04/02/24	05/02/24	06/02/24	07/02/24						
RAMIPRIL		6				Review								
Dose 2.5 mg	Route ORAL	(8)	X	X	X	☐								
		12												
Notes	Start Date 02/02/24	14												
Prescriber – sign + print		18												
P. Smith PAUL SMITH		22												

Medicine (Approved Name)		Time	02/02/24	03/02/24	04/02/24	05/02/24	06/02/24	07/02/24						
DALTEPARIN		6												
Dose 5000 units	Route SC	8												
		12												
Notes VTE prophylaxis. Anti-factor Xa levels every 5/7	Start Date 02/02/24	14				Pre and post dose levels due								
Prescriber – sign + print		(18)		FD				☐						
P. Smith PAUL SMITH		22												

Medicine (Approved Name)		Time	02/02/24	03/02/24	04/02/24	05/02/24	06/02/24	07/02/24						
CO-AMOXICLAV (1000 mg/200 mg)		6												
Dose 600 mg	Route IV	(8)		FD										
		12												
Notes Pyelonephritis - 14 days treatment r/v renal function r/v daily re. oral switch	Start Date 02/02/24	14												
Prescriber – sign + print		(18)		FD										
P. Smith PAUL SMITH		22												

Medicine (Approved Name)		Time												
		6												
Dose	Route	8												
		12												
Notes	Start Date	14												
Prescriber – sign + print		18												
		22												

Medicine (Approved Name)		Time												
		6												
Dose	Route	8												
		12												
Notes	Start Date	14												
Prescriber – sign + print		18												
		22												

Medicine (Approved Name)		Time												
		6												
Dose	Route	8												
		12												
Notes	Start Date	14												
Prescriber – sign + print		18												
		22												

Fig. 6.13 Prescription and administration record (regular therapy) for Mark White.

FLUID PRESCRIPTION CHART

Hospital/Ward: WGH MAU **Consultant:** DR OLAG

Weight: 50 kg (ESTIMATED) **Height:** 164 cm (ESTIMATED)

Name of Patient: MARK WHITE

Hospital Number: 456488932

D.O.B: 14/04/1949

Date/ Time	FLUID / ADDED DRUGS	VOLUME / DOSE	ROUTE	RATE	PRESCRIBER – SIGN AND PRINT
02/02/24 19.00	SODIUM CHLORIDE 0.9%	500 mL	IV	Over 15 min	P. Smith PAUL SMITH
02/02/24 19.25	GLUCOSE 10%	250 mL	IV	Over 30 min	P. Smith PAUL SMITH
	INSULIN (ACTRAPID)	10 units			
02/02/24 19.25	SODIUM CHLORIDE 0.9%	500 mL	IV	Over 15 min	P. Smith PAUL SMITH

Fig. 6.14 Fluid prescription chart for Mark White.

Name: DAVID OLDFIELD

Date of Birth: 12/10/1946

REGULAR THERAPY

PRESCRIPTION	Date → Time ↓		02/02/24	03/02/24										

Medicine (Approved Name): SENNA
Dose: 15 mg | **Route:** ORAL
Notes: | **Start Date:** 02/02/24
Prescriber – sign + print: P. Smith PAUL SMITH

Time		02/02/24	03/02/24										
6													
8													
12													
14													
18													
(22)		FD											

Medicine (Approved Name): DALTEPARIN
Dose: 5000 units | **Route:** SC
Notes: | **Start Date:** 02/02/24
Prescriber – sign + print: P. Smith PAUL SMITH

Time		02/02/24	03/02/24										
6													
8													
12													
14													
(18)		FD											
22													

Medicine (Approved Name):
Dose: |
Notes: | **Start Date:**
Prescriber – sign + print:

Time													
6													
8													
12													
14													
18													
22													

Medicine (Approved Name):
Dose: | **Route:**
Notes: | **Start Date:**
Prescriber – sign + print:

Time													
6													
8													
12													
14													
18													
22													

Medicine (Approved Name):
Dose: | **Route:**
Notes: | **Start Date:**
Prescriber – sign + print:

Time													
6													
8													
12													
14													
18													
22													

Medicine (Approved Name):
Dose: | **Route:**
Notes: | **Start Date:**
Prescriber – sign + print:

Time													
6													
8													
12													
14													
18													
22													

Fig. 6.15 Prescription and administration record (regular therapy) for David Oldfield.

FLUID PRESCRIPTION CHART

Hospital/Ward: WGH ONCOLOGY	**Consultant:** DR MORRIS	**Name of Patient:** DAVID OLDFIELD
Weight: 80 kg	**Height:** 176 cm	**Hospital Number:** 432907155
		D.O.B: 12/10/1946

Date/ Time	FLUID / ADDED DRUGS	VOLUME / DOSE	ROUTE	RATE	PRESCRIBER – SIGN AND PRINT
02/02/24 18.00	SODIUM CHLORIDE 0.9%	1 L	IV	166 mL/h	P. Smith PAUL SMITH
03/02/24 00.00	SODIUM CHLORIDE 0.9%	1 L	IV	166 mL/h	P. Smith PAUL SMITH
03/02/24 09.00	SODIUM CHLORIDE 0.9% DISODIUM PAMIDRONATE	500 mL 90 mg	IV	250 mL/h	P. Smith PAUL SMITH

Fig. 6.16 Fluid prescription chart for David Oldfield.

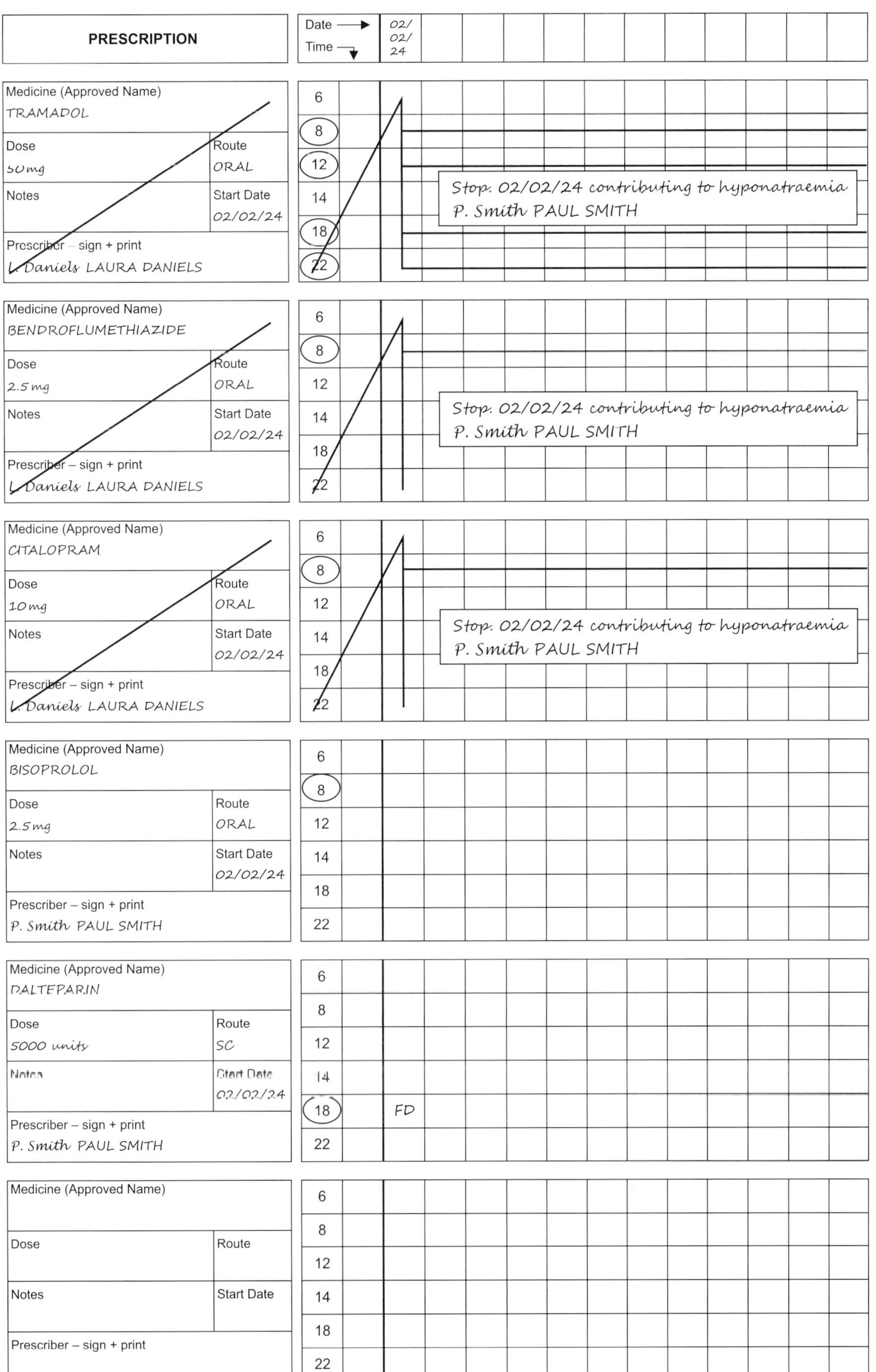

Name: *OMAR SHAH*

Date of Birth: *02/02/1954*

REGULAR THERAPY

PRESCRIPTION	Date → / Time ↓	02/02/24

Medicine (Approved Name): *TRAMADOL*
Dose: *50 mg* | Route: *ORAL*
Notes | Start Date: *02/02/24*
Prescriber – sign + print: *L. Daniels LAURA DANIELS*
Times: 6, (8), (12), 14, (18), (22)
Stop. 02/02/24 contributing to hyponatraemia P. Smith PAUL SMITH

Medicine (Approved Name): *BENDROFLUMETHIAZIDE*
Dose: *2.5 mg* | Route: *ORAL*
Notes | Start Date: *02/02/24*
Prescriber – sign + print: *L. Daniels LAURA DANIELS*
Times: 6, (8), 12, 14, 18, 22
Stop. 02/02/24 contributing to hyponatraemia P. Smith PAUL SMITH

Medicine (Approved Name): *CITALOPRAM*
Dose: *10 mg* | Route: *ORAL*
Notes | Start Date: *02/02/24*
Prescriber – sign + print: *L. Daniels LAURA DANIELS*
Times: 6, (8), 12, 14, 18, 22
Stop. 02/02/24 contributing to hyponatraemia P. Smith PAUL SMITH

Medicine (Approved Name): *BISOPROLOL*
Dose: *2.5 mg* | Route: *ORAL*
Notes | Start Date: *02/02/24*
Prescriber – sign + print: *P. Smith PAUL SMITH*
Times: 6, (8), 12, 14, 18, 22

Medicine (Approved Name): *DALTEPARIN*
Dose: *5000 units* | Route: *SC*
Notes | Start Date: *02/02/24*
Prescriber – sign + print: *P. Smith PAUL SMITH*
Times: 6, 8, 12, 14, (18) *FD*, 22

Medicine (Approved Name):
Dose | Route
Notes | Start Date
Prescriber – sign + print
Times: 6, 8, 12, 14, 18, 22

Fig. 6.17 Prescription and administration record (regular therapy) for Omar Shah.

FLUID PRESCRIPTION CHART

Hospital/Ward: WGH MAU	**Consultant:** DR WILKINS	**Name of Patient:** OMAR SHAH
Weight: 60 kg	**Height:** 169 cm	**Hospital Number:** 549309293
		D.O.B: 02/02/1954

Date/ Time	FLUID / ADDED DRUGS	VOLUME / DOSE	ROUTE	RATE	PRESCRIBER – SIGN AND PRINT
02/02/24 21.30	SODIUM CHLORIDE 3% (monitor sodium regularly)	1L	IV	60 mL/h	P. Smith PAUL SMITH
	Stopped as sodium now 126 03/02/24 P. Smith PAUL SMITH				

Fig. 6.18 Fluid prescription chart for Omar Shah.

PRESCRIPTION AND ADMINISTRATION RECORD

Standard Chart

Hospital/Ward: WGH GENERAL SURGERY **Consultant:** MR SMITH **Weight:** 52 kg **Height:** 155 cm **If re-written, date:** **DISCHARGE PRESCRIPTION** **Date completed:-** **Completed by:-**	**Name of Patient:** ABIGAEL YU **Hospital Number:** 908236125 **D.O.B.:** 30/08/1983

OTHER MEDICINE CHARTS IN USE	
Date	Type of Chart

PREVIOUS ADVERSE REACTIONS This section must be completed before any medicine is given		Completed by (sign & print)	Date
None known ☒		P. Smith PAUL SMITH	01/02/24
Medicine/Agent	Description of Reaction		

CODES FOR NON-ADMINISTRATION OF PRESCRIBED MEDICINE

If a dose is not administered as prescribed, initial and enter a code in the column with a circle drawn round the code according to the reason as shown below. **Inform the responsible doctor in the appropriate timescale.**

1. Patient refuses
2. Patient not present
3. Medicines not available – CHECK ORDERED
4. Asleep/drowsy
5. Administration route not available – CHECK FOR ALTERNATIVE
6. Vomiting/nausea
7. Time varied on doctor's instructions
8. Once only/as required medicine given
9. Dose withheld on doctor's instructions
10. Possible adverse reaction/side effect

ONCE-ONLY

Date	Time	Medicine (Approved Name)	Dose	Route	Prescriber – Sign + Print	Time Given	Given By
02/02/24	15.00	HYDROCORTISONE	100 mg	IV	P. Smith PAUL SMITH	15.10	KO

OXYGEN

Start Date	Start Time	Route Mask (%)	Route Prongs (L/min)	Prescriber – Sign + Print	Administered by	Stop Date	Stop Time

Fig. 6.19 Prescription and administration record (standard chart) for Abigael Yu.

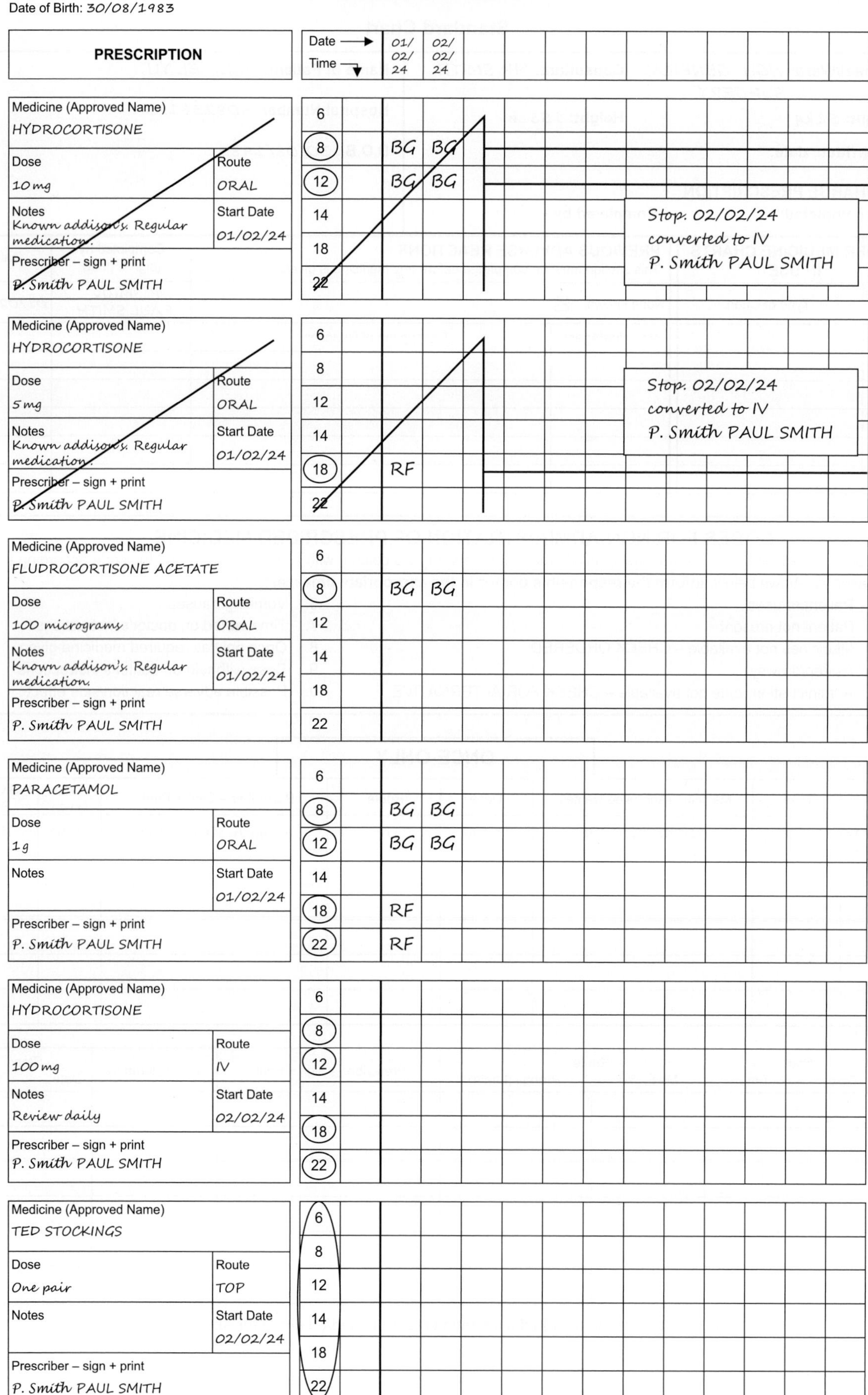

Name: ABIGAEL YU

Date of Birth: 30/08/1983

REGULAR THERAPY

PRESCRIPTION	Time ↓ / Date →	01/02/24	02/02/24
Medicine (Approved Name): HYDROCORTISONE	6		
Dose: 10 mg; Route: ORAL	(8)	BG	BG
Notes: Known addison's. Regular medication. Start Date: 01/02/24	(12)	BG	BG
Prescriber – sign + print: P. Smith PAUL SMITH	14		
	18		
	22		

Stop: 02/02/24 converted to IV P. Smith PAUL SMITH

PRESCRIPTION	Time	01/02/24	02/02/24
Medicine (Approved Name): HYDROCORTISONE	6		
Dose: 5 mg; Route: ORAL	8		
Notes: Known addison's. Regular medication. Start Date: 01/02/24	12		
Prescriber – sign + print: P. Smith PAUL SMITH	14		
	(18)	RF	
	22		

Stop: 02/02/24 converted to IV P. Smith PAUL SMITH

PRESCRIPTION	Time	01/02/24	02/02/24
Medicine (Approved Name): FLUDROCORTISONE ACETATE	6		
Dose: 100 micrograms; Route: ORAL	(8)	BG	BG
Notes: Known addison's. Regular medication. Start Date: 01/02/24	12		
Prescriber – sign + print: P. Smith PAUL SMITH	14		
	18		
	22		

PRESCRIPTION	Time	01/02/24	02/02/24
Medicine (Approved Name): PARACETAMOL	6		
Dose: 1 g; Route: ORAL	(8)	BG	BG
Notes: ; Start Date: 01/02/24	(12)	BG	BG
Prescriber – sign + print: P. Smith PAUL SMITH	14		
	(18)	RF	
	(22)	RF	

PRESCRIPTION	Time		
Medicine (Approved Name): HYDROCORTISONE	6		
Dose: 100 mg; Route: IV	(8)		
Notes: Review daily; Start Date: 02/02/24	(12)		
Prescriber – sign + print: P. Smith PAUL SMITH	14		
	(18)		
	(22)		

PRESCRIPTION	Time		
Medicine (Approved Name): TED STOCKINGS	(6		
Dose: One pair; Route: TOP	8		
Notes: ; Start Date: 02/02/24	12		
Prescriber – sign + print: P. Smith PAUL SMITH	14		
	18		
	22)		

Fig. 6.20 Prescription and administration record (regular therapy) for Abigael Yu.

Name: ABIGAEL YU

Date of Birth: 30/08/1983

REGULAR THERAPY

PRESCRIPTION

Date → / Time ↓	01/02/24	02/02/24										

Medicine (Approved Name): DALTEPARIN

Dose: 5000 units | Route: SC

Notes: | Start Date: 02/02/24

Prescriber – sign + print: P. Smith PAUL SMITH

Time													
6													
8													
12													
14													
(18)													
22													

Medicine (Approved Name):

Dose: | Route:

Notes: | Start Date:

Prescriber – sign + print:

Time													
6													
8													
12													
14													
18													
22													

Medicine (Approved Name):

Dose: | Route:

Notes: | Start Date:

Prescriber – sign + print:

Time													
6													
8													
12													
14													
18													
22													

Medicine (Approved Name):

Dose: | Route:

Notes: | Start Date:

Prescriber – sign + print:

Time													
6													
8													
12													
14													
18													
22													

Medicine (Approved Name):

Dose: | Route:

Notes: | Start Date:

Prescriber – sign + print:

Time													
6													
8													
12													
14													
18													
22													

Medicine (Approved Name):

Dose: | Route:

Notes: | Start Date:

Prescriber – sign + print:

Time													
6													
8													
12													
14													
18													
22													

Fig. 6.21 Prescription and administration record (regular therapy) for Abigael Yu.

FLUID PRESCRIPTION CHART

Hospital/Ward: WGH GENERAL SURGERY **Consultant:** MR SMITH **Weight:** 52 kg **Height:** 155 cm	**Name of Patient:** ABIGAEL YU **Hospital Number:** 908236125 **D.O.B:** 30/08/1983

Date/ Time	FLUID / ADDED DRUGS	VOLUME / DOSE	ROUTE	RATE	PRESCRIBER – SIGN AND PRINT
02/02/24 15.00	SODIUM CHLORIDE 0.9%	500 mL	IV	Over 15 min	P. Smith PAUL SMITH
02/02/24 15.30	SODIUM CHLORIDE 0.9%	1 L	IV	1000 mL/h	P. Smith PAUL SMITH

Fig. 6.22 Fluid prescription chart for Abigael Yu.

PRESCRIPTION AND ADMINISTRATION RECORD

Standard Chart

Hospital/Ward: WGH A&E	Consultant: DR ROGERS	Name of Patient: MATTHEW SOUTHERN
Weight: 75 kg	Height: 178 cm	Hospital Number: 444829012
If re-written, date:		D.O.B.: 02/02/1947
DISCHARGE PRESCRIPTION Date completed:-	Completed by:-	

OTHER MEDICINE CHARTS IN USE		PREVIOUS ADVERSE REACTIONS This section must be completed before any medicine is given		Completed by (sign & print)	Date
Date	Type of Chart	None known ☒		P. Smith PAUL SMITH	27/10/24
		Medicine/Agent	Description of Reaction		

CODES FOR NON-ADMINISTRATION OF PRESCRIBED MEDICINE

If a dose is not administered as prescribed, initial and enter a code in the column with a circle drawn round the code according to the reason as shown below. **Inform the responsible doctor in the appropriate timescale.**

1. Patient refuses
2. Patient not present
3. Medicines not available – CHECK ORDERED
4. Asleep/drowsy
5. Administration route not available – CHECK FOR ALTERNATIVE
6. Vomiting/nausea
7. Time varied on doctor's instructions
8. Once only/as required medicine given
9. Dose withheld on doctor's instructions
10. Possible adverse reaction/side effect

ONCE-ONLY

Date	Time	Medicine (Approved Name)	Dose	Route	Prescriber – Sign + Print	Time Given	Given By
27/10/24	14.00	PROPRANOLOL	80 mg	ORAL	P. Smith PAUL SMITH	14.00	FR
27/10/24	14.10	PARACETAMOL	1 g	ORAL	P. Smith PAUL SMITH	14.10	FR
27/10/24	14.20	FUROSEMIDE	40 mg	IV	P. Smith PAUL SMITH	14.25	FR
27/10/24	14.30	CARBIMAZOLE	10 mg	ORAL	P. Smith PAUL SMITH	14.30	FR
27/10/24	15.30	AQUEOUS IODINE SOLUTION (IODINE 5%, POTASSIUM IODIDE 10%) dilute well in water or milk	0.3 mL	ORAL	P. Smith PAUL SMITH	15.40	FR

OXYGEN	Start Date	Start Time	Route Mask (%)	Route Prongs (L/min)	Prescriber – Sign + Print	Administered by	Stop Date	Stop Time
	27/10/24	13.50	15L/min via NON-REBREATHER MASK		P. Smith PAUL SMITH	GH 13.53	27/10/24	15.00
	27/10/24	15.05	40% via FACE MASK		P. Smith PAUL SMITH	AF 15.10		

Fig. 6.23 Prescription and administration record (standard chart) for Matthew Southern.

Name: MATTHEW SOUTHERN

Date of Birth: 02/02/1947

REGULAR THERAPY

PRESCRIPTION	Date → / Time ↓	27/10/24												
Medicine (Approved Name) PROPRANOLOL	6													
Dose 80 mg · **Route** ORAL	8													
Notes · **Start Date** 27/10/24	12													
Prescriber – sign + print P. Smith PAUL SMITH	14													
	18	FD												
	22	FD												
Medicine (Approved Name) PARACETAMOL	6													
Dose 1 g · **Route** ORAL	8													
Notes · **Start Date** 27/10/24	12													
Prescriber – sign + print P. Smith PAUL SMITH	14													
	18	FD												
	22	FD												
Medicine (Approved Name) CARBIMAZOLE	6													
Dose 10 mg · **Route** ORAL	8													
Notes · **Start Date** 27/10/24	12													
Prescriber – sign + print P. Smith PAUL SMITH	14													
	18	FD												
	22	FD												
Medicine (Approved Name) DALTEPARIN	6													
Dose 5000 units · **Route** SC	8													
Notes · **Start Date** 27/10/24	12													
Prescriber – sign + print P. Smith PAUL SMITH	14													
	18	FD												
	22													
Medicine (Approved Name) AQUEOUS IODINE SOLUTION (IODINE 5%, POTASSIUM IODIDE 10%)	6													
Dose 0.3 mL · **Route** ORAL	8													
Notes Dilute well in water or milk · **Start Date** 27/10/24	12													
Prescriber – sign + print P. Smith PAUL SMITH	14													
	18													
	22	FD												
Medicine (Approved Name)	6													
Dose · **Route**	8													
Notes · **Start Date**	12													
Prescriber – sign + print	14													
	18													
	22													

Fig. 6.24 Prescription and administration record (regular therapy) for Matthew Southern.

Name: *HARRIET PHIPPS*

Date of Birth: *12/02/1947*

REGULAR THERAPY

PRESCRIPTION

Date → / Time ↓	02/02/24												

Medicine (Approved Name) *LEVOTHYROXINE SODIUM*	
Dose *25 micrograms*	Route *ORAL*
Notes	Start Date *02/02/24*
Prescriber – sign + print *P. Smith PAUL SMITH*	

Time													
6													
(8)	FD												
12													
14													
18													
22													

Medicine (Approved Name)	
Dose	Route
Notes	Start Date
Prescriber – sign + print	

Time													
6													
8													
12													
14													
18													
22													

Medicine (Approved Name)	
Dose	Route
Notes	Start Date
Prescriber – sign + print	

Time													
6													
8													
12													
14													
18													
22													

Medicine (Approved Name)	
Dose	Route
Notes	Start Date
Prescriber – sign + print	

Time													
6													
8													
12													
14													
18													
22													

Medicine (Approved Name)	
Dose	Route
Notes	Start Date
Prescriber – sign + print	

Time													
6													
8													
12													
14													
18													
22													

Medicine (Approved Name)	
Dose	Route
Notes	Start Date
Prescriber – sign + print	

Time													
6													
8													
12													
14													
18													
22													

Fig. 6.25 Prescription and administration record (regular therapy) for Harriet Phipps.

Obstetrics and Gynaecology

7

Samuel Lockley, Matthew G. Wood

Chapter Outline

Station 7.1: Preterm Labour
Station 7.2: Bleeding in Pregnancy
Station 7.3: Preeclampsia
Station 7.4: Hyperemesis Gravidarum
Station 7.5: Urinary Tract Infection in Pregnancy

STATION 7.1: PRETERM LABOUR

You are the junior doctor currently rotating through obstetrics and gynaecology. You have been asked to see a new admission to the labour ward. Anne Seymour is a 29-year-old, 32 weeks into her first pregnancy, who attends with her husband. She has presented with a 10-hour history of acute intermittent abdominal pain which is becoming more frequent and more painful.

Patient Details

Name:	Anne Seymour
DOB:	27/03/95
Hospital number:	2103914534
Weight:	65 kg
Height:	1.6 m
Consultant:	Dr Roy
Hospital/Ward:	LGH Ward 4
Current medications:	None
Allergies:	No known drug allergies
Admission date:	22/10/24

Differential Diagnosis of Abdominal Pain in Pregnancy

NONOBSTETRIC CAUSES

- Renal colic
- Urinary tract infection
- Pyelonephritis
- Gallstones/cholecystitis
- Pancreatitis
- Gastritis
- Appendicitis

OBSTETRIC CAUSES

- Musculoskeletal ('stretching') pain
- Braxton–Hicks contractions
- Preterm labour
- Severe preeclampsia
- Placental abruption
- Uterine rupture

INITIAL ASSESSMENT

AIRWAY, BREATHING, CIRCULATION

- All patients, even those who appear stable, require an ABC assessment. This can, however, be done very quickly in patients that are not acutely unwell.

'The patient is sitting up on a bed talking to her partner when you enter the room. She looks a little uncomfortable but not unwell. The midwife shows you the admission observations she has recorded. The patient has a RR of 15/min, oxygen saturations of 99% on room air, pulse 95 bpm, a blood pressure of 120/80 mmHg, capillary refill time (CRT) <2 seconds and a temperature of 36.9°C.'

You identify that the patient is currently stable, allowing for a full history to be taken followed by examination.

HISTORY

A history and examination focused on eliminating potential differential diagnoses will quickly identify the likely diagnosis.

'The pains have the character of a tightening feeling across the abdomen. Initially they were coming every 30 minutes lasting about 10 seconds, now they are coming at least every 10 minutes, lasting up to a minute and are becoming more painful. Anne now has to stop what she is doing when the pain comes on. There are no symptoms of infection, no symptoms of preeclampsia, fetal movements have been normal and there has been no vaginal blood loss. Anne's pregnancy has been uneventful up to this point. The only other important fact noted from the history was that the patient thinks she had a procedure on her cervix about a year ago following an abnormal smear.'

The history of the pains is consistent with contractions which are increasing in frequency and intensity. There is a possibility that the patient also had a large loop excision of the transformation zone (LLETZ), which is a risk factor for preterm labour.

EXAMINATION

- Assess pallor, the pulse and CRT.
- Abdominal examination:
  - Identify areas of tenderness.
  - Measure symphysis–fundal height (SFH).
  - Palpate the uterus to identify tenderness and tightening.
  - Assess fetal lie, presentation and engagement using 'Leopold manoeuvres'.
- Speculum examination:
  - Always look at previous scans to confirm there is no placenta praevia before undertaking a pelvic examination.
  - Assess vulva and vagina for any abnormalities, blood or liquor in the vagina.
  - Obtain a good view of the cervix assessing cervical length, dilatation and presence of blood, fluid or membranes expectorating through the os.
  - Take a high vaginal swab (HVS).
- If 30+0 weeks pregnant or more, consider transvaginal ultrasound measurement of cervical length as a prognostic indicator to determine likelihood of birth within 48 hours; women are unlikely to be in preterm labour if the cervical length is 15 mm or more.
- If a transvaginal ultrasound measurement of cervical length is not appropriate, a fetal fibronectin swab can be taken from the posterior fornix of the vagina.

Fetal Fibronectin

- Simple bedside test used between 22 and 35 weeks' gestation.
- A testing swab is taken from the vagina at the same time as the speculum examination.
- A negative result suggests there is a 99% chance the patient will not labour in the next 14 days, but clinical judgement must be used when interpreting the result.
- Bleeding, recent intercourse, previous speculum examination and use of lubrication can all produce false-positive results.

'Heart rate is 80 bpm, CRT is 2 seconds. The abdomen is soft with no specific areas of tenderness. SFH 31 cm, uterus is initially soft but tightenings are palpable, and there is no uterine tenderness. Fetus is in a longitudinal lie, cephalic presentation, three-fifths palpable.

Normal vulva and vagina, no blood or liquor seen. The cervix is posterior, 1 cm long, 1 cm dilated, no membranes or fluid leak seen. High vaginal swab taken and sent to microbiology. Fibronectin was positive'.

The examination findings support the diagnosis of threatened preterm labour.

In obstetrics there are two patients:
- Assess maternal well-being first.
- Never forget to assess fetal well-being as well.

INITIAL INVESTIGATIONS

- **Urinalysis:** Rule out urinary tract infection (UTI).
- **Bloods:** To assess for signs of infection and to be prepared for delivery complications such as postpartum haemorrhage. Full blood count (FBC), C-reactive protein (CRP), urea and electrolytes (U&Es), group and save (Table 7.1).
- Check previous results for Group B *Streptococcus* carrier status.
- **Cardiotocography (CTG)**: To assess fetal well-being and frequency of contractions.

In most instances these investigations will have been carried out by the midwife prior to your arrival.

'In this case, urinalysis was normal, fetal heart tracing was normal and the tocograph showed 1–2 contractions every 10 minutes. Bloods were normal.'

INITIAL MANAGEMENT

Management Summary of Preterm Labour

- Treat any potential cause of preterm labour, e.g. infection (bacterial vaginosis, candidiasis and urinary tract infections are all associated with an increased risk of preterm labour).
- Administer corticosteroids.
- Magnesium sulphate for fetal neuroprotection.
- Tocolytic medication.
- Continuous CTG monitoring.
- Neonatal team involvement.

- Treat any potentially reversible cause of preterm labour:
  - Chase bloods and microbiology results. Regularly reassess the patient for signs of infection and have a low threshold for commencing treatment.
- Optimise conditions for delivery.

Table 7.1 Mrs Seymour's Blood Results

PARAMETER	VALUE	NORMAL RANGE (UNITS)
WCC	8 × 10^9/L	4–11 (×10^9/L)
Neutrophil	6 × 10^9/L	2–7.5 (×10^9/L)
Lymphocyte	2 × 10^9/L	1.4–4 (×10^9/L)
Platelet	300 × 10^9/L	150–400 (×10^9/L)
Haemoglobin	150 g/L	Men: 135–177 (g/L) Women: 115–155 (g/L)
CRP	3 mg/L	0–5 (mg/L)
Urea	2.5 mmol/L	2.5–6.7 (mmol/L)
Creatinine	79 µmol/L	79–118 (µmol/L)
Sodium	136 mmol/L	135–146 (mmol/L)
Potassium	5 mmol/L	3.5–5.0 (mmol/L)
eGFR	>60 ml/min	>60 (mL/min)

CRP, C-reactive protein; *eGFR*, estimated glomerular filtration rate; *WCC*, white cell count.

- Give betamethasone 12 mg IM, followed by a further dose 12 to 24 hours later to help mature the fetal lungs.
- Obtain intravenous (IV) access.
- Prescribe a tocolytic agent, e.g. nifedipine (immediate release (IR) preparation).
- Initial loading dose of 20 mg PO then maintenance dose of 10 to 20 mg PO TDS.
- The purpose of the nifedipine is to attempt to prolong the pregnancy to allow the corticosteroids to take effect.
- Magnesium sulfate should be offered for viable pregnancies before 30 weeks' gestation for fetal neuroprotection and should be considered up to 33 weeks' and 6 days' gestation (the loading and maintenance dosage are the same as used in the treatment of severe preeclampsia/eclampsia—see Section 7.3)
- Neonatal team involvement:
  - Confirm that the neonatal unit has a cot for this premature delivery; otherwise, an intrauterine transfer to another hospital may be needed.
  - Neonatal team to discuss likely management of the neonate with Anne and her husband.
- Venous thromboembolism (VTE) prophylaxis:
  - Low-molecular-weight heparin (LMWH) should be avoided as there is a risk the patient will go on to labour. Encourage adequate hydration and mobilisation, but this is a low-risk patient anyway.
  - If VTE prophylaxis is required in a high-risk patient, consider unfractionated heparin.

Keep the Patient Informed

- This is a very stressful time for parents with a lot of information for them to take in. Make sure you allow time to answer their questions. Keep your explanations simple.
- If you are unsure about how to answer a question, be honest and tell the patient you don't know the answer, but go and find a senior obstetrician or neonatologist who does.
- There is nothing worse for the patient than being given contradictory information.

Prescribe (Figs 7.1 and 7.2)

Corticosteroids:

- BETAMETHASONE 12 mg IM STAT (and repeated 12–24 hours later)

NIFEDIPINE (IR) 20 mg PO loading dose followed by NIFEDIPINE (IR) 10–20 mg PO TDS

OUTCOME

- If the contractions settle and there are no signs of infection or fetal compromise, Anne will be able to go home and continue the pregnancy.
- If there is any sign of fetal distress, delivery may be expedited (by either vaginal delivery or caesarean section).
- If Anne goes into established preterm labour despite our efforts to delay or prevent this, she will require antibiotics to reduce the risk of neonatal infection (benzylpenicillin 3 g loading dose followed by benzylpenicillin 1.5 g 4-hourly until birth).
- If Anne goes on to deliver despite attempts to prevent preterm labour, then we have prepared as well as possible for the preterm delivery.

HANDING OVER TO THE NIGHT TEAM

'Mrs Seymour presented to labour ward at 32 weeks' gestation in preterm labour. This is her first pregnancy, and there is a possible history of a large loop excision of the transformation zone last year. There are no symptoms of infection, no symptoms of preeclampsia, fetal movements have been normal and there has been no vaginal blood loss. Anne's pregnancy had been uneventful up to this point.

Mrs Seymour is haemodynamically stable, and initial bloods are normal. The CTG shows a normal fetal heart rate, and 1–2 contractions every 10 minutes. Two doses of betamethasone have been given and nifedipine has been started. The neonatal team is aware of the patient, and mum has been counselled about the likely fetal outcomes.

Please review Ms Seymour in a few hours; she may deliver today or tomorrow. If she is found to have gone into established labour, please commence antibiotic prophylaxis and consider magnesium sulphate for fetal neuroprotection, as per the preterm labour protocol. If there are any signs of fetal distress, delivery may need to be expedited.'

STATION 7.2: BLEEDING IN PREGNANCY

You are the junior doctor working in the emergency department. You are asked to urgently review Susan Cox, a 32-year-old who states she is 12 weeks pregnant and has presented with heavy vaginal bleeding.

Patient Details

Name:	Susan Cox
DOB:	21/03/92
Hospital number:	2103914531
Weight:	65 kg
Height:	1.5 m
Consultant:	Dr Roy
Hospital/Ward:	LGH ED
Current medications:	None
Allergies:	No known drug allergies
Admission date:	22/10/24

Bleeding in Pregnancy Differential Diagnosis

- Miscarriage:
  - Threatened (bleeding, os closed). May progress to complete miscarriage
  - Inevitable (bleeding, os open ± visible products)
  - Complete (bleeding settled, products passed, os closed)
- Ectopic pregnancy (classically presents 5–10/40 weeks)
- Cervical ectropion
- Cervical cancer
- Later gestation (>18/40 weeks) also:
  - Placenta praevia
  - Vasa praevia
  - Placental abruption
  - Labour (term or preterm)

Initial Assessment and Management Summary

- Resuscitate using an ABCDE approach
- 2 × large-bore cannula
- FBC, clotting, U&E, G&S and cross-match
- IV fluid resuscitation
- Regular assessment
- Consider:
  - Blood products
  - Medication to stop bleeding
  - Early specialist input

Holistic Practice

- Your focus should be the physical well-being of your patient.
- Do not neglect the psychological stress for the patient.
- Keep yourself and the environment as calm as possible.
- Offer support and allow a relative to sit with the patient when appropriate.

INITIAL ASSESSMENT

AIRWAY

- Assess patency of the airway.

'The patient is comfortably able to talk to you; there is no obvious airway problem.'

BREATHING

- Respiratory rate and oxygen saturations.
- Assess work of breathing.
- Perform a brief respiratory examination.

'RR 20/min, oxygen saturations are 97% on room air. The patient is speaking in full sentences. There is good air entry bilaterally on auscultation.'

No action is required for airway or breathing.

CIRCULATION

- Assess haemodynamic status by measuring pulse, blood pressure (BP) and CRT. Attach the patient to a three-lead electrocardiogram (ECG) and a noninvasive BP monitor set to recheck BP every 5 minutes.
- Additionally, make an initial assessment of the current blood loss. This only needs to be a crude assessment by looking at the patient and the paraphernalia around the room. For example, the patient may have some blood-soaked sanitary pads to show you, there may be some tennis-ball-sized blood clots on the bed that the patient has just passed or there may be blood all over the patient's clothing and blood may be all over the bed and dripping onto the floor.

'The patient's heart rate is 134 bpm, with a BP of 100/60 mmHg and CRT of 3 seconds. I note a heavily blood-stained incontinence pad underneath the patient, but I can't see active blood loss on this inspection.'

This patient is tachycardic and hypotensive with evidence of blood loss. She is at risk of further blood loss and hypotensive shock.

Obtain IV access with two large-bore cannulas, taking bloods at the same time. Prescribe and commence IV fluids. Prepare to catheterise the patient.

Prescribe (Figs 7.3–7.5)

Fluid:
- SODIUM CHLORIDE 0.9% 500 mL (over 15 min)

DISABILITY

- Assess the patient's Glasgow Coma Scale (GCS) or AVPU (is the patient Alert? If not, do they respond to Verbal or Painful stimuli? Or are they Unresponsive?) level.
- Check capillary blood glucose.

'The patient is GCS 15 (E4, M6, V5), blood glucose is 5.1 mmol/L.'

EXPOSURE

- Examine the abdomen, assess for areas of tenderness and for a palpable mass consistent with a uterus. (At 12 weeks of gestation the uterus may just be palpable above the pubic bone.)
- Check the temperature.
- Perform a speculum examination. With a lubricated Cusco speculum, attempt to locate the cervix and assess the current active blood loss. Gauze wrapped on sponge holder forceps will likely be needed to remove clots and blood in the vagina to visualise the cervix. The important points to assess are:
  - Extent of active bleeding
  - Cervical os open or closed (open suggests miscarriage inevitable)
  - Are products of conception visible at the os (if so try to remove with a sponge holder)
- A digital vaginal examination (PV) can be performed (ensure you know there is no placenta praevia first as this is a contraindication to PV) to assess whether

the cervical os is open when it has been difficult to visualise, and to assess size, position and mobility of the uterus.

- Catheterisation can be done after pelvic examination.

'The patient's abdomen is soft with mild tenderness suprapubically and a mass consistent with a 12-week-sized uterus is palpable suprapubically. On pelvic examination, there were two tennis-ball-sized blood clots removed from the vagina, an open cervix was seen with fresh blood trickling through the os, no products of conception seen. Temperature is 37°C.'

Your working diagnosis after your initial assessment is an inevitable miscarriage with active blood loss and a haemodynamically compromised patient.

Undertaking a Pelvic Exam

- Obtain verbal consent.
- Wear gloves.
- Always have a chaperone.
- All equipment close to hand—speculum, lubrication, sponge holder forceps, gauze.
- Adequate examination light/torch.

INITIAL INVESTIGATIONS

- **Bloods (Table 7.2):**
  - FBC—Assess for anaemia (may be falsely reassuring in an acute bleed prior to fluid resuscitation). Raised white cell count (WCC) can suggest infection, which may be a cause, or complication, of miscarriage. Decreased platelets with active heavy bleeding are suggestive of consumptive loss/disseminated intravascular coagulation (DIC) requiring further investigation of clotting and replacement of platelets.

Table 7.2 Ms Cox's Blood Results

PARAMETER	VALUE	NORMAL RANGE (UNITS)
WCC	10×10^9/L	4–11 ($\times 10^9$/L)
Neutrophil	7×10^9/L	2–7.5 ($\times 10^9$/L)
Lymphocyte	2×10^9/L	1.4–4 ($\times 10^9$/L)
Platelet	250×10^9/L	150–400 ($\times 10^9$/L)
Haemoglobin	**100 g/L**	**Men: 135–177 (g/L)** **Women: 115–155 (g/L)**
PT	12 seconds	11.5–13.5 seconds
APTT	35 seconds	26–37 seconds
CRP	4 mg/L	0–5 (mg/L)
Urea	2.5 mmol/L	2.5–6.7 (mmol/L)
Creatinine	79 µmol/L	79–118 (µmol/L)
Sodium	138 mmol/L	135–146 (mmol/L)
Potassium	4 mmol/L	3.5–5.0 (mmol/L)
eGFR	>60 mL/min	>60 (mL/min)

Data in bold signifies results that are outside the normal laboratory range.
APTT, Activated partial thromboplastin time; *CRP*, C-reactive protein; *eGFR*, estimated glomerular filtration rate; *PT*, prothrombin time; *WCC*, white cell count.

  - Clotting—Raised prothrombin time (PT)/activated partial thromboplastin time (APTT) with active bleeding needs urgent discussion with haematology and consideration of replacement of clotting factors with fresh frozen plasma (FFP) or cryoprecipitate.
  - U&Es—Baseline renal function should the patient require surgery under general anaesthesia.
  - Lactate—Can be obtained on bloods sent to the lab or using a bedside venous blood gas. Raised lactate can be a marker of hypoxia due to hypoperfusion and can help guide resuscitation.
  - CRP—Additional marker of infection (Table 7.2).
  - Group, save and cross-match 2 units—Blood product replacement should be considered if haemoglobin <70 g/L, haemoglobin <80 g/L in a symptomatic patient, or if bleeding is heavy >1.5 L and ongoing. If surgical management is undertaken, rhesus-negative patients (over 12 weeks' gestation) will require anti-D prophylaxis.

'Haemoglobin is 100 g/L, and the rest of the blood tests are normal.'

INITIAL MANAGEMENT

- Fluid resuscitation.
- Reduce the blood loss.
- Refer for definitive specialist management.

FLUID RESUSCITATION

- Reassess the heart rate and BP after the first fluid bolus has been infused.
- Continually reassess heart rate, BP and urine output. Remember, inserting two large-bore cannula allows two bags of IV fluid to be rapidly infused. These patients could have lost a significant amount of blood prior to admission and can lose a lot of their circulating volume very quickly:
  - If the patient is not stabilised after 2 to 3 L of IV fluid, it is important to refer to an intensivist/anaesthetist for support.
  - Significant blood loss (>2 L) is associated with anaemia and a consumption of platelets and clotting factors leading to a coagulopathy. Further fluid resuscitation with colloid or crystalloid will lead to a dilution of remaining red cells, platelets and clotting factors. Early recognition and replacement of packed red cells, platelets and FFP or cryoprecipitate reduce the risk of coagulopathy developing.
- With obstetric patients in particular (16 weeks and above), blood loss can escalate very quickly. All maternity units have a major obstetric haemorrhage (MOH) protocol, usually triggered by an estimated loss of around 1.5 L. Triggering the MOH protocol informs the multiple members of staff, including obstetricians, anaesthetists, porters and the haematology laboratory, so that blood products can be prepared and brought to where the patient is as quickly as possible.

REDUCE THE BLOOD LOSS

- There are several medications that can be given to increase uterine muscle tone which causes constriction of the blood vessels transecting the myometrium, thereby reducing the blood loss.
- First-line medication is ergometrine 500 micrograms with oxytocin 5 units (Syntometrine 1 mL) given by intramuscular injection. A second dose can be repeated after 10 minutes if bleeding persists:
  - Both ergometrine and oxytocin can also be given by slow IV infusion.
  - Care should be given using ergometrine IV and should be avoided entirely in patients with a history of hypertension as it can cause a severe hypertensive crisis.
- If bleeding is still uncontrolled after two doses of Syntometrine, senior help is needed urgently for definitive management. However, further treatments are available:
  - Misoprostol (prostaglandin E analogue) comes in tablet form which can be given orally, rectally or vaginally. Rectal administration is usually preferred as the vaginal absorption can be reduced by blood loss and the oral route is more likely to cause the side effects of vomiting and diarrhoea. This is an unlicensed use of misoprostol. A commonly used dose is 800 micrograms PR.
  - Carboprost (prostaglandin F analogue) can be given 250 micrograms by intramuscular injection repeated at 15-minute intervals to a maximum of eight doses (caution should be used in patients with asthma, as carboprost can induce bronchospasm in such patients).
  - Further to the previous uterotonic medications, tranexamic acid (an antifibrinolytic) can also be considered to reduce blood loss—in an emergency situation such as this, 1 g is typically administered intravenously over 10 minutes.
- VTE prophylaxis:
  - In this acute setting, the risk of haemorrhage is significant so pharmacological prophylaxis should be avoided.
  - Prescribe TED stockings and maintain adequate hydration.
  - After definitive management of the haemorrhage, LMWH should be considered.

Prescribe (see Figs 7.3–7.5)

SYNTOMETRINE (ERGOMETRINE 500 MICROGRAMS/ OXYCTOCIN 5 units in 1 mL) 1 mL IM STAT
Further fluids, SODIUM CHLORIDE 0.9% 500 mL (over 15 minutes)
Mechanical thromboprophylaxis:
- TED STOCKINGS 1 pair TOP

The patient is stable after this. Therefore, prescribe maintenance fluids (25–30 ml/kg), but be prepared to adjust the rate in response to observations and clinical reviews. Keep the patient nil by mouth (NBM) as may need to go to theatre.

Prescribe (see Figs 7.3–7.5)

Further fluids:
- SODIUM CHLORIDE 0.9% 1 L with 20 mmol KCl at 81 mL/h

HANDING OVER THE PATIENT

Refer for definitive specialist management:
- Have all relevant information to hand before making the referral:
  - Patient history—The definitive management is likely to be surgical so include past surgical and medical history, medication history, allergies and the last time the patient ate or drank.
  - Examination and findings, most recent observations and ABCDE reassessment.
  - Available investigation results.

'Hello am I speaking to the Obs & Gynae on-call doctor? I am Doctor…in A&E. I have a patient with probable miscarriage I would like to refer to be reviewed urgently by you.

The patient's name is Susan Cox. She is 32 years old and 12 weeks pregnant. She has attended this evening with heavy PV loss. This is her first pregnancy. On admission, she had a heart rate of 130 bpm, blood pressure 100/60 mmHg with a prolonged CRT. I have examined her, finding an open cervix with fresh vaginal bleeding but no products seen. I would estimate that the patient has lost about 500 mL in the department.

We have inserted two large-bore cannula, given 2 L IV fluid and have started a third litre. Bloods have been sent for FBC, clotting, U&Es, lactate, group and save, and 2 units have been cross-matched. Hb has come back at 100 g/L, platelets and clotting are normal.

We have given one dose of IM Syntometrine and the bleeding now appears to have reduced. Heart rate is now 100 bpm and blood pressure is 110/70 mmHg.

She has no previous past medical, surgical or obstetric history; she is on no medications and has no allergies. She last ate or drank about 4 hours ago.

I feel we have stabilised the patient's condition but would appreciate your input on her ongoing management of her miscarriage. Is there anything else you would like us to do prior to your arrival?'

The admitting obstetrics and gynaecology team will then review the patient and most likely offer the patient a surgical evacuation of retained products of conception under general anaesthesia. (Anti-D immunoglobulin administration will be required after the procedure if the patient is rhesus negative.)

STATION 7.3: PREECLAMPSIA

You are the junior doctor working in obstetrics. You are asked to review Michelle Fisher, a 37-year-old who is 34 weeks pregnant in her first pregnancy, attending with a persistent headache. Her BP is also raised.

Patient Details

Name:	Michelle Fisher
DOB:	01/02/87
Hospital number:	2103914527
Weight:	65 kg
Height:	1.5 m
Consultant:	Dr Roy
Hospital/Ward:	LGH Ward 4
Current medications:	None
Allergies:	No known drug allergies
Admission date:	22/10/24

Differential Diagnosis of Headache in Pregnancy

- Simple headache
- Migraine
- Cluster headache
- Meningitis
- Raised intracranial pressure
- Intracranial haemorrhage
- Preeclampsia
- Venous sinus thrombosis

Differential Diagnosis of Hypertension in Pregnancy

- Preeclampsia
- Gestational hypertension
- Chronic hypertension
- Hyperthyroidism
- Incorrect size of BP cuff
- White coat syndrome

INITIAL ASSESSMENT

AIRWAY

- Assess patency of the airway.

'Michelle is sitting talking to the midwife on your arrival. There is no obvious airway problem.'

No action required.

BREATHING

- Respiratory rate and oxygen saturations.
- Assess work of breathing.

'RR 14/min, oxygen saturations are 98% on room air. The patient is speaking in full sentences. There are no acute breathing concerns.'

No action required.

CIRCULATION

- Assess haemodynamic status by measuring pulse, BP and CRT. The patient's heart rate is 80 bpm with a BP of 165/111 mmHg and CRT of 2 seconds. This patient has severe hypertension. This will need treatment. Coupled with a headache, an important diagnosis to exclude is preeclampsia. Check urine dipstick, take bloods and establish IV access.

DISABILITY

- Assess the patient's GCS or AVPU (is the patient Alert? If not, do they respond to Verbal or Painful stimuli? Or are they Unresponsive?) level.
- Complete a full neurological examination if there are concerns of intracranial pathology/infection.
- To assess for signs of preeclampsia:
  - Check reflexes to identify hyperreflexia.
  - Check for abnormal clonus (three or more beats).
  - Undertake fundoscopy to assess for papilloedema.
- Check capillary blood glucose.

'The patient is GCS 15, blood glucose is 4.8 mmol/L. Reflexes are brisk, there is 1 beat of clonus, and fundoscopy appears normal. No other abnormality on gross neurological examination.'

EXPOSURE

- Examine the abdomen, assess for areas of tenderness (particularly epigastric tenderness which is associated with preeclampsia).
- Examine the abdomen obstetrically, measuring SFH, assess uterine tone and tenderness, assess fetal lie, presentation and engagement.
- Check the temperature. Look for periorbital oedema.

'The patient's abdomen is soft with no areas of abdominal or loin tenderness. The uterus is soft, nontender. Fetus is in a longitudinal lie, cephalic presentation, four-fifths palpable. The SFH is 30 cm, which is small for gestation. Temperature is 37°C.'

Hypertension in Pregnancy

NICE categorises gestational hypertension into two groups:

- Hypertension (140/90–159/109)
- Severe hypertension (160/110 or above)

An elevation of either the systolic or diastolic BP is required to diagnose hypertension.

Risk Factors for Preeclampsia

- First pregnancy
- Age >40
- BMI >35 at booking
- Family history of preeclampsia
- Multiple pregnancy
- Chronic hypertension
- Chronic kidney disease
- Diabetes
- Autoimmune disease
- Previous pregnancy with either:
  - hypertension
  - preeclampsia
  - placental abruption

Preeclampsia can cause significant fluid shift from intravascular to extracellular spaces which can cause significant oliguria. It is important not to blindly give fluid challenges to these patients as the likely outcome is no change in intravascular volume with worsening fluid shift, which can result in severe pulmonary and or cerebral oedema. A senior obstetrician's input should be sought for fluid balance concerns.

INITIAL INVESTIGATIONS

- **Urinalysis:**
  - ++ protein or above is significant proteinuria, which should then be quantified either by sending a sample for protein–creatinine ratio (PCR) or collecting a 24-hour urine sample for protein quantification.
  - Leucocytes and nitrites on urinalysis are suggestive of a UTI, and a midstream urine (MSU) should be sent for culture and sensitivities. A UTI could be the cause of proteinuria.
  - Ketones on urinalysis could indicate poor nutrition and hydration which could be a differential cause of a headache.
- **Blood tests (Table 7.3):**
  - FBC—Baseline Hb in case delivery is required, and platelets can be reduced in complications of preeclampsia (e.g. HELLP syndrome: haemolysis, elevated liver enzymes, low platelets).
  - Group and save—Taken in case of expedited delivery.
  - U&Es—Kidney disease in isolation can cause hypertension and proteinuria, and preeclampsia also affects end organs such as the kidneys.
  - Liver function tests (LFTs)—Elevated liver enzymes are also part of HELLP syndrome, and acute fatty liver and acute liver failure are also complications of preeclampsia.
  - CRP—Suggestive of infective cause of symptoms.
  - Other blood tests that may be considered:
    - Lactate dehydrogenase (LDH)—Additional marker of haemolysis which may occur in HELLP.
    - Clotting—If platelets low, previous history of clotting abnormalities or very large proteinuria (>3 g/day).
    - IV access for ongoing management.
- CTG—Assess fetal well-being and any uterine activity.
- Request an obstetric ultrasound scan to assess further fetal well-being and development. Request assessments of growth, liquor volume and umbilical artery Dopplers. (If not known also ask for placental location as this could affect mode of delivery.) These tests will help to determine any need for an expedited delivery for fetal reasons.

'Urinalysis shows protein++, a sample is sent for PCR. FBC, U&Es, LFTs and CRP are all normal. Urine PCR is raised at 35 mg/mmol. (An abnormal PCR is >30 mg/mmol, abnormal 24 h urine collection is >300 mg protein.) Group and save has been sent. CTG was normal. An ultrasound has been requested.'

Table 7.3 Ms Fisher's Blood Results

PARAMETER	VALUE	NORMAL RANGE (UNITS)
WCC	10 × 10⁹/L	4–11 (×10⁹/L)
Neutrophil	5 × 10⁹/L	2–7.5 (×10⁹/L)
Lymphocyte	4 × 10⁹/L	1.4–4 (×10⁹/L)
Platelet	200 × 109/L	150–400 (×10⁹/L)
Haemoglobin	150 g/L	Men: 135–177 (g/L) Women: 115–155 (g/L)
PT	12 seconds	11.5–13.5 seconds
APTT	34 seconds	26–37 seconds
CRP	4 mg/L	0–5 (mg/L)
Urea	2.7 mmol/L	2.5–6.7 (mmol/L)
Creatinine	79 µmol/L	79–118 (µmol/L)
Sodium	140 mmol/L	135–146 (mmol/L)
Potassium	4 mmol/L	3.5–5.0 (mmol/L)
eGFR	>60 mL/min	>60 (mL/min)
Bilirubin	10 µmol/L	<17 (µmol/L)
ALT	30 IU/L	<40 (IU/L)
ALP	110 IU/L	39–117 (IU/L)

ALP, Alkaline phosphatase; *ALT,* alanine transaminase; *APTT,* activated partial thromboplastin time; *CRP,* C-reactive protein; *eGFR,* estimated glomerular filtration rate; *PT,* prothrombin time; *WCC,* white cell count.

DIAGNOSIS

Hypertension with proteinuria in pregnancy should be treated as preeclampsia, and other causes ruled out. Further investigation results and ongoing monitoring will further help to confirm the diagnosis and the severity of the condition. Always complete the initial assessment by taking a full history from the patient and review the antenatal notes for additional risk factors and previous scan results. The current working diagnosis is severe preeclampsia (preeclampsia with severe hypertension).

Some maternity units utilise either fullPIERS (Preeclampsia Integrated Estimate of Risk) or PREP-S (Prediction model for Risks of complications in Early-onset Preeclampsia—Survival analysis model) risk scores to calculate the risk of adverse maternal outcomes within 48 hours. These scores can help to risk stratify patients and highlight those at the highest risk of associated complications.

MANAGEMENT

- **Stabilise the patients (mother and fetus):**
  - Control hypertension.
  - Level 2/high dependency unit (HDU) monitoring.

- Consider anticonvulsant therapy.
- Antenatal corticosteroids.
- Symptom management.
- Fetal monitoring.

- **Control hypertension:**
  - The biggest risks of uncontrolled hypertension in pregnancy are cerebrovascular haemorrhage and an eclamptic seizure. However, BP should not be lowered too quickly. Aim for BPs of 130–150/80–100 mmHg initially.
  - Labetalol, nifedipine and methyldopa (Table 7.4) are the three oral antihypertensive medications recommended for pregnancy by the National Institute for Health and Care Excellence (NICE).
  - Usually labetalol is the first-line medication used; however, this should be avoided if the patient is allergic or has severe asthma.
  - If after using one medication to its maximum dose the BP is still not controlled and there are no contraindications, one of the alternative therapies can be tried, and all three can be used simultaneously.
  - When prescribing nifedipine, you should specify if you are requesting the sustained release or immediate release preperation.
  - Labetalol and hydralazine can be given intravenously in severe hypertension of pregnancy if the patient's BP is unresponsive to oral antihypertensive medications.
  - Monitor the BP closely when administering hydralazine (particularly the initial IV bolus), as it can cause profound hypotension. If the BP is lowering before the whole bolus dose is given, stop giving the bolus and document how much has actually been given.
- **VTE prophylaxis:**
  - LMWH should be avoided acutely as there is a risk the patient will need imminent delivery.
  - However, preeclampsia is a risk factor for VTE. Prescribe TED stockings and encourage mobilisation.

Prescribe (Figs 7.6 and 7.7)

Antihypertensive:
- LABETALOL 200 mg PO STAT

Blood pressure 60 min later was 160/100 mmHg

Antihypertensive:
- NIFEDIPINE (SR) 10 mg PO STAT

Mechanical thromboprophylaxis:
- TED STOCKINGS 1 pair TOP

- **Level 2/HDU monitoring:**
  - Adequate staffing levels and training to manage this type of patient
  - Continuous BP monitoring
  - Thirty-minute observations of heart rate, respiratory rate, saturations and at least 4 hourly temperature
  - Fluid input/output monitoring:
    - Assess current level of dehydration/fluid overload.
    - Aim to restrict total fluid in (including any infusions) to 80 mL/h. Due to the multisystem involvement and increased vascular permeability associated with preeclampsia, patients are at risk of fluid overload and severe pulmonary oedema.
    - Monitor urine output and consider catheterisation if the patient is not passing urine regularly. A normal minimum urine output is around 0.5 mL/kg per hour, but in preeclampsia, due to fluid shift to the extravascular space, some oliguria is not uncommon. With input from anaesthetic colleagues, a careful balance must be reached to avoid pulmonary or cerebral oedema and also underperfusion of the kidneys. Sequential renal function blood tests will help in this regard.

'After initial doses of labetalol and nifedipine the blood pressure is now stable at 140/90 mmHg. All other observations have been normal. The patient is fluid restricted and currently has a urine output of 20 mL/h. The consultant obstetrician has been informed and is currently happy with the blood pressure and fluid

Table 7.4 Drugs Used to Control Acute Hypertension in Pregnancy

	FIRST-LINE THERAPY			ALTERNATIVE/SEVERE ASTHMA		
	DRUG	**DOSE**	**ROUTE**	**DRUG**	**DOSE**	**ROUTE**
First dose	Labetalol	200 mg	PO	Nifedipine	10 mg	PO
If BP high after 60 minutes	Labetalol	200 mg	PO	Nifedipine	10 mg	PO
If BP high after further 60 minutes	Labetalol	50 mg	IV bolus	Hydralazine	5–10 mg	Slow IV
	Then labetalol infusion 20 mg/h, doubled every 30 minutes if required to maximum dose 160 mg/h			Then hydralazine infusion 50–150 micrograms/ minute, dose dependent on blood pressure		

BP, Blood pressure; *IV*, intravenous.

status, but would like the patient to remain in an HDU setting and the blood tests rechecked 24 hours after they were first taken.'

- **Consider medication to increase seizure threshold:**
  - Magnesium should be given if the patient is having or has had an eclamptic seizure.
  - It can be considered if the patient has severe preeclampsia and their condition appears to be deteriorating or not improving despite treatment, or if delivery is anticipated within 24 hours.
  - It is given as a 4 g IV bolus over 15 minutes, followed by an infusion of 1 g/h for 24 hours (a further 2 g bolus can be given if there are recurrent seizures).
  - Magnesium overdose is rare but a recognised risk of therapy. Regular monitoring for loss of deep tendon reflexes, patient agitation and a lowering respiratory rate should be undertaken to diagnose toxicity early. If there are any concerns:
    - Stop the infusion.
    - Start cardiac monitoring (risk of arrhythmia).
    - Request a serum magnesium level.
- Administer 10 mL of 10% calcium gluconate slowly IV if there are signs of arrhythmia, respiratory depression or the serum magnesium level is at the toxic level. Further boluses may be given depending on response.

'The patient's condition including blood pressure is currently stable, so the consultant does not wish to give magnesium at this time.'

ANTENATAL CORTICOSTEROIDS

- With a diagnosis of severe preeclampsia, the patient is most likely to need delivery within the next few days (earlier if there is deterioration). At 34 weeks' gestation, there is a risk of prematurity. Giving corticosteroids can help mature the fetal lungs by increasing production of surfactant and reduce neonatal complications.
- Give betamethasone 12 mg IM, followed by a further dose 12 hours later.

Prescribe (see Figs 7.6 and 7.7)

Corticosteroids:

- BETAMETHASONE 12 mg IM STAT (and repeated in 12 h)

PARACETAMOL 1 g PO QDS

Giving Corticosteroids? Think: Inform the Neonatal Team

- Whenever there is a possibility of preterm delivery, it is essential to inform the neonatal team so they can:
  - Prepare their unit.
  - Discuss with patient the likely neonatal management and outcome.
- If there are no neonatal beds available then an intrauterine transfer may be needed.

SYMPTOM MANAGEMENT

- Never forget the patient. She presented with a persistent headache. To optimise the patient's well-being and ability to engage with the situation and make decisions about her ongoing care, it is important to treat the pain.
- Analgesia in pregnancy is discussed in the UTI in pregnancy section.

FETAL MONITORING

- There are always two patients to consider in obstetrics. If either is compromised during the pregnancy, then there can be an indication to deliver.
- Monitor fetal well-being by monitoring fetal movements felt by the mother.
- CTG should be done if there are concerns about fetal movement or there is a significant change in the mother's condition (e.g. sudden hypertension or hypotension), and most senior obstetricians ask for at least a daily CTG even in stable patients.
- Review any previous ultrasound scans and any performed during the admission.

'Fetal movements have remained normal during the admission and CTGs performed have been normal. The ultrasound scan shows estimated fetal weight is just below the 10th centile, with normal liquor volume and normal umbilical artery Dopplers.'

PRESENTING YOUR FINDINGS TO THE ON-CALL OBSTETRIC CONSULTANT

'Michelle Fisher is 37 years old. She is a primigravida, 34 weeks into her first pregnancy. She booked as low risk and has had an uneventful pregnancy so far. She presented today with a persistent frontal headache. Blood pressure on admission was 165/111 mmHg, with 2+ protein on urinalysis. Urine PCR is 35 mg/mmol, but blood tests are all normal.

No other symptoms or signs of preeclampsia were identified on examination. I have given a dose of labetalol 200 mg and a further dose of nifedipine 10 mg and the blood pressure is now 140/90 mmHg. Urine output is 20 mL/h, but other observations are normal. The patient's headache has been eased with paracetamol.

Michelle has not had any concerns with fetal movements and admission CTG was normal. However, on examination SFH measured 30 cm so I arranged a growth scan which shows estimated fetal weight is just below the 10th centile with normal liquor and Dopplers. I have given the first dose of betamethasone with the next dose prescribed for 12 hours later. I have checked with the neonatal unit and they can accommodate a neonate at this gestation if expedited delivery is required.

My diagnosis is preeclampsia with a small for gestational age fetus.'

OUTCOME

The patient was admitted with severe preeclampsia. She has been stabilised. The fetus is small for gestational age on ultrasound scan, which may indicate intrauterine growth restriction. The fetus has been optimised for delivery with corticosteroids.

The obstetric consultant will need to discuss with Michelle in detail about the risks and benefits of continuing the pregnancy or delivering. They will also need to discuss ongoing antihypertensive therapy and the most appropriate mode of delivery in this situation.

STATION 7.4: HYPEREMESIS GRAVIDARUM

You are the junior doctor working as part of the obstetrics and gynaecology team. You are asked by your registrar to review a new admission to the ward who has been referred in by a local general practitioner. Miss Rachel Jones is a 23-year-old who believes she is around 8 weeks pregnant in her first pregnancy. She has been suffering from nausea and vomiting for the past few weeks, but over the last 3 days she says she has been unable keep any food or drink down.

Patient Details

Name:	Rachel Jones
DOB:	21/10/01
Hospital number:	2103914761
Weight:	65 kg
Height:	1.6 m
Address:	41 Westminister Street, Newhampton, CA4 5AY
Consultant:	Dr Roy
Hospital/Ward:	Day Case Unit, Greg General Hospital, Recroft, Southerland Tel: 01965 456 259
Current medications:	None
Allergies:	No known drug allergies
Admission date:	22/10/24

Initial Differential Diagnosis of Hyperemesis Gravidarum

- Infection: gastroenteritis, UTI, appendicitis, LRTI
- Gastrointestinal: GORD, peptic ulceration, liver disease
- Hyperthyroidism
- Diabetic ketoacidosis
- Psychiatric: bulimia nervosa, anxiety
- Raised intracranial pressure

Nausea and vomiting in early pregnancy are very common (around 60% of pregnancies are affected). This is generally known as 'morning sickness'. The cause is not fully understood but a popular theory is that the hormone human chorionic gonadotrophin (HCG), which is maximally raised in the first 8 to 12 weeks of pregnancy, has a direct stimulatory effect on the chemoreceptor trigger zone and vomiting centres of the midbrain. Vomiting beyond 20 weeks of gestation is unlikely to be due to hyperemesis and close attention should be made to find an alternative cause.

Hyperemesis gravidarum is thought to affect 0.3% to 3.6% of pregnancies. The Royal College of Obstetricians and Gynaecologists specifies that simple nausea and vomiting of pregnancy becomes hyperemesis gravidarum when there is a triad of more than 5% prepregnancy weight loss, dehydration and electrolyte imbalance. If not managed carefully, these patients are at risk of refeeding syndrome.

INITIAL ASSESSMENT

- Using an ABCDE approach, ensure the patient is stable.
- Identify any alternative cause of the patient's symptoms (hyperemesis gravidarum is a diagnosis of exclusion).
- Establish the severity of the patient's symptoms, the degree of dehydration and identifying risks for refeeding.

HISTORY

- Confirm gestation/last menstrual period (LMP).
- Use history of presenting complaint and systematic enquiry to elicit any additional symptoms that may support a different diagnosis to hyperemesis gravidarum.
- Obstetric history, medical history, drug history and social history may identify other relevant information relevant to both the diagnosis and subsequent management.

'During your initial assessment you identify that the patient is stable. She has taken the last 3 days off work as a result of these symptoms, vomiting at least every hour, more frequently if she tries to eat or drink. There are no infective symptoms or symptoms to suggest any of the other differential diagnoses. She has no significant past medical history.'

EXAMINATION

- **Observations:** Heart rate, BP, respiratory rate, oxygen saturations and temperature.
- **Cardiac:** Pulse, CRT and mucous membranes.
- **Respiratory:** Rule out clinically evident lower respiratory tract infection.
- **Abdominal:** Abdominal tenderness, renal angle tenderness, bowel sounds and masses (uterus may be palpable from 12 weeks' gestation).
- **Neurological:** A gross assessment of gait and conscious level (assessed during the history taking) will be adequate, but if there are any concerns regarding raised intracranial pressure, then a full neurological exam should be undertaken.

- **Exposure:** Examine any other area of relevance highlighted from the history. In particular, examine the legs for signs of deep vein thrombosis (DVT) (pregnancy and dehydration are both independent risk factors).

'On examination you identify that Rachel has dry mucous membranes. However, the rest of the examination and observations are entirely normal.'

INITIAL INVESTIGATIONS

- **Blood tests (Table 7.5):** FBC, U&Es, LFTs, amylase, CRP, thyroid stimulating hormone and glucose. These tests rule out causes of vomiting and assess the severity of dehydration (haematocrit and U&Es).
- **Urinalysis:**
  - Leucocytes and nitrites are suggestive of infection; send an MSU for microscopy, culture and sensitivities.
  - Ketones demonstrate starvation (metabolism of fatty acids and amino acids rather than glucose).
  - Glucose may suggest gestational diabetes mellitus or a renal pathology.
- **Urinary pregnancy test:** To confirm the patient's report of being pregnant.
- **Weight:** 5% to 10% loss of body weight may indicate severe dehydration and the patient may be at increased risk of metabolic disturbance.
- **Ultrasound scan:** Identifies twin or molar pregnancy, both of which can cause significantly elevated HCG levels causing severe hyperemesis.
- **Other investigations** to consider if the patient is unwell:
  - Arterial blood gas (occasionally severe starvation can cause ketoacidosis)
  - ECG (assess for cardiac cause of a persistent tachycardia despite rehydration)
  - Chest radiography (CXR) (assess for respiratory infection/cardiomyopathy)
  - Endoscopy (if there is a strong suspicion of a significant upper gastrointestinal (GI) bleed, small haematemesis is likely to be caused by a Mallory–Weiss tear)

'The patient provided a small volume of urine for analysis which looks concentrated. Urinalysis showed +++ ketones, was pregnancy test positive, but was otherwise normal. Her weight is 68 kg which indicates a 5% decrease from her normal prepregnancy weight. Blood tests and ultrasound have been requested. At this time you see no indication to request any of the additional investigations.'

Table 7.5 Miss Jones's Blood Results

PARAMETER	VALUE	NORMAL RANGE (UNITS)
WCC	11 × 10^9/L	4–11 (×10^9/L)
Neutrophil	4 × 10^9/L	2–7.5 (×10^9/L)
Lymphocyte	4 × 10^9/L	1.4–4 (×10^9/L)
Platelet	220 × 10^9/L	150–400 (×10^9/L)
Haemoglobin	140 g/L	Men: 135–177 (g/L) Women: 115–155 (g/L)
CRP	3 mg/L	0–5 (mg/L)
Urea	3.2 mmol/L	2.5–6.7 (mmol/L)
Creatinine	80 µmol/L	79–118 (µmol/L)
Sodium	142 mmol/L	135–146 (mmol/L)
Potassium	4.5 mmol/L	3.5–5.0 (mmol/L)
eGFR	>60 mL/min	>60 (mL/min)
Bilirubin	12 µmol/L	<17 (µmol/L)
ALT	32 IU/L	<40 (IU/L)
ALP	100 IU/L	39–117 (IU/L)
Glucose	4.5 mmol/L	4.5–5.6 (mmol/L) (fasting)

ALP, Alkaline phosphatase; *ALT*, alanine transaminase; *CRP*, C-reactive protein; *eGFR*, estimated glomerular filtration rate; *WCC*, white cell count.

DIAGNOSIS

'You are awaiting the blood and ultrasound results, but in the meantime as you have not identified another cause for the patient's symptoms, you make your provisional diagnosis of hyperemesis gravidarum and begin treatment.'

INITIAL MANAGEMENT

Management Summary of Hyperemesis Gravidarum

- Rehydration
- Antiemetics
- Prevent refeeding syndrome (if at risk)
- Encourage oral intake
- Return of normal metabolism

Most UK hospitals treat hyperemesis as a day case admission, usually admitting patients in the morning, treating and then discharging the patient home roughly 8 hours later the same day. Only if the treatment aims cannot be achieved or the patient has severe hyperemesis would an admission be considered.

REHYDRATION

- Obtain IV access (if not already achieved when taking bloods).
- Crystalloid IV fluid can then be prescribed:
  - The aim is to infuse at least 2 L during the admission and then to assess if further hydration is required (as patients are normally fit and well with good renal function, each litre can be prescribed over 1–2 hours without risk of fluid overload).
  - 0.9% sodium chloride is usually the preferred choice—additional potassium can be added to these fluids if required.

'You prescribe 1 L of 0.9% sodium chloride over 1 hour, then a second litre over 2 hours.'

Prescribe (Figs 7.8 and 7.9)

Fluids:

- SODIUM CHLORIDE 0.9% 1 L 1000 mL/h then SODIUM CHLORIDE 0.9% 1 L 500 mL/h

ANTIEMETICS

- As with many of the medications used in pregnancy, the antiemetics that are used are generally some of the older classes of drug which have been given to pregnant women for years without evidence of detriment to the fetus (Table 7.6).
- The first-line medications used in hyperemesis act either as histamine H_1 receptor antagonists (promethazine and cyclizine) or as central dopamine receptor antagonists (chlorpromazine and prochlorperazine). If one first-line agent alone is not effective, then combination therapy with two first-line agents can be considered (one histamine receptor antagonist with one dopamine receptor antagonist) before utilising second-line agents. Route of administration can be decided based on the patient's current symptoms, so usually the first dose is parenteral, and subsequent doses can be given orally if vomiting has subsided.
- The second-line medications are ondansetron and metoclopramide. These can be used in addition to, or as an alternative to, the first-line medications. Ondansetron is a serotonin receptor antagonist with an associated small increased risk of fetal orofacial clefts when used in the first 12 weeks of pregnancy. Metoclopramide has antidopamine properties (acting both centrally and also to encourage gastric emptying) and has the rare extrapyramidal side effects of dystonia, resulting in facial and skeletal muscle spasms and, in extreme cases, oculogyric crisis. These extrapyramidal side effects are more likely in young females. Both second-line side effects are rare but serious and therefore these medications should be used with caution when appropriate.
- Once vomiting has been brought under control, the subsequent antiemetic used should be given as an oral dose.
- There are further antiemetics that can be prescribed, but it is advisable to seek consultant input prior to their use because there is limited evidence about the safety of their use in pregnancy.
- Gastro-oesophageal reflux can be an important contributing factor to both the initial cause of vomiting and perpetuating hyperemesis. Histamine antagonists such as ranitidine (150 mg BD) and the proton pump inhibitor omeprazole (20 mg OD) can both safely be given orally in pregnancy.

'You prescribe cyclizine 50 mg TDS with the option of intravenous or oral route. (IV given first as patient is symptomatic.) After 2 hours the patient is no longer vomiting but still reporting significant nausea and is unwilling to try to take an oral diet. You then prescribe prochloperazine 5 mg TDS orally in addition to the cyclizine. The patient takes this orally, does not vomit it back and after another hour or so is feeling better.'

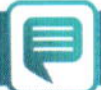
Prescribe (see Figs 7.8 and 7.9)

Antiemetics:

- CYCLIZINE 50 mg TDS PO/IV and PROCHLORPERAZINE 5 mg TDS PO

REFEEDING COMPLICATIONS

- Severe hyperemesis and prolonged starvation are rare, as is significant vitamin deficiency in the UK. However, there are some at risk groups, e.g. patients with inflammatory bowel disease, patients with low or very high body mass index (BMI), patients with alcohol use disorder, patients with substance use disorder and patients with no fixed abode. Patients admitted to hospital with a history of prolonged starvation, severe hyperemesis or at risk of vitamin deficiency should be given vitamin B_1 (thiamine) prior to attempting eating again or receiving IV fluids containing carbohydrates. An appropriate oral thiamine replacement regimen is a dose of 50 mg PO OD. In severe cases, IV B vitamin complexes are also available.
- Thiamine is used in carbohydrate metabolism. When subclinical thiamine deficiency is not treated and carbohydrates are given (e.g. IV glucose), the thiamine in the body is quickly depleted, resulting in death of astrocytes and neuronal cell death, resulting quickly in Wernicke's encephalopathy (classically a triad of confusion, ataxia and nystagmus, but any of these symptoms in isolation should alert the clinician to the diagnosis). Urgent repeated doses of IV B vitamin complex (and specialist medical input) are then required to prevent permanent brain damage and progression to Korsakoff's psychosis, and ultimately death. Therefore, glucose is NOT given in fluid replacement.
- Patients at risk of vitamin deficiency are also at risk of refeeding syndrome. As a result of prolonged starvation, ions usually in high concentration in intracellular fluid and low concentrations in extracellular fluid (magnesium, phosphate, potassium and calcium) shift out of cells to maintain the extracellular concentrations. When feeding is recommenced, increased carbohydrate levels cause an increased release of insulin. Insulin drives these ions back into the intracellular space resulting in dangerously low extracellular concentrations that can cause seizures, arrhythmias, heart failure, confusion, coma and death. To prevent this, it is important to regularly take blood to monitor these electrolyte levels and give IV replacement in a timely manner. These patients also require high dependency staffing and close attention to fluid balance.

Table 7.6 Antiemetics Commonly Used in Pregnancy

LINE	MEDICATION	ROUTE				FREQUENCY
		PO	IM	IV	BUCCAL	
First	Cyclizine	50 mg	50 mg	50 mg	–	TDS
First	Promethazine	12.5–25 mg	12.5–25 mg	12.5–25 mg	–	TDS
First	Prochlorperazine	5–10 mg	12.5 mg	12.5 mg	3 mg	TDS
First	Chlorpromazine	10–25 mg	10–25 mg	10–25 mg		QDS
Second	Metoclopramide	10 mg	10 mg	10 mg	–	TDS
Second	Ondansetron	4–8 mg	–	8 mg	–	BD

BD, Bis die (twice daily); *IM*, Intramuscular; *IV*, intravenous; *PO*, per oram (orally); *QDS*, quater die sumendus (four times daily); *TDS*, ter die sumendus (three times daily).

'There is nothing from the patient's history or examination to concern you about refeeding syndrome in Rachel's case. Her FBC, U&Es, LFTs and CRP are all now back and are all normal providing further reassurance that refeeding should not be a concern and that other causes of vomiting are unlikely in this case.'

ENCOURAGE ORAL INTAKE

- For most patients presenting with hyperemesis, complications of refeeding will not be an issue. As soon as the nausea and vomiting are under control, it is essential to encourage oral intake to return the patient to normal function. Advise the patient to take small amounts of food and liquid initially, building up first the frequency of the small amounts, and then gradually the quantity. The theory is that the stomach does not become too full (due to gastric stasis) and the chemoreceptor trigger zone is not excited because food is ingested in lower concentrations.

RETURN OF NORMAL METABOLISM

- Once the patient has been rehydrated with IV fluid, has stopped vomiting and has begun to ingest food, normal metabolism will resume. Evidence of this will be that the patient produces dilute urine, demonstrating adequate rehydration, and a reduction in the concentration of ketones on urinalysis will indicate that normal glucose metabolism has resumed.
- At this point, any outstanding investigations can be reviewed, and the patient can then be discharged, usually with 1 to 2 weeks supply of the oral version of the antiemetic used to control the patient's symptoms on admission. The patient should be advised to take the medication regularly for a few days and then gradually reduce the frequency of use. If symptoms return, she should restart the medication at the original dose promptly to prevent worsening of symptoms and the need for readmission. If the patient was also symptomatic of gastro-oesophageal reflux she should also be given antacid medication.

'Rachel began eating and drinking small amounts once her symptoms were under control. After a couple more hours, Rachel was feeling much better and was keen to go home. You review the outstanding investigation results which show that Rachel has a normal TSH level, and the ultrasound scan confirms a single intrauterine pregnancy. You send Rachel home with a 1-week prescription of cyclizine 50 mg TDS PO and prochlorperazine 5 mg TDS PO, with advice to reduce the frequency of medication use after a few days if symptoms remain controlled, but to return to the dosing regimen at discharge if symptoms return.'

Prescribe (Fig. 7.10)

CYCLIZINE 50 mg PO TDS 7 DAYS
PROCHLORPERAZINE 5 mg PO TDS 7 DAYS

VTE PROPHYLAXIS

- Rachel has been treated as a day case. She has attended dehydrated but this has been corrected. No additional prophylaxis is required in her case.
- If a hyperemesis patient requires admission, the risk factors of pregnancy and dehydration would warrant consideration of LMWH, TED stockings, rehydration and encouragement of mobilisation.
- Remember to write up regular medications, including folic acid, if the patient is admitted. Thiamine replacement may also be considered in severe cases.

Remember: Thromboprophylaxis

- Patients with severe hyperemesis are at risk of VTE if they are dehydrated, pregnant and immobile.
- Prescribe thromboprophylaxis if admitted to the ward.

HANDING OVER THE PATIENT TO PRIMARY CARE: DISCHARGE SUMMARY

'Rachel Jones was admitted at 8 weeks gestation with hyperemesis gravidarum. She was treated with IV fluids and antiemetics, which quickly resolved her symptoms. FBC, U&Es, LFTs, CRP and TFTs were all normal. USS demonstrated a single intrauterine pregnancy of 8/40 weeks gestation.

The patient has been discharged home with a 7-day supply of cyclizine 50 mg PO TDS and prochlorperazine

5 mg PO TDS. We have advised her gradually to reduce the frequency of cyclizine use, but quickly to restart at the full dose if symptoms return.

The patient has been advised to contact yourselves to arrange a booking visit with your practice's midwife.'

STATION 7.5: URINARY TRACT INFECTION IN PREGNANCY

Chantelle Symonds is a 19-year-old who is 22 weeks into her first pregnancy. She attends the emergency department complaining of pain on passing urine, associated with lower abdominal discomfort for the last 2 days.

Patient Details

Name:	Chantelle Symonds
DOB:	21/10/05
Hospital number:	2103914353
Weight:	65 kg
Height:	1.6 m
Address:	46 Worcester Street, Carlisle, CA3 5YY
Consultant:	Dr Roy
Hospital/Ward:	Emergency department (Greg General Hospital, Recroft, Southerland, Tel 01965 456 259)
Current medications:	None
Allergies:	No known drug allergies
Attendance date:	22/11/24

Differential Diagnosis of Abdominal Pain in Pregnancy

- UTI
- Renal colic
- Pyelonephritis
- Appendicitis
- Musculoskeletal pain
- Preterm labour
- Placental abruption

Very few medications have been tested in pregnancy during prelicensing trials. Almost all the evidence for safety in pregnancy is based on long-term observational studies. For this reason a large number of sources will emphasise, with regards to pregnancy and breastfeeding, 'not known to be harmful, manufacturer advises avoid.' However, a large number of medications are used during pregnancy where the clinician and patient assess the available evidence and balance the benefit of treating against the risk of not treating. The UK Teratology Information Service (UKTIS) provides up to date evidence and advice for the use of medicines in pregnancy.

INITIAL ASSESSMENT

- This patient is currently well, and a quick ABCD assessment can be done. By watching the patient walk into the room, sit down and start making appropriate conversation, you can be confident the patient has an unobstructed airway, breathing without difficulty, a circulation capable of maintaining walking and conversation and a fully perfused alert brain.

HISTORY

- Find out more information about the presenting problem, to suggest a diagnosis.

'Stinging and burning sensation when passing urine in the pubic region, associated with an aching suprapubic pain which is worse just before urination and relieved by it. No loin or back pains; pains not affected by movement. No other associated symptoms and nothing elicited on systemic review. Good fetal movements, no vaginal fluid loss and no contraction or tightening like pains. No medical history of note, this is the patient's first pregnancy which has been uncomplicated so far with a normal anomaly scan 2 weeks ago. She takes no medications, has no allergies, and no relevant social history. The patient says this feels just like a urine infection which she wants treated because it is painful'.

EXAMINATION

- Measure heart rate, BP and temperature.
- Abdominal examination:
  - Identify areas of tenderness.
  - Assess specifically for uterine tenderness and tightening.
- Consider speculum examination if any concerns of preterm labour or vaginal fluid loss.

'The patient's heart rate is 70 bpm, with a BP of 120/70 mmHg, a CRT of 2 seconds, and a normal temperature. The abdomen is soft with mild suprapubic tenderness only, no guarding, no peritonism. There is no renal angle tenderness. The uterus is the correct size for gestation and is not tender. Bowel sounds normal.'

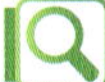

Remember

In pregnancy, due to the enlargement of the uterus, other abdominal structures are moved away from their usual positions, so pathology may present with atypical signs and symptoms.

INVESTIGATIONS

- **Hand-held Doppler to listen to fetal heart:**
  - Confirmation of fetal well-being is usually the most important concern for the patient. However, do not attempt this unless you are trained to do so, failure to find a fetal heart (which eventually is found to be present) causes significant emotional distress.
- **Urinalysis:** If positive for leucocytes or nitrites, send an MSU sample for microscopy, culture and sensitivities.

- **Blood tests** are not routinely indicated in diagnosing a UTI.

'Fetal heart rate 140 bpm. Urinalysis was positive for leucocytes and nitrites, with a trace of protein and blood. An MSU sample has been sent.'

You are confident to make the diagnosis of a UTI, and there is no evidence of pyelonephritis or systemic sepsis.

MANAGEMENT

There are two key aims of management:

- Provide symptomatic (pain) relief.
- Treat the infection.

The management options to discuss with the patient are:

- Do nothing: The advantage of doing nothing is there is no risk of causing harm with treatments, and the body may naturally kill the infection. However, the risk of doing nothing is that, in pregnancy, the body's immune system is less effective against infection. This could mean the infection worsens and causes a patient to become very unwell, and severe infection could affect the development of the fetus or contribute to preterm labour.
- Advise on nonpharmacological measures: Simple nonpharmacological methods such as encouraging adequate hydration and drinking cranberry juice to help treat the infection are advantageous because they are unlikely to cause direct harm, but there is less evidence to support their effectiveness compared to medication.
- Pharmacological management: Medication is the management most likely to treat both the pain and the symptoms. All medications have potential side effects but careful selection of the most appropriate prescription for the patient can be sought.

> Wherever possible, it is important to offer patients the information they need to make an informed decision about their own treatment, recognising that they should be full and equal participants in healthcare and concordant with the decisions affecting their own care (shared decision-making).

PRESCRIBING ANALGESIA

Follow the World Health Organization (WHO) analgesic ladder (Table 7.7) to select the most appropriate level of analgesia, but be aware of the contraindications in pregnancy.

PRESCRIBING ANTIBIOTICS

Choice of antibiotics should be based on specific patient requirements (e.g. severity of condition, likely pathogen, allergies, concurrent medication), local prescribing guidelines from local microbiologists and taking into account specific medication side effect and risk profiles.

NICE recommends the following antibiotic options for uncomplicated UTI in pregnancy:

- Nitrofurantoin:
  - First-line medication—patients should be less than 36 weeks pregnant (risk of fetal haemolysis during labour and the early postnatal period if given beyond this gestation)
  - Dose 50 mg PO QDS for 7 days (note treatment duration is usually extended in pregnancy compared to nonpregnant patients)
- Amoxicillin:
  - A penicillin derivative
  - A second-line antibiotic option for UTI in pregnancy
  - Not known to be harmful in pregnancy but always ask about previous allergy
  - Dose 500 mg PO TDS for 7 days (note treatment duration is usually extended in pregnancy compared to nonpregnant patients)
- Cefalexin:
  - A cephalosporin; risk of hypersensitivity reaction in patients with severe penicillin allergy
  - A second-line antibiotic option for UTI in pregnancy
  - Not known to be harmful in pregnancy
  - Dose 500 mg PO QDS for 7 days

'After discussion with the patient you both decide the best management course would be to try nitrofurantoin and paracetamol prescribed as described above. You advise the patient that you will follow up the MSU result and contact her in 3–4 days if this indicates a

Table 7.7 Analgesia in Pregnancy

Paracetamol	Not known to be harmful in pregnancy. Dose 500 mg–1 g PO every 4 hours (max dose 4 g daily)
NSAIDs, e.g. ibuprofen, naproxen, diclofenac	Manufacturers advise to avoid in pregnancy. Risk of premature closure of the ductus arteriosus and pulmonary hypertension in the neonate
Codeine phosphate	Not known to be harmful in pregnancy. Like all opioid analgesia, caution is advised in labour due to potential neonatal respiratory depression. With prolonged use, there is also risk of neonatal withdrawal syndrome. Dose 30–60 mg PO every 4 hours (max dose 240 mg daily)
Tramadol	Manufacturer advises avoid in pregnancy, embryo-toxic in animal studies
Morphine	Not known to be harmful in pregnancy (caution in labour, see codeine). Dose dependent on route of administration (can be given oral, IM, IV) and patient characteristics

IM, Intramuscular; *IV*, intravenous; *PO*, per oram (orally); *NSAID*, non-steroidal antiinflammatory drug.

more appropriate antibiotic choice. You also advise the patient to come back in 3 days if the symptoms have not improved or earlier if symptoms worsen.'

Prescribe (Fig. 7.11)

Antibiotics:

- NITROFURANTOIN 50 mg PO QDS for 7 DAYS

- Always advise the patient on what to do if initial treatment fails or their condition deteriorates.
- Keep organised and follow up any investigations ordered.

'Three days later the midstream urine report arrives. An E. coli species is isolated in the urine. Sensitivities show that it is resistant to nitrofurantoin, amoxicillin and cefalexin but sensitive to ciprofloxacin, doxycycline and trimethoprim.'

It is important to check the contraindications to any medication before prescribing:

- Ciprofloxacin:
  - Quinolones
  - Avoid in pregnancy, have caused arthropathy in animal studies
- Doxycycline:
  - Tetracycline
  - Avoid in pregnancy, effects on skeletal development in first trimester, fetal teeth discouloration in later pregnancy
- Trimethoprim:
  - Folate antagonist
  - Teratogenic in first trimester, manufacturer advises avoid in pregnancy

If the antibiotics found to be sensitive were not appropriate to use for the patient (for example contraindicated in pregnancy or patient allergy), it is worth contacting the microbiology laboratory to ask them to identify other sensitivities and discuss the options with the consultant microbiologist.

REFERRING THE PATIENT FOR SPECIALIST OPINION—CONSULTANT MICROBIOLOGIST

'I am ringing for some advice on the ongoing management of a patient. The patient is Chantelle Symonds, a 19-year-old who is 22 weeks pregnant in her first pregnancy. She is normally fit and well. She presented to me 3 days ago with symptoms suggestive of a UTI, with a supporting urinalysis result. The patient was clinically well. I sent the patient home with an outpatient prescription for a 7-day course of nitrofurantoin 50 mg QDS and sent an MSU to the lab. Unfortunately, the sensitivities have come back showing that the E. coli is resistant to the nitrofurantoin, and the antibiotics which it is sensitive to are contraindicated in pregnancy.'

Even the usually simple task of treating a UTI can cause difficulty in pregnancy. It is important to consider all the factors when prescribing, using local and national guidance where available. Do no harm; if you are unsure of anything when prescribing in pregnancy, then seek advice.

Be aware that other antibiotics are potentially useful for the management of UTI in pregnancy but have certain caveats:

- Nitrofurantoin: avoid at term (beyond 36 weeks' gestation).
- Co-amoxiclav: avoid at term, risk of neonatal necrotising enterocolitis.
- Metronidazole: manufacturer advises avoid high doses.

In this case, the consultant microbiologist advises you that local prescribing guidelines support the use of trimethoprim at a dose of 200 mg twice a day for 7 days for pregnant patients beyond the first trimester.

You contact the patient and explain the MSU result. The patient is still symptomatic, so you prescribe trimethoprim as an outpatient prescription following the local guidelines and again ask the patient to contact you after 3 days of treatment if there is no improvement.

Prescribe (Fig. 7.12)

Antibiotics:

- TRIMETHOPRIM 200 mg BD PO for 7 DAYS

FURTHER READING

British National Formulary (BNF). Obstetrics, 2012. https://bnf.nice.org.uk/treatment-summaries/obstetrics/ (Last accessed 12/09/24).

National Institute for Health and Care Excellence, 2018. Biomarker tests to help diagnose preterm labour in women with intact membranes. National Institute for Health and Care Excellence—Diagnostic Guidance 33. https://www.nice.org.uk/guidance/dg33/chapter/3-The-diagnostic-tests (Last accessed 12/9/24).

National Institute for Health and Care Excellence, 2018. Urinary tract infection (lower): antimicrobial prescribing. National Institute for Health and Care Excellence – NICE guideline 109. https://www.nice.org.uk/guidance/ng109/resources/urinary-tract-infection-lower-antimicrobial-prescribing-pdf-66141546350533 (Last accessed 12/9/24).

National Institute for Health and Care Excellence, 2021. Neonatal infection: antibiotics for prevention and treatment. National Institute for Health and Care Excellence – NICE guideline 195. https://www.nice.org.uk/guidance/ng195/chapter/Recommendations#intrapartum-antibiotics (Last accessed 12/9/24).

National Institute for Health and Care Excellence, 2019. Hypertension in pregnancy: diagnosis and management. National Institute for Health and Care Excellence – NICE guideline 133 (Last updated: 17 April 2023). https://www.nice.org.uk/guidance/ng133/resources/hypertension-in-pregnancy-diagnosis-and-management-pdf-66141717671365 (Last accessed 12/9/24).

Royal College of Obstetricians and Gynaecologists, 2016. Prevention and management of postpartum haemorrhage. Royal College of Obstetricians and Gynaecologists—green-top guidelines No. 52. https://obgyn.onlinelibrary.wiley.com/doi/full/10.1111/1471-0528.14178 (Last accessed 12/9/24).

Royal College of Obstetricians and Gynaecologists, 2016. The management of nausea and vomiting of pregnancy and hyperemesis gravidarum. Royal College of Obstetricians and Gynaecologists – Green-top Guideline No. 69. https://www.rcog.org.uk/media/y3fen1x1/gtg69-hyperemesis.pdf (Last accessed 12/9/24).

Royal College of Obstetricians and Gynaecologists, 2016. Care of women presenting with suspected preterm prelabour rupture of membranes from 24+0 weeks of gestation. Royal College of Obstetricians and Gynaecologists. Green-top Guideline No. 73. https://obgyn.onlinelibrary.wiley.com/doi/pdf/10.1111/1471-0528.15803 (Last accessed 12/9/24).

UK teratology information service: Best use of medicines in pregnancy. Webpage. https://www.medicinesinpregnancy.org/ (Last accessed 12/9/24).

PRESCRIPTION CHARTS

PRESCRIPTION AND ADMINISTRATION RECORD

Standard Chart

Hospital/Ward: LGH WARD 4 **Consultant:** DR ROY	**Name of Patient:** ANNE SEYMOUR
Weight: 65 kg **Height:** 1.6 m	**Hospital Number:** 2103914534
If re-written, date:	**D.O.B:** 27/03/1995
DISCHARGE PRESCRIPTION **Date completed:-** **Completed by:-**	

OTHER MEDICINE CHARTS IN USE		PREVIOUS ADVERSE REACTIONS This section must be completed before any medicine is given		Completed by (sign & print)	Date
Date	Type of Chart	None known ☒		S. Lockley S. LOCKLEY	22/10/24
		Medicine/Agent	Description of Reaction		

CODES FOR NON-ADMINISTRATION OF PRESCRIBED MEDICINE

If a dose is not administered as prescribed, initial and enter a code in the column with a circle drawn round the code according to the reason as shown below. **Inform the responsible doctor in the appropriate timescale.**

1. Patient refuses
2. Patient not present
3. Medicines not available – CHECK ORDERED
4. Asleep/drowsy
5. Administration route not available – CHECK FOR ALTERNATIVE
6. Vomiting/nausea
7. Time varied on doctor's instructions
8. Once only/as required medicine given
9. Dose withheld on doctor's instructions
10. Possible adverse reaction/side effect

ONCE-ONLY

Date	Time	Medicine (Approved Name)	Dose	Route	Prescriber – Sign + Print	Time Given	Given By
22/10/24	19.30	BETAMETHASONE	12 mg	IM	S. Lockley S. LOCKLEY	19.30	YP
22/10/24	19.30	NIFEDIPINE (IR)	20 mg	PO	S. Lockley S. LOCKLEY	19.30	YP
23/10/24	07.30	BETAMETHASONE	12 mg	IM	S. Lockley S. LOCKLEY	07.35	YP

OXYGEN	Start Date	Start Time	Route Mask (%)	Route Prongs (L/min)	Prescriber – Sign + Print	Administered by	Stop Date	Stop Time

Fig. 7.1 Prescription and administration record (standard chart) for Anne Seymour.

Name: ANNE SEYMOUR
Date of Birth: 27/03/1995

REGULAR THERAPY

PRESCRIPTION	Date → / Time ↓	22/10/24	23/10/24										
Medicine (Approved Name): NIFEDIPINE (IR)	(6)		PD										
Dose: 10 mg / Route: PO	8												
	(12)		FD										
Notes / Start Date: 22/10/24	16												
	(18)												
Prescriber – sign + print: M. Wood M. WOOD	24												
Medicine (Approved Name)	6												
Dose / Route	8												
	12												
Notes / Start Date	16												
	18												
Prescriber – sign + print	24												
Medicine (Approved Name)	6												
Dose / Route	8												
	12												
Notes / Start Date	16												
	18												
Prescriber – sign + print	24												
Medicine (Approved Name)	6												
Dose / Route	8												
	12												
Notes / Start Date	16												
	18												
Prescriber – sign + print	24												
Medicine (Approved Name)	6												
Dose / Route	8												
	12												
Notes / Start Date	16												
	18												
Prescriber – sign + print	24												
Medicine (Approved Name)	6												
Dose / Route	8												
	12												
Notes / Start Date	16												
	18												
Prescriber – sign + print	24												

Fig. 7.2 Prescription and administration record (regular therapy) for Anne Seymour.

PRESCRIPTION AND ADMINISTRATION RECORD

Standard Chart

Hospital/Ward: LGH WARD 7	Consultant: DR ROY	Name of Patient: SUSAN COX
Weight: 65 kg	Height: 1.5 m	Hospital Number: 2103914531
If re-written, date:		D.O.B.: 21/03/1992
DISCHARGE PRESCRIPTION Date completed:-	Completed by:-	

OTHER MEDICINE CHARTS IN USE	
Date	Type of Chart

PREVIOUS ADVERSE REACTIONS This section must be completed before any medicine is given		Completed by (sign & print)	Date
None known ☒		S. Lockley S. LOCKLEY	22/10/24
Medicine/Agent	Description of Reaction		

CODES FOR NON-ADMINISTRATION OF PRESCRIBED MEDICINE

If a dose is not administered as prescribed, initial and enter a code in the column with a circle drawn round the code according to the reason as shown below. **Inform the responsible doctor in the appropriate timescale.**

1. Patient refuses
2. Patient not present
3. Medicines not available – CHECK ORDERED
4. Asleep/drowsy
5. Administration route not available – CHECK FOR ALTERNATIVE
6. Vomiting/nausea
7. Time varied on doctor's instructions
8. Once only/as required medicine given
9. Dose withheld on doctor's instructions
10. Possible adverse reaction/side effect

ONCE-ONLY

Date	Time	Medicine (Approved Name)	Dose	Route	Prescriber – Sign + Print	Time Given	Given By
22/10/24	19.30	SYNTOMETRINE (ERGOMETRINE 500 micrograms/OXYTOCIN 5 units in 1mL)	1 mL	IM	S. Lockley S. LOCKLEY	19.30	YP
22/10/24	19.30	TRANEXAMIC ACID	1g	IV	S. Lockley S. LOCKLEY	19.30	YP

OXYGEN	Start		Route		Prescriber – Sign + Print	Administered by	Stop	
	Date	Time	Mask (%)	Prongs (L/min)			Date	Time

Fig. 7.3 Prescription and administration record (standard chart) for Susan Cox.

Name: SUSAN COX

Date of Birth: 21/03/1992

REGULAR THERAPY

PRESCRIPTION		Date → / Time ↓	22/10/24	23/10/24										
Medicine (Approved Name): TED STOCKINGS		6												
Dose: 1 pair	Route: TOP	8												
Notes	Start Date: 22/10/24	12												
Prescriber – sign + print: M. Wood M. WOOD		16												
		18	FD	FD										
		24												
Medicine (Approved Name)		6												
Dose	Route	8												
Notes	Start Date	12												
Prescriber – sign + print		16												
		18												
		24												
Medicine (Approved Name)		6												
Dose	Route	8												
Notes	Start Date	12												
Prescriber – sign + print		14												
		18												
		22												
Medicine (Approved Name)		6												
Dose	Route	8												
Notes	Start Date	12												
Prescriber – sign + print		14												
		18												
		22												
Medicine (Approved Name)		6												
Dose	Route	8												
Notes	Start Date	12												
Prescriber – sign + print		14												
		18												
		22												
Medicine (Approved Name)		6												
Dose	Route	8												
Notes	Start Date	12												
Prescriber – sign + print		14												
		18												
		22												

Fig. 7.4 Prescription and administration record (regular therapy) for Susan Cox.

FLUID PRESCRIPTION CHART

Hospital/Ward: LGH WARD 7	**Consultant:** DR ROY	**Name of Patient:** SUSAN COX
		Hospital Number: 2103914531
Weight: 65 kg	**Height:** 1.5 m	**D.O.B:** 21/03/1992

Date/ Time	FLUID / ADDED DRUGS	VOLUME / DOSE	ROUTE	RATE	PRESCRIBER – SIGN AND PRINT
22/10/24 19.30	SODIUM CHLORIDE 0.9%	500 mL	IV	Over 15 min	M. Wood M. WOOD
22/10/24 19.45	SODIUM CHLORIDE 0.9%	500 mL	IV	Over 15 min	M. Wood M. WOOD
22/10/24 20.10	SODIUM CHLORIDE 0.9%	1000 mL	IV	81 mL/h	M. Wood M. WOOD
	POTASSIUM CHLORIDE	20 mmol			

Fig. 7.5 Fluid prescription chart for Susan Cox.

PRESCRIPTION AND ADMINISTRATION RECORD

Standard Chart

Hospital/Ward: LGH WARD 4 **Consultant:** DR ROY	**Name of Patient:** MICHELLE FISHER
Weight: 65 kg **Height:** 1.5 m	**Hospital Number:** 2103914527
If re-written, date:	**D.O.B.:** 01/02/1987
DISCHARGE PRESCRIPTION **Date completed:-** **Completed by:-**	

OTHER MEDICINE CHARTS IN USE		PREVIOUS ADVERSE REACTIONS This section must be completed before any medicine is given		Completed by (sign & print)	Date
Date	Type of Chart	None known ☒		S. Lockley S. LOCKLEY	22/10/24
		Medicine/Agent	Description of Reaction		

CODES FOR NON-ADMINISTRATION OF PRESCRIBED MEDICINE

If a dose is not administered as prescribed, initial and enter a code in the column with a circle drawn round the code according to the reason as shown below. **Inform the responsible doctor in the appropriate timescale.**

1. Patient refuses
2. Patient not present
3. Medicines not available – CHECK ORDERED
4. Asleep/drowsy
5. Administration route not available – CHECK FOR ALTERNATIVE
6. Vomiting/nausea
7. Time varied on doctor's instructions
8. Once only/as required medicine given
9. Dose withheld on doctor's instructions
10. Possible adverse reaction/side effect

ONCE-ONLY

Date	Time	Medicine (Approved Name)	Dose	Route	Prescriber – Sign + Print	Time Given	Given By
22/10/24	19.30	LABETALOL	200 mg	PO	S. Lockley S. LOCKLEY	19.30	YP
22/10/24	20.30	NIFEDIPINE (SR)	10 mg	PO	S. Lockley S. LOCKLEY	20.30	YP
22/10/24	20.10	BETAMETHASONE	12 mg	IM	S. Lockley S. LOCKLEY	20.10	YP
23/10/24	08.10	BETAMETHASONE	12 mg	IM	S. Lockley S. LOCKLEY	08.10	YP

OXYGEN	Start Date	Start Time	Route Mask (%)	Route Prongs (L/min)	Prescriber – Sign + Print	Administered by	Stop Date	Stop Time

Fig. 7.6 Prescription and administration record (standard chart) for Michelle Fisher.

Name: *MICHELLE FISHER*

Date of Birth: *01/02/1987*

REGULAR THERAPY

PRESCRIPTION	Date → Time ↓		*22/10/24*	*23/10/24*										
Medicine (Approved Name): *PARACETAMOL*	6													
Dose: *1g* / Route: *PO*	8													
Notes: / Start Date: *22/10/24*	12													
Prescriber – sign + print: *M.Wood M. WOOD*	16													
	18													
	24		*FD*											
Medicine (Approved Name): *TED STOCKINGS*	6													
Dose: *1 pair* / Route: *TOP*	8													
Notes: / Start Date: *22/10/24*	12													
Prescriber – sign + print: *M.Wood M. WOOD*	16													
	18		*FD*											
	24													
Medicine (Approved Name)	6													
Dose / Route	8													
Notes / Start Date	12													
Prescriber – sign + print	14													
	18													
	22													
Medicine (Approved Name)	6													
Dose / Route	8													
Notes / Start Date	12													
Prescriber – sign + print	14													
	18													
	22													
Medicine (Approved Name)	6													
Dose / Route	8													
Notes / Start Date	12													
Prescriber – sign + print	14													
	18													
	22													
Medicine (Approved Name)	6													
Dose / Route	8													
Notes / Start Date	12													
Prescriber – sign + print	14													
	18													
	22													

Fig. 7.7 **Prescription and administration record (regular therapy) for Michelle Fisher.**

Name: RACHEL JONES
Date of Birth: 21/10/2001

REGULAR THERAPY

PRESCRIPTION

Medicine (Approved Name): CYCLIZINE
Dose: 50 mg | Route: PO
Notes: | Start Date: 22/10/24
Prescriber – sign + print: M. Wood M. WOOD

Time		22/10/24	23/10/24										
6													
(8)		FD											
12													
(16)		FD											
18													
22	(24)	FD											

Medicine (Approved Name): PROCHLORPERAZINE
Dose: 5 mg | Route: PO
Notes: | Start Date: 22/10/24
Prescriber – sign + print: M. Wood M. WOOD

Time		22/10/24	23/10/24										
6													
(8)		FD											
12													
(16)		FD											
18													
22	(24)	FD											

Medicine (Approved Name):
Dose: | Route:
Notes: | Start Date:
Prescriber – sign + print:

Time													
6													
8													
12													
14													
18													
22													

Medicine (Approved Name):
Dose: | Route:
Notes: | Start Date:
Prescriber – sign + print:

Time													
6													
8													
12													
14													
18													
22													

Medicine (Approved Name):
Dose: | Route:
Notes: | Start Date:
Prescriber – sign + print:

Time													
6													
8													
12													
14													
18													
22													

Medicine (Approved Name):
Dose: | Route:
Notes: | Start Date:
Prescriber – sign + print:

Time													
6													
8													
12													
14													
18													
22													

Fig. 7.8 Prescription and administration record (regular therapy) for Rachel Jones.

FLUID PRESCRIPTION CHART

Hospital/Ward: DAY CASE UNIT	**Consultant:** DR ROY	**Name of Patient:** RACHEL JONES
		Hospital Number: 2103914761
Weight: 65 kg	**Height:** 1.6 m	**D.O.B:** 21/10/2001

Date/ Time	FLUID / ADDED DRUGS	VOLUME / DOSE	ROUTE	RATE	PRESCRIBER – SIGN AND PRINT
22/10/24 08.30	SODIUM CHLORIDE 0.9%	1000 mL	IV	1000 mL/h	M. Wood M. WOOD
22/10/24 09.30	SODIUM CHLORIDE 0.9%	1000 mL	IV	500 mL/h	M. Wood M. WOOD

Fig. 7.9 Fluid prescription chart for Rachel Jones.

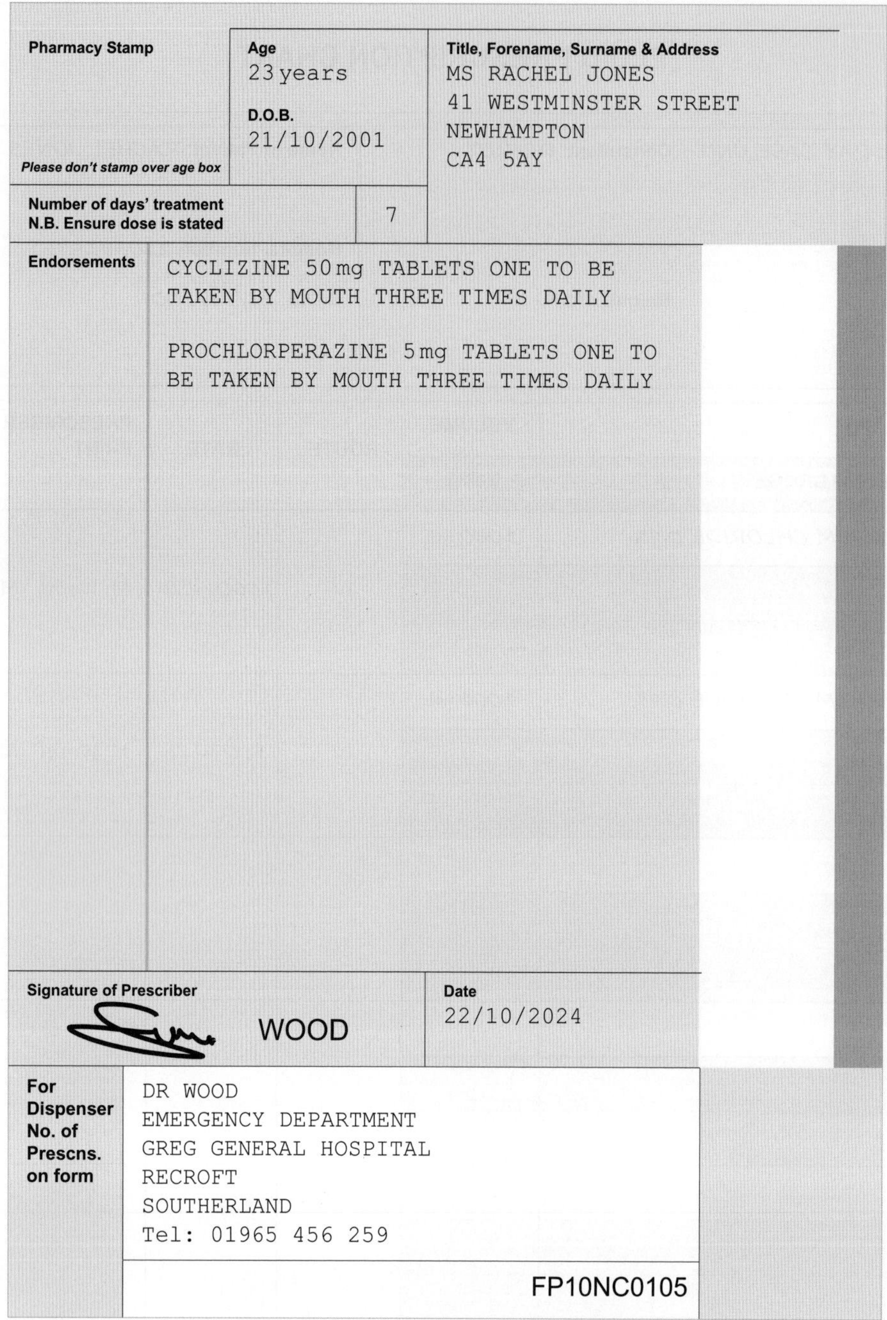

Pharmacy Stamp

Please don't stamp over age box

Age
23 years

D.O.B.
21/10/2001

Title, Forename, Surname & Address
MS RACHEL JONES
41 WESTMINSTER STREET
NEWHAMPTON
CA4 5AY

Number of days' treatment
N.B. Ensure dose is stated
7

Endorsements

CYCLIZINE 50 mg TABLETS ONE TO BE TAKEN BY MOUTH THREE TIMES DAILY

PROCHLORPERAZINE 5 mg TABLETS ONE TO BE TAKEN BY MOUTH THREE TIMES DAILY

Signature of Prescriber
WOOD

Date
22/10/2024

For Dispenser
No. of Prescns. on form

DR WOOD
EMERGENCY DEPARTMENT
GREG GENERAL HOSPITAL
RECROFT
SOUTHERLAND
Tel: 01965 456 259

FP10NC0105

Fig. 7.10 Prescription form for Rachel Jones.

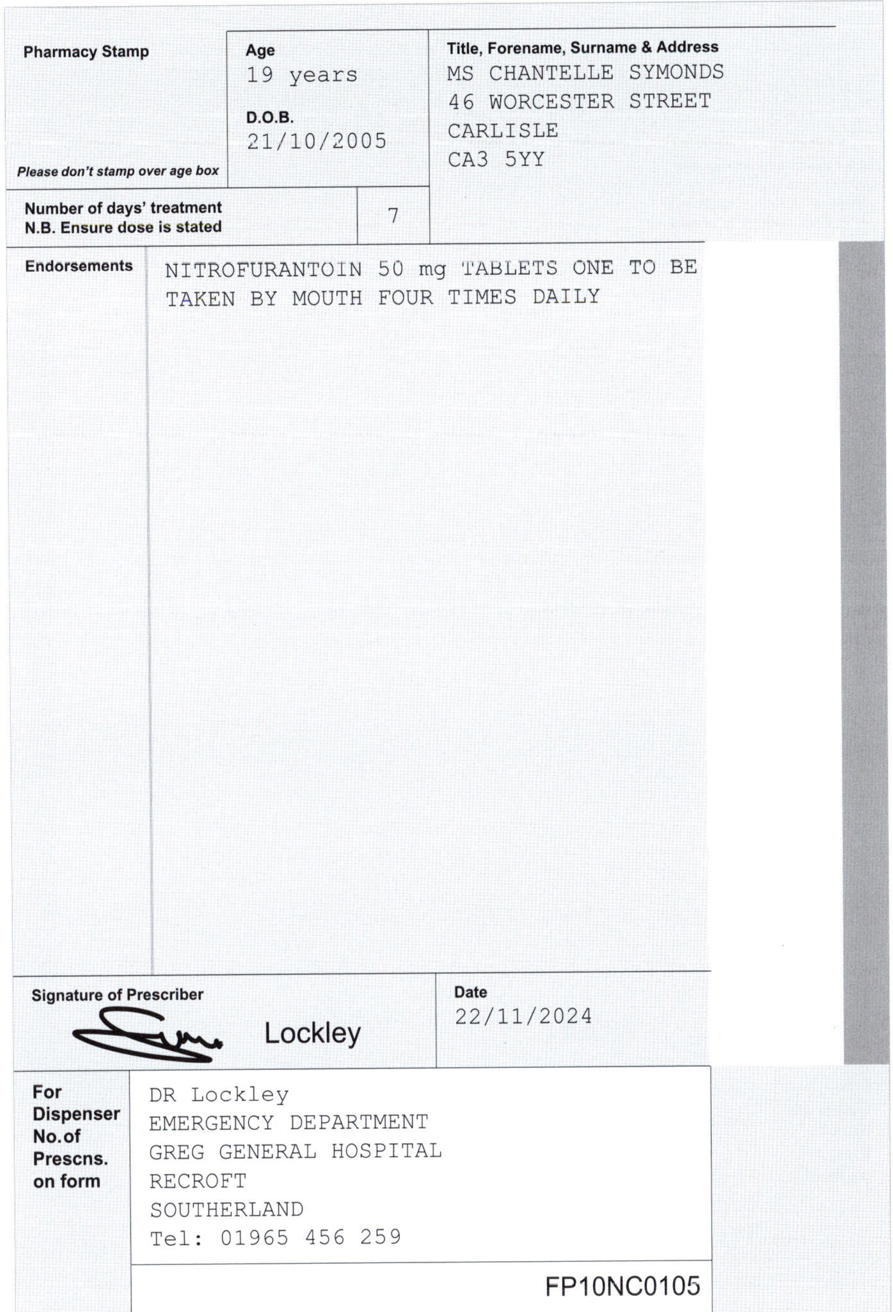

Pharmacy Stamp

Please don't stamp over age box

Age
19 years

D.O.B.
21/10/2005

Title, Forename, Surname & Address
MS CHANTELLE SYMONDS
46 WORCESTER STREET
CARLISLE
CA3 5YY

Number of days' treatment
N.B. Ensure dose is stated
7

Endorsements

NITROFURANTOIN 50 mg TABLETS ONE TO BE
TAKEN BY MOUTH FOUR TIMES DAILY

Signature of Prescriber
Lockley

Date
22/11/2024

For Dispenser No.of Prescns. on form

DR Lockley
EMERGENCY DEPARTMENT
GREG GENERAL HOSPITAL
RECROFT
SOUTHERLAND
Tel: 01965 456 259

FP10NC0105

Fig. 7.11 First prescription form for Chantelle Symonds.

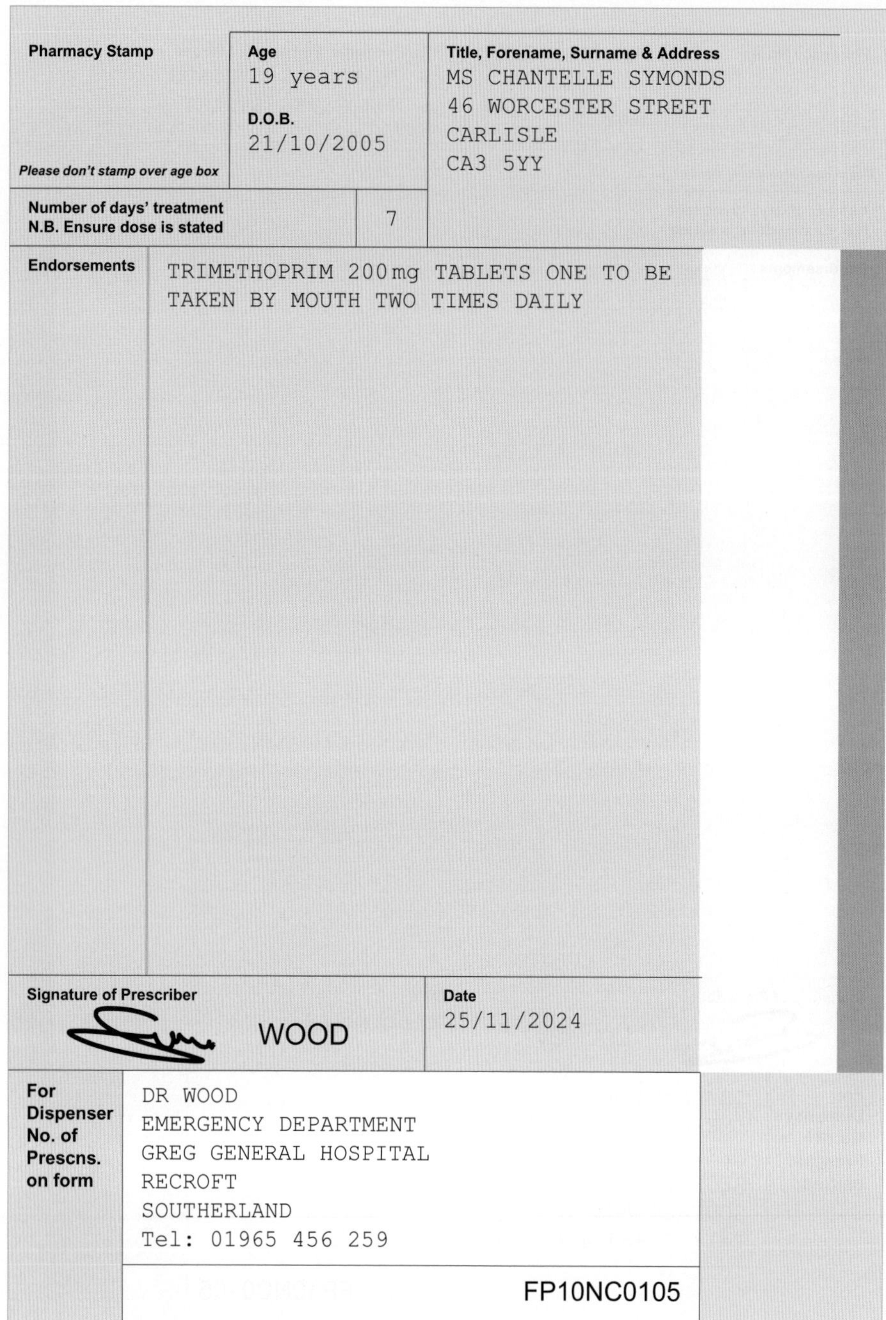

Pharmacy Stamp

Please don't stamp over age box

Age
19 years

D.O.B.
21/10/2005

Title, Forename, Surname & Address
MS CHANTELLE SYMONDS
46 WORCESTER STREET
CARLISLE
CA3 5YY

Number of days' treatment
N.B. Ensure dose is stated
7

Endorsements

TRIMETHOPRIM 200 mg TABLETS ONE TO BE TAKEN BY MOUTH TWO TIMES DAILY

Signature of Prescriber
WOOD

Date
25/11/2024

For Dispenser No. of Prescns. on form

DR WOOD
EMERGENCY DEPARTMENT
GREG GENERAL HOSPITAL
RECROFT
SOUTHERLAND
Tel: 01965 456 259

FP10NC0105

Fig. 7.12 Second prescription form for Chantelle Symonds.

General Surgery

8

Ali B.A.K. Al-Hadithi

Chapter Outline

Station 8.1: Venous Thromboembolism (VTE) Prophylaxis
Station 8.2: Acute Pancreatitis
Station 8.3: Intestinal Obstruction
Station 8.4: Diabetes in the Surgical Patient With Osteomyelitis
Station 8.5: Postoperative Fluid Loss

STATION 8.1: VENOUS THROMBOEMBOLISM (VTE) PROPHYLAXIS

You are the surgical junior doctor. A 23-year-old woman (Nicole Smith 05/03/01) is brought to the emergency department with periumbilical pain that has radiated to the right iliac fossa. She also has a fever. She is on the oral contraceptive pill (OCP) and previously her mother had a deep vein thrombosis (DVT). Your registrar has reviewed the patient and has decided that this patient requires an appendicectomy tomorrow. She has normal renal function, raised C-reactive protein (CRP) and raised white cell count (WCC). The registrar wants you to start regular painkillers (paracetamol and codeine), intravenous (IV) fluids and IV antibiotics (cefuroxime and metronidazole). Please also perform a VTE prophylaxis assessment and prescribe the appropriate treatment.

Patient Details

Name:	Nicole Smith
DOB:	05/03/01
Hospital number:	1208973948
Weight:	60 kg
Height:	1.6 m
Consultant:	Mr King
Hospital/Ward:	WGH Ward 3
Current medications:	Oral contraceptive pill only
Allergies:	No known drug allergies
Admission date:	22/09/24

Stop all antiplatelets prior to procedures/operations to prevent bleeding, ideally 10 days ($t_{½}$ of platelets).

Patients on warfarin should have it stopped before the procedure and bridged with LMWH. If INR is significantly raised, consider reversal with Vitamin K and take advice from haematology. Recommence all anticoagulation as soon as bleeding risk is minimal (which will vary depending on the procedure).

THROMBOPROPHYLAXIS

All patients admitted to hospital require a VTE prophylaxis assessment.

ASSESSMENT OF VENOUS THROMBOSIS RISK FACTORS

Surgical patients are at increased risk of VTE if they have one or more of the following risk factors:

1. Age >60
2. Dehydration
3. Obesity (body mass index (BMI) >30)
4. Known thrombophilias
5. Critical care admission
6. Pregnancy or postpartum
7. Varicose veins with phlebitis
8. Oestrogen therapy (hormone replacement therapy, oral contraceptive therapy)
9. Active cancer or chemotherapy
10. Reduced mobility
11. Personal or family history of DVT
12. Significant medical comorbidities
13. Surgical procedures taking longer than 90 minutes in theatre
14. Acute admission with infection/inflammation/intraabdominal condition

GENERAL MEASURES TO REDUCE VTE RISK

1. Keep the patient well hydrated.
2. Encourage early mobilisation.
3. Utilise regional rather than general anaesthesia.

VTE prophylaxis (pharmacological or mechanical) does not need to be routinely offered to all surgical patients. For example, it is not indicated in a patient undergoing a surgical procedure with local anaesthesia by local infiltration with no limitation of mobility.

However, most surgical patients at increased risk of VTE (by the previous criteria) should receive mechanical VTE prophylaxis as well as pharmacological (unless contraindicated).

MECHANICAL THROMBOPROPHYLAXIS

Prescribing Mechanical Thromboprophylaxis

There are several types of mechanical VTE prophylaxis available. Graduated compression stockings, e.g. TED stockings, are the most common. Other possible options used less commonly are intermittent pneumatic compression (thigh or knee), and foot impulse devices.

Contraindications to Mechanical VTE Prophylaxis

Possible contraindications to mechanical VTE prophylaxis:

1. Peripheral arterial disease, be it suspected or proven
2. Peripheral arterial bypass graft
3. Severe leg oedema
4. Peripheral neuropathy
5. Deformity or unusual shape to prevent correct fitting
6. Allergies to materials
7. Ulcers/wounds/cellulitis

PHARMACOLOGICAL THROMBOPROPHYLAXIS

Risk of Bleeding on VTE Prophylaxis

Potential contraindications to pharmacological VTE prophylaxis:

1. Active bleeding
2. On oral anticoagulants
3. Significant procedure-related bleeding risk
4. Acute stroke: haemorrhagic or large infarct
5. Untreated inherited or acquired bleeding disorders (e.g. haemophilia, Von Willebrand disease)
6. Platelets <75 × 10^9/L or abnormal clotting screen
7. Blood pressure (BP) >230 mmHg systolic or >120 mmHg diastolic
8. Lumbar puncture/epidural/spinal anaesthesia in previous 4 hours or within next 12 hours
9. Heparin-induced thrombocytopenia

Offer patient and/or families information on:

1. Risks and possible consequence of VTE
2. Importance of VTE prophylaxis and its possible side effects
3. The correct use of VTE prophylaxis
4. How patients themselves can reduce their risk of VTE

In those whom thromboprophylaxis is felt not indicated, this should be reassessed on a daily basis while in hospital.

PRESCRIBING PHARMACOLOGICAL THROMBOPROPHYLAXIS

The option depends on renal function.

If renal function is normal, prescribe subcutaneous low-molecular-weight heparin (LMWH)/factor Xa inhibitor (e.g. enoxaparin, or dalteparin, or fondaparinux).

Several possible variants occur in reduced renal function, so consult your local hospital formulary. Both the definition of reduced renal function and the management will vary from trust to trust.

Two example protocols:

- Definition of reduced renal function: estimated glomerular filtration rate (eGFR) <30 mL/min.
  - Action in reduced renal function: prescribe subcutaneous unfractionated heparin instead of LMWH.
- Definition of reduced renal function: eGFR <20 mL/min.
  - Action in reduced renal function: a standard dose of dalteparin can be prescribed, but anti-factor Xa levels need to be monitored. The peak level is measured 4 hours postdose and trough level immediately predose. This should be done every 4 to 5 days while on LMWH. Peaks >0.6 and troughs >0.3 anti-Xa units/mL indicate a need for dose reduction.

PATIENT'S RISK FACTORS AND BLEEDING RISK

1. Nicole is a surgical patient.
2. She is an acute admission with an inflammatory/infective/intraabdominal condition.
3. She currently is using the OCP, which promotes a prothrombotic state.
4. She has a family history of DVTs, which gives her a theoretical risk of thrombosis.
5. She potentially could be a critical care admission if she becomes septic.
6. If she has a complicated appendicectomy, her procedure could potentially take longer than 90 minutes.

Nicole has no bleeding risk factors. Therefore, in addition to mechanical VTE prophylaxis, pharmacological prophylaxis is required as her VTE risk is high.

Prescribe (Figs 8.1 and 8.2)

Pharmacological VTE Prophylaxis:

- DALTEPARIN 5000 units SC OD

Mechanical VTE Prophylaxis:

- TED STOCKINGS 1 pair TOP CONT

Analgesia:

- PARACETAMOL 1 g PO QDS and CODEINE PHOSPHATE 30 mg PO QDS

Antibiotics:

- CEFUROXIME 750 mg IV (over 30 minutes) TDS and METRONIDAZOLE 500 mg IV (over 20–30 minutes) TDS

IV Fluids:

- SODIUM CHLORIDE 0.9% 1000 mL (with 40 mmol KCl) at 85 mL/h, followed by GLUCOSE 5% 1000 mL (with 20 mmol KCl) at 85 mL/h, followed by GLUCOSE 5% 1000 mL (with 20 mmol KCl) at 85 mL/h. Note this is based on 30 ml/kg of fluid, and approximately 60 mmol K a day.

Note that the patient will need to be fasted preoperatively. Policy for this will vary between units. Once a time for surgery is settled, the patient, for instance, would not be allowed water or oral medications for 4 hours preoperatively.

ADDITIONAL VTE PROPHYLAXIS EXAMPLES: SEE PRESCRIBE BOXES IN MARGIN (DRUG CHARTS NOT SHOWN)

- Mr Smith is a 58-year-old gentleman with pancreatic cancer admitted for a Whipple's resection. He is known to have peripheral arterial disease and has normal renal function.

Prescribe Example 1

Pharmacological VTE Prophylaxis (e.g. ENOXAPARIN 40 mg OD SC) but do not give mechanical VTE prophylaxis due to peripheral artery disease

- Mrs Mercury is a 59-year-old woman with cholecystitis secondary to gallstones. She is scheduled for an emergency cholecystectomy. She has chronic kidney disease (eGFR 20 mL/min).

Prescribe Example 2

Subcutaneous unfractionated heparin (e.g. HEPARIN 5000 units BD SC) and mechanical VTE prophylaxis (e.g. TED STOCKINGS 1 pair TOP CONT)

STATION 8.2: ACUTE PANCREATITIS

You are the surgical junior doctor in the emergency department. A 42-year-old woman, Jane, with a background of gallstones presents with severe epigastric pain radiating to the back. She has vomited on multiple occasions and feels that she is becoming more breathless. Please assess her and commence appropriate management.

Patient Details

Name:	Jane Smith
DOB:	05/03/82
Hospital number:	J345789
Weight:	85 kg
Height:	1.6 m
Consultant:	Mr King
Hospital/Ward:	BFH Surgical
Current medications:	None
Allergies:	No known drug allergies
Admission date:	22/09/24

Differential Diagnosis of Epigastric Pain

- Peptic ulcer disease
- Oesophagitis
- Perforated peptic ulcer
- Symptomatic gallstones
- Acute pancreatitis
- Dissecting aortic aneurysm
- Small bowel obstruction
- Myocardial infarction

Causes of Acute Pancreatitis

- Gallstones (40%)
- Alcohol (40%)
- Idiopathic (10%)
- Post-endoscopic retrograde cholangiopancreatography (ERCP)
- Hyperlipidaemia
- Viral (mumps, coxsackie)
- Drugs (azathioprine, tamoxifen, corticosteroids, valproate, aminosalicylates)
- Autoimmune (vasculitides)

Complications of Pancreatitis

- Early: shock, acute respiratory distress syndrome (ARDS), systemic inflammatory response syndrome (SIRS), hypocalcaemia, renal failure, hyperglycaemia, retroperitoneal haemorrhage
- Late: pseudocyst formation, pancreatic abscess formation, necrotising pancreatitis, recurrent pancreatitis, pancreatic cancer

INITIAL ASSESSMENT

AIRWAY

- Assess the patency of her airway. Does she have any vomitus obstructing her airway?

'The airway is secure and patent as she is responding to questions.'

Continue to monitor the airway but no intervention currently required.

BREATHING

- Assess the rate and depth of respiration. Is she using her accessory muscles for respiration? Check oxygen saturations. Auscultate her chest: does she have any degree of lung impairment, crackles or wheeze?

'RR 28/min and oxygen saturations are 91% pre-oxygen therapy. She is using her accessory muscles of respiration. She has reduced air entry and crackles are heard throughout both lung fields bilaterally with some wheeze. She is complaining that she cannot catch her breath.'

This patient is tachypnoeic and unable to maintain normal saturations. She requires high-flow oxygen on a nonrebreather mask and optimisation of pain control.

CIRCULATION

- Assess her capillary refill time (CRT), pulse and BP. Check her mucous membranes and assess her hydration status by looking at her tongue and skin turgor.

'HR 115 bpm, BP 90/60 mmHg and CRT 3 seconds peripherally. Her hands are moist and cool with a thready pulse. Her mucous membranes are dry. Her eyes appear sunken. Her heart sounds are normal with no murmurs.'

This patient is intravascularly depleted. She needs aggressive fluid resuscitation. Two large-bore IV cannulae (14 or 16 G) should be inserted (while simultaneously taking bloods) and a fluid challenge should be given (e.g. over 15 minutes). A urinary catheter should be inserted to assess end-organ perfusion.

DISABILITY

- Assess her Glasgow Coma Scale (GCS) and her blood glucose levels.

'She has normal neurological function with a 15/15 GCS and her last blood glucose was 10 mmol/L.'

No action is currently required.

Prescribe (Figs 8.3–8.5)

High-flow oxygen:
- 15 L/min OXYGEN via NONREBREATHER MASK

Analgesia:
- MORPHINE 5 to 10 mg IV (titrate to response)

Antiemetic:
- CYCLIZINE 50 mg IV STAT (to reduce morphine-related vomiting)

Fluid bolus:
- SODIUM CHLORIDE 0.9% 500 mL IV (over 15 minutes)

EXPOSURE

- Examine the abdomen as this is the source of the pain. Does she have any bruising around the flanks or periumbilical region? Does she have any tenderness on palpation? Are there any signs of peritonism, such as rebound, guarding or percussion-induced pain? Assess for flank tenderness. Measure temperature.

'This woman does not have any ecchymosis in the flank (Grey–Turner's sign) or periumbilical (Cullen's sign) area. Her abdomen is soft but extremely tender throughout, mainly around the epigastric region. There is voluntary guarding but no abdominal distension or percussion tenderness. Her bowel sounds are present and her temperature is 37.5°C.'

INITIAL INVESTIGATIONS

- **Arterial blood gas (ABG)**: A metabolic acidosis is characterised by a low pH and bicarbonate with an increasingly negative base excess and elevated lactate. She may be compensating her pH by hyperventilating; a low CO_2 would confirm this.
- **Bloods**: Full blood count (FBC), urea and electrolyte (U&E), CRP, liver function test (LFT), amylase, lactate dehydrogenase (LDH), calcium, coagulation profile and blood glucose. A raised amylase, 3 times its upper limit, is highly sensitive for acute pancreatitis. Assess her LFTs; a raised alkaline phosphatase (ALP) and bilirubin may be due to a stone in her common bile duct (CBD) and this could be causing pancreatitis. A CRP is a good surrogate to assess inflammation. A raised WCC may indicate infection (sometimes upper abdominal pain can be caused by a lower lobe pneumonia or abdominal sepsis) but may be raised purely due to pancreatitis. A dropping Hb may be a sign of retroperitoneal haemorrhage. Additional bloods listed are used for severity scoring (Table 8.1).
- **Imaging**: A chest radiography (CXR) is important to assess any element of ARDS. Diffuse bilateral pulmonary infiltrates are indicative of severe pancreatitis and that the need for respiratory support may be pending. No free air under the diaphragm reduces the likelihood of perforation. An ultrasound is important as this can determine the cause and severity of the pancreatitis; 40% of pancreatitides is due to gallstones. The presence of stones and a dilated CBD is a good indicator of its cause. However, a nondilated CBD does not exclude gallstones as the cause of pancreatitis. If there are doubts about the diagnosis, a contract computed tomography (CT) abdomen scan can provide evidence of pancreatitis.

'ABG shows a pH of 7.32, $PaCO_2$ 4 kPa, PaO_2 10 kPa, HCO_3 18 mmol/L, lactate 3 mmol/L and BE is –4 mmol/L. Hb 135 g/L, CRP 250 mg/L, WCC 18 × 10^9/L, amylase 477 IU/L, bilirubin 50 μmol/L, ALT 45 IU/L, ALP 200 IU/L, potassium 4 mmol/L, sodium 138 mmol/L, creatinine 175 μmol/L and urea 16.5 mmol/L (eGFR 36 mL/min). Initial Imrie score is 2 (WCC and urea). CXR shows mild bilateral pulmonary infiltrates, no free air under the diaphragm. USS shows multiple gallstones with a CBD diameter of 12 mm. The pancreas is markedly inflamed, but no obvious collections.'

INITIAL MANAGEMENT

Management Summary: Acute Pancreatitis

- Aggressive resuscitation
- Assessment of disease severity
- Early ITU involvement in severe pancreatitis
- Imaging to identify aetiology and severity
- Early nutritional support
- Avoid antibiotics unless infection identified
- Treatment in specific aetiology (i.e. ERCP)

- **Get help early**: Intensive **therapy** unit (ITU) team **and** senior surgical team members.
- **Airway and breathing support**: High-flow oxygen with a nonrebreather mask to maintain oxygen saturation >94%.
- **Analgesia**: Opioids early to prevent any splinting of diaphragm due to pain. Patients generally require patient-controlled analgesia (PCA) to control the pain; the ITU team will help you with this but you can start with a regular oral morphine preparation.
- **Fluid support**: Monitor intravascular fluid volume with serial creatinine and urine output. Patients

Table 8.1 Miss Smith's Blood Results and ABG Result

PARAMETER	VALUE	NORMAL RANGE (UNITS)
WCC	**18 × 10⁹/L**	**4–11 (×10⁹/L)**
Neutrophil	**12 × 10⁹/L**	**2–7.5 (×10⁹/L)**
Lymphocyte	4 × 10⁹/L	1.4–4 (×10⁹/L)
Platelet	300 × 10⁹/L	150–400 (×10⁹/L)
Haemoglobin	135 g/L	Men: 135–177 (g/L) Women: 115–155 (g/L)
PT	12 seconds	11.5–13.5 seconds
APTT	30 seconds	26–37 seconds
CRP	**250 mg/L**	**0–5 (mg/L)**
Urea	**16.5 mmol/L**	**2.5–6.7 (mmol/L)**
Creatinine	**175 μmol/L**	**79–118 (μmol/L)**
Sodium	138 mmol/L	135–146 (mmol/L)
Potassium	4 mmol/L	3.5–5.0 (mmol/L)
eGFR	**36 mL/min**	**>60 (mL/min)**
Bilirubin	**50 μmol/L**	**<17 (μmol/L)**
ALT	**45 IU/L**	**<40 (IU/L)**
ALP	**200 IU/L**	**39–117 (IU/L)**
Amylase	**477 IU/L**	**25–125 (IU/L)**
LDH	460 IU/L	240–480 (IU/L)
Glucose	5.6 mmol/L	4.5–5.6 (mmol/L) (fasting)
Calcium (corrected)	2.20 mmol/L	2.20–2.67 (mmol/L)
Albumin	40 g/L	35–50 (g/L)
Lactate	3 mmol/L	0.6–2.4 (mmol/L)
pH	**7.32**	**7.35–7.45**
$PaCO_2$	**4 kPa**	**4.8–6.1 (kPa)**
HCO_3	**18 mmol/L**	**22–26 (mmol/L)**
PaO_2	**10 kPa**	**10.6–13.3 (kPa) on air**
BE	**−4 mmol/L**	**±2 (mmol/L)**

Data in bold signifies results that are outside the normal laboratory range. *ABG,* Arterial blood gas; *ALP,* alkaline phosphatase; *ALT,* alanine transaminase; *BE,* base excess; *CRP,* C-reactive protein; *eGFR,* estimated glomerular filtration rate; *WCC,* white cell count.

with severe pancreatitis normally need >5 L within the first 24 hours due to third space loss (the space between tissues where fluid does not normally collect). They may require central access for BP monitoring and accurate fluid balance.

- **Nutrition**: Acute pancreatitis is a catabolic event and promotes nutritional deterioration. Early feeding plays an important role in accelerating recovery. Start with oral fluids and avoid fatty foods. Nasogastric (NG)/nasojejunal (NJ) feeds may be required if unable to tolerate oral feeds. Total parenteral nutrition (TPN) is used for specific indications, such as a paralytic ileus.
- **Supportive**: VTE prophylaxis as guided by trust guidelines, both mechanical and pharmacological.
- The patient should be placed nil by mouth (NBM) given the severe pain and vomiting. Oral medications (plus fluid and diet) can be restarted as soon as the patient can tolerate them. This could be after as little as a day if the pancreatitis is mild but may be several weeks in severe cases.

Modified Glasgow Score (IMRIE)

- Age >55 years
- WCC >15 × 10⁹/L
- Blood glucose >10 mmol/L
- AST or ALT >200 IU/L
- LDH >600 IU/L
- Serum urea >16 mmol/L
- Serum Ca^{2+} <2 mmol/L
- Serum albumin <32 g/L
- PaO_2 <7.9 kPa on air

A score ≥3 is indicative of severe pancreatitis and carries a 40% mortality. In this case, the score is 2 due to the WCC of 18 × 10⁹/L and urea of 16.5 mmol/L.

Prescribe (see Figs. 8.3–8.5)

Proton pump inhibitor:

- ESOMEPRAZOLE 40 mg IV (over 10–30 minutes) OD

Thromboprophylaxis:

- DALTEPARIN 5000 units OD SC and TED STOCKINGS TOP CONT

Regular analgesia:

- MORPHINE 5 mg 4 HOURLY IV (with antiemetic, e.g. CYCLIZINE 50 mg IV TDS)

REASSESSMENT

It is essential to continue monitoring these patients as they can deteriorate rapidly. Early and continued disease scoring (at least every 24 hours) with the modified Glasgow score (Imrie) is helpful. A score of 3 and greater signifies severe disease. The important aspects to consider early are pain control, fluid resuscitation and diagnostic/therapeutic tools to aid in diagnosing and treating the underlying condition. If no improvement, high-resolution CT scan would be necessary to look for complications such as pseudocyst formation, and in the event of positive findings, the case would need to be managed at a specialist pancreatic centre.

'After initial fluid resuscitation and analgesia, Miss Smith is more stable. Airway is patent, RR is 18/min, saturating 100% on 15 L/min oxygen. The patient is less dehydrated with HR 80 bpm, BP 110/75 mmHg and CRT <2 seconds. Urine output is 0.4 mL/kg/h. No further vomiting. Pain is still severe, rated at 7/10 despite morphine regularly.'

Oxygen should be titrated down while maintaining saturations above 94%. The patient has responded well to a fluid bolus. However, ongoing fluids will be required as the patient is currently NBM. On top of this, the patient has an acute kidney injury (AKI), and is slightly tachycardic with a poor urine output, so fluids should be given at a faster rate than maintenance requirements. Fluid requirements will need to be assessed frequently. Anaesthetic input is likely needed for pain review: a PCA is probably now required.

Prescribe (see Figs 8.3–8.5)

Further fluids:

- SODIUM CHLORIDE 0.9% 1 L with 20 mmol KCL at 500 mL/h

OXYGEN:

- 8 L/min via MASK

STOP

Initial oxygen prescription

HANDING OVER THE PATIENT

'Miss Smith is a 42-year-old woman with acute pancreatitis. She presented with severe epigastric pain and dehydration. She has been stabilised with regular morphine and paracetamol analgesia, a 500 mL sodium chloride 0.9% bolus and oxygen therapy.

Admission ABG showed a lactic acidosis, pH of 7.32, $PaCO_2$ 4 kPa, HCO_3 18 mmol/L, lactate 3 mmol/L, BE –4 mmol/L. Amylase is 477 IU/L. There is evidence of cholestasis with a bilirubin 50 µmol/L, ALP 200 IU/L and prerenal AKI with creatinine 175 µmol/L and urea 16.5 mmol/L. Blood glucose is normal. CXR shows mild bilateral pulmonary infiltrates with no free air under the diaphragm.

She has had early scorings (currently Imrie 2) pancreatitis and an USS has demonstrated gallbladder disease with a dilated CBD. Her pancreas is moderately inflamed but appears uncomplicated.

She is currently haemodynamically stable. Her urine output is approximately 0.4 mL/kg/h. Current observations are: RR 18/min, oxygen saturations 95% on 8 L/min oxygen, HR 80 bpm, BP 110/75 mmHg, apyrexial with 7/10 pain.

She has been placed nil by mouth and is on intravenous fluids. IV morphine is being used to control pain with cyclizine as an antiemetic. An ERCP referral has been made for the gallstones.

The plan is to continue 500 mL/h of sodium chloride 0.9% for the next 4 hours and discuss with the anaesthetic team about starting a PCA to optimise pain control. She needs to be discussed with the ITU team. She also will require a fluid review, repeat bloods and a repeat blood gas later this evening.'

STATION 8.3: INTESTINAL OBSTRUCTION

You are the surgical junior doctor on-call clerking in the emergency department. You are asked to see Julio, a 62-year-old man who presents with colicky abdominal pain and distension associated with nausea and vomiting. On closer questioning, you realise he has not opened his bowels for the past 3 days and has had an appendicectomy for a perforated appendix 40 years ago.

Patient Details

Name:	Julio Smith
DOB:	05/03/62
Hospital number:	J345333
Weight:	70 kg
Height:	1.6 m
Consultant:	Mr Sing
Hospital/Ward:	GDH Surgical
Current medications:	None
Allergies:	Penicillin (rash)
Admission date:	22/09/24

Differential Diagnosis of Causes of Intestinal Obstruction

- Small bowel: Adhesions/bands, hernia (inguinal, femoral, incisional), strictures, volvulus, neoplasia
- Large bowel: Constipation, neoplasia, volvulus, strictures
- Ileus: Metabolic disturbances

Cardinal Features of Intestinal Obstruction

- Pain
- Vomiting
- Abdominal distension
- Constipation

These vary depending on the location and aetiology of the obstruction. Anatomically higher obstructions are more likely to cause vomiting, while lower obstructions tend to have greater abdominal distension.

Complications of Bowel Obstruction

- Visceral perforation
- Electrolyte derangement
- AKI
- Infection

INITIAL ASSESSMENT

AIRWAY

- Assess the patency of his airway. Does he have any vomitus obstructing his airway?

'The airway is patent.'

No additional airway support is required.

BREATHING

- Assess the rate and depth of respiration. Assess his work of breathing and his oxygen saturations. Percuss the lung fields. Auscultate to assess air entry or presence of crackles.

'RR 20/min, oxygen saturation 96% in room air. He has slightly reduced air entry bilaterally and minimal crackles at the base. He is complaining of worsening abdominal pain on deep inspiration.'

The patient is saturating well in air but there is possible evidence of atelectasis or aspiration pneumonia. Abdominal distension and pain can cause atelectasis, which will impair proper ventilation and perfusion. Prescribe analgesia and order a CXR.

CIRCULATION

- Assess the haemodynamic stability by assessing the pulse, BP, CRT, skin temperature and mucous membranes.

'HR 110 bpm, BP 110/90 mmHg, CRT 3 seconds and mucous membranes are pink and dry. During the past 48 hours, he mentions that he has passed less urine and that it appears concentrated.'

This man will require two large-bore IV cannulae (with bloods taken simultaneously) and a fluid challenge. Reassessment should occur immediately after. The best way to assess his response is by assessing his urine output and vital signs. A narrow pulse pressure is a good indicator of an intravascularly depleted patient.

DISABILITY

- Assess the patient's consciousness using the GCS. Is the patient confused or agitated? What's the capillary glucose reading?

'This man's GCS is E4, M6, V4 = 14/15. He seems a bit confused and his blood glucose currently is 7 mmol/L.'

His confusion is probably due to his depleted intravascular volume or due to infection. These should be thoroughly assessed as well as considering other potential causes of confusion, e.g. metabolic disturbances.

EXPOSURE

- Expose and examine this gentleman's abdomen and hernial orifices thoroughly. Complete the assessment by doing a digital rectal examination. Pay extra attention to any signs of peritonism as this may indicate a perforated viscous.

'The abdomen is generally distended, particularly centrally, and he has an appendicectomy scar in the right iliac fossa. On palpation his abdomen is tender but there is no local tenderness, guarding or rigidity. On percussion his abdomen is tympanic and his bowels sounds are hyperactive. The rectal and hernial examination was unremarkable.'

This patient has the cardinal signs of intestinal obstruction. It is important to rule out any hernias as this is a common cause of obstruction; check previous incision sites. Rigidity, guarding and absent/reduced bowel sounds are features of perforation or strangulation and would indicate a surgical emergency.

Prescribe (Figs 8.6–8.8)

Analgesia:
- MORPHINE 5 to 10 mg (titrate to response) IV STAT

Antiemetic:
- CYCLIZINE 50 mg IV STAT

Fluid challenge:
- 500 mL SODIUM CHLORIDE 0.9% (over 15 minutes)

INITIAL INVESTIGATIONS

- **Bloods:** FBC, CRP, electrolytes, coagulation, amylase, LFTs, group and save. Raised WCC and CRP may indicate perforation or strangulation. A raised creatinine and urea can indicate an AKI due to dehydration. Electrolyte disturbances can cause a nonmechanical cause of intestinal obstruction. A raised amylase may indicate this is pancreatitis (presenting as an ileus). Abdominal pain may be due to gallstones/liver dysfunction. A group and save and coagulation screen should also be sent if you think the patient may require surgical intervention (Table 8.2).
- **ABG:** An acidosis on ABG with a raised lactate may indicate ischaemia secondary to strangulation.
- **Erect CXR:** Identifies any free air under the diaphragm with intestinal perforation. Assess if there is any evidence of aspiration pneumonia such as consolidation.
- **AXR:** Assessing for dilated loops of bowel. Small bowel obstruction has complete bands through the bowel wall called plica circularis (or valvulae conniventes). Large bowel dilatation is markedly larger and has haustra. Small bowel tends to be more central, whereas large bowel tends to be more peripheral. A CT scan will be able to definitely say where the obstruction might be and might identify a secondary cause, e.g. an obstructing tumour.
- **Urine dipstick:** To assess for evidence of a UTI. Offer testing for β-hCG in female patients to check for pregnancy.

'ABG is normal. WCC 8 × 10⁹/L, CRP 7 mg/L, sodium 138 mmol/L, potassium 4.1 mmol/L, urea 12 mmol/L and creatinine 130 μmol/L (eGFR 53 mL/min); other bloods are normal. Erect CXR shows no free air under the diaphragm and no abnormalities in the lung zones. AXR shows multiple centrally positioned dilated bowel loops. The bowel loops appear to be of small bowel as the valvulae conniventes are seen. The maximum diameter is 5 cm.'

INITIAL MANAGEMENT

Management of Intestinal Obstruction

- GI decompression (NG)
- Keep NBM
- Fluid and electrolyte restoration
- Timely treatment of obstruction

Table 8.2 Mr Smith's Blood Results and ABG Result

PARAMETER	VALUE	NORMAL RANGE (UNITS)
WCC	8 × 10^9/L	4–11 (×10^9/L)
Platelet	300 × 10^9/L	150–400 (×10^9/L)
Haemoglobin	140 g/L	Men: 135–177 (g/L) Women: 115–155 (g/L)
PT	13 seconds	11.5–13.5 seconds
APTT	32 seconds	26–37 seconds
CRP	**7 mg/L**	**0–5 (mg/L)**
Urea	**12 mmol/L**	**2.5–6.7 (mmol/L)**
Creatinine	**130 µmol/L**	**79–118 (µmol/L)**
Sodium	138 mmol/L	135–146 (mmol/L)
Potassium	4.1 mmol/L	3.5–5.0 (mmol/L)
eGFR	**53 mL/min**	**>60 (mL/min)**
Bilirubin	7 µmol/L	<17 (µmol/L)
ALT	20 IU/L	<40 (IU/L)
ALP	100 IU/L	39–117 (IU/L)
Amylase	100 IU/L	25–125 (IU/L)
Calcium (corrected)	2.20 mmol/L	2.20–2.67 (mmol/L)
Albumin	40 g/L	35–50 (g/L)
pH	7.40	7.35–7.45
$PaCO_2$	5 kPa	4.8–6.1 (kPa)
HCO_3	25 mmol/L	22–26 (mmol/L)
PaO_2	12 kPa	10.6–13.3 (kPa) on air
BE	−1 mmol/L	±2 (mmol/L)

Data in bold signifies results that are outside the normal laboratory range. *ABG*, Arterial blood gas; *ALP*, alkaline phosphatase; *ALT*, alanine transaminase; *BE*, base excess; *CRP*, C-reactive protein; *eGFR*, estimated glomerular filtration rate; *WCC*, white cell count.

- **Airway support:** Airway patent in this case, with no intervention required.
- **Supplementary oxygen:** If saturations <94%.
- **Decompression:** This patient should be made NBM and have a large-bore NG tube inserted to encourage free drainage of stomach contents.
- **Fluid resuscitation:** This patient requires two large-bore IV access points and a fluid bolus due to being significantly dehydrated. His gastric/NG losses should be matched with an isotonic crystalloid. He will also require his normal maintenance fluid. As he is NBM, all fluid will be given IV. Minimum urine output should be 0.5 mL/kg per hour and ideally around 1 mL/kg per hour.
- **Medications:** Patient will require regular analgesia and a centrally acting antiemetic (e.g. cyclizine). Medications that promote gastric emptying (e.g. domperidone) should be avoided as this may exacerbate the patient's symptoms or cause a perforation. Withhold any nephrotoxic drugs if the patient has AKI.
- **VTE thromboprophylaxis:** The patient is at an increased risk of thromboembolic event, so should be considered for pharmacological thromboprophylaxis as per local guidelines. Measure renal function before prescribing thromboprophylaxis if there is a concern about significant kidney injury.

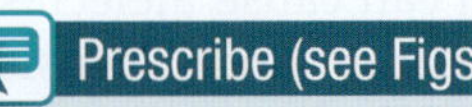

Prescribe (see Figs 8.6–8.8)

Regular antiemetic:
- CYCLIZINE 50 mg IV TDS

Thromboprophylaxis:
- ENOXAPARIN 40 mg SC OD
- TED STOCKINGS CONT TOP

Regular analgesia:
- MORPHINE 5 mg (titrate to response) IV 4 hourly

Further fluids:
- 1 L SODIUM CHLORIDE 0.9% with 20 mmol KCl at 250 mL/h

REASSESSMENT

- After NG decompression along with a fluid bolus, the patient is reassessed.

'The patient looks mildly improved. The airway is patent, RR 18/min, oxygen saturation is 97% on room air. His breathing is satisfactory and his abdomen continues to be distended. HR 70 bpm, BP 120/75 mmHg, CRT 2 seconds and urine output 1 mL/kg/h. NG has drained 1.5 L of bilious fluid. After one dose of morphine, pain is well controlled on regular paracetamol.'

The patient has responded well to a fluid bolus but has ongoing losses with significant bilious aspirates. Another fluid bolus is not necessary at the moment but fluids will be needed at a rate faster than maintenance fluid to replace bilious and insensible losses. Fluid requirements will need to be assessed frequently.

HANDING OVER THE PATIENT

'Julio Smith is a 62-year-old patient with a previous appendicectomy who has now presented with a 3-day history of signs and symptoms of bowel obstruction. On his initial assessment, he was dehydrated and in pain. He has been stabilised with an NG tube and given a 500 mL fluid bolus and analgesia/antiemetics. AXR demonstrated small bowel obstruction with no evidence of perforation. Bloods show evidence of AKI with urea 12 mmol/L and creatinine 130 µmol/L. He is currently haemodynamically stable with good urine output. Oxygen saturations are 95% on room air.

Julio is currently on 250 mL/h of sodium chloride 0.9%. The patient is awaiting a CT abdomen to determine the level of the obstruction. Please do a fluid review and reexamine the abdomen later this evening.'

Indications for Operative Intervention

- Visceral perforation
- Signs of peritoneal irritation
- Irreducible/strangulated hernia
- Deteriorating patient
- Failure to resolve within 48 hours

STATION 8.4: DIABETES IN THE SURGICAL PATIENT WITH OSTEOMYELITIS

You are the junior doctor on a general surgical ward. The patient is a 67-year-old man with type 2 diabetes, normally only on metformin, who requires a below-knee amputation for his infected and gangrenous right foot. Please assess the patient and instigate the appropriate management plan in preparation for theatre tomorrow.

Patient Details

Name:	Adam Smith
DOB:	05/03/57
Hospital number:	J345400
Weight:	70 kg
Height:	1.6 m
Consultant:	Mr Wood
Hospital/Ward:	CGH Surgical
Current medications:	Metformin 500 mg PO TDS (for diabetes)
Allergies:	No known drug allergies
Admission date:	22/09/24

Complications of Diabetes Mellitus

MICROVASCULAR DISEASE
- Retinopathy
- Nephropathy
- Neuropathy

MACROVASCULAR DISEASE
- Coronary heart disease
- Cerebral vascular disease
- Peripheral vascular disease

Symptoms of Diabetes

- Polyuria/polydipsia
- Unintentional weight loss
- Worsening blurred vision
- Recurrent infections
- Lethargy/weakness
- Sensory loss

INITIAL ASSESSMENT

AIRWAY

- Assess patency of the airway. Does he have any stridor?

  'The airway is patent'.

  No additional airway support is required.

BREATHING

- Assess the rate and depth of respiration. Assess his work of breathing and his oxygen saturations. Percuss the different lung zones for any abnormalities. Auscultate the lungs to assess air entry or presence of crackles.

  'The respiratory rate is 28/min with saturations of 96%. He is taking deep breaths, and is in visible pain with accessory muscles of breathing apparent. Despite his tachypnoea, he has good air entry with no crackles or wheeze.'

  No additional breathing support is required.

CIRCULATION

- Assess the haemodynamic stability by measuring pulse, BP, CRT, skin temperature and assessing the mucous membranes.

  'HR 110 bpm, BP 120/70 mmHg, CRT 3 seconds and mucous membranes are pink and moist. His distal peripheries are clammy and sweaty with thready pulses.'

This man will require IV access, bloods and a fluid bolus. A reassessment should occur immediately after. Urinary catheterisation should be considered to monitor his urinary output.

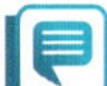

Prescribe (Figs 8.9–8.11)

Fluid challenge:
- 500 mL SODIUM CHLORIDE 0.9% (over 15 minutes)

DISABILITY

- Assess the patient's level of consciousness using the GCS. Is the patient confused or agitated? What is the capillary glucose reading?

  'This patient's GCS is E4, M6, V4 = 14/15. He seems a bit confused and his blood glucose currently is 16 mmol/L (post-fluid challenge).'

His confusion is probably due to being septic with uncontrolled hyperglycaemia. He will require a variable rate IV insulin infusion (VRIII) to control the blood glucose. Note that blood glucose is often corrected just with adequate crystalloid (nonglucose) resuscitation, but in this case, it is inadequate, and a VRIII is required anyway preoperatively. (Note VRIII was previously called a sliding scale regimen.)

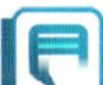

Prescribe (see Figs 8.9–8.11)

Write on front of drug chart:
VRIII regimen (shown in Table 8.3).
Note the blood glucose values, rate of insulin infusion and coprescribed fluids vary between hospitals; consult local guidelines.

EXPOSURE

- Examine this gentleman ensuring adequate exposure of all possible sites of infection. Examine for both macrovascular and microvascular complications of diabetes. Assess his core body temperature for pyrexia.

Table 8.3 VRIII Regimen

BLOOD GLUCOSE (MMOL/L) (TARGET RANGE 6–10 MMOL/L)	INSULIN (ACTRAPID) INFUSION (UNITS/H = ML/H)
>20	5
15–19.9	4
10–14.9	3
7–9.9	2
4–6.9	1
<3.9	0.5

VRIII fluids = glucose 5%/sodium chloride 0.45%/ potassium chloride 0.15% 1000 mL 125 mL/h. 50 units of insulin (Actrapid) is made up in 50 mL of sodium chloride 0.9% to give a concentration of 1 unit/mL of insulin. This means that 1 unit/h of insulin equates to 1 mL/h.

'His right foot and distal leg are markedly erythematous, malodorous, swollen and red with exudative pyogenic material oozing from the foot. The patient has no sensations below the knee. His core temperature is 38.5°C and there are no other sites of infection.'

Commence antipyretics to reduce his temperature. Swab the wound for microscopy, culture and sensitivity (M/C/S) and dress the wound appropriately until formal surgical intervention tomorrow.

INITIAL INVESTIGATIONS

- **Bloods:** FBC, U&Es, CRP, blood culture, serum glucose, ketones. Look for evidence of infection, assess renal function and hydration status. Serum glucose is important to assess the severity of hyperglycaemia (Table 8.4).

Table 8.4 Mr Smith's Blood Results and ABG Result

PARAMETER	VALUE	NORMAL RANGE (UNITS)
WCC	**25 × 10⁹/L**	**4–11 (×10⁹/L)**
Neutrophil	**18 × 10⁹/L**	**2–7.5 (×10⁹/L)**
Lymphocyte	4 × 10⁹/L	1.4–4 (×10⁹/L)
Platelet	200 × 10⁹/L	150–400 (×10⁹/L)
Haemoglobin	135 g/L	Men: 135–177 (g/L) Women: 115–155 (g/L)
CRP	**267 mg/L**	**0–5 (mg/L)**
Urea	**9.3 mmol/L**	**2.5–6.7 (mmol/L)**
Creatinine	**120 µmol/L**	**79–118 (µmol/L)**
Sodium	135 mmol/L	135–146 (mmol/L)
Potassium	4.9 mmol/L	3.5–5.0 (mmol/L)
eGFR	**54 mL/min**	**>60 (mL/min)**
Lactate	**2.8 mmol/L**	**0.6–2.4 (mmol/L)**
Glucose	**13 mmol/L**	**4.5–5.6 (mmol/L)**
pH	**7.28**	**7.35–7.45**
PaO_2	12 kPa	10.6–13.3 (kPa) on air
$PaCO_2$	**4 kPa**	**4.8–6.1 (kPa)**
HCO_3	**20 mmol/L**	**22–26 (mmol/L)**
BE	**−4 mmol/L**	**±2 (mmol/L)**

Data in bold signifies results that are outside the normal laboratory range. *ABG*, Arterial blood gas; *BE*, base excess; *CRP*, C-reactive protein; *eGFR*, estimated glomerular filtration rate; *WCC*, white cell count.

- **ABG:** An acute metabolic acidosis is indicated by a low pH, a normal/reduced pCO_2 and reduced bicarbonate/base excess. Tachypnoea may result in low pCO_2 (respiratory compensation for metabolic acidosis).
- **Wound swab:** Used to identify the organism and guide correct antibiotic treatment. Organism resistance is growing, especially in diabetic patients as they tend to have had more courses of treatment and hospital admissions.
- **CXR and foot/leg X-rays:** Baseline CXR should be completed to rule out any other focus of infections and identify any cardiomegaly. Limb X-rays determine the presence and extent of any osteomyelitis.
- **Electrocardiogram (ECG):** To assess for ischaemic heart disease. Diabetic patients can have a silent myocardial infarction (MI) due to autonomic neuropathy.
- **Urine dipstick:** Look for ketones in the urine if blood ketone testing is not available. A urine dipstick can also pick up a possible UTI.

'Arterial blood gas shows a pH 7.28, $PaCO_2$ of 4.0 kPa, PaO_2 12 kPa, HCO_3 20 mmol/L, BE −4.0 mmol/L, lactate 2.8 mmol/L. Hb is 135 g/L, WCC 25 × 10⁹/L, neutrophils 18 × 10⁹/L. Sodium 135 mmol/L, potassium 4.9 mmol/L, urea 9.3 mmol/L, creatinine 120 µmol/L (eGFR = 54 mL/min), CRP 267 mg/L, glucose 13 mmol/L. Wound swab/blood culture microscopy shows Gram-negative rods. Leg X-rays show osteomyelitic changes to the distal tibia. ECG and CXR are normal. Urine dipstick shows no glucose and no ketones.'

INITIAL MANAGEMENT

Management Summary: Unwell Diabetic Patients

- Fluid resuscitation
- Early variable rate insulin infusion regimen and stop other hypoglycaemics
- Empirical antibiotics
- Identify focus of infection: Blood, wound, urine culture
- Monitor electrolytes and urine output
- Early diabetic team involvement
- Blood gas and urine dipstick

- **Airway support:** The airway is patent in this case, with no intervention required.
- **Supplementary oxygen**: If saturations <94%.
- **Fluid support**: All patients require maintenance fluids while NBM. Insensible losses will be increased due to being septic. Urine output should be monitored with a urinary catheter in unwell patients, aiming for a minimum rate of 0.5 mL/kg per hour. This patient required a fluid bolus due to being dehydrated and responded well to it.
- Since this patient is getting 3 L of fluid every 24 hours through the VRIII and has received a 500 mL bolus, if he is not clinically dehydrated anymore,

maintenance fluids are accounted for, and further resuscitation fluid is not currently required. Fluid balance needs to be carefully monitored. Further crystalloid fluids at a later stage (via a second line to the insulin infusion) may be necessary. Note that with the VRIII, the fluid is generally not changed if the blood glucose drops or increases. The blood glucose is unlikely to fluctuate dramatically in this clinical situation and it avoids unnecessarily changing between different fluid bags.

- **Blood glucose:** All non-diet-controlled diabetic patients (type 1 or 2) requiring major surgery (unable to eat and drink for >4 hours after surgery) will need to start a VRIII preoperatively.
- In this scenario, as the patient is septic with elevated blood glucose readings, a VRIII should be commenced as soon as possible. The regimen involves drawing up 50 units of human soluble insulin in 50 mL of sodium chloride 0.9% in a syringe-pump. This will give a concentration of 1 unit/mL of insulin. Repeated blood glucose levels are required to be tested hourly and rate adjusted accordingly. Glucose 5% with sodium chloride 0.45% and with potassium chloride 0.15% at a rate of 125 mL/h should be used with the VRIII regimen. If the serum potassium is low, use the potassium chloride 0.30% instead of 0.15% solution.
- The goal is to maintain the blood glucose levels between 6 and 10 mmol/L.
- All patients with type 2 diabetes should stop their oral hypoglycaemics when on VRIII. Metformin ideally should be stopped as it may cause lactic acidosis. It should be restarted once eating and drinking safely.
- If this were an elective procedure in a well patient (with non-diet controlled diabetes), then the VRIII could be delayed. If they were on the morning list, they could fast from midnight and could be started on a VRIII from the early morning (e.g. 0600) of the day of the procedure. If they are on the afternoon list (ideally this should not be the case), they could fast from the early morning (e.g. 0700) and commence the VRIII in the late morning (e.g. 1100).
- Patients having minor operations (able to eat within 4 hours after surgery or day cases) do not require a VRIII regimen unless stated otherwise. Patients with diabetes should omit their morning short-acting insulin but continue with their long-acting insulin on the day of the operation. For patients having minor operations, oral hypoglycaemics such as metformin and glitazones should be continued as normal but sulphonylureas and gliptins should not be taken on the morning of the operation.
- Diet controlled diabetes patients do not require any form of treatment for either minor or major surgery as they are not at significantly increased risk of glucose instability.
- **Empirical antibiotics:** Antibiotics should be commenced (as per trust guidelines) immediately once cultures are taken. These antibiotics vary from trust to trust; however, all patients should be treated as suspected methicillin-resistant *Staphylococcus aureus* (MRSA) positive until confirmed negative. After 48 hours, blood culture results can tailor antibiotic therapy. One option would be teicoplanin (Gram-positive cover), fusidic acid (MRSA cover) and piperacillin/tazobactum (broad-spectrum antibiotic).
- **Analgesia:** Start with simple analgesia and titrate upwards as required.
- **VTE prophylaxis:** Commence pharmacological prophylaxis if there are no contraindications, adjusted to renal function. Mechanical prophylaxis is contraindicated due to neuropathy and infection.
- **Potassium monitoring:** This will have to be monitored closely: if it falls significantly, the fluid would need to be changed to sodium chloride 0.45% and glucose 5% with potassium chloride 0.3%.

Prescribe (see Figs 8.9–8.11)

Thromboprophylaxis:
- ENOXAPARIN 40 mg SC OD

Regular analgesia:
- PARACETAMOL 1 g PO QDS

Antibiotics
- TEICOPLANIN 800 mg IV (over 30 minutes) STAT then BD on DAY 1, OD from DAY 2 and PIPERACILLIN/TAZOBACTAM 4.5 g IV (over 30 minutes) STAT the TDS and FUSIDIC ACID 750 mg PO STAT then TDS

REASSESSMENT

- The patient is reassessed after a fluid bolus, commencement of the VRIII, supplemental oxygen and empirical antibiotics.

'The patient looks significantly better. Airway is patent. RR 20/min, oxygen saturations are 95% on air with mild accessory muscle of respiration use. The chest is clear. HR 80 bpm, BP 140/80 mmHg and CRT <1 second. Glucose is now 9 mmol/L on the VRIII.'

Note: All oral regular medications should resume as normal once the patient is able to eat and drink safely. VRIII regimens may continue for some time postoperatively due to the effects of stress hormones. Fine control can be best achieved with a variable rate IV insulin infusion. The decision to stop the VRIII depends on the trend of stable blood glucose control.

HANDING OVER THE PATIENT

'Mr Smith is a 67-year-old with type 2 diabetes with probable osteomyelitis/infected right foot awaiting a below right knee amputation tomorrow. He presented with an infected foot with associated osteomyelitis and sepsis.

He has required supplementary oxygen to maintain adequate oxygen saturations. In terms of circulation, he was significantly dehydrated requiring a fluid bolus. Blood glucose was high, so a VRIII regimen was also started.

Currently, he is much improved. RR 20/min, oxygen saturations are 95% on air. He is haemodynamically stable, well hydrated, and glucose has been maintained within normal limits.

Investigations showed an initial partially compensated metabolic acidosis. His WCC was 25 × 10^9/L and neutrophils 18 × 10^9/L with a CRP of 267 mg/L.

The plan is to transfer to the ward in a side room due to infection risk, keep NBM, continue on the VRIII regimen and IV antibiotics. Most recent blood glucose is stable.

He will require hourly blood glucose checks and insulin adjusted accordingly. Repeat ABG should be done prior to his operation in the morning; he is already first on the list in view of his diabetes. Keep an eye on his urine output to make sure he is properly rehydrated and please do a fluid review later this evening.'

STATION 8.5: POSTOPERATIVE FLUID LOSS

You are the junior doctor on call covering the wards. You have been asked by the surgical ward nurse to prescribe some fluids for a postoperative patient. The patient is Jake, a 62-year-old man who underwent a lobectomy of the left lung yesterday.

Patient Details

Name:	Jake Smith
DOB:	05/03/62
Hospital number:	J345600
Weight:	75 kg
Height:	1.6 m
Consultant:	Mr Walker
Hospital/Ward:	REI Surgical
Current medications:	Paracetamol 1 g PO QDS, ibuprofen 400 mg PO TDS, morphine IV PCA (started postoperatively for analgesia) Enoxaparin 40 mg SC OD and TED stocking one pair TOP continuous (started this admission for thromboprophylaxis) Cyclizine 50 mg PO TDS (started this admission to reduce morphine-related nausea) Esomeprazole 20 mg PO OD (started this admission to reduce ibuprofen-related gastric irritation)
Allergies:	No known drug allergies
Admission date:	22/09/24

INITIAL ASSESSMENT

AIRWAY

- Assess patency of the airway. Does he have any stridor? Is his trachea central?

'The airway is patent and his trachea is central.'

No additional airway support is required.

BREATHING

- Assess the rate and depth of respiration. Assess his work of breathing and his oxygen saturations. Percuss the different lung zones for dullness or hyperresonance. Auscultate the lungs to assess air entry or presence of crackles. Check the chest drain is functioning normally (Is it swinging/bubbling? Does it look blocked?).

'RR 20/min, oxygen saturation at 100% with an 8 L/min oxygen face mask. There is a chest drain on the left side which has drained 300 mL of haemoserous fluid in the last 6 hours (500 mL in 24 hours). He has reduced air entry at the base of the left lung with dullness to percussion. He is complaining of pain on deep inspiration.'

Given these, it is unlikely he has a pneumothorax; however, there may be a haemothorax. A CXR should be done to exclude these problems. Avoid any splinting due to pain by prescribing appropriate analgesia. Supplementary oxygen should be given to maintain oxygen saturations above 94%.

CIRCULATION

- Assess the haemodynamic stability by assessing the pulse, BP, CRT and mucous membranes. Check the vital signs records and assess the trends rather than isolated findings. Also note the patient's urine output and fluid input for the past 24 hours.

'HR 110 bpm, BP 110/90 mmHg, CRT 3 seconds and mucous membranes are pale and dry.'

This man will require IV access, bloods and a fluid bolus. Give the fluid bolus as 500 mL followed by reassessment.

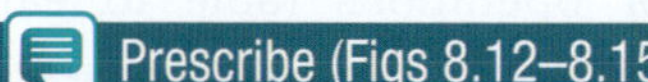

Fluid challenge:
- 500 mL SODIUM CHLORIDE 0.9% (over 15 minutes)

OXYGEN:
- OXYGEN, e.g. 8 L/min via MASK

DISABILITY

- Assess the patient's consciousness using the GCS. Is the patient confused or agitated? What's the capillary glucose reading?

'This man's GCS is E4, M6, V4 = 14/15. He seems a bit confused and his blood glucose currently is 7 mmol/L.'

His confusion is probably due to his depleted intravascular volume, although other causes such as infection need to be considered. He appears to have ongoing pain despite his prescribed analgesia.

EXPOSURE

- Expose and examine this gentleman thoroughly and examine all possible sources of bleeding. Have a proper assessment of his fluid balance. Assess all drains and their respective volume over the past 24 hours. Assess his core body temperature for pyrexia as this is a cause of an increased insensible loss.

'As noted before, this man has a chest drain and it has drained 500 mL of serosanguineous fluid in the past 24 hours. His urine output for the day has been approximately 800 mL. His oral input has been 800 mL. His fluid balance works out to be negative 500 mL plus insensible losses. His temperature is normal.'

Surgical drains are an important component of measuring fluid balance. Do not forget to check them.

INITIAL INVESTIGATIONS

- **Bloods**: FBC, U&Es, CRP. Look for evidence of anaemia or drop in Hb. Assess renal function and hydration status. A group and save and a coagulation screen should also be sent if you think the patient is bleeding. CRP trend may suggest possible infection (Table 8.5).
- **ABG:** Quick investigation to assess acid–base status, arterial $PaCO_2$ and PaO_2 levels. It also gives an approximate Hb, electrolyte, lactate and glucose level.

Table 8.5 Mr Smith's Blood Results and ABG Result

PARAMETER	VALUE	NORMAL RANGE (UNITS)
WCC	8 × 10^9/L	4–11 (×10^9/L)
Platelet	200 × 10^9/L	150–400 (×10^9/L)
Haemoglobin	**93 g/L**	**Men: 135–177 (g/L)** **Women: 115–155 (g/L)**
CRP	**7 mg/L**	**0–5 (mg/L)**
Urea	**14 mmol/L**	**2.5–6.7 (mmol/L)**
Creatinine	**160 μmol/L**	**79–118 (μmol/L)**
eGFR	**41 mL/min**	**>60 (mL/min)**
Sodium	134 mmol/L	135–146 (mmol/L)
Potassium	**5.2 mmol/L**	**3.5–5.0 (mmol/L)**
pH	7.36	7.35–7.45
PaO_2	12 kPa	10.6–13.3 (kPa) on air
$PaCO_2$	4.9 kPa	4.8–6.1 (kPa)
HCO_3	23 mmol/L	22–26 (mmol/L)
BE	1 mmol/L	±2 (mmol/L)

Data in bold signifies results that are outside the normal laboratory range. *ABG*, Arterial blood gas; *BE*, base excess; *CRP*, C-reactive protein; *eGFR*, estimated glomerular filtration rate; *WCC*, white cell count.

- **CXR**: Will demonstrate the presence of a haemothorax or pneumothorax. 250 mL of blood in the pleural space is required before anything is seen on a CXR. 750 mL of blood will fill half of a lung field; it appears as a diffuse opacification or white-out and loss of the costophrenic angles.
- **ECG:** To look for any cardiac abnormalities.

'ABG shows a pH of 7.36, $PaCO_2$ 4.9 kPa, PaO_2 12 kPa and HCO_3 23 mmol/L. Hb 93 g/L, WCC 8 × 10^9/L, CRP 7 mg/L, urea 14 mmol/L, creatinine 160 μmol/L and eGFR 41 mL/min (baseline Hb 110 g/L, baseline urea 7 mmol/L and creatinine 80 μmol/L). CXR shows a correctly placed chest drain with no haemo/pneumothorax. ECG is normal.'

INITIAL MANAGEMENT

- **Airway support:** Airway patent in this case with no intervention required.
- **Supplementary oxygen**: Maintain oxygen supplementation aiming for SpO_2 94% to 98%.
- **Gastric protection**: A proton pump inhibitor (PPI) is often given to ITU patients, particularly if taking ibuprofen for analgesia, to reduce risk of ulcers. The patient is already on esomeprazole.
- **Analgesia**: Paracetamol, opioids and ibuprofen (with daily U&Es and gastric protection) can be used. Regular and PRN morphine can be used to ensure good control but a PCA system can be used to allow the patient to titrate morphine to pain. Speak to the anaesthetic team about increasing analgesia via a PCA and ensure he is on appropriate additional medications. The patient is already on paracetamol, ibuprofen and a morphine PCA (with regular cyclizine). Ibuprofen should be stopped in this case due to worsening renal function.
- **Haemoglobin level**: Transfusion thresholds vary between surgeons and surgical units. A threshold of 70 to 80 g/L for transfusion is typical. A higher haemoglobin is generally aimed for in patients with ischaemic heart disease or peripheral vascular disease. Aiming for a haemoglobin above 90 g/L might be reasonable with a history of angina. Each unit of blood is approximately 250 mL and raises the Hb by 10 g/L. This patient does not require a transfusion at present as the haemoglobin is 93 g/L.
- **Ensure on appropriate thromboprophylaxis:** He should be on mechanical VTE prophylaxis. Consider withholding enoxaparin if there are signs of active bleeding. In this case, there is no strong evidence of active bleeding: only 500 mL has drained in 24 hours, there is no haemothorax on the CXR and the fluid is haemoserous rather than frank blood.
- **Ensure appropriate fluid balance:** Prescribing 100 mL/h of fluid over 24 hours (plus a 500 mL fluid challenge) will ensure appropriate fluid

balance. Maintenance fluids would need to be given plus replenishment of the 500 mL fluid deficit (and insensible losses). This will need to be continually reassessed to consider stopping IV fluids when the patient is more stable and drinking well.

REASSESSMENT

- After a fluid bolus and commencement of maintenance fluid, the patient is reassessed.

'The patient looks significantly improved. The airway is patent. RR 18/min and oxygen saturation is 97% on 2 L/min nasal cannula oxygen. There continues to be crackles at the base of the right lung but air entry is fine. HR 70 bpm, BP 120/75 mmHg, CRT is 2 seconds and urine output 0.8 mL/kg/h. Patient GCS is 15/15 with a blood glucose of 6 mmol/L.'

Prescribe (see Figs 8.12–8.15)

Maintenance fluids:

- 500 mL SODIUM CHLORIDE 0.9% with 20 mmol KCl IV at 100 mL/h

OXYGEN:

- 2 L/min via NASAL CANNULAE

STOP

Previous oxygen prescription

Ibuprofen and esomeprazole (since gastric protection no longer required)

HANDING OVER THE PATIENT

'Mr Smith is a 62-year-old patient who is 1 day postop left lung upper lobectomy (for lung cancer) with anaemia and dehydration.

On his initial assessment he was pale, dehydrated and in significant pain. He has been stabilised with a 500 mL sodium chloride 0.9% bolus. Analgesia-wise, he is on regular paracetamol and a morphine PCA. Ibuprofen has been stopped due to worsening renal function. Postoperative CXR shows no further bleeding in the chest and no pneumothorax. Bloods showed a haemoglobin of 93 g/L, so he has not been transfused. He is currently haemodynamically stable with good urine output.

The plan is to continue on maintenance IV fluids and to monitor this patient's vital signs, keeping close attention to the heart rate and BP. If these worsen, repeat FBC and U&E should be sent to see if the patient is actively bleeding. The on-call surgical registrar is aware of the patient and is happy to be contacted if there are any further concerns. The anaesthetist is coming later this evening to review the morphine PCA and optimise analgesia.'

FURTHER READING

Ayman, G, Dhatariya, K Dhesi, J. et al. Guideline for Perioperative Care for People with Diabetes Mellitus Undergoing Elective and Emergency Surgery. Centre for Perioperative Care, 2021. Available from: https://cpoc.org.uk/guidelines-resources-guidelines-resources/guideline-diabetes (Last accessed: 12 September 2024).

Catena, F, De Simone, B, Coccolini, F, et al., 2019. Bowel obstruction: a narrative review for all physicians. *World J Emerg Surg*. 29, 14–20.

Goodchild G, Chouhan M, Johnson GJ. Practical guide to the management of acute pancreatitis. *Frontline Gastroenterology* 2019;10:292–299. https://fg.bmj.com/content/10/3/292 (Last accessed: 12 September 2024).

Mederos, MA, Reber, HA, Girgis, MD, 2021. Acute pancreatitis: a review. *JAMA*. 325, 382–390.

National Collaborating Centre for Acute Care for NICE, 2018. Venous thromboembolism in over 16s: reducing the risk of hospital-acquired deep vein thrombosis or pulmonary embolism. https://www.nice.org.uk/guidance/ng89. (Last accessed 12/09/24).

PRESCRIPTION CHARTS

Name: *NICOLE SMITH*
Date of Birth: *5/3/2001*

REGULAR THERAPY

PRESCRIPTION	Date ▶ / Time ▼	*22/04/24*											
Medicine (Approved Name) *PARACETAMOL*	(6)												
Dose *1 g* — Route *ORAL*	8												
Notes — Start Date *22/09/24*	(12)												
	14												
Prescriber – sign + print *John Meyer JOHN MEYER*	(18)	*FD*											
	22 (24)	*FD*											
Medicine (Approved Name) *CODEINE PHOSPHATE*	(6)												
Dose *30 mg* — Route *ORAL*	8												
Notes — Start Date *22/09/24*	(12)												
	14												
Prescriber – sign + print *John Meyer JOHN MEYER*	(18)	*FD*											
	22 (24)	*FD*											
Medicine (Approved Name) *CEFUROXIME*	(6)												
Dose *750 mg* — Route *IV*	8												
Notes *For infected appendicitis review after 48 h. Over 30 mins* — Start Date *22/09/24*	12												
	(14)												
Prescriber – sign + print *John Meyer JOHN MEYER*	18												
	(22)	*FD*											
Medicine (Approved Name) *METRONIDAZOLE*	(6)												
Dose *500 mg* — Route *IV*	8												
Notes *For infected appendicitis review after 48 h. Over 20–30 mins* — Start Date *22/09/24*	12												
	(14)												
Prescriber – sign + print *John Meyer JOHN MEYER*	18												
	(22)	*FD*											
Medicine (Approved Name) *DALTEPARIN*	6												
Dose *5000 units* — Route *SC*	8												
Notes — Start Date *22/09/24*	12												
	14												
Prescriber – sign + print *John Meyer JOHN MEYER*	(18)	*FD*											
	22												
Medicine (Approved Name) *TED STOCKINGS*	(6												
Dose *1 pair* — Route *TOP*	8												
Notes — Start Date *22/09/24*	12												
	14												
Prescriber – sign + print *John Meyer JOHN MEYER*	18	*FD*											
	22)												

Fig. 8.1 Prescription and administration record (regular therapy) for Nicole Smith.

FLUID PRESCRIPTION CHART

Hospital/Ward: WGH WARD 3	**Consultant:** MR KING	**Name of Patient:** NICOLE SMITH **Hospital Number:** 1208973948
Weight: 60 kg	**Height:** 1.6 m	**D.O.B:** 05/03/2001

Date/ Time	FLUID / ADDED DRUGS	VOLUME / DOSE	ROUTE	RATE	PRESCRIBER – SIGN AND PRINT
22/09/24	SODIUM CHLORIDE 0.9%	1000 mL			
19.30	POTASSIUM CHLORIDE	40 mmol	IV	85 mL/h	J. Meyer JOHN MEYER
23/09/24	GLUCOSE 5%	1000 mL			
07.30	POTASSIUM CHLORIDE	20 mmol	IV	85 mL/h	J. Meyer JOHN MEYER

Fig. 8.2 Fluid prescription chart for Nicole Smith.

PRESCRIPTION AND ADMINISTRATION RECORD

Standard Chart

Hospital/Ward: BFH SURGICAL **Consultant:** MR KING	**Name of Patient:** JANE SMITH
Weight: 85kg **Height:** 1.6m	**Hospital Number:** J345789
If re-written, date:	**D.O.B:** 05/03/1982
DISCHARGE PRESCRIPTION **Date completed:-** **Completed by:-**	

OTHER MEDICINE CHARTS IN USE		PREVIOUS ADVERSE REACTIONS This section must be completed before any medicine is given		Completed by (sign & print)	Date
Date	Type of Chart	None known ☒		J. Meyer JOHN MEYER	22/09/24
		Medicine/Agent	Description of Reaction		

CODES FOR NON-ADMINISTRATION OF PRESCRIBED MEDICINE

If a dose is not administered as prescribed, initial and enter a code in the column with a circle drawn round the code according to the reason as shown below. **Inform the responsible doctor in the appropriate timescale.**

1. Patient refuses
2. Patient not present
3. Medicines not available – CHECK ORDERED
4. Asleep/drowsy
5. Administration route not available – CHECK FOR ALTERNATIVE
6. Vomiting/nausea
7. Time varied on doctor's instructions
8. Once only/as required medicine given
9. Dose withheld on doctor's instructions
10. Possible adverse reaction/side effect

ONCE-ONLY

Date	Time	Medicine (Approved Name)	Dose	Route	Prescriber – Sign + Print	Time Given	Given By
22/09/24	19.30	MORPHINE (titrate to response)	5 to 10 mg	IV	J. Meyer JOHN MEYER	19.30	JS (10mg)
22/09/24	19.30	CYCLIZINE	50mg	IV	J. Meyer JOHN MEYER	19.30	JS

OXYGEN	Start Date	Start Time	Route Mask (%)	Route Prongs (L/min)	Prescriber – Sign + Print	Administered by	Stop Date	Stop Time
	22/09/24	19.30	15L/min via NON-REBREATHER MASK		J. Meyer JOHN MEYER	JS	22/09/24	20.30
	22/09/24	20.30	8L/min via MASK		J. Meyer JOHN MEYER	JS		

Fig. 8.3 Prescription and administration record (standard chart) for Jane Smith.

Name: *JANE SMITH*
Date of Birth: *05/03/1982*

REGULAR THERAPY

PRESCRIPTION		
Medicine (Approved Name): *ESOMEPRAZOLE*		
Dose: *40 mg*	Route: *IV*	
Notes: *over 10–30 mins*	Start Date: *22/09/24*	
Prescriber – sign + print: *John Meyer JOHN MEYER*		

Time		22/09/24	23/09/24	24/09/24									
6													
(8)			FD										
12													
14													
18													
22													

PRESCRIPTION		
Medicine (Approved Name): *MORPHINE*		
Dose: *5 mg*	Route: *IV*	
Notes:	Start Date: *22/09/24*	
Prescriber – sign + print: *John Meyer JOHN MEYER*		

Time		22/09/24	23/09/24	24/09/24									
6	(2)		FD										
8	(6)		FD										
12	(10)		FD										
(14)			FD										
(18)			FD										
(22)		FD	FD										

PRESCRIPTION		
Medicine (Approved Name): *TED STOCKINGS*		
Dose: *One pair*	Route: *TOP*	
Notes:	Start Date: *22/09/24*	
Prescriber – sign + print: *John Meyer JOHN MEYER*		

Time (all circled)		22/09/24	23/09/24	24/09/24									
6													
8													
12													
14													
18		FD	FD										
22													

PRESCRIPTION		
Medicine (Approved Name): *DALTEPARIN*		
Dose: *5000 units*	Route: *SC*	
Notes:	Start Date: *22/09/24*	
Prescriber – sign + print: *John Meyer JOHN MEYER*		

Time		22/09/24	23/09/24	24/09/24									
6													
8													
12													
14													
(18)		FD	FD										
22													

PRESCRIPTION		
Medicine (Approved Name): *CYCLIZINE*		
Dose: *50 mg*	Route: *IV*	
Notes:	Start Date: *22/09/24*	
Prescriber – sign + print: *John Meyer JOHN MEYER*		

Time		22/09/24	23/09/24	24/09/24									
(6)			FD										
8													
12													
(14)			FD										
18													
(22)		FD	FD										

PRESCRIPTION		
Medicine (Approved Name):		
Dose:	Route:	
Notes:	Start Date:	
Prescriber – sign + print:		

Time													
6													
8													
12													
14													
18													
22													

Fig. 8.4 Prescription and administration record (regular therapy) for Jane Smith.

FLUID PRESCRIPTION CHART

Hospital/Ward: BFH SURGICAL	**Consultant:** MR KING	**Name of Patient:** JANE SMITH
		Hospital Number: J345789
Weight: 85 kg	**Height:** 1.6 m	**D.O.B:** 05/03/1982

Date/ Time	FLUID / ADDED DRUGS	VOLUME / DOSE	ROUTE	RATE	PRESCRIBER – SIGN AND PRINT
22/09/21 19.30	SODIUM CHLORIDE 0.9%	500 mL	IV	Over 15 min	J. Meyer JOHN MEYER
22/09/24 20.00	SODIUM CHLORIDE 0.9%	1 L	IV	500 mL/h	J. Meyer JOHN MEYER
	POTASSIUM CHLORIDE	20 mmol			

Fig. 8.5 Fluid prescription chart for Jane Smith.

PRESCRIPTION AND ADMINISTRATION RECORD

Standard Chart

Hospital/Ward: GDH SURGICAL **Consultant:** MR SING	**Name of Patient:** JULIO SMITH
Weight: 70 kg **Height:** 1.6 m	**Hospital Number:** J345333
If re-written, date:	**D.O.B:** 05/03/1962
DISCHARGE PRESCRIPTION **Date completed:-** **Completed by:-**	

OTHER MEDICINE CHARTS IN USE		PREVIOUS ADVERSE REACTIONS This section must be completed before any medicine is given		Completed by (sign & print)	Date
Date	Type of Chart	None known ☐			
	None	Medicine/Agent	Description of Reaction		
22/09/24		PENICILLIN	RASH	J. Meyer JOHN MEYER	22/09/24

CODES FOR NON-ADMINISTRATION OF PRESCRIBED MEDICINE

If a dose is not administered as prescribed, initial and enter a code in the column with a circle drawn round the code according to the reason as shown below. **Inform the responsible doctor in the appropriate timescale.**

1. Patient refuses
2. Patient not present
3. Medicines not available – CHECK ORDERED
4. Asleep/drowsy
5. Administration route not available – CHECK FOR ALTERNATIVE
6. Vomiting/nausea
7. Time varied on doctor's instructions
8. Once only/as required medicine given
9. Dose withheld on doctor's instructions
10. Possible adverse reaction/side effect

ONCE-ONLY

Date	Time	Medicine (Approved Name)	Dose	Route	Prescriber – Sign + Print	Time Given	Given By
22/09/24	19.30	MORPHINE (titrate to response)	5 to 10 mg	IV	J. Meyer JOHN MEYER	19.30	JS (5 mg)
22/09/24	19.30	CYCLIZINE	50 mg	IV	J. Meyer JOHN MEYER	19.30	JS

OXYGEN	Start Date	Start Time	Route Mask (%)	Route Prongs (L/min)	Prescriber – Sign + Print	Administered by	Stop Date	Stop Time

Fig. 8.6 Prescription and administration record (standard chart) for Julio Smith.

Name: JULIO SMITH

Date of Birth: 5/3/1962

REGULAR THERAPY

PRESCRIPTION	

Date → / Time ↓		22/09/24	23/09/24										

Medicine (Approved Name)	
MORPHINE	
Dose: 5 mg	Route: IV
Notes:	Start Date: 22/09/24
Prescriber – sign + print: John Meyer JOHN MEYER	

Time		22/09/24	23/09/24										
6	2		QW										
8	6		QW										
12	10		QW										
14	14		QW										
18			QW										
22		QW	QW										

Medicine (Approved Name)	
ESOMEPRAZOLE	
Dose: 40 mg	Route: IV
Notes: Over 10-30 mins	Start Date: 22/09/24
Prescriber – sign + print: John Meyer JOHN MEYER	

Time		22/09/24	23/09/24										
6													
8			QW										
12													
14													
18													
22													

Medicine (Approved Name)	
ENOXAPARIN	
Dose: 40 mg	Route: SC
Notes:	Start Date: 22/09/24
Prescriber – sign + print: John Meyer JOHN MEYER	

Time		22/09/24	23/09/24										
6													
8													
12													
14													
18		QW	QW										
22													

Medicine (Approved Name)	
TED STOCKINGS	
Dose: One pair	Route: TOP
Notes:	Start Date: 22/09/24
Prescriber – sign + print: John Meyer JOHN MEYER	

Time		22/09/24	23/09/24										
6													
8													
12													
14													
18		QW	QW										
22													

Medicine (Approved Name)	
CYCLIZINE	
Dose: 50 mg	Route: IV
Notes:	Start Date: 22/09/24
Prescriber – sign + print: John Meyer JOHN MEYER	

Time		22/09/24	23/09/24										
6													
8			QW										
12													
14			QW										
18													
22	24	QW	QW										

Medicine (Approved Name)	
Dose:	Route:
Notes:	Start Date:
Prescriber – sign + print:	

Time													
6													
8													
12													
14													
18													
22													

Fig. 8.7 Prescription and administration record (regular therapy) for Julio Smith.

FLUID PRESCRIPTION CHART

Hospital/Ward: GDH SURGICAL	**Consultant:** MR SING	**Name of Patient:** JULIO SMITH
		Hospital Number: J345333
Weight: 70 kg	**Height:** 1.6 m	**D.O.B:** 05/03/1962

Date/Time	FLUID / ADDED DRUGS	VOLUME / DOSE	ROUTE	RATE	PRESCRIBER – SIGN AND PRINT
22/09/24 20.00	SODIUM CHLORIDE 0.9%	500 mL	IV	Over 15 min	J. Meyer JOHN MEYER
22/09/24 20.30	SODIUM CHLORIDE 0.9%	1 L	IV	250 mL/h	J. Meyer JOHN MEYER
	POTASSIUM CHLORIDE	20 mmol			

Fig. 8.8 Fluid prescription chart for Julio Smith.

PRESCRIPTION AND ADMINISTRATION RECORD

Standard Chart

Hospital/Ward: CGH SURGICAL	**Consultant:** MR WOOD	**Name of Patient:** ADAM SMITH
Weight: 70 kg	**Height:** 1.6 m	**Hospital Number:** J345400
If re-written, date:		**D.O.B:** 5/3/1957
DISCHARGE PRESCRIPTION **Date completed:-**	**Completed by:-**	

OTHER MEDICINE CHARTS IN USE		PREVIOUS ADVERSE REACTIONS This section must be completed before any medicine is given		Completed by (sign & print)	Date
Date	Type of Chart	None known ☒		J. Meyer JOHN MEYER	22/09/24
		Medicine/Agent	Description of Reaction		

CODES FOR NON-ADMINISTRATION OF PRESCRIBED MEDICINE

If a dose is not administered as prescribed, initial and enter a code in the column with a circle drawn round the code according to the reason as shown below. **Inform the responsible doctor in the appropriate timescale.**

1. Patient refuses
2. Patient not present
3. Medicines not available – CHECK ORDERED
4. Asleep/drowsy
5. Administration route not available – CHECK FOR ALTERNATIVE
6. Vomiting/nausea
7. Time varied on doctor's instructions
8. Once only/as required medicine given
9. Dose withheld on doctor's instructions
10. Possible adverse reaction/side effect

ONCE-ONLY

Date	Time	Medicine (Approved Name)	Dose	Route	Prescriber – Sign + Print	Time Given	Given By
22/09/24	09.30	TEICOPLANIN (over 30 mins)	400 mg	IV	J. Meyer JOHN MEYER	09.30	JS
22/09/24	09.30	PIPERACILLIN/TAZOBACTAM (over 30 mins)	4.5g	IV	J. Meyer JOHN MEYER	09.30	JS
22/09/24	09.30	FUSIDIC ACID	750 mg	ORAL	J. Meyer JOHN MEYER	09.30	JS
22/09/24	09.30	50 units INSULIN (ACTRAPID) IN 50 mL SODIUM CHLORIDE 0.9%	AS VARIABLE RATE INSULIN INFUSION BELOW	IV	J. Meyer JOHN MEYER	09.40	JS

BLOOD GLUCOSE (mmol/L) (target range 6–10 mmol/L)	INSULIN (ACTRAPID) INFUSION (UNITS/HOUR = mL/h)
>20	5
15–19.9	4
10–14.9	3
7–9.9	2
4–6.9	1
<3.9	0.5

Fig. 8.9 Prescription and administration record (standard chart) for Adam Smith.

Name: ADAM SMITH

Date of Birth: 5/3/1957

REGULAR THERAPY

PRESCRIPTION	Date → / Time ↓	22/09/24	23/09/24									

Medicine (Approved Name): PARACETAMOL	Time	22/09/24	23/09/24									
Dose: 1g — Route: ORAL	(6)		FD									
Notes: — Start Date: 22/09/24	8											
Prescriber – sign + print: John Meyer JOHN MEYER	(12)	FD	FD									
	14											
	(18)	FD	FD									
	(22)	FD	FD									

Medicine (Approved Name): TEICOPLANIN	Time	22/09/24	23/09/24									
Dose: 400 mg — Route: IV	(6)		FD									
Notes: Loading dose: Day 1—400 mg bd thereafter 400 mg OD. For infected wound review in 48 h. Give over 30 mins — Start Date: 22/09/24	8											
Prescriber – sign + print: John Meyer JOHN MEYER	12											
	14											
	(18)	FD	X	X	X	X	X	X	X	X	X	X	X
	22											

Medicine (Approved Name): PIPERACILLIN/TAZOBACTAM	Time	22/09/24	23/09/24									
Dose: 4.5g — Route: IV	(6)		FD									
Notes: For infected wound. Review at 48 h. Give over 30 mins — Start Date: 22/09/24	8											
Prescriber – sign + print: John Meyer JOHN MEYER	12											
	(14)	FD	FD									
	18											
	(22)	FD	FD									

Medicine (Approved Name): FUSIDIC ACID	Time	22/09/24	23/09/24									
Dose: 750 mg — Route: ORAL	(6)		FD									
Notes: For infected wound review in 48 h — Start Date: 22/09/24	8											
Prescriber – sign + print: John Meyer JOHN MEYER	12											
	(14)	FD	FD									
	18											
	(22)	FD	FD									

Medicine (Approved Name): ENOXAPARIN	Time	22/09/24	23/09/24									
Dose: 40 mg — Route: SC	6											
Notes: — Start Date: 22/09/24	8											
Prescriber – sign + print: John Meyer JOHN MEYER	12											
	14											
	(18)	FD	FD									
	22											

Medicine (Approved Name):	Time											
Dose: — Route:	6											
Notes: — Start Date:	8											
Prescriber – sign + print:	12											
	14											
	18											
	22											

Fig. 8.10 Prescription and administration record (regular therapy) for Adam Smith.

FLUID PRESCRIPTION CHART

Hospital/Ward: CGH SURGICAL	Consultant: MR WOOD	Name of Patient: ADAM SMITH
		Hospital Number: J345400
Weight: 70 kg	Height: 1.6 m	D.O.B: 5/3/1957

Date/Time	FLUID / ADDED DRUGS	VOLUME / DOSE	ROUTE	RATE	PRESCRIBER – SIGN AND PRINT
22/09/24 09.30	SODIUM CHLORIDE 0.9%	500 mL	IV	Over 15 min	J. Meyer JOHN MEYER
22/09/24 11.00	GLUCOSE 5%/SODIUM CHLORIDE 0.45%/ POTASSIUM CHLORIDE 0.15%	1000 mL	IV	125 mL/h	J. Meyer JOHN MEYER
22/09/24 19.00	GLUCOSE 5%/SODIUM CHLORIDE 0.45%/ POTASSIUM CHLORIDE 0.15%	1000 mL	IV	125 mL/h	J. Meyer JOHN MEYER

Fig. 8.11 Fluid prescription chart for Adam Smith.

PRESCRIPTION AND ADMINISTRATION RECORD

Standard Chart

Hospital/Ward: REI SURGICAL **Consultant:** MR WALKER	**Name of Patient:** JAKE SMITH
Weight: 75 kg **Height:** 1.6 m	**Hospital Number:** J345600
If re-written, date:	**D.O.B:** 5/3/1962
DISCHARGE PRESCRIPTION **Date completed:-** **Completed by:-**	

OTHER MEDICINE CHARTS IN USE		PREVIOUS ADVERSE REACTIONS This section must be completed before any medicine is given		Completed by (sign & print)	Date
Date	Type of Chart	None known ☒		J. Meyer JOHN MEYER	22/09/24
22/09/24	MORPHINE PCA CHART	Medicine/Agent	Description of Reaction		

CODES FOR NON-ADMINISTRATION OF PRESCRIBED MEDICINE

If a dose is not administered as prescribed, initial and enter a code in the column with a circle drawn round the code according to the reason as shown below. **Inform the responsible doctor in the appropriate timescale.**

1. Patient refuses
2. Patient not present
3. Medicines not available – CHECK ORDERED
4. Asleep/drowsy
5. Administration route not available – CHECK FOR ALTERNATIVE
6. Vomiting/nausea
7. Time varied on doctor's instructions
8. Once only/as required medicine given
9. Dose withheld on doctor's instructions
10. Possible adverse reaction/side effect

ONCE-ONLY

Date	Time	Medicine (Approved Name)	Dose	Route	Prescriber – Sign + Print	Time Given	Given By

OXYGEN	Start Date	Start Time	Route Mask (%)	Route Prongs (L/min)	Prescriber – Sign + Print	Administered by	Stop Date	Stop Time
	23/09/24	19.30	8L/min via MASK		J. Meyer JOHN MEYER	JS	23/09/24	20.30
	23/09/24	20.30		2L/min via NASAL CANNULAE	J. Meyer JOHN MEYER	JS		

Fig. 8.12 Prescription and administration record (standard chart) for Jake Smith.

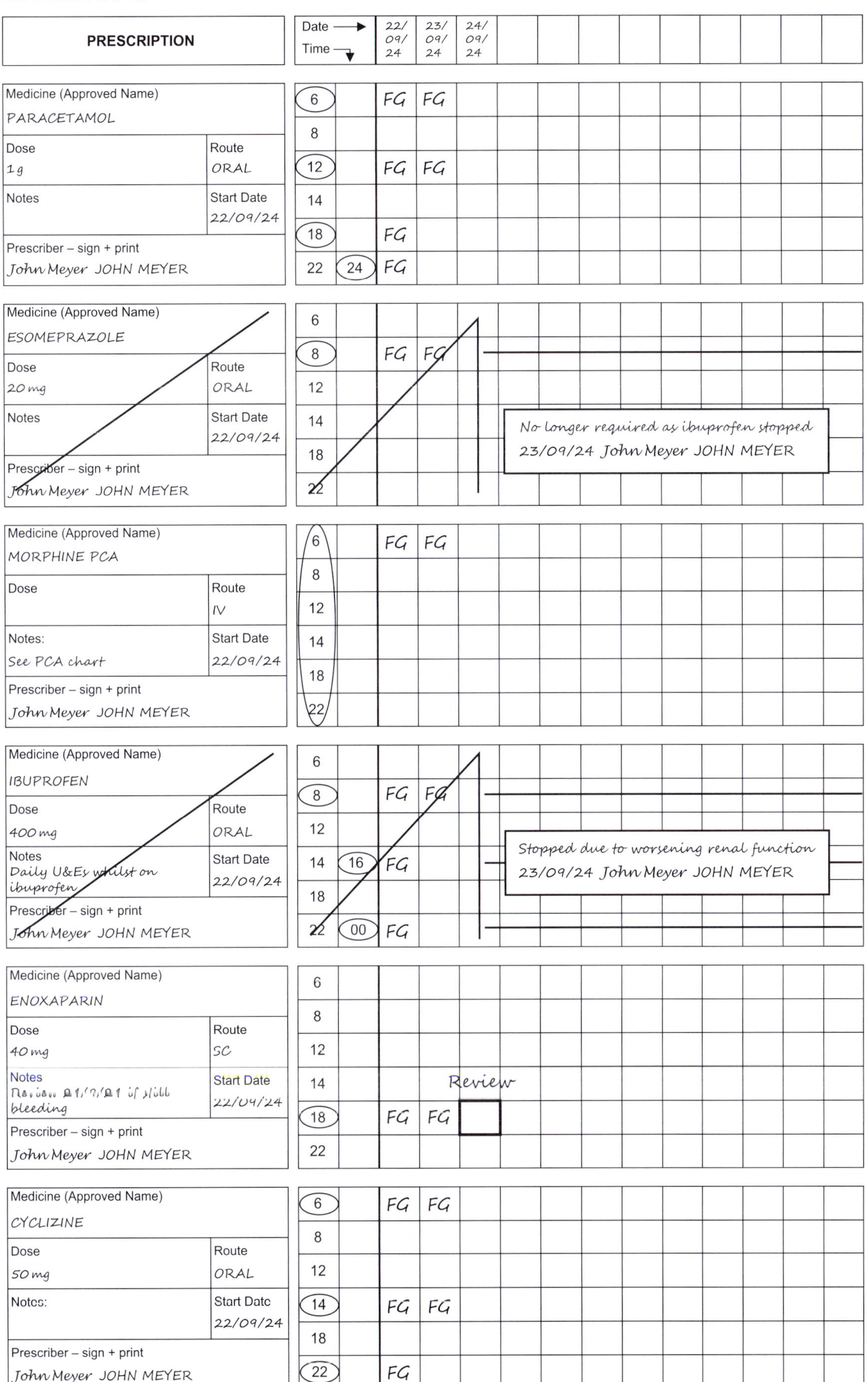

Name: JAKE SMITH
Date of Birth: 5/3/1962

REGULAR THERAPY

PRESCRIPTION

Medicine (Approved Name): PARACETAMOL
Dose: 1g | Route: ORAL
Notes: | Start Date: 22/09/24
Prescriber – sign + print: John Meyer JOHN MEYER

Time		22/09/24	23/09/24	24/09/24
6		FG	FG	
8				
12		FG	FG	
14				
18		FG		
22	24	FG		

Medicine (Approved Name): ESOMEPRAZOLE
Dose: 20 mg | Route: ORAL
Notes: | Start Date: 22/09/24
Prescriber – sign + print: John Meyer JOHN MEYER

Time		22/09/24	23/09/24	24/09/24
6				
8		FG	FG	
12				
14				
18				
22				

No longer required as ibuprofen stopped 23/09/24 John Meyer JOHN MEYER

Medicine (Approved Name): MORPHINE PCA
Dose: | Route: IV
Notes: See PCA chart | Start Date: 22/09/24
Prescriber – sign + print: John Meyer JOHN MEYER

Time		22/09/24	23/09/24	24/09/24
6		FG	FG	
8				
12				
14				
18				
22				

Medicine (Approved Name): IBUPROFEN
Dose: 400 mg | Route: ORAL
Notes: Daily U&Es whilst on ibuprofen | Start Date: 22/09/24
Prescriber – sign + print: John Meyer JOHN MEYER

Time		22/09/24	23/09/24	24/09/24
6				
8		FG	FG	
12				
14	16	FG		
18				
22	00	FG		

Stopped due to worsening renal function 23/09/24 John Meyer JOHN MEYER

Medicine (Approved Name): ENOXAPARIN
Dose: 40 mg | Route: SC
Notes: [illegible] bleeding | Start Date: 22/04/24
Prescriber – sign + print: John Meyer JOHN MEYER

Time		22/09/24	23/09/24	24/09/24
6				
8				
12				
14				Review
18		FG	FG	
22				

Medicine (Approved Name): CYCLIZINE
Dose: 50 mg | Route: ORAL
Notes: | Start Date: 22/09/24
Prescriber – sign + print: John Meyer JOHN MEYER

Time		22/09/24	23/09/24	24/09/24
6		FG	FG	
8				
12				
14		FG	FG	
18				
22		FG		

Fig. 8.13 Prescription and administration record (regular therapy) for Jake Smith (part 1).

Name: JAKE SMITH

Date of Birth: 05/03/1962

REGULAR THERAPY

PRESCRIPTION

Medicine (Approved Name): TED STOCKINGS

Dose: 1 pair | Route: TOP

Notes: | Start Date: 22/09/24

Prescriber – sign + print: J. Meyer JOHN MEYER

Date → / Time ↓		22/09/24	23/09/24										
(6)													
(8)		NH	NH										
(12)													
(14)													
(18)													
(22)													

Medicine (Approved Name):

Dose: | Route:

Notes: | Start Date:

Prescriber – sign + print:

Time													
6													
8													
12													
14													
18													
22													

Medicine (Approved Name):

Dose: | Route:

Notes: | Start Date:

Prescriber – sign + print:

Time													
6													
8													
12													
14													
18													
22													

Medicine (Approved Name):

Dose: | Route:

Notes: | Start Date:

Prescriber – sign + print:

Time													
6													
8													
12													
14													
18													
22													

Medicine (Approved Name):

Dose: | Route:

Notes: | Start Date:

Prescriber – sign + print:

Time													
6													
8													
12													
14													
18													
22													

Medicine (Approved Name):

Dose: | Route:

Notes: | Start Date:

Prescriber – sign + print:

Time													
6													
8													
12													
14													
18													
22													

Fig. 8.14 Prescription and administration record (regular therapy) for Jake Smith (part 2).

FLUID PRESCRIPTION CHART

Hospital/Ward: REI SURGICAL	Consultant: MR WALKER	Name of Patient: JAKE SMITH
		Hospital Number: J345600
Weight: 75 kg	Height: 1.6 m	D.O.B: 5/3/1962

Date/ Time	FLUID / ADDED DRUGS	VOLUME / DOSE	ROUTE	RATE	PRESCRIBER – SIGN AND PRINT
23/09/24 19.30	SODIUM CHLORIDE 0.9%	500 mL	IV	Over 15 min	J. Meyer JOHN MEYER
23/09/24 19.45	SODIUM CHLORIDE 0.9%	500 mL	IV	100 mL/h	J. Meyer JOHN MEYER
	POTASSIUM CHLORIDE	20 mmol			

Fig. 8.15 Fluid prescription chart for Jake Smith.

Paediatrics

9

Alexandra Richards, Zeshan Qureshi

Chapter Outline

Station 9.1: Acute Bronchiolitis
Station 9.2: Respiratory Distress in the Newborn
Station 9.3: Acute Exacerbation of Asthma
Station 9.4: Infective Exacerbation of Cystic Fibrosis
Station 9.5: Gastroenteritis
Station 9.6: Sickle Cell Chest Crisis
Station 9.7: Idiopathic Nephrotic Syndrome

STATION 9.1: ACUTE BRONCHIOLITIS

You are a junior doctor working in the emergency department. A 6-month-old baby, Layla James, has presented with a 3-day history of cough, runny nose and difficulty in breathing. Today she has become more breathless and is not tolerating feeds. Please assess the baby and instigate appropriate management.

Patient Details

Name:	Layla James
DOB:	02/04/24
Hospital number:	L3439402
Weight:	7 kg
Consultant:	Dr Wi
Hospital/Ward:	BGH Paediatric ward
Current medications:	Nil
Allergies:	None known
Admission date:	12/10/24

Initial Differential Diagnosis of Respiratory Distress

- Respiratory: Bronchiolitis, pertussis, foreign body inhalation, aspiration of food/milk, pneumothorax, pneumonia
- Cardiac: Heart failure
- Musculoskeletal: Chest deformity, e.g. pectus excavatum
- Gastrointestinal: Gastro-oesophageal reflux

Complications of Bronchiolitis

- Secondary bacterial infection
- Respiratory distress syndrome (RDS)
- Dehydration
- Syndrome of inappropriate secretion of antidiuretic hormone (SIADH)

INITIAL ASSESSMENT

AIRWAY

- Is the airway patent? Has the baby had any cyanosis or apnoeas?

'The airway is patent, with no obvious obstruction. No apnoeas or cyanotic spells are seen or reported.'

No additional airway support is required.

BREATHING

- Assess respiratory rate, oxygen saturations and work of breathing. Auscultate for air entry and additional sounds, such as wheeze and crepitations.
- In significant respiratory distress, feeding is usually affected. Assess hydration and ask about feeding. If breastfeeding, assess length of feeds and enquire about quality of latching and sucking. If bottle-feeding, assess total volume taken during each feed.

'RR 70/min, oxygen saturations are 90% with intercostal recessions, tracheal tug, nasal flaring and abdominal breathing. Crackles are heard throughout the lung fields bilaterally with an occasional wheeze and reduced air entry at the lung bases. The child is breastfed only and normally feeds for 15 minutes every 3 hours but today has only managed to feed for 5 minutes in 6 hours.'

Do not forget that crepitations could be a sign of heart failure.

Given these observations, you give supplementary oxygen as the oxygen saturations are persistently less than 90%. If the baby deteriorates further or the saturations do not improve despite oxygen support, consider noninvasive ventilation measures such as HHFNC or CPAP. Reassess following any intervention.

This baby will require admission due to increased work of breathing and inadequate oral intake. The National Institute for Health and Care Excellence (NICE) guidelines criteria for admission in bronchiolitis are as follows:

- Apnoeas
- Exhaustion

- Inadequate oral fluid intake (50%–75% of usual volume)
- Persisting severe respiratory distress, e.g. grunting, marked chest recession or a respiratory rate of over 70 breaths/minute

Prescribe (Figs 9.1 and 9.2)

OXYGEN:
- 2 L via NASAL CANNULAE or SIMPLE FACE MASK

Fluid bolus:
- 70 mL (10 mL/kg) SODIUM CHLORIDE 0.9% IV (over 15 minutes)

CIRCULATION

- Assess haemodynamic stability by measuring pulse, blood pressure (BP) and capillary refill time (CRT).
- Assess hydration status by looking at the mucous membranes, baseline observations (particularly heart rate, CRT, temperature and conscious state) and skin turgor. Assess the eyes and fontanelles and ask about the number of wet nappies and whether this has changed from the normal daily amount.
- Perform a cardiovascular examination to exclude evidence of heart failure. In a baby, you would pay attention to gallop rhythm, a heart murmur, hepatomegaly, peripheral oedema and ascites. Crackles in the lung may not be bronchiolitis; they may be a sign of left-sided heart failure.

'HR 180 bpm, BP 60/40 mmHg and CRT 4 seconds centrally. The anterior fontanelle and eyes are slightly sunken and the mucous membranes are dry. Layla has only had one wet nappy today, when usually she would have had three by this time. Cardiovascular exam shows normal heart sounds with no murmurs or hepatomegaly.'

The baby has signs of dehydration and, therefore, they will require intravenous (IV) access and a fluid bolus, given as 10 mL/kg, followed by reassessment. Bloods and a blood gas can be sent at the same time.

DISABILITY

- Assess the patient's level of consciousness using AVPU (is the patient Alert? If not, do they respond to Verbal or Painful stimuli? Or are they Unresponsive?). Check glucose levels.

'The baby is alert and has blood sugar of 6.5 mmol/L.'

EXPOSURE

- Expose the baby and look for other possible sources of infection. Measure the temperature. Feel the abdomen. Certain abdominal pathologies, e.g. intestinal obstruction, may cause diaphragmatic splinting and subsequent respiratory distress.

'Temperature is 37.5°C and examination is otherwise normal.'

INITIAL INVESTIGATIONS

- **Capillary blood gas:** An acute respiratory acidosis is indicated by a low pH, a raised $PaCO_2$ and a normal bicarbonate/base excess. A raised lactate or a reduction in the base excess indicates a metabolic acidosis, possibly secondary to infection or hypoperfusion. Note: PaO_2 is of little use on a capillary gas. Blood gases are helpful to assess for worsening respiratory distress and in impending respiratory failure.
- **Bloods:** Full blood count (FBC), urea and electrolytes (U&Es), C-reactive protein (CRP). Look for evidence of infection; assess renal function and hydration status (Table 9.1).
- **Nasopharyngeal aspirate (or combined nose and throat swabs):** Used to detect respiratory syncytial virus (RSV), a common cause of bronchiolitis. A patient with confirmed RSV should be isolated in a side room.
- **Chest radiography (CXR):** Will potentially show patchy changes consistent with bronchiolitis or pneumonia (though these are difficult to differentiate radiologically). Other respiratory pathology such as pneumothorax can be ruled out. The cardiac shadow may be suggestive of congenital heart disease (such as cardiomegaly or a boot-shaped heart in tetralogy of Fallot), which is an important differential. A CXR is not always required and is reserved for atypical symptoms, concerns about pneumothoraces or superadded infection and if intubation or admission to critical care is needed.
- **Weight:** Important for fluid calculations (Box 9.1).

Table 9.1 Layla's Blood Test Results and ABG

PARAMETER	VALUE	NORMAL RANGE (UNITS FOR 6-MONTH-OLDS)
Haemoglobin	145 g/L	105–150 (g/L)
WCC	**15 × 10⁹/L**	**6–14 (×10⁹/L)**
Neutrophil	**8 × 10⁹/L**	**3.7–6.7 (×10⁹/L)**
Lymphocyte	**4.5 × 10⁹/L**	**1.7–4.1 (×10⁹/L)**
Platelet	160 × 10⁹/L	150–400 (×10⁹/L)
CRP	**20 mg/L**	**0.8–11.2 (mg/L)**
Urea	**9.3 mmol/L**	**1.8–6.4 (mmol/L)**
Creatinine	**45 µmol/L**	**2.65–44.2 (µmol/L)**
Sodium	**131 mmol/L**	**134–144 (mmol/L)**
Potassium	4.0 mmol/L	3.5–5.6 (mmol/L)
pH	**7.28**	**7.35–7.45**
$PaCO_2$	**7.5 kPa**	**4.7–6.0 (kPa)**
HCO_3	22 mmol/L	22–26 (mmol/L)
BE	−0.5 mmol/L	±2 mmol/L

Data in bold signifies results that are outside the normal laboratory range. *ABG*, Arterial blood gas; *BE*, base excess; *CRP*, C-reactive protein; *WCC*, white cell count.

'Capillary blood gas shows a respiratory acidosis with no metabolic compensation. pH 7.28, $PaCO_2$ of 7.5 kPa, HCO_3 22 mmol/L, BE −0.5 mmol/L. Hb is 145 g/L, WCC 15 × 10^9/L, neutrophils 8 × 10^9/L, lymphocytes 4.5 × 10^9/L. Na 131 mmol/L, urea 9.3 mmol/L, creatinine 45 µmol/L. CRP is 20 mg/L. Nasal assay is positive for RSV. CXR shows diffuse patchy changes in both lung fields. Weight is 7 kg.'

INITIAL MANAGEMENT

Bronchiolitis Management

- Acute: Minimal handling, supplementary oxygen (if saturations <92%), consider the need for humidified high-flow nasal cannula (HHFNC, e.g. Optiflow), continuous positive airway pressure (CPAP) or intubation.
- Adequate hydration: Children may require NG feeding or IV fluids.
- Prophylaxis: High-risk babies may benefit from monoclonal antibody treatment (e.g. Palivizumab). However, this can only be initiated by a specialist.

- **Airway support:** No airway intervention is required in this case. Indications for intubation include frequent apnoeas/cyanotic spells or worsening respiratory distress despite optimal supportive treatment.
- **Supplementary oxygen**: If persistent oxygen saturations <90% in children aged over 6 weeks or <92% for children under 6 weeks or with underlying comorbidities.
- **Fluid support**: This baby required a fluid bolus as they were significantly dehydrated. Moderate to severe respiratory distress will impair normal feeding. Depending on the degree of respiratory distress, feeding support may take one of two forms. Nasogastric (NG) feeds allow milk to be put in the stomach with less interruption in breathing than breast or bottle feeds. Smaller feed volumes can be given to minimise gastric distension by increasing feed frequency, ensuring total daily volume is the same. If the baby is too unwell to tolerate NG feeds, maintenance IV fluids can be given.
- Feed requirements would need to be calculated based on weight and the Holliday-Segar formula. For a weight of 7 kg, 700 mL/day is required for maintenance fluid (7 × 100 mL/kg per day) (Box 9.1). SIADH may develop in children with acute respiratory problems, indicated by low serum sodium as in this case. Giving full maintenance fluids may cause the sodium to fall dangerously. Therefore, two-thirds maintenance fluid of sodium chloride 0.9% with glucose 5% would be given rather than full maintenance fluid. Two-thirds maintenance of 700 mL = 466 mL/24 hours, prescribed as 19.4 mL/h.

REASSESSMENT

- Following treatment, the patient is reassessed.

Box 9.1 Calculating 24-Hour Volume Requirements

- 100 mL/kg for the first 10 kg
- 50 mL/kg for the next 10 kg
- 20 mL for every kg over 20 kg

  e.g. if 25 kg:
  100 × 10 for first 10 kg
  50 × 10 for second 10 kg
  20 × 5 for the 5 kg left
  =1600 mL/24 h

'Layla has significantly improved. Her airway is patent. RR 55/min, oxygen saturations are 95%, on 2 L of nasal cannula oxygen with mild intercostal recession and nasal flaring. Crackles are heard throughout the lung fields bilaterally but air entry is much improved. HR 140 bpm, BP 90/60 mmHg, CRT 1 second centrally.'

Prescribe (see Figs 9.1 and 9.2)

Two-thirds maintenance fluids:

- SODIUM CHLORIDE 0.9%/ GLUCOSE 5% IV (19.4 mL/h)

HANDING OVER THE PATIENT

'Layla James is a 6-month-old with RSV positive bronchiolitis.

She presented with significant respiratory distress and reduced feeding following a 3-day history of coryzal symptoms. She was given supplementary oxygen and her saturations improved to 95%. In terms of circulation, she was significantly dehydrated and required a fluid bolus, which she responded to. Currently, she has a RR 55/min, oxygen saturations are 95% on 2 L of nasal cannula oxygen and there is only mild respiratory distress. She is haemodynamically stable and more hydrated.

Investigations show an initial respiratory acidosis, with a pH 7.28, $PaCO_2$ 7.5 kPa, BE −0.5 mmol/L on capillary gas. She initially was hyponatraemic with a Na^+ of 131 mmol/L and dehydrated (urea 9.3 mmol/L, creatinine 45 µmol/L). CRP 20 mg/L. CXR shows diffuse patchy changes in both lung fields consistent with bronchiolitis.

The plan is to transfer to the ward and keep her nil by mouth (NBM) on two-thirds maintenance IV fluids. High-flow humidified nasal cannula (HHFNC) oxygen may be beneficial. She will need a repeat capillary gas, U&Es and blood sugar later this evening. Supplementary oxygen should be continued to keep saturations above 94%.'

STATION 9.2: RESPIRATORY DISTRESS IN THE NEWBORN

You are a junior doctor working on a postnatal ward. You are called to assess a baby (male infant Khan) who is 12 hours old with a rapid respiratory rate. He was born by emergency C-section following failure to progress at 38 + 4 weeks' gestation. Mum had antibiotics during labour due to fever. The baby was born in good condition and no immediate resuscitation was required.

Patient Details

Name:	Male infant Khan
DOB:	12/10/24
Hospital number:	XS3439960469
Weight:	3.5 kg
Consultant:	Dr Wi
Hospital/Ward:	BGH Postnatal Ward
Current medications:	Nil
Allergies:	None known
Admission date:	12/10/24

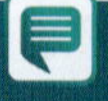

Differential Diagnosis of Respiratory Distress in a Newborn

- Congenital pneumonia. Risk factors include prolonged rupture of membranes, maternal pyrexia and maternal Group B *Streptococcus* colonisation.
- Meconium aspiration syndrome. Meconium may be passed in utero due to distress and aspirated prior to delivery.
- RDS, most common in prematurity due to surfactant deficiency. Gestational diabetes increases risk at term.
- Transient tachypnoea of the newborn is common after caesarean and resolves over several hours.
- Pneumothorax.
- Congenital heart disease.
- Congenital diaphragmatic hernia.

Complications of Respiratory Distress

- Respiratory failure
- Pneumothorax
- Poor feeding with hypoglycaemia
- Persistent pulmonary hypertension of the newborn (PPHN)

INITIAL ASSESSMENT

AIRWAY

- Assess patency of the airway. Is there any sign of meconium staining that might indicate aspiration?

'The airway is patent and the baby can cry. There is no evidence of meconium staining.'

The baby does not require any airway support.

BREATHING

- Observe the baby for signs of respiratory distress, including grunting, nasal flaring, tracheal tug, intercostal and subcostal recessions. Assess for cyanosis and request oxygen saturation monitoring.
- Assess respiratory rate as tachypnoea is the earliest sign of respiratory distress.
- It is very difficult to assess respiratory pathology in newborns by auscultating the chest and subtle signs such as reduced air entry may signify significant pathology.
- Assess quality of feeding as respiratory distress will impair this and regular feeds are important to prevent hypoglycaemia.

'The baby is pink but has increased work of breathing with grunting, nasal flaring, tracheal tug and subcostal and intercostal recessions. Air entry is good throughout the chest with no added sounds. His respiratory rate is 70/min and his oxygen saturations are 92%. The baby has been unable to latch to the breast for the last 6 hours due to an increased work of breathing.'

Given these, the baby needs respiratory support and further investigations. He will need admission to the special care baby unit (SCBU) and supplemental oxygen, which can be given as ambient oxygen in the incubator or via nasal cannula.

CIRCULATION

- Assess heart rate, plus central and peripheral perfusion with CRT.
- Assess for evidence of underlying cardiac abnormality by auscultating for murmurs, feeling for a heave and displaced apex beat and feeling for femoral pulses (which may indicate coarctation of the aorta if weak).

'HR 160 bpm, CRT 2 seconds centrally. The apex is felt at fourth intercostal space, lateral to the midclavicular line. The heart sounds are normal with no audible murmurs. Both femoral pulses are palpable.'

DISABILITY

- Assess the baby's conscious level using AVPU as described (is the patient Alert? If not, do they respond to Verbal or Painful stimuli? Or are they Unresponsive?) Check glucose levels.

'The baby responds only to handling. The baby's blood sugar is 1.7 mmol/L.'

The baby will require a bolus of glucose, given as 2 mL/kg of glucose 10%.

Prescribe (Figs 9.3–9.6)

Oxygen:
- 1 L/min via NASAL CANNULAE

Glucose:
- 7 mL (2 mL/kg) GLUCOSE 10% IV (over 5 minutes)

EXPOSURE

- Expose the baby and look for clues towards other possible causes of respiratory distress, including other congenital problems that may be associated with underlying lung pathology. Measure the baby's temperature as newborns can get cold very quickly, especially when unwell or hypoglycaemic.

- A brief antenatal history is important including abnormal antenatal scan results, gestation and maternal factors such as gestational diabetes or medication. A birth history may elucidate risk factors for infection such as maternal pyrexia or known colonisation with Group B *Streptococcus*.

'The antenatal history was unremarkable. However, the mother mentions that she had a temperature during labour and prolonged rupture of membranes. The baby's temperature is 36.2°C and extended examination is otherwise normal.'

INITIAL INVESTIGATIONS

- **Capillary blood gas:** An acute respiratory acidosis is indicated by a low pH, a raised $PaCO_2$ and a normal bicarbonate/base excess. A raised lactate and/or reduced base excess indicate a metabolic acidosis, which may be secondary to sepsis or reduced perfusion.
- **Bloods:** FBC, U&Es, CRP and blood culture, looking for evidence of infection. Blood cultures should be taken before starting antibiotics. Neonatal jaundice may be more pronounced in unwell newborns, so a baseline serum bilirubin (SBR) should be taken. Group and save is normally taken early to minimise delays should this baby develop sepsis and require transfusion of packed red cells or platelets (Table 9.2).
- **CXR:** May show focal consolidation due to congenital pneumonia (secondary to maternal chorioamnionitis). Patchy shadowing with evidence of air trapping may indicate meconium aspiration. Hyperexpansion with a ground-glass appearance is typical of surfactant deficiency (RDS), while overloaded lung fields with cardiomegaly may be due to underlying congenital heart disease. Spontaneous pneumothorax should be excluded.
- **Weight:** Important for drug and fluid calculations. This should also be plotted on a newborn growth chart. Note: prematurity should be taken into consideration when plotting weights.

'Capillary blood gas shows a pH 7.22, $PaCO_2$ of 8.2 kPa, HCO_3 18 mmol/L, BE −4 mmol/L. Hb is 190 g/L, WCC 36 × 10^9/L, neutrophils 22 × 10^9/L. CRP is 75 mg/L. Bilirubin is 95 mg/dL, which plots below the threshold for phototherapy. CXR shows lobar left-sided consolidation consistent with congenital pneumonia. The weight is 3.5 kg, which plots on the fiftieth centile.'

Table 9.2 Male Infant Khan's Blood Test Results and ABG

PARAMETER	VALUE	NORMAL RANGE (UNITS)
Haemoglobin	190 g/L	150–240 (g/L)
WCC	**36 × 10^9/L**	**9.1–34 (×10^9/L)**
Neutrophils	**22 × 10^9/L**	**5.6–21 (× 10^9/L)**
Lymphocytes	**10 × 10^9/L**	**2.6–9.9 (× 10^9/L)**
Platelet	145 × 10^9/L	84–478 (× 10^9/L)
CRP	**75 mg/L**	**0.8–15.8 (mg/L)**
Urea	4 mmol/L	1.1–4.3 (mmol/L)
Creatinine	40 µmol/L	2.65–44.2 (µmol/L)
Sodium	131 mmol/L	133–146 (mmol/L)
Potassium	4.0 mmol/L	3.5–5.5 (mmol/L)
Bilirubin	95 mg/dL	<150 (phototherapy) <200 (exchange transfusion) (mg/dL)
pH	**7.22**	**7.35–7.45**
$PaCO_2$	**8.2 kPa**	**4.7–6.0 (kPa)**
HCO_3	**18 mmol/L**	**22–26 (mmol/L)**
BE	**−4 mmol/L**	**±2 (mmol/L)**

Data in bold signifies results that are outside the normal laboratory range.
ABG, Arterial blood gas; *BE*, base excess; *CRP*, C-reactive protein; *WCC*, white cell count.

Congenital Pneumonia Management

- Breathing: Supplementary oxygen, or respiratory support as required including CPAP and ventilation
- Antibiotics: Initially broad, e.g. benzylpenicillin and gentamicin
- Supportive care: May include an incubator, IV or NG fluids and close monitoring

INITIAL MANAGEMENT

Management Summary: Respiratory Distress

- Respiratory support: oxygen as required. Escalation to invasive ventilation (e.g. HHFNC, CPAP or intubation) may be considered if necessary.
- Consider sepsis: obtain IV access, blood cultures, and lactate. Measure urine output. Give IV antibiotics, IV fluids and oxygen, if needed.
- Rehydration: IV fluids, or an oral fluid challenge.

- **Supplementary oxygen**: If saturations <94%. The baby is placed prone as this reduces the work of breathing. If the baby is premature or hypothermic, they may be placed in an incubator or on the resuscitare for warmth.
- **Antibiotics:** Broad-spectrum antibiotics are given intravenously to cover most common pathogens, which commonly arise from the mother's genital tract such as Group B *Streptococcus*, Gram-negative enterococci and bacilli. Benzylpenicillin and gentamicin are a combination favoured by many neonatal units. Refer to local unit guidelines.
- Gentamicin requires regular monitoring of trough levels to avoid dose-dependent toxicity such as renal impairment (temporary) and ototoxicity causing sensorineural hearing loss (permanent). Trough levels are usually taken before the second dose.
- Positive blood cultures with sensitivities may allow more focused antibiotic therapy depending on the organisms grown.

Box 9.2 Calculating 24-Hour Volume Requirements in Neonates

- Birth to day 1: 50–60 mL/kg
- Day 2: 70–80 mL/kg
- Day 3: 80–100 mL/kg
- Day 4: 100–120 mL/kg
- Days 5 to 28: 120–150 mL/kg

This is a guideline and should be altered depending on fluid balance and blood sugars.

- **Glucose bolus:** This is given quickly as a 2 mL/kg bolus of glucose 10%. The sugar must be reassessed within 30 minutes in case a further bolus is required.
- **Fluid support**: As the baby has significantly increased work of breathing, even NG feeding is contraindicated as a stomach full of milk will splint the diaphragm.
- **IV fluids:** In neonates, this is usually glucose 10% to prevent hypoglycaemia as newborns have a higher glucose requirement than children (Box 9.2). The sugar will need to be monitored regularly.
- In the first few days until physiological diuresis occurs, electrolytes such as Na^+ and K^+ are not required.
- Hourly fluid infusion rate is calculated as weight × 60 mL/24 hours. 3.5 kg × 60 mL/kg per 24 hours = 8.8 mL/h.
- **Vitamin K:** All newborns are given intramuscular (IM) vitamin K at birth to prevent haemorrhagic disease of the newborn, which can otherwise present with significant and potentially catastrophic bleeding in the first few months of life. In healthy babies, who are low risk for bleeding disorders, some centres prefer to use oral vitamin K (phytomenadione), which is prescribed in two to three doses.
- **Lumbar puncture:** In babies where there is clinical suspicion of meningitis, sepsis or the CRP is significantly raised (thresholds will vary between units, but >10–20 mg/L is typical), a lumbar puncture should be considered.

Prescribe (see Figs 9.3–9.6)

VITAMIN K 1 mg IM STAT

Antibiotics:

- BENZYLPENICILLIN (50 mg/kg) 175 mg IV (over 30 minutes) BD and GENTAMICIN (5 mg/kg) 17.5 mg IV OD

Maintenance fluids:

- GLUCOSE 10% (60 mL/kg/day) 500 mL IV 8.8 mL/h

REASSESSMENT

- After a glucose bolus, supplemental oxygen and antibiotics, the baby is reassessed.

'The baby looks more alert and the airway remains patent. RR 65/min, oxygen saturations are 97% on 1 L nasal cannula oxygen. The grunting has stopped but the work of breathing remains high. HR 160 bpm, BP 62/28 mmHg, CRT 1 second centrally. Glucose is now 3.6 mmol/L and the temperature is 37.0°C.'

HANDING OVER THE PATIENT

'Baby Khan is a term newborn, currently 18 hours old, being treated for congenital pneumonia.

They were born by emergency caesarean for maternal chorioamnionitis. There were no other antenatal concerns. The baby developed respiratory distress over the first 12 hours of life and required admission to SCBU.

From a respiratory point of view, they are on 1 L oxygen via nasal cannula. The initial gas showed a mixed acidosis and CXR shows congenital pneumonia. The baby initially required a glucose bolus for hypoglycaemia and now remains NBM on 60 mL/kg/day glucose 10% with stable sugars. The bloods are also suggestive of infection and, therefore, we have started benzylpenicillin and gentamicin. The bilirubin level is below the treatment line. We have given IM vitamin K. The parents have been updated.

The plan is to wean oxygen as tolerated, repeat a capillary gas, continue antibiotics for 5 days, chase blood cultures and repeat FBC, U&Es, SBR and CRP in the morning. The baby will require a lumbar puncture now that he is stable in view of the raised CRP. Gentamicin levels are due to be taken before the third dose.'

STATION 9.3: ACUTE EXACERBATION OF ASTHMA

You are a junior doctor in the emergency department. A 6-year-old named Tania has presented with a 3-day history of coryzal symptoms, shortness of breath and a wheeze. This is her first wheezing episode. Today she is becoming progressively more breathless. Please assess Tania and instigate appropriate management.

Patient Details

Name:	Tania Keya
DOB:	23/05/18
Hospital number:	XD11324059
Weight:	20 kg
Consultant:	Dr Wi
Hospital/Ward:	BGH Paediatric ward
Current medications:	Nil
Allergies:	None known
Admission date:	15/11/24

Complications of Asthma

- Pneumothorax
- Infective/noninfective asthma exacerbation
- Poor growth/failure to thrive
- Medication-related side effects, especially with oral corticosteroids, e.g. thin skinning, candida infection, adrenal suppression, weakened immunity

Exacerbation of Asthma Management

- Supplementary oxygen
- Inhaled or nebulised bronchodilators, e.g. salbutamol, ipratropium bromide, magnesium
- IV medications including salbutamol, aminophylline and magnesium sulfate
- Oral corticosteroids

INITIAL ASSESSMENT

AIRWAY

- Assess patency of the airway.

'The airway is patent with no obstruction. There is obvious wheeze and no stridor.'

BREATHING

- Assess respiratory rate, oxygen saturations and work of breathing. Auscultate for air entry and wheeze.
- Assess whether the child can talk in full sentences. If not, asking them to count to 10 is a good marker of reserve and can be repeated after intervention to assess response.

'RR 50/min, oxygen saturations are 88% with marked intercostal and subcostal recessions, tracheal tug and abdominal breathing. On auscultation, there is minimal wheeze and reduced air entry throughout with a very long expiratory phase. The child is not able to talk in full sentences and can count to two only.'

Given these features are consistent with life-threatening asthma, you give high-flow oxygen via a non-rebreathe facemask and nebulised salbutamol with ipratropium bromide (also known as Atrovent). Reassess following any intervention.

Prescribe (Figs 9.7 and 9.8)

High-flow OXYGEN:
- 100% via NONREBREATHE FACE MASK

Nebulisers:
- SALBUTAMOL 5 mg NEB (driven with oxygen) STAT and IPRATROPIUM BROMIDE 250 micrograms NEB (driven with oxygen) STAT

PREDNISOLONE 40 mg PO solution

Consider adding MAGNESIUM SULFATE 150 mg NEB in children presenting with saturations <92%.

CIRCULATION

- Assess haemodynamic stability by measuring pulse, BP and CRT. Assess hydration status by looking at the mucous membranes, skin turgor and ask about urine output.
- Note that hypotension is a sign of life-threatening asthma.

'HR 120 bpm, BP 110/65 mmHg, CRT 1 second. Cardiovascular examination is normal.'

Tania is haemodynamically stable. However, given the severity of the asthma attack, it is worth getting IV access early for a blood gas and in case IV medication is required.

DISABILITY

- Assess the patient's level of consciousness using AVPU (is the patient Alert? If not, do they respond to Verbal or Painful stimuli? Or are they Unresponsive?). Check glucose levels; it may be high due to stress associated with respiratory distress.

'Tania responds to voice and has blood sugar of 9.2 mmol/L.'

EXPOSURE

- Examine for signs that might differentiate between viral wheeze and asthma, including signs of atopy and eczema. Measure the temperature.

'Temperature is 37.7°C and examination is otherwise normal.'

INITIAL INVESTIGATIONS

- **Capillary blood gas:** Not routinely performed unless life-threatening features which are not responding to treatment. Moderate to severe wheeze may show a respiratory alkalosis (with low $PaCO_2$) due to hyperventilation. However, a life-threatening attack with silent chest may show decompensation with respiratory acidosis (high $PaCO_2$) due to reduced ventilation.
- **Bloods:** Not routinely performed unless life-threatening features which are not responding to treatment. FBC, U&Es, CRP may suggest an infectious aetiology. If the child requires high-dose and frequent salbutamol, potassium should be monitored (Table 9.3).
- **CXR:** Not routinely performed unless there are signs of subcutaneous emphysema, pneumothorax, lobar collapse or consolidation and/or life-threatening asthma which is not responding to treatment.
- **Peak flow:** Children above the age of 5 may be able to perform this.
- **Weight:** Important for drug calculations.

'Capillary blood gas shows decompensation with respiratory acidosis, pH 7.22, $PaCO_2$ of 8.9 kPa, HCO_3 22 mmol/L, BE –0.5 mmol/L. Bloods are otherwise unremarkable. CXR shows hyperexpansion with flattened diaphragm, with some bilateral streaky shadows consistent with mucous plugging. Weight is 14 kg.'

INITIAL MANAGEMENT

- **Airway support:** No airway intervention is required in this case at present. Life-threatening cases refractory to treatment occasionally require intubation; however, this is rare.

Table 9.3 Tania's Blood and ABG Results

PARAMETER	VALUE	NORMAL RANGE (UNITS)
Haemoglobin	120 g/L	115–145 (g/L)
WCC	8 × 10^9/L	4–12 (×10^9/L)
Platelet	160 × 10^9/L	150–400 (×10^9/L)
CRP	4 mg/L	0.6–7.9 (mg/L)
Urea	5.3 mmol/L	2.5–6.7 (mmol/L)
Creatinine	45 μmol/L	2.65–52.2 (μmol/L)
Sodium	138 mmol/L	134–144 (mmol/L)
Potassium	4.2 mmol/L	3.3–4.6 (mmol/L)
pH	**7.22**	**7.35–7.45**
$PaCO_2$	**8.9 kPa**	**4.7–6.0 (kPa)**
HCO_3	22 mmol/L	22–26 (mmol/L)
BE	−0.5 mmol/L	±2 (mmol/L)

Data in bold signifies results that are outside the normal laboratory range.
ABG, Arterial blood gas; *BE*, base excess; *CRP*, C-reactive protein; *WCC*, white cell count.

- **Supplementary oxygen:** If saturations <94% or life-threatening asthma.
- **Inhaled bronchodilators:** Inhaled β_2 agonists are first line. In mild to moderate wheeze with no oxygen requirement, 4 to 10 puffs of salbutamol may be given via a metered dosed inhaler and spacer device and repeated as required. If wheezing is severe with oxygen requirement, it may be given by nebuliser. Doses can be repeated as required and back-to-back treatment (also known as 'burst therapy') is given in the initial management of moderate to life-threatening cases.
- If there is poor response, you may initially consider adding ipratropium bromide nebulisers (mixed in with the beta-2 agonists). Ipratropium can be used as repeated doses every 4 to 6 hours. Magesium nebulisers can also be given in severe cases.
- **IV treatment:** If the wheeze is severe with poor response to inhaled bronchodilators or the patient is requiring inhaled treatment more frequently than every hour, IV treatment may be considered. Both salbutamol and aminophylline infusions require the child to have cardiac monitoring for arrhythmia, which is best done on a high dependency unit. IV options include:
  - Loading IV salbutamol 15 micrograms/kg (followed by a continuous infusion 1–5 micrograms/kg per minute)
  - Loading IV aminophylline 5 mg/kg (followed by a continuous infusion 1 mg/kg per hour)
  - IV magnesium sulfate 40 mg/kg (max. 2 g)

In this case, the patient, due to continued poor response, ends up having back-to-back nebulisers, a magnesium bolus, a salbutamol bolus followed by an infusion of IV salbutamol.

In order to prescribe the salbutamol infusion, you must first make up the infusion as per your IV handbook (e.g. Box 9.3).

Box 9.3 Calculating Salbutamol Infusion Rate

Dilute 10 mg salbutamol up to 50 mL with sodium chloride 0.9%.

You must then calculate the rate in order to deliver 1 microgram/kg per minute:

10 mg in 50 mL gives 200 micrograms/mL, so 1 mL/h delivers 200 micrograms/h, or 3.33 micrograms/min. This child is 20 kg and so 1 microgram/kg/min is equal to 20 micrograms/min.

Therefore, to achieve 1 microgram/kg/minute divide 20 by 3.33 and prescribe a rate of 6 mls/min.

Silent Chest

The absence of wheeze with quiet breath sounds is a sign of life-threatening asthma. As the child responds to treatment and air entry improves, the wheeze will initially become more prominent.

- **Fluid support**: May be required if the child is too breathless to drink or needs electrolyte correction. This should be kept to two-thirds maintenance if given to avoid hyponatraemia secondary to SIADH.
- **Oral corticosteroids**: Asthma exacerbations are commonly treated with short courses of oral corticosteroids. There is evidence that suggests preschool children with mild to moderate viral wheezing disorders do not benefit from oral corticosteroids, unless there is a personal or family history of atopy, or interval symptoms suggestive of asthma. However, it is still recommended to give oral corticosteroids to children with moderate to severe wheeze without a diagnosis of asthma and children who require admission to hospital. It is important to note how many courses of steroids the child has had in the last year.

Prescribe (see Figs 9.7 and 9.8)

Back-to-back nebulisers:
- SALBUTAMOL 5 mg NEB (driven with oxygen) STAT, IPRATROPIUM BROMIDE 250 micrograms NEB (driven with oxygen) STAT

Followed by SALBUTAMOL 2.5 mg NEB (driven with oxygen) STAT and IPRATROPIUM BROMIDE 250 micrograms NEB (driven with oxygen) STAT

MAGNESIUM SULFATE 150 mg NEB (driven with oxygen) STAT

Magnesium bolus:
- MAGNESIUM SULFATE 800 mg (40 mg/kg) IV (over 20 minutes) STAT

Salbutamol bolus:
- SALBUTAMOL (15 micrograms/kg [maximum dose 250 micrograms]) 250 micrograms IV (over 5 minutes) STAT

Salbutamol infusion:
- 10 mg SALBUTAMOL in 50 mL SODIUM CHLORIDE 0.9%, at a rate of 6 mL/min (1 microgram/kg/minute)

REASSESSMENT

- After salbutamol and ipratropium bromide nebulisers, you reassess quickly and, because of poor response, give a magnesium sulfate and salbutamol bolus. A salbutamol infusion is then started with good effect.

'Tania has improved. Her airway remains patent. RR 40/min, oxygen saturations are 95%. She has moderate intercostal recession and her tracheal tug has improved. The air entry throughout the chest has improved markedly with more prominent polyphonic expiratory wheeze. HR 150 bpm, BP 115/70 mmHg, CRT 1 second centrally.'

HANDING OVER THE PATIENT

'Tania is a 6-year-old girl with an acute exacerbation of asthma.

She presented with significant respiratory distress, hypoxia and silent chest. She initially had only minimal response to inhaled bronchodilators despite back-to-back nebulisers. She has been treated with an IV bolus of salbutamol and with magnesium sulfate, with significant improvement in air entry. She remains on 100% oxygen. In terms of circulation, she is stable but tachycardic due to the salbutamol. She does not require IV fluids and well hydrated.

Her initial gas showed decompensation with respiratory acidosis. This has now improved. Initial bloods were normal with no signs of pneumonia. CXR shows hyperinflation with streaky bilateral changes consistent with a viral infection.

The plan is to transfer to HDU for ongoing management, including a salbutamol infusion, cardiac monitoring and oxygen. She will need to continue inhaled bronchodilators and they can be appropriately tapered. She will need repeat U&Es to exclude hypokalaemia and review in a few hours. She will also require further investigations for asthma in the future.'

STATION 9.4: INFECTIVE EXACERBATION OF CYSTIC FIBROSIS

You are a junior doctor on the paediatric ward. A 16-year-old named Imogen with cystic fibrosis (CF) has been admitted directly from respiratory clinic. She has had increasing shortness of breath and has been increasingly productive of sputum. Her recent lung function tests have deteriorated. Please assess her and instigate appropriate management.

Patient Details

Name:	Imogen Saunders
DOB:	02/04/08
Hospital number:	XD11324059
Weight:	39 kg
Consultant:	Dr Wi
Hospital/Ward:	BGH Paediatric ward
Current medications:	Creon 10000 (pancreatin) 2 capsules oral TDS and Creon 10000 (pancreatin) 1 capsule oral BD (with snacks) (for cystic fibrosis-related pancreatic insufficiency) Ranitidine 150 mg oral BD and domperidone 10 mg oral TDS (for cystic fibrosis-related gastro-oesophageal reflux) Dalivit (vitamin A, B, C and D) 1 mL oral OD (for cystic fibrosis related nutritional deficiency)
Allergies:	None known
Admission date:	01/11/24

Differential Diagnosis of Infective Exacerbation of CF

- Younger children: *Staphylococcus/Haemophilus*
- Older children: *Pseudomonas*, *Burkholderia cepacian*
- Allergic bronchopulmonary aspergillosis (ABPA)

Complications of Cystic Fibrosis

- Meconium ileus (newborn)
- Infective exacerbations
- Cor pulmonale
- Pancreatic exocrine insufficiency
- Diabetes
- Cirrhosis
- Constipation and distal intestinal obstruction syndrome
- Infertility/subfertility

INITIAL ASSESSMENT

AIRWAY

- Assess patency of the airway.

'The airway is patent.'

BREATHING

- Assess respiratory rate, oxygen saturations and work of breathing. Auscultate the chest; you may hear widespread wheeze and crackles. Look for a focal area with reduced air entry or increased crepitations.

'RR 22/min, oxygen saturations are 96% with no increased work of breathing. Crackles and wheeze are heard bilaterally. The left base has reduced air entry with marked coarse crepitations. The cough is productive of sputum which is green.'

There is no need for oxygen or respiratory support. Some CF patients have an element of bronchospasm and, if the patient feels tight or wheezy, they may have symptomatic relief from inhaled bronchodilators.

CIRCULATION

- Assess haemodynamic stability by measuring pulse, BP and CRT.
- Perform a cardiovascular examination. It is important to be confident in excluding right-sided heart failure as this is a poor prognostic sign. Palpate for right ventricular heave and displaced apex beat. Auscultate for a loud second heart sound and inspect for raised jugular venous pressure (JVP) and peripheral or sacral oedema.

'HR 70 bpm, BP 116/72 mmHg, CRT 2 seconds centrally. Cardiovascular examination is unremarkable with no evidence of cor pulmonale.'

DISABILITY

- Assess the patient's level of consciousness using AVPU (is the patient Alert? If not, do they respond to Verbal or Painful stimuli? Or are they Unresponsive?). Check glucose levels as many older children with CF have diabetes associated with pancreatic endocrine insufficiency.

'Imogen is alert and has blood sugar of 8 mmol/L.'

EXPOSURE

- Perform a systems examination to exclude other pathology. She may have other complications of her CF that need attention during her admission.
- Look for central venous access; many children with CF have a central or peripheral line for recurrent courses of IV antibiotics and/or blood sampling. Review the line site for signs of line infection such as erythema or tenderness.
- Record her temperature in view of likely infectious aetiology.
- Perform an abdominal examination. Some patients require overnight feeding to aid caloric intake and so they may have a gastrostomy. Look for evidence of nutrient deficiency such as koilonychia and look for reduced fat mass and muscle bulk. She may be on pancreatic supplements. If the dose is insufficient, she may be symptomatic with steatorrhoea.
- Assess for abdominal pain, masses and bilious vomiting as older children with CF are prone to distal intestinal obstruction syndrome (DIOS).
- Some teenagers with CF go on to develop liver disease. Assess for jaundice, hepatomegaly and stigmata of chronic liver disease.

'Temperature is 38.2°C. She has a Hickman line in situ; the site looks healthy. Abdominal examination reveals a large laparotomy scar which she tells you is from meconium ileus surgery as a newborn. She looks slim with evidence of reduced subcutaneous fat. She has no gastrostomy. She is taking pancreatic supplements and vitamins and has no steatorrhoea. She has no evidence of DIOS or liver disease.'

INITIAL INVESTIGATIONS

- **Sputum culture/cough swab:** Ensure this is repeated and enquire about the most recent results. Positive growth and sensitivities may guide your management and colonisation with *Pseudomonas* or staphylococcus is important.
- **Bloods:** FBC, U&Es, LFTs, CRP. Look for evidence of infection. Note significant eosinophilia may point to ABPA. If this is suspected, consider sending specific IgE/IgG which may be raised in ABPA. Send sputum samples for aspergillus if suspected (Table 9.4).
- **Spirometry:** This is performed regularly in CF clinic and with exacerbations. An acute deterioration often points to infectious exacerbation. Note that CF can show both obstructive problems due to thick mucus in the airways or bronchospasm and a restrictive defect due to lung damage. Peak flow rate is a useful bedside test.
- **CXR:** Chest X-ray may be helpful if there are focal signs. It should be compared to previous films. Look for focal consolidation and widespread changes.
- **Height and weight:** Important for drug calculations and planning nutritional support.

'Her last sputum culture was 4 months ago and grew Pseudomonas, for which she has monthly cycles of nebulised tobramycin. Her blood tests show WCC 15 × 10^9/L, neutrophils 11.2 × 10^9/L, eosinophils 0.4 × 10^9/L, CRP 32 mg/L. She had spirometry today in clinic showing reduced FVC and reduced FEV_1 with normal FEV_1/FVC ratio. Chest X-ray shows left basal consolidation. Her weight is 39 kg and plots on the 2nd centile for weight. Her height is 158 cm and plots on the 25th centile for height.'

Table 9.4 Imogen's Blood Test Results

PARAMETER	VALUE	NORMAL RANGE (UNITS)
Haemoglobin	140 g/L	120–150 (g/L)
WCC	**15 × 10^9/L**	**3.2–11 (× 10^9/L)**
Neutrophils	**11.2 × 10^9/L**	**2.0–7.5 (× 10^9/L)**
Lymphocyte	3 × 10^9/L	1.4–4 (× 10^9/L)
Eosinophils	0.4 × 10^9/L	0.4–4.0 (× 10^9/L)
Platelet	145 × 10^9/L	120–400 (× 10^9/L)
CRP	**32 mg/L**	**0.6–8.1 (mg/L)**
Urea	5.4 mmol/L	2.5–6.4 (mmol/L)
Creatinine	70 µmol/L	27.4–77.8 (µmol/L)
Sodium	139 mmol/L	135–145 (mmol/L)
Potassium	4.2 mmol/L	3.3–4.6 (mmol/L)
ALT	17 IU/L	5–45 (IU/L)
ALP	82 IU/L	39–117 (IU/L)
Bilirubin	14 µmol/L	<17 (µmol/L)

Data in bold signifies results that are outside the normal laboratory range.
ALP, Alkaline phosphatase; *ALT,* alanine transaminase; *CRP,* C-reactive protein; *WCC,* white cell count.

INITIAL MANAGEMENT

Management of Infective Exacerbation of Cystic Fibrosis

- Supplementary oxygen
- Aggressive antibiotics
- Physiotherapy
- Nutritional support

- **Supplementary oxygen**: If saturations <94%.
- **Antibiotics:** Infective exacerbations are treated aggressively to prevent ongoing infective and inflammatory damage to the lungs and prevent accelerated loss of lung function. Positive sputum cultures with sensitivities allow antibiotic courses to be tailored to exacerbations. In this case, she is colonised with *Pseudomonas* so the treatment should cover for this. Typically, if treating pseudomonas, dual therapy is used with a broad-spectrum β-lactam or cephalosporin and an aminoglycoside. Imogen is to be started on piperacillin–tazobactam and amikacin IV.
- Patients with CF often have increased clearance rates of antibiotics, especially aminoglycosides, so often increased or more frequent doses are used and levels monitored closely as patients may have variable clearance rates. Note your hospital pharmacy may have its own protocol specifically for patients with CF.
- Treatment is continued until the symptoms of the exacerbation (such as reduced lung function or increased sputum) have resolved, which can often be 10 days to 3 weeks. Some patients may require long-term prophylactic antibiotics once recovered.
- **Physiotherapy:** All patients with CF undergo daily physiotherapy regimens. During exacerbations, these should be intensified and often in-hospital physiotherapy teams will be involved with this.
- **Corticosteroids:** While not used for infectious exacerbations, if the deterioration is due to ABPA, the patient should receive high dose systemic corticosteroids.
- **Nutrition**: Optimising nutrition is important both for exacerbations and long-term preservation of lung function. Admissions allow the hospital team to review nutrition and liaise closely with dieticians to ensure the patient is on optimum doses of pancreatic supplements as well as assess the need for nutritional adjuncts like overnight NG feeding.
- **Other medication:** CF patients are often on many different medications that will need to continue in hospital. Make sure these are prescribed appropriately. They commonly include:
  - **Multivitamins:** Micronutrient supplementation, especially of fat-soluble vitamins A, D, E and K, is important in all CF patients.
  - **Pancreatic enzyme supplements Creon 10000 (pancreatin):** Most CF patients have pancreatic exocrine dysfunction, so replacement of these enzymes allows better absorption and aids in symptomatic control of steatorrhoea.
  - **Ranitidine/domperidone:** CF patients are more likely to suffer gastro-oesophageal reflux disease and this can be exacerbated by the intensive chest physiotherapy they receive.
  - **Mucolytics (e.g. Domase alfa):** Breaks up DNA in pulmonary secretions, reducing viscosity. It may improve pulmonary function in children over 5 years with forced vital capacity (FVC) >40% predicted.
  - **Inhaled bronchodilators:** May have a role if the patient is responsive or has concurrent asthma.
  - **Insulin:** CF patients may develop diabetes in their teens due to pancreatic endocrine insufficiency. They will require insulin replacement in order to prevent the long-term sequelae of diabetes.
  - **Cystic fibrosis transmembrane conductance regulator (CFTR) modulators:** These are a class of drugs designed to improve the production and/or function of the CFTR molecule. One modulator is the triple therapy called Kaftrio (elexacaftor–tezacaftor–ivacaftor).

Prescribe (Figs 9.9–9.11)

Antibiotics:
- PIPERACILLIN/TAZOBACTAM 4.5 g IV (over 30 minutes) TDS and AMIKACIN 390 mg (10 mg/kg) IV TDS

Multivitamins:
- Dalivit (vitamin A, B, C and D) 1 mL PO OD

Pancreatic enzyme supplements:
- Creon 10000 (pancreatin) PO 2 capsules TDS (with meals), 1 capsule BD (with snacks)

Reflux medication:
- DOMPERIDONE 10 mg PO TDS and RANITIDINE 150 mg PO BD

Mucolytics:
- DORNASE ALFA 2500 units (2.5 mg) NEB OD

REASSESSMENT

- After several days of regular physiotherapy, IV antibiotics and optimising her nutrition, the patient is reviewed.

'Imogen looks and feels better. Airway is patent. RR 16/min, oxygen saturations are 97% in air. She has fewer crackles and wheeze and the air entry at the left base has improved. She is still producing an increased amount of sputum. HR 68 bpm, BP 118/74 mmHg, CRT <2 seconds centrally. Cardiovascular examination is unremarkable.'

HANDING OVER THE PATIENT

'Imogen is a 16-year-old girl with infective exacerbation of cystic fibrosis. She is known to be colonised with Pseudomonas.

She presented with increased shortness of breath, worsening production of green sputum and deterioration in her lung function. From a respiratory point of view, she has not required support but has had intensive physiotherapy. She has been having IV piperacillin/tazobactam and amikacin via her central line and is now on day 5 of treatment.

Sputum sample repeated this admission has again grown Pseudomonas which is amikacin sensitive. Her initial bloods showed raised inflammatory markers and her CXR showed left-sided infection.

During her admission she has also had review of her nutrition and her glycaemic control, which are satisfactory. The local cystic fibrosis team are involved with her inpatient care.

The plan is to continue her antibiotics for 2 weeks until her exercise tolerance has returned to normal for her and her sputum production decreases. She will require ongoing physiotherapy during this time and repeat spirometry before discharge.'

STATION 9.5: GASTROENTERITIS

You are a junior doctor in the emergency department. A 2-month-old baby, Brychan, is brought in with a 3-day history of diarrhoea. Today he has started vomiting his feeds and is becoming sleepier and less interested in feeding. Please assess the baby and instigate appropriate management.

Patient Details

Name:	Brychan Matthews
DOB:	09/08/24
Hospital number:	SDE1939102
Weight:	6 kg
Consultant:	Dr Wi
Hospital/Ward:	BGH Paediatric ward
Current medications:	Nil
Allergies:	None known
Admission date:	14/10/24

Differential Diagnosis of Acute Diarrhoea

- Genitourinary: Urinary tract infection (UTI)
- Gastrointestinal: Overflow diarrhoea, gastroenteritis, intussusception
- Drugs: Laxatives, antibiotics (such as macrolides)

Complications of Gastroenteritis

- Dehydration
- Acute kidney injury
- Sepsis
- Electrolyte disturbances
- Lactose intolerance
- Haemolytic uraemic syndrome (if *Escherichia coli* O157)

INITIAL ASSESSMENT

AIRWAY

- Assess patency of the airway.

'The airway is patent with no obstruction.'

BREATHING

- Assess respiratory rate. Tachypnoea could be a sign of underlying metabolic acidosis (a late sign) or another diagnosis.

'RR 30/min, oxygen saturations are 100%, no signs of increased work of breathing. The chest is clear on auscultation.'

CIRCULATION

- Measure heart rate, BP and CRT. Signs of dehydration include dry mucous membranes with decreased urine output. Ask the parent/carer about the number wet nappies and whether this is different to a normal daily amount.
- Red flag signs of dehydration include tachycardia, tachypnoea, reduced skin turgor, sunken eyes and fontanelles.
- Signs of shock include cool extremities, mottled skin, prolonged CRT, weak pulses and reduced consciousness. Hypotension in children is a late sign suggestive of decompensated shock and is preterminal.

'HR 180 bpm, BP 84/52 mmHg. The baby has had only one slightly wet nappy today; yesterday they were reduced in frequency. On examination, there are dry mucous membranes but skin turgor is normal and CRT is 2 seconds centrally. The baby is pink and peripherally warm with strong femoral pulses; there is no evidence of hypovolaemic shock.'

This baby is dehydrated and needs rehydration but is not shocked and does not require urgent fluid boluses. Therefore, this can be performed with an oral fluid challenge initially.

DISABILITY

- Assess the patient's conscious level using AVPU (is the patient Alert? If not, do they respond to Verbal or Painful stimuli? Or are they Unresponsive?). Check glucose levels as babies require very regular feeds and are unable to maintain a normal blood sugar when starved, especially when acutely unwell.

'The baby is alert and has blood sugar of 4.2 mmol/L.'

EXPOSURE

- A full examination to exclude any other potential cause for the symptoms. Fully expose to ensure there are no rashes and look for other possible sources of infection. It is sensible to exclude a urinary tract infection (UTI) as this can present with diarrhoea and vomiting, especially if the child is febrile. Measure the temperature.

- Examine the abdomen carefully. A painful abdomen with guarding or a palpable mass may suggest a surgical cause such as intussusception. True bilious vomit (dark green) is highly suggestive of obstruction and usually requires a surgical opinion. The presence of blood or mucus in the diarrhoea is suggestive of nonviral causes or surgical pathology and warrants further investigation. Absent bowel sounds may suggest ileus or obstruction.

'Temperature is 38.2°C. Clean catch urine dip was positive for 2+ ketones and 1+ protein, but negative for white cells and nitrites. The abdomen shows mild gaseous distension, with active bowel sounds. It is not tender and there is no guarding or masses on palpation. The vomit is light yellow and the diarrhoea offensive, watery and green without blood or mucus. There are no signs suggestive of infection due to another cause or surgical pathology.'

- Given that there are no signs suspicious of sepsis, a nonviral cause or a surgical problem, this child does not need further investigation but does require treatment for dehydration.
- Urine dipstick is not sensitive for excluding UTI in children under 3 years. Even if the dipstick result is reassuring, it should always be sent urgently to microbiology for formal microscopy if a UTI is suspected. If the microscopy is negative for white cells, it is very unlikely to be a UTI. Children who are starved will have urinary ketones due to ketogenesis.

INITIAL INVESTIGATIONS

- In simple cases of viral gastroenteritis, no investigations are indicated but it is important to recognise when they are.
- **Bloods:** Bloods are not done routinely. However, if IV fluids are required, U&Es and lab glucose should be sent. They should also be sent if there is clinical suspicion of hypernatraemic dehydration. This is more likely if the child is less than 3 months, is abnormally drowsy or has jittering, increased muscle tone or convulsions.
- **Stool sample for microscopy:** Not routinely indicated but should be considered if the diarrhoea is not improving by 7 days, if there is blood or mucus in the stool or if the child has recently been abroad. It should also be performed if there is doubt about the diagnosis or evidence of sepsis, or if the child is immunocompromised.
- **Evidence of sepsis:** If the child is shocked and there is evidence of infection elsewhere, or the history of vomiting is not sufficient to cause the level of shock, then the child should have a blood gas, blood culture and FBC, CRP and U&Es to look for evidence of septicaemia. A full septic screen would include urine microscopy, chest X-ray and consideration of lumbar puncture. If sepsis is suspected, you should not wait for these results before starting broad-spectrum antibiotics.
- **Weight:** Important for fluid calculations.

'The child has no clinical evidence of hypernatraemia and does not require IV fluids. There are no signs to suggest a diagnosis other than viral gastroenteritis. As he has only had diarrhoea for 3 days and there is no blood or mucus in the stool, it is not appropriate to investigate at this time. His weight is 6 kg.'

INITIAL MANAGEMENT

Gastroenteritis Management

- Exclusion of other pathology
- Rehydration with enteral hypoosmolar solution (such as Dioralyte Relief) or IV fluids if required.

- **Airway support:** Airway **patent** in this case with no intervention required.
- **Rehydration and maintenance fluids:** Oral rehydration is preferable if the patient does not require a fluid bolus. This should be given as an oral rehydration solution (240–250 mOsm/L), such as Dioralyte. In a small child, this should be given slowly into the mouth with a syringe (e.g. 1 mL/kg every 10 minutes) or via an NG tube (NGT) to reduce the risk of vomiting the fluids.
- If there are ongoing losses, it is sensible to complete an accurate fluid input/output chart—nappies can be weighed to achieve this. This will help flag up if ongoing losses are likely to require further replacement.
- **IV fluids:** Are indicated if the patient is shocked, persistently vomits the oral fluids despite NGT or deteriorates on the oral regimen. Close monitoring of electrolytes should be performed every 24 hours, or 8 to 12 hourly if they are abnormal. Fluids would normally be given as sodium chloride 0.9%/glucose 5% or glucose 10%, dependent on age. The decision to use hypotonic fluids (i.e. sodium chloride 0.45%) should be made by a senior doctor. IV potassium supplementation is likely to be required and should be added when the serum potassium levels are known.
- **Feeding advice:** Breastfeeding should continue alongside fluid replacement as tolerated. Solid food should be avoided until rehydration is completed.
- **Other therapies:** Antidiarrhoeal medications should not be used.

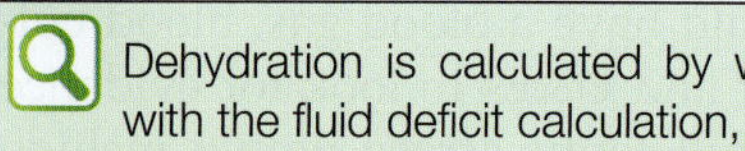

Dehydration is calculated by weight loss or clinically with the fluid deficit calculation, given over 48 hours:

- Fluid deficit (in L) = % dehydration × preillness weight (kg) / 100
  e.g. a 7-kg child who is 5% dehydrated has a water deficit of 350 mL.
- Fluid deficit (in L) = preillness weight (kg) – current weight (kg)
  e.g. a 7-kg child now weighs 6.5 kg has a fluid deficit of 500 mL.

If a child is dehydrated but able to tolerate enteral fluids (PO/NG), then 50 mL/kg over 4 hours fluid deficit is calculated. In this child, we can use NG fluids, as calculated in the following:

50 mL/kg × 6 kg = 300 mL over 4 hours, or 75 mL/h

The child should also be given full maintenance fluids (including whilst the replacement fluids are given and then continues afterwards). Full maintenance for this child is 600 mL over 24 hours, or 25 mL/h.

You should prescribe 100 (75 + 25) mL/h Dioralyte via NGT for 4 hours or if not tolerated/available, IV sodium chloride 0.9%/glucose 5%.

Then continue on 25 mL/h until recovered.

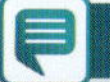

Prescribe (Fig. 9.12)

Rehydration fluid:

- Dioralyte 2 sachets in 400 mL WATER, 100 mL/h via NGT

Maintenance fluid:

- Dioralyte 1 sachet in 200 mL WATER, 25 mL/h via NGT

REASSESSMENT

- After 2 hours of rehydration, the patient is reassessed.

'The baby has improved significantly. The RR is 30/min, oxygen saturations are 100% in air. HR 156 bpm, BP 86/54 mmHg, CRT 1 second centrally. Mucous membranes are moist. He has tolerated the fluids without vomiting. He has had one further episode of diarrhoea. Urine microscopy has confirmed the absence of white cells.'

HANDING OVER THE PATIENT

'Brychan is a 2-month-old with viral gastroenteritis.

He presented with 3 days of diarrhoea and 1 day of vomiting. Respiratory system is stable. With regards to circulation, he was initially dehydrated requiring replacement over 4 hours with Dioralyte, which was well tolerated via NG tube. Blood sugars have been stable. He is now much improved and well hydrated.

As there are no signs to suggest another underlying pathology or nonviral cause for his diarrhoea, I have not ordered investigations other than urine microscopy, which was negative.

The plan is to transfer him to the ward in a cubicle until normal feeding is established and tolerated. He will continue on Dioralyte full maintenance fluids via NG tube. He is allowed to breastfeed on top of this if able. His fluid input and output will be monitored with a fluid balance chart; if his diarrhoeal losses are large, his fluids may need to be increased.'

STATION 9.6: SICKLE CELL CHEST CRISIS

You are a junior doctor in the emergency department. A 10-year-old boy named Jimiyu is brought into resus with shortness of breath, chest pain and fever. He is known to have sickle cell disease. Please assess him and instigate appropriate management.

Patient Details

Name:	Jimiyu Abosi
DOB:	05/02/14
Hospital number:	GF54034930
Weight:	23 kg
Consultant:	Dr Wi
Hospital/Ward:	BGH Paediatric ward
Current medications:	Penicillin V 250 mg oral BD (prophylaxis for pneumococcal infection)
Allergies:	None known
Admission date:	15/11/24

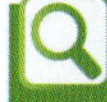

Diagnostic Criteria for Acute Chest Crisis in Sickle Cell

New infiltrate seen on CXR *AND* one of the following:

- Chest pain
- Fever >38.5°C
- Tachypnoea, wheeze or cough
- Hypoxaemia

Causes of Chest Pain in a Child

- Musculoskeletal, e.g. trauma
- Gastro-oesophageal reflux
- Pneumothorax
- Pneumonia
- Sickle cell chest crisis
- Costochondritis
- Cardiac abnormality, e.g. pericarditis, arrhythmia

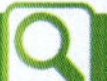

Complications of Acute Chest Crisis

- Respiratory failure requiring ventilation
- Pulmonary embolism or infarction
- Cerebrovascular events
- Peripheral vaso-occlusive crisis

INITIAL ASSESSMENT

AIRWAY

- Assess patency of the airway.

'The airway is patent with no obstruction.'

BREATHING

- Assess respiratory rate, oxygen saturations and work of breathing. Auscultate for crepitations and air entry and specifically for signs of bronchospasm such as wheeze.
- Ask about pain on breathing, as pleuritic pain may cause the patient to take shallow breaths, worsening hypoxia and hypoventilation.

'RR 45/min, oxygen saturations 87%, with tracheal tug and intercostal recessions. He is sat upright leaning forward on his hands. On auscultation, he has reduced air entry on the left base with crackles and wheeze bilaterally. There is a pleural rub on the left. He is talking in broken sentences and says his chest is painful. You note he is coughing intermittently. His mother notes he has a history of asthma.'

Given these, you give supplementary facemask oxygen (to keep saturations >92%). You also initiate regular inhaled salbutamol.

CIRCULATION

- Assess haemodynamic stability by measuring pulse, BP and CRT (centrally and peripherally). Assess hydration status by looking at mucous membranes and skin turgor. Perform a cardiovascular examination and look for haemodynamic signs of anaemia.

'HR 140 bpm, BP 105/52 mmHg, he has CRT 3 seconds centrally. He has dry mucous membranes and good skin turgor. He looks pale with a systolic flow murmur 2/6 heard at the left sternal edge.'

He has signs of dehydration and poor perfusion and will require IV access and a fluid bolus of sodium chloride 0.9% 10 mL/kg followed by reassessment. Bloods including cross-match, blood culture and a blood gas can be sent at the same time.

DISABILITY

- Assess the patient's level of consciousness using AVPU (is the patient Alert? If not, do they respond to Verbal or Painful stimuli? Or are they Unresponsive?). Check glucose levels. Assess for pain, as this can be severe and needs addressing early.

'Fever 38.7°C, responds to voice, he seems confused and agitated. You ask about pain and he says his chest hurts.'

You give him antipyretics and first-line analgesia. You will have to assess response to pain relief shortly. The pain is severe, so you give morphine as well as paracetamol.

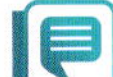

Prescribe (Figs 9.13–9.15)

OXYGEN therapy:
- 15 L 100% OXYGEN via NONREBREATHE MASK

Bronchodilator:
- SALBUTAMOL 2.5 mg NEB (driven with oxygen) STAT

Fluid bolus:
- SODIUM CHLORIDE 0.9% 230 mL (10 mL/kg) IV (over 20 min)

Analgesia:
- PARACETAMOL 480 mg PO STAT and MORPHINE 2.3 mg (0.1 mg/kg) IV STAT.

EXPOSURE

- Expose and examine further. Look for signs of infection including meningitis, chest and abdominal signs. Do not forget ears and throat as possible sources.
- Look for signs of systemic sickle cell disease. Look in the eyes for anaemia and jaundice. The patient may have a large spleen but by this age the spleen may be small and fibrotic (autosplenectomy).
- Look for other signs of vaso-occlusive crisis, including examining hands and feet for dactylitis and other joints for erythema, pain and tenderness and reduced range of movement.

'Temperature is 38.7°C. He has no signs of infection other than his chest as described earlier. He has pale conjunctivae and is mildly icteric. He has a 2 cm spleen and no hepatomegaly with a soft, nontender abdomen. He has some swelling and tenderness of his fingers and left elbow, which is warm to touch.'

INITIAL INVESTIGATIONS

- **Capillary blood gas:** May show signs of respiratory compromise with hypoventilation and a high $PaCO_2$. He may also have a metabolic acidosis with negative base excess if there is significant tissue hypoxia. Most blood gas machines will also give haemoglobin, which may be useful for early ordering of cross-matched blood if a transfusion is required.
- **Bloods:** FBC may show leucocytosis and anaemia, you should also ask for a reticulocyte count. Take U&Es as IV fluids will be required. Send a CRP and blood culture. Take an urgent group and save and consider cross-match if significant anaemia is suspected. A sickle cell index may be helpful (which measures the percentage of haemoglobin cells that are sickling) in guiding transfusion decisions (Table 9.5).
- **CXR:** May show atelectasis and signs of lobar consolidation.
- **Joint X-ray:** May be considered if there is localised joint pain or erythema/swelling present to help exclude pathological fractures or bone destruction from recurrent crises.

Table 9.5 Jimiyu's Blood and ABG Results

PARAMETER	VALUE	NORMAL RANGE (UNITS)
Haemoglobin	**65 g/L**	**115–145 (g/L)**
WCC	**17 × 10^9/L**	**4–12 (× 10^9/L)**
Neutrophil	**12 × 10^9/L**	**2.5–7.4 (× 10^9/L)**
Lymphocyte	2 × 10^9/L	1.2–3.5 (× 10^9/L)
Platelet	160 × 10^9/L	150–400 (× 10^9/L)
CRP	**67 mg/L**	**0.6–7.9 (mg/L)**
Urea	5.7 mmol/L	2.5–6.7 (mmol/L)
Creatinine	70 µmol/L	27.4–77.8 (µmol/L)
Sodium	139 mmol/L	135–145 (mmol/L)
Potassium	4.1 mmol/L	3.3–4.6 (mmol/L)
pH	**7.23**	**7.35–7.45**
$PaCO_2$	**8.0 kPa**	**4.7–6.0 (kPa)**
HCO_3	23 mmol/L	22–26 (mmol/L)
BE	−0.5 mmol/L	±2 mmol/L

Data in bold signifies results that are outside the normal laboratory range. *ABG*, Arterial blood gas; *BE*, base excess; *CRP*, C-reactive protein; *WCC*, white cell count.

- **Other cultures:** Consider urine and stool samples if clinically indicated.
- **Weight:** Important for fluid and drug calculations.

'Capillary blood gas shows a respiratory acidosis from hypoventilation with a pH 7.23, $PaCO_2$ of 8 kPa, BE −0.5 mmol/L. Hb is 65 g/L, WCC 17 × 10^9/L, neutrophils 12 × 10^9/L. CRP is 67 mg/L, with normal U&Es. CXR shows left-sided opacification with air bronchograms and loss of the left heart border. There are also streaky changes at both bases consistent with atelectasis. His weight is 23 kg.'

INITIAL MANAGEMENT

Management Summary: Sickle Cell Chest Crisis

- Resuscitate using an ABCDE approach
- IV antibiotics
- Analgesia
- Antipyretics
- Bronchodilators
- Oxygen as required
- Incentive spirometry
- Consider transfusion

Acute Chest Syndrome Management

The aim is to reverse any factors that may contribute to deoxygenation the sickle haemoglobin (HbS) to minimise sickling, improve blood flow and prevent tissue hypoxia.

- **Airway support:** None required in this case at present. Severe cases may require noninvasive ventilation (CPAP or bilevel positive airway pressure (Bi-PAP)) and sometimes intubation.
- **Oxygen:** Should be given to keep saturations >92%. Note deoxygenation of the sickle haemoglobin (HbS) causes increased sickling and worsening of vaso-occlusive disease.
- **Incentive spirometry:** Should be performed 2-hourly with a healthcare professional to prevent atelectasis from hypoventilation. This is effort dependent and so relies on good analgesia.
- **Bronchodilators:** Should be used regularly during a chest crisis if wheeze is present, especially in known asthmatics.
- **Analgesia/antipyretics:** Should always include simple analgesia including regular paracetamol and consideration of non-steroidal antiinflammatory drugs (NSAIDs). However, a patient with acute chest crisis may have severe pain and require opiates as well. If regular opiates are required, it may be worth considering a patient-controlled analgesia (PCA) or nurse-controlled analgesia (NCA) in younger children to prevent oversedation.
- **Antibiotics:** As infection is a common cause for acute chest crisis, antibiotics are recommended. Normally, a broad-spectrum cephalosporin is used alongside a macrolide for atypical cover. *Chlamydia* and *mycoplasma* are common causes.

IV Antibiotics

IV antibiotics are given to achieve high serum concentrations. However, the bioavailability of most macrolide antibiotics is the same IV as orally so, unless the patient is strictly NBM, these are normally given orally.

- **Fluids:** Once any dehydration has been corrected, you should maintain euvolaemia with full maintenance fluids (either IV or oral) (Box 9.4). A fluid balance chart will be helpful to ensure you are meeting this goal.
- **Transfusion:** Transfusion can be used to increase oxygen carriage in the blood and improve tissue hypoxia. Indications for transfusion include SpO_2 <92% in room air, multiorgan failure or if the haematocrit 10% to 20% lower than the patient's normal haematocrit. The patient should be transfused to a haematocrit of 30%, or a Hb of 110 g/L (Box 9.5) Please note some hospitals will have separate transfusion charts (with a pre transfusion checklist) and this must be prescribed on the appropriate chart.

Box 9.4 Full maintenance fluid must be calculated as below (weight is 23 kg)

First 10 kg body weight = 100 mL/kg × 10 kg = 1000 mL

Second 10 kg body weight = 50 mL/kg × 10 kg = 500 mL

Remainder of body weight = 20 mL/kg × 3 kg = 60 mL

This gives the total fluid requirement for a 24-hour period = 1560 mL

Prescribe 1560 mL/24 h = 65 mL/h.

Box 9.5 Transfusion Calculation

Change in Hb required [Desired Hb – Actual Hb] × 0.4 mL/ kg.

So, in this patient, if the Hb is 65 g/L and required Hb is 110 g/L, he will need:

(110 – 65) × 0.4 mL × 23 kg = 414 mL packed red cells.

- Blood must be used within 4 hours of coming from the fridge, so is often transfused over 3 to 4 hours.
- **Partial exchange transfusion:** This involves removing the patient's sickled haemoglobin and replacing with packed red cells to reduce the total percentage of HbS to <30% of the total haemoglobin. Indications include progressive chest crisis, multilobar disease and severe hypoxia.
- **Corticosteroids:** The role of IV corticosteroids is unclear as they can be helpful acutely but have been shown to be associated with an increased relapse rate. If considering corticosteroids, you should refer to local policies or specialist advice.
- **Intensive care:** Acute chest crisis is a potentially life-threatening condition with significant associated mortality. For moderate to severe cases, early referral to intensive care may be appropriate, especially as in paediatrics this frequently involves transfer to another centre.

REASSESSMENT

- After supplemental oxygen, inhaled bronchodilators, a fluid bolus, analgesia, antibiotics and blood transfusion, the patient is reassessed.

'Jimiyu looks to have improved. His airway is patent. RR 35/min, oxygen saturations are 97% in 100% facemask oxygen. He has intercostal recession but is no longer having to use all his accessory muscles. The wheeze has improved but he still has reduced air entry on the left with crackles. HR 114 bpm, BP 110/72 mmHg, he has a CRT 2 seconds centrally. He has moist mucous membranes. He looks less pale and his flow murmur has disappeared. He is alert and his temperature has come down to 37.6°C. He says his pain is well controlled at present.'

Prescribe (see Figs 9.13–9.15)

Antibiotics:
- CEFUROXIME 460 mg (20 mg/kg) IV TDS and AZITHROMYCIN 200 mg PO OD

Bronchodilators:
- SALBUTAMOL 2.5 mg NEB (driven with air or oxygen) 4 HOURLY

Regular analgesia/antipyretic:
- PARACETAMOL 480 mg PO QDS

Maintenance fluid:
- SODIUM CHLORIDE 0.9%/GLUCOSE 5% (with 10 mmol KCl) 500 mL IV 65 mL/h

Red cells:
- PACKED RED CELLS 414 mL IV (given over 3 h at 138 mL/h)

WITHHOLD

Penicillin V (since on treatment antibiotics)

HANDING OVER THE PATIENT

'Jimiyu is a 10-year-old boy with acute chest crisis secondary to sickle cell disease.

He presented with significant respiratory distress, fever and chest pain. Respiratory wise, he has required facemask oxygen and regular inhaled salbutamol. In terms of circulation, he initially was poorly perfused requiring a fluid bolus. He has also been given a blood transfusion for anaemia. His pain has been controlled with paracetamol and IV morphine; he has a history of asthma so has not been given NSAIDs. He has been started on cefuroxime and azithromycin. Currently, he is much improved. RR 35/min, oxygen saturations are 97% on 100% facemask oxygen. He is haemodynamically stable and his perfusion has improved.

Initial blood gas showed a respiratory acidosis, with a pH 7.23, $PaCO_2$ 8 kPa, BE –0.5 mmol/L. Initial Hb was 65 g/L, WCC 17 × 10^9/L and CRP was raised at 67 mg/L. CXR shows new focal infiltrates at the left base with bibasal atelectasis.

He has been reviewed by the consultant who does not feel he needs HDU at this time. The plan is to transfer him to the ward on oxygen with regular inhaled bronchodilators and incentive spirometry. He is on full maintenance IV fluids. He will need assessment for further analgesia and consideration of PCA if regular opiates are required. He will need a repeat capillary gas and FBC when the transfusion has finished. Supplementary oxygen should be continued to keep saturations above 92%.'

STATION 9.7: IDIOPATHIC NEPHROTIC SYNDROME

You are a junior doctor in the child assessment unit. A 6-year-old boy named Charlie has been referred by his GP with swelling around his eyes, for which he has been given antihistamines with no response. He has now developed abdominal distension. Please assess him and instigate appropriate management.

Patient Details

Name:	Charlie Manning
DOB:	12/07/18
Hospital number:	SDE1939493
Weight:	18 kg
Height:	106 cm
Consultant:	Dr Wi
Hospital/Ward:	BGH Paediatric ward
Current medications:	Nil
Allergies:	None known
Admission date:	01/11/24

Initial Differential Diagnosis of Oedema

- Glomerulonephritis
- Renal failure
- Heart failure
- Liver failure
- Hypothyroidism
- Protein losing enteropathy
- Angioedema
- Anaphylaxis

Acute Complications of Nephrotic Syndrome

- Hypovolaemia
- Hyponatraemia
- Pleural effusions
- Ascites with peritonitis
- Septicaemia
- Venous thromboembolism
- If atypical cause may develop renal failure, nephritis and hypertension with seizures

INITIAL ASSESSMENT

AIRWAY

- Assess patency of the airway. Is there any neck swelling that could cause airway obstruction?

'The airway is patent with no obstruction. He has no neck swelling or masses.'

No additional airway support is required.

BREATHING

- Assess respiratory rate, oxygen saturations and work of breathing. Auscultate for air entry and percuss for pleural effusions.
- Assess for focal signs of superadded infection such as crepitations or focal reduction in air entry.

'RR 18/min, oxygen saturations are 100%, with no evidence of increased work of breathing. There are no focal signs but air entry is slightly reduced at the bases bilaterally. There is slight dullness to percussion at the bases.'

Given there are no signs of respiratory compromise, he does not need intervention at present but may need a chest X-ray for possible basal effusions.

CIRCULATION

- Patients with nephrotic syndrome may be significantly intravascularly depleted despite peripheral oedema. Assess haemodynamic stability by measuring pulse rate, BP and CRT (centrally and peripherally). Also assess hydration status by looking for sunken eyes and looking at mucous membranes and skin turgor. Ask about urine output and fluid intake.
- Perform a cardiovascular examination to exclude heart failure as a primary cause. Assess for heaves and thrills, displaced apex beat and auscultate for murmurs. Signs of heart failure may include a gallop rhythm (added 3rd/4th heart sound), raised JVP and hepatomegaly.

'HR 98 bpm, BP 104/64 mmHg, CRT 2 seconds centrally. He has no signs of dehydration with good skin turgor and normal mucous membranes. He has been passing a lot of urine and drinking a lot of water. Cardiovascular examination is normal with normal heart sounds and no signs of heart failure, normal JVP and no hepatomegaly.'

He is haemodynamically stable at present without dehydration, so needs no immediate fluid resuscitation.

DISABILITY

- Assess the patient's level of consciousness using AVPU (is the patient Alert? If not, do they respond to Verbal or Painful stimuli? Or are they Unresponsive?). Check glucose levels.
- Assess for headache as patients with nephritis can develop hypertension causing severe headache and even reduced consciousness and seizures.

'He is alert and happy with a blood sugar of 5.1 mmol/L.'

EXPOSURE

- Expose the child looking for the extent of the oedema. Commonly affected sites include around the feet and calves, sacrum and abdomen. Be careful to exclude venous thromboembolism if calf swelling is painful, red or unilateral, as patients with nephrotic syndrome are prothrombotic (due to renal loss of antithrombin III).
- Perform an abdominal examination as ascites with peritonitis can cause significant morbidity and needs urgent attention (due to static fluid in the abdomen and relative immunodeficiency due to renal loss of immunoglobulin and complement). There may be a distended abdomen or oedematous anterior abdominal wall. Palpate gently for tenderness; if there is any tenderness, look for signs of peritonitis such as guarding. If there is distension, examine for ascites with fluid thrill or shifting dullness. Palpate for organomegaly and lymphadenopathy. There may be significant oedema of the genitalia.
- Measure the temperature as a marker of superadded infection, which should be investigated and treated aggressively if suspected.

Diagnostic Criteria (All Three Are Required)

1. Oedema
2. Hypoalbuminaemia of <30 g/L
3. Nephrotic range proteinuria, either PCR >300 mg/mmol or urinary protein excretion >50 mg/kg per day

'Charlie has periorbital oedema and peripheral oedema up to his knees. There are no signs of venous thromboembolism. His abdomen is distended and he has signs of ascites including shifting dullness and fluid thrill. His abdomen is nontender with no evidence of peritonitis. He has no organomegaly. His temperature is 36.8°C and he has no signs of superadded infection.'

INITIAL INVESTIGATIONS

- **Urinalysis:** Initial dipstick can be helpful and would be expected to show 3+ of protein or more. It is also useful to exclude haematuria (which might suggest nephritis or more atypical nephrotic syndrome) and exclude urine infection.
- For diagnostic purposes, formal urinalysis is required. Nephrotic range proteinuria is defined as urinary protein excretion >50 mg/kg per day on 24-hour urine collection. A urine PCR of >300 mg protein/mmol creatinine on a single urine sample is also considered nephrotic range and is helpful when 24-hour collection is difficult or impractical.
- **Bloods:** Hypoalbuminaemia of <30 g/L is another diagnostic criterion for nephrotic syndrome. It is important to check U&Es and estimated glomerular filtration rate (GFR) to exclude renal impairment, which would suggest an atypical cause requiring specialist review. Hyponatraemia is common and electrolytes may need close monitoring, especially if the child requires rehydration. Other initial tests include FBC, inflammatory markers and blood cultures for superadded infection. The FBC may show thrombocytosis. Hyperlipidaemia is common. Some centres suggest checking complement levels initially as low C3/C4 can suggest atypical causes for nephrotic syndrome that may require further investigation including biopsy (Table 9.6).
- **Weight:** Very important for accurate prescribing. Daily weights will also help guide fluid management in patients who are intravascularly depleted. For these patients, strict input/output monitoring should be performed.
- **Height:** Important for calculating body surface area which is required for prescribing in nephrotic syndrome.
- **CXR:** Indicated for respiratory compromise; may demonstrate bilateral pleural effusions.

'Charlie meets diagnostic criteria for nephrotic syndrome with peripheral oedema, a raised protein–creatinine ratio of 370 mg/mmol and hypoalbuminaemia of 19 g/L. His urine dipstick also shows 4+ protein. Microscopy shows no red cells or white cells. He has normal urea and creatinine. Sodium is 135 mmol/L, potassium is 4.6 mmol/L. FBC shows thrombocytosis and there is no evidence of infection with normal WCC and normal inflammatory markers. Total cholesterol and triglycerides are raised, C3/C4 are normal. He has no features or findings of atypical nephrotic syndrome. His weight is 18 kg and his height 106 cm.'

Table 9.6 Charlie's Bloods

PARAMETER	VALUE	NORMAL RANGE (UNITS)
Haemoglobin	125 g/L	115–145 (g/L)
WCC	9 × 10^9/L	3.2–11 (× 10^9/L)
Platelet	**440 × 10^9/L**	**150–400 (× 10^9/L)**
Protein/ creatinine ratio	**370 mg/mmol**	**<300 (mg/mmol)**
Albumin	**19 g/L**	**35–56 (g/L)**
Sodium	135 mmol/L	134–144 (mmol/L)
Potassium	4.6 mmol/L	3.3–4.6 (mmol/L)
C3	1.25 g/L	0.75–1.65 (g/L)
C4	0.45 g/L	0.20–0.60 (g/L)
Cholesterol	**7.5 mmol/L**	**3.5–6.5 (mmol/L)**
HDL cholesterol	1.2 mmol/L	0.8–1.8 (mmol/L)
LDL cholesterol	**5.5 mmol/L**	**<4 (mmol/L)**
Triglycerides	**3.2 mmol/L**	**0.5–1.7 (mmol/L)**
Urea	6 mmol/L	2.5–6.7 (mmol/L)
Creatinine	50 µmol/L	2.65–52.2 (µmol/L)

Data in bold signifies results that are outside the normal laboratory range. *HDL*, High-density lipoprotein; *LDL*, low-density lipoprotein; *WCC*, white cell count.

Atypical Features

Presence of atypical features at presentation would require specialist advice before starting treatment, i.e. await specialist input before giving any corticosteroids:

- Macroscopic haematuria
- Hypertension
- Renal impairment
- Low C3/C4
- Age less than 1 year
- Age more than 10 years

INITIAL MANAGEMENT

Management Summary: Nephrotic Syndrome

- Confirm diagnosis with urinalysis, plasma albumin, urinary protein, urine protein–creatinine ratio (PCR)
- Look for atypical features
- High-dose corticosteroids
- Early identification of infection
- Careful fluid management

- **Corticosteroids:** Provided there are no atypical features present at diagnosis to suggest aetiology other than minimal change disease, most children are treated empirically with oral corticosteroids which are started at a high dose and slowly weaned. You should refer to your local trust or tertiary centre protocol but a typical regimen is likely to start at 60 mg/m² body surface area of prednisolone once per day for 4 to 6 weeks until remission, followed by a slow weaning regimen of alternate day prednisolone over several months. A maximum dose of 80 mg per day can be given.

> Body surface area (m^2) can be calculated by: √ (height in cm × weight in kg/3600)
> For Charlie, this equals the square root of (106 cm × 18 kg / 3600) = 0.73 m^2
> The initial dose of prednisolone is 60 mg/m^2 = 60 mg × 0.73 m^2. This equals 43.8 mg once daily (often rounded to the nearest 5 mg)
> You prescribe 45 mg oral OD.

- Weaning regimens can be followed provided the child goes into remission and does not relapse as the corticosteroids are weaned.
- **Fluid management:** Fluid management can be complex in nephrotic syndrome. Children may be well and just need input/output monitoring, or may be intravascularly deplete requiring IV replacement (resuscitation and maintenance) with close attention paid to electrolytes, fluid balance and daily weights. As such, fluid management should be overseen by an experienced paediatrician. Some basic principles in nephrotic syndrome include:
  - Fluid resuscitation for hypovolaemia should be discussed with seniors urgently. Often albumin infusions are used on specialist advice (since hypoalbuminaemia in these patients causes a fluid shift from circulating fluid into extravascular space).
  - Salt restriction may be used to treat oedema as the patient may have a high total body sodium (note the kidneys retain sodium when intravascularly deplete).
  - Fluid restriction has a role in patients who are not volume depleted and can be helpful in reducing oedema.
  - Diuretics: The role of diuretics is controversial but may be useful for severe oedema. Intravascular volume depletion is a contraindication to diuretics. Furosemide is sometimes used in conjunction with albumin infusions in severe cases with respiratory compromise or massive ascites.
- **Infection:** Due to loss of immunoglobulin, children are at risk of infection from encapsulated bacteria such as streptococcus pneumoniae. Prophylactic antibiotics are not given but infection should be treated promptly. The pneumococcal vaccine should be considered. Children can also be at risk of varicella and so vaccination should be considered for those with negative varicella titres.
- **Hypercoagulability**: Prophylactic anticoagulation is not commonly offered but risk should be minimised by mobilisation and prompt management of hypovolaemia, volume depletion and sepsis. Anticoagulation with heparin may be used if thrombosis occurs.

Definitions in Nephrotic Syndrome

- Remission: Dipstick shows no protein for three consecutive days
- Relapse: Urine protein 2+ or more for three consecutive days
- Frequent relapse: Two or more episodes of relapse in first 6 months of treatment

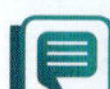

Prescribe (Fig. 9.16)

Corticosteroids:
- PREDNISOLONE 45 mg (60 mg/m^2) PO OD

REASSESSMENT

- After several days of prednisolone, dietary salt restriction and fluid balance monitoring, the patient is reassessed.

'Charlie looks significantly improved. Airway remains patent. RR 18/min, oxygen saturations are 100% in air. Air entry at the lung bases has improved with resolution of percussion dullness. HR 100 bpm, BP 102/58 mmHg, CRT 1 second centrally, 2 seconds peripherally. He remains well hydrated. His periorbital oedema has resolved and his peripheral oedema is improving. His ascites has reduced in size and his abdomen remains nontender. He remains afebrile and there is no evidence of thromboembolism.'

HANDING OVER THE PATIENT

'Charlie is a 6-year-old boy with first presentation of nephrotic syndrome.

He presented 3 days ago with periorbital oedema, peripheral oedema and ascites. There were initially signs consistent with small pleural effusions but Charlie did not require respiratory support. In terms of circulation, he had no evidence of volume depletion or dehydration and was haemodynamically stable without hypertension. His blood sugar was normal. He had no abdominal pain or evidence of peritonitis, no evidence of infection and no evidence of venous thromboembolism.

Investigations confirmed the diagnosis of nephrotic syndrome with albumin of 19 g/L and PCR of 370 mg/mmol. He had no haematuria and no evidence of renal failure or infection on his initial blood tests. Complement levels were normal.

As he has no atypical features, he was initially treated for idiopathic nephrotic syndrome with salt restriction and oral prednisolone at 60 mg/m² once daily. He remains stable and his oedema is improving.

The plan is to continue his current corticosteroid treatment for 1 month with ongoing review of his urinary protein losses. His parents are being trained on how and when to dipstick his urine to help detect relapse. The plan is for him to be discharged later this week.'

FURTHER READING

BTS/Sign Guidelines, 2019. Asthma. Available at: https://www.brit-thoracic.org.uk/quality-improvement/guidelines/asthma/ (Last accessed 12.09.24).

Geeky Medics, 2023. Paediatric intravenous (IV) fluid prescribing. Available at: https://geekymedics.com/intravenous-iv-fluid-prescribing-in-paediatrics/ (Last accessed 12.09.24).

NHSGGC Paediatrics for Health Professionals, 2023. Sickle cell protocol. Available at: https://www.clinicalguidelines.scot.nhs.uk/nhsggc-guidelines/nhsggc-guidelines/haematologyoncology/sickle-cell-protocol/ (Last accessed 12.09.24).

Niaudet, P., 2022. Treatment of idiopathic nephrotic syndrome in children. https://www.uptodate.com/contents/treatment-of-idiopathic-nephrotic-syndrome-in-children (Last accessed 12.09.24).

NICE Guidelines, 2009. Diarrhoea and vomiting caused by gastroenteritis in under 5s: diagnosis and management. Available at: https://www.nice.org.uk/guidance/cg84/chapter/Recommendations#assessing-dehydration-and-shock-2 (Last accessed 12.09.24).

NICE Guidelines, 2020. Intravenous fluid therapy in children and young people in hospital. Available at: https://www.nice.org.uk/guidance/ng29/chapter/Recommendations#fluid-resuscitation-2 (Last accessed 12.09.24).

NICE Guidelines, 2021. Neonatal infection: antibiotics for prevention and treatment. Available at: https://www.nice.org.uk/guidance/ng195 (Last accessed 12.09.24).

NICE Guidelines, 2021. Bronchiolitis in children: diagnosis and management. Available at: https://www.nice.org.uk/guidance/ng9 (Last accessed 12.09.24).

NICE Guidelines, 2023. Scenario: child gastroenteritis. Available at: https://cks.nice.org.uk/topics/gastroenteritis/management/child-gastroenteritis/ (Last accessed 12.09.24).

PRESCRIPTION CHARTS

PRESCRIPTION AND ADMINISTRATION RECORD
Standard Chart

Hospital/Ward: BGH PAEDIATRIC WARD **Consultant:** DR WI	**Name of Patient:** LAYLA JAMES
Weight: 7kg **Height:**	**Hospital Number:** L3439402
If re-written, date:	**D.O.B.:** 2/4/2024
DISCHARGE PRESCRIPTION **Date completed:-** **Completed by:-**	

OTHER MEDICINE CHARTS IN USE		PREVIOUS ADVERSE REACTIONS This section must be completed before any medicine is given		Completed by (sign & print)	Date
Date	Type of Chart	None known ☒		P. Smith PAUL SMITH	12/10/24
		Medicine/Agent	Description of Reaction		

CODES FOR NON-ADMINISTRATION OF PRESCRIBED MEDICINE

If a dose is not administered as prescribed, initial and enter a code in the column with a circle drawn round the code according to the reason as shown below. **Inform the responsible doctor in the appropriate timescale.**

1. Patient refuses
2. Patient not present
3. Medicines not available – CHECK ORDERED
4. Asleep/drowsy
5. Administration route not available – CHECK FOR ALTERNATIVE
6. Vomiting/nausea
7. Time varied on doctor's instructions
8. Once only/as required medicine given
9. Dose withheld on doctor's instructions
10. Possible adverse reaction/side effect

ONCE-ONLY

Date	Time	Medicine (Approved Name)	Dose	Route	Prescriber – Sign + Print	Time Given	Given By

OXYGEN	Start		Route		Prescriber – Sign + Print	Administered by	Stop	
	Date	Time	Mask (%)	Prongs (L/min)			Date	Time
	12/10/24	12.00		2L/min via NASAL CANNULAE	P. Smith PAUL SMITH	KP		

Fig. 9.1 Prescription and administration record (standard chart) for Layla James.

FLUID PRESCRIPTION CHART

Hospital/Ward: BGH PAEDIATRIC WARD	Consultant: DR WI	Name of Patient: LAYLA JAMES
		Hospital Number: L3439402
Weight: 7kg	Height:	D.O.B: 2/4/2024

Date/ Time	FLUID / ADDED DRUGS	VOLUME / DOSE	ROUTE	RATE	PRESCRIBER – SIGN AND PRINT
12/10/24 12.00	SODIUM CHLORIDE 0.9% (10 mL/kg)	70mL	IV	Over 15 min	P. Smith PAUL SMITH
12/10/24 13.00	SODIUM CHLORIDE 0.9%/GLUCOSE 5%	500 mL	IV	19.4 mL/h	P. Smith PAUL SMITH

Fig. 9.2 Fluid prescription chart for Layla James.

PRESCRIPTION AND ADMINISTRATION RECORD

Standard Chart

Hospital/Ward: BGH SCBU **Consultant:** DR WI	**Name of Patient:** MALE INFANT KHAN
Weight: 3.5 kg **Height:**	**Hospital Number:** XS349960469
If re-written, date:	**D.O.B:** 12/10/2024
DISCHARGE PRESCRIPTION **Date completed:-** **Completed by:-**	

OTHER MEDICINE CHARTS IN USE		**PREVIOUS ADVERSE REACTIONS** This section must be completed before any medicine is given		Completed by (sign & print)	Date
Date	Type of Chart	None known ☒		P. Smith PAUL SMITH	12/10/24
		Medicine/Agent	Description of Reaction		

CODES FOR NON-ADMINISTRATION OF PRESCRIBED MEDICINE

If a dose is not administered as prescribed, initial and enter a code in the column with a circle drawn round the code according to the reason as shown below. **Inform the responsible doctor in the appropriate timescale.**

1. Patient refuses
2. Patient not present
3. Medicines not available – CHECK ORDERED
4. Asleep/drowsy
5. Administration route not available – CHECK FOR ALTERNATIVE
6. Vomiting/nausea
7. Time varied on doctor's instructions
8. Once only/as required medicine given
9. Dose withheld on doctor's instructions
10. Possible adverse reaction/side effect

ONCE-ONLY

Date	Time	Medicine (Approved Name)	Dose	Route	Prescriber – Sign + Print	Time Given	Given By
12/10/24	02.00	VITAMIN K	1 mg	IM	P. Smith PAUL SMITH	02.10	DF

	Start		Route		Prescriber – Sign + Print	Administered by	Stop	
	Date	Time	Mask (%)	Prongs (L/min)			Date	Time
OXYGEN	12/10/24	02.00	Oxygen 1 L/min via NASAL CANNULAE		P. Smith PAUL SMITH	FG		

Fig. 9.3 Prescription and administration record (standard chart) for male infant Khan.

Name: MALE INFANT KHAN

Date of Birth: 12/10/2024

REGULAR THERAPY

PRESCRIPTION		Date → Time ↓		12/10/24											
Medicine (Approved Name) BENZYLPENICILLIN		6	(2)	FD											
Dose 175 mg	Route IV	8													
		12													
Notes 50 mg/kg/dose. For pneumonia. Review at 48 h Given over 30 mins	Start Date 12/10/24	(14)		FD											
Prescriber – sign + print P. Smith PAUL SMITH		18													
		22													
Medicine (Approved Name) GENTAMICIN		6	(2)												
Dose	Route	8													
		12													
Notes See gentamicin chart	Start Date 12/10/24	14													
Prescriber – sign + print P. Smith PAUL SMITH		18													
		22													
Medicine (Approved Name)		6													
Dose	Route	8													
		12													
Notes	Start Date	14													
Prescriber – sign + print		18													
		22													
Medicine (Approved Name)		6													
Dose	Route	8													
		12													
Notes	Start Date	14													
Prescriber – sign + print		18													
		22													
Medicine (Approved Name)		6													
Dose	Route	8													
		12													
Notes	Start Date	14													
Prescriber – sign + print		18													
		22													
Medicine (Approved Name)		6													
Dose	Route	8													
		12													
Notes	Start Date	14													
Prescriber – sign + print		18													
		22													

Fig. 9.4 Prescription and administration record (regular therapy) for male infant Khan.

FLUID PRESCRIPTION CHART

Hospital/Ward: BGH SCBU **Consultant:** DR WI

Weight: 3.5 kg **Height:**

Name of Patient: MALE INFANT KHAN

Hospital Number: XS349960469

D.O.B: 12/10/2024

Date/ Time	FLUID / ADDED DRUGS	VOLUME / DOSE	ROUTE	RATE	PRESCRIBER – SIGN AND PRINT
12/10/24 02.00	GLUCOSE 10% (2mL/kg)	7 mL	IV	Over 5 min	P. Smith PAUL SMITH
12/10/24 02.05	GLUCOSE 10% (60 mL/kg/day)	500 mL	IV	8.8 mL/h	P. Smith PAUL SMITH

Fig. 9.5 Fluid prescription chart for male infant Khan.

Name: *MALE INFANT KHAN*
Date of Birth: *12/10/2024*

THERAPY REQUIRING LEVEL MONITORING

PRESCRIPTION	
Medicine (Approved Name) *GENTAMICIN*	
Dose *17.5 mg*	Route *IV*
Notes *GENTAMICIN (5 mg/kg)*	Start Date *12/10/24*
Prescriber–sign + print *P. Smith PAUL SMITH*	

Date → Time ↓		12/10/2024			13/10/2024			14/10/2024			15/10/2024			16/10/2024		
		Time Level taken	Level result	Given by (and time)	Time Level taken	Level result	Given by (and time)	Time Level taken	Level result	Given by (and time)	Time Level taken	Level result	Given by (and time)	Time Level taken	Level result	Given by (and time)
6	(2)			*DS 02.00*												
8					*Pre-dose level due*											
12																
14																
18																
22																

PRESCRIPTION	
Medicine (Approved Name)	
Dose	Route
Notes	Start Date
Prescriber–sign + print	

Date → Time ↓																
		Time Level taken	Level result	Given by (and time)	Time Level taken	Level result	Given by (and time)	Time Level taken	Level result	Given by (and time)	Time Level taken	Level result	Given by (and time)	Time Level taken	Level result	Given by (and time)
6																
8																
12																
14																
18																
22																

Fig. 9.6 Prescription and administration record (gentamicin chart) for male infant Khan.

PRESCRIPTION AND ADMINISTRATION RECORD

Standard Chart

Hospital/Ward: BGH PAEDIATRIC WARD **Consultant:** DR WI	**Name of Patient:** TANIA KEYA
Weight: 20kg **Height:**	**Hospital Number:** XD11324059
If re-written, date:	**D.O.B:** 23/05/2018
DISCHARGE PRESCRIPTION **Date completed:-** **Completed by:-**	

OTHER MEDICINE CHARTS IN USE		PREVIOUS ADVERSE REACTIONS This section must be completed before any medicine is given		Completed by (sign & print)	Date
Date	Type of Chart	None known ☒		P. Smith PAUL SMITH	15/11/24
		Medicine/Agent	Description of Reaction		

CODES FOR NON-ADMINISTRATION OF PRESCRIBED MEDICINE

If a dose is not administered as prescribed, initial and enter a code in the column with a circle drawn round the code according to the reason as shown below. **Inform the responsible doctor in the appropriate timescale.**

1. Patient refuses
2. Patient not present
3. Medicines not available – CHECK ORDERED
4. Asleep/drowsy
5. Administration route not available – CHECK FOR ALTERNATIVE
6. Vomiting/nausea
7. Time varied on doctor's instructions
8. Once only/as required medicine given
9. Dose withheld on doctor's instructions
10. Possible adverse reaction/side effect

ONCE-ONLY

Date	Time	Medicine (Approved Name)	Dose	Route	Prescriber – Sign + Print	Time Given	Given By
15/11/24	11.00	SALBUTAMOL (driven with oxygen)	5 mg	NEB	P. Smith PAUL SMITH	11.00	FD
15/11/24	11.00	IPRATROPIUM BROMIDE (driven with oxygen)	250 micrograms	NEB	P. Smith PAUL SMITH	11.00	FD
15/11/24	11.10	SALBUTAMOL (driven with oxygen)	5 mg	NEB	P. Smith PAUL SMITH	11.10	FD
15/11/24	11.10	PREDNISOLONE	40 mg	PO	P. Smith PAUL SMITH	11.10	FD
15/11/24	11.10	IPRATROPIUM BROMIDE (driven with oxygen)	250 micrograms	NEB	P. Smith PAUL SMITH	11.10	FD
15/11/24	11.20	SALBUTAMOL (driven with oxygen)	5 mg	NEB	P. Smith PAUL SMITH	11.20	FD
15/11/24	11.20	IPRATROPIUM BROMIDE (driven with oxygen)	250 micrograms	NEB	P. Smith PAUL SMITH	11.20	FD
15/11/24	11.25	MAGNESIUM SULFATE (driven with oxygen)	150 mg	NEB	P. Smith PAUL SMITH	11.40	FD
15/11/24	11.30	MAGNESIUM SULFATE (40 mg/kg over 20 mins)	800 mg	IV	P. Smith PAUL SMITH	11.50	FD
15/11/24	11.50	SALBUTAMOL (15 micrograms/kg over 5 mins)	250 micrograms	IV	P. Smith PAUL SMITH	12.10	FD

OXYGEN	Start Date	Start Time	Route Mask (%)	Route Prongs (L/min)	Prescriber – Sign + Print	Administered by	Stop Date	Stop Time
	15/11/24	11.00	100% via NON-REBREATHE FACE MASK		P. Smith PAUL SMITH	FD		

Fig. 9.7 Prescription and administration record (standard chart) for Tania Keya.

FLUID PRESCRIPTION CHART

Hospital/Ward: BGH PAEDIATRIC WARD	Consultant: DR WI	Name of Patient: TANIA KEYA
		Hospital Number: XD11324059
Weight: 20 kg	Height:	D.O.B: 23/05/2018

Date/ Time	FLUID / ADDED DRUGS	VOLUME / DOSE	ROUTE	RATE	PRESCRIBER – SIGN AND PRINT
15/11/24 12.00	SODIUM CHLORIDE 0.9%	50 mL	IV	6 mL/min	P. Smith PAUL SMITH
	SALBUTAMOL (1 microgram/kg/min)	10 mL			

Fig. 9.8 Fluid prescription chart for Tania Keya.

Name: *IMOGEN SAUNDERS*
Date of Birth: *02/04/2008*

REGULAR THERAPY

PRESCRIPTION

Date → / Time ↓		01/11/24											

Medicine (Approved Name)	
PIPERACILLIN/TAZOBACTAM	
Dose: *4.5g*	Route: *IV*
Notes: *For chest infection 14 days given over 30 mins*	Start Date: *01/11/24*
Prescriber – sign + print: *P. Smith PAUL SMITH*	

Time		01/11/24											
(6)		*FD*											
8													
12													
(14)		*FD*											
18													
(22)		*FD*											

Medicine (Approved Name)	
AMIKACIN	
Dose:	Route:
Notes: *See amikacin chart*	Start Date: *01/11/24*
Prescriber – sign + print: *P. Smith PAUL SMITH*	

Time		01/11/24											
(6)													
8													
12													
(14)													
18													
(22)													

Medicine (Approved Name)	
DORNASE ALFA	
Dose: *2500 units (2.5 mg)*	Route: *NEB*
Notes: *1 hour before physio*	Start Date: *01/11/24*
Prescriber – sign + print: *P. Smith PAUL SMITH*	

Time		01/11/24											
6													
(8)		*FD*											
12													
14													
18													
22													

Medicine (Approved Name)	
CREON 10000 (PANCREATIN)	
Dose: *2 capsules*	Route: *ORAL*
Notes: *With meals*	Start Date: *01/11/24*
Prescriber – sign + print: *P. Smith PAUL SMITH*	

Time		01/11/24											
6													
(8)		*FD*											
(12)		*FD*											
14													
(18)		*FD*											
22													

Medicine (Approved Name)	
CREON 10000 (PANCREATIN)	
Dose: *1 capsule*	Route: *ORAL*
Notes: *With snacks*	Start Date: *01/11/24*
Prescriber – sign + print: *P. Smith PAUL SMITH*	

Time		01/11/24											
6													
8													
12													
(14)		*FD*											
18													
22	(20)	*FD*											

Medicine (Approved Name)	
RANITIDINE	
Dose: *150 mg*	Route: *ORAL*
Notes: *2 hours before food*	Start Date: *01/11/24*
Prescriber – sign + print: *P. Smith PAUL SMITH*	

Time		01/11/24											
(6)		*FD*											
8													
12													
14													
18	(16)	*FD*											
22													

Fig. 9.9 Prescription and administration record (regular therapy) for Imogen Saunders.

Name: *IMOGEN SAUNDERS*
Date of Birth: *02/04/2008*

REGULAR THERAPY

PRESCRIPTION

Medicine (Approved Name)		Date → / Time ↓		01/11/24											
DOMPERIDONE		(6)		FD											
Dose: *10 mg*	Route: *ORAL*	8													
		12													
Notes	Start Date: *01/11/24*	(14)		FD											
Prescriber – sign + print		18													
P. Smith PAUL SMITH		(22)		FD											

Medicine (Approved Name)		Time		01/11/24											
DALIVIT (VITAMINS A, B, C AND D)		(6)		FD											
Dose: *1 mL*	Route: *ORAL*	8													
		12													
Notes	Start Date: *01/11/24*	14													
Prescriber – sign + print		18													
P. Smith PAUL SMITH		22													

Medicine (Approved Name)		Time													
		6													
Dose	Route	8													
		12													
Notes	Start Date	14													
Prescriber – sign + print		18													
		22													

Medicine (Approved Name)		Time													
		6													
Dose	Route	8													
		12													
Notes	Start Date	14													
Prescriber – sign + print		18													
		22													

Medicine (Approved Name)		Time													
		6													
Dose	Route	8													
		12													
Notes	Start Date	14													
Prescriber – sign + print		18													
		22													

Medicine (Approved Name)		Time													
		6													
Dose	Route	8													
		12													
Notes	Start Date	14													
Prescriber – sign + print		18													
		22													

Fig. 9.10 Prescription and administration record (standard chart) for Imogen Saunders.

Name: *IMOGEN SAUNDERS*
Date of Birth: *02/04/2008*

THERAPY REQUIRING LEVEL MONITORING

PRESCRIPTION	
Medicine (Approved Name) *AMIKACIN*	
Dose *390 mg*	Route *IV*
Notes *10 mg/kg for chest infection for 14 days*	Start Date *01/11/24*
Prescriber–sign + print *P. Smith PAUL SMITH*	

Date → / Time ↓	1/11/2024			2/11/2024			3/11/2024			4/11/2024			5/11/2024		
	Time Level taken	Level result	Given by (and time)	Time Level taken	Level result	Given by (and time)	Time Level taken	Level result	Given by (and time)	Time Level taken	Level result	Given by (and time)	Time Level taken	Level result	Given by (and time)
(6)			*FD 06.00*												
8					*Pre-dose level due*										
12															
(14)			*FD 14.00*												
18															
(22)			*FD 22.00*												

PRESCRIPTION	
Medicine (Approved Name)	
Dose	Route
Notes	Start Date
Prescriber–sign + print	

Date → / Time ↓															
	Time Level taken	Level result	Given by (and time)	Time Level taken	Level result	Given by (and time)	Time Level taken	Level result	Given by (and time)	Time Level taken	Level result	Given by (and time)	Time Level taken	Level result	Given by (and time)
6															
8															
12															
14															
18															
22															

Fig. 9.11 Prescription and administration record (Amikacin therapy) for Imogen Saunders.

ORAL FLUID PRESCRIPTION CHART

Hospital/Ward: BGH PAEDIATRIC WARD	Consultant: DR WI	Name of Patient: Brychan MATTHEWS
		Hospital Number: SDE1939102
Weight: 6 kg	Height:	D.O.B: 09/08/2024

Date/ Time	FLUID / ADDED DRUGS	VOLUME / DOSE	ROUTE	RATE	PRESCRIBER – SIGN AND PRINT
14/10/24 12.00	WATER	400 mL	NG	100 mL/h via nasogastric tube	P. Smith PAUL SMITH
	DIORALYTE	2 sachets			
14/10/24 16.00	WATER	200 mL	NG	25 mL/h via nasogastric tube	P. Smith PAUL SMITH
	DIORALYTE	1 sachet			

Fig. 9.12 **Oral fluid prescription chart for Brychan Matthews.** Note: In some hospitals, there may be a separate chart for oral fluids and nasogastric (or enteral) feeding but in others this must be prescribed on the standard fluid chart noting very clearly the route of administration.

PRESCRIPTION AND ADMINISTRATION RECORD

Standard Chart

Hospital/Ward: BGH PAEDIATRIC WARD **Consultant:** DR WI	**Name of Patient:** JIMIYU ABOSI
Weight: 23 kg **Height:**	**Hospital Number:** GF54034930
If re-written, date:	**D.O.B:** 05/02/2014
DISCHARGE PRESCRIPTION **Date completed:-** **Completed by:-**	

OTHER MEDICINE CHARTS IN USE		PREVIOUS ADVERSE REACTIONS This section must be completed before any medicine is given		Completed by (sign & print)	Date
Date	Type of Chart	None known ☒		P. Smith PAUL SMITH	15/11/24
		Medicine/Agent	Description of Reaction		

CODES FOR NON-ADMINISTRATION OF PRESCRIBED MEDICINE

If a dose is not administered as prescribed, initial and enter a code in the column with a circle drawn round the code according to the reason as shown below. **Inform the responsible doctor in the appropriate timescale.**

1. Patient refuses
2. Patient not present
3. Medicines not available – CHECK ORDERED
4. Asleep/drowsy
5. Administration route not available – CHECK FOR ALTERNATIVE
6. Vomiting/nausea
7. Time varied on doctor's instructions
8. Once only/as required medicine given
9. Dose withheld on doctor's instructions
10. Possible adverse reaction/side effect

ONCE-ONLY

Date	Time	Medicine (Approved Name)	Dose	Route	Prescriber – Sign + Print	Time Given	Given By
15/11/24	14.15	SALBUTAMOL (driven with oxygen)	2.5 mg	NEB	P. Smith PAUL SMITH	14.15	FR
15/11/24	14.20	PARACETAMOL	480mg	ORAL	P. Smith PAUL SMITH	14.20	FR
15/11/24	14.45	MORPHINE (0.1 mg/kg titrate to response)	2.3 mg	IV	P. Smith PAUL SMITH	14.50	FR (2.3 mg)

OXYGEN	Start Date	Start Time	Route Mask (%)	Route Prongs (L/min)	Prescriber – Sign + Print	Administered by	Stop Date	Stop Time
	15/11/24	14.00	15L 100% OXYGEN via NON-REBREATHE MASK		P. Smith PAUL SMITH	FR		

Fig. 9.13 Prescription and administration record (standard chart) for Jimmy Abosi.

Name: JIMIYU ABOSI

Date of Birth: 05/02/2014

REGULAR THERAPY

PRESCRIPTION

Medicine (Approved Name): CEFUROXIME
Dose: 460 mg | **Route:** IV
Notes: 20 mg/kg/dose. For sickle cell chest crisis. Review after 48 h | **Start Date:** 15/11/24
Prescriber – sign + print: P. Smith PAUL SMITH

Date → / Time ↓		15/11/24	16/11/24										
(6)			FG										
8													
12													
(14)		FG	FG										
18													
(22)		FG											

Medicine (Approved Name): AZITHROMYCIN
Dose: 200 mg | **Route:** ORAL
Notes: For sickle cell chest crisis review after 48 h | **Start Date:** 15/11/24
Prescriber – sign + print: P. Smith PAUL SMITH

Date → / Time ↓		15/11/24	16/11/24										
6													
8													
12													
(14)		FG	FG										
18													
22													

Medicine (Approved Name): PARACETAMOL
Dose: 480 mg QDS | **Route:** ORAL
Notes: | **Start Date:** 15/11/24
Prescriber – sign + print: P. Smith PAUL SMITH

Date → / Time ↓		15/11/24	16/11/24										
6	(02)		FG										
(8)			FG										
12													
(14)		x	FG										
18													
22	(20)	FG											

Medicine (Approved Name): SALBUTAMOL
Dose: 2.5 mg | **Route:** NEB
Notes: Driven with air or oxygen | **Start Date:** 15/11/24
Prescriber – sign + print: P. Smith PAUL SMITH

Date → / Time ↓		15/11/24	16/11/24										
6	(04)		FG										
(8)			FG										
(12)			FG										
14	(16)	x											
18	(20)	FG											
22	(24)	FG											

Medicine (Approved Name):
Dose: | **Route:**
Notes: | **Start Date:**
Prescriber – sign + print:

Date → / Time ↓													
6													
8													
12													
14													
18													
22													

Medicine (Approved Name):
Dose: | **Route:**
Notes: | **Start Date:**
Prescriber – sign + print:

Date → / Time ↓													
6													
8													
12													
14													
18													
22													

Fig. 9.14 Prescription and administration record (regular therapy chart) for Jimmy Abosi.

FLUID PRESCRIPTION CHART

Hospital/Ward: BGH PAEDIATRIC WARD	Consultant: DR WI	Name of Patient: JIMIYU ABOSI
		Hospital Number: GF54034930
Weight: 23 kg	Height: 1 m	D.O.B: 05/02/2014

Date/ Time	FLUID / ADDED DRUGS	VOLUME / DOSE	ROUTE	RATE	PRESCRIBER – SIGN AND PRINT
15/11/24 14.00	SODIUM CHLORIDE 0.9% (10 mL/kg)	230 mL	IV	Over 20 min	P. Smith PAUL SMITH
15/11/24 14.30	SODIUM CHLORIDE 0.9% /GLUCOSE 5%	500 mL	IV	65 mL/h	P. Smith PAUL SMITH
	POTASSIUM CHLORIDE	10 mmol			
15/11/24 15.00	PACKED RED CELLS	414 mL	IV	138 mL/h	P. Smith PAUL SMITH

Fig. 9.15 Fluid prescription chart for Jimiyu Abosi. Note blood prescriptions are often done on a separate prescription chart.

Name: *CHARLIE MANNING*

Date of Birth: *12/07/2018*

REGULAR THERAPY

PRESCRIPTION	Date → Time ↓		01/11/24											

Medicine (Approved Name): *PREDNISOLONE*														
Dose: *45 mg* / Route: *ORAL*	6													
Notes: *60 mg/m²* / Start Date: *01/11/24*	8													
Prescriber – sign + print: *P. Smith PAUL SMITH*	(12)		*SQ*											
	14													
	18													
	22													

Medicine (Approved Name)	6													
Dose / Route	8													
Notes / Start Date	12													
Prescriber – sign + print	14													
	18													
	22													

Medicine (Approved Name)	6													
Dose / Route	8													
Notes / Start Date	12													
Prescriber – sign + print	14													
	18													
	22													

Medicine (Approved Name)	6													
Dose / Route	8													
Notes / Start Date	12													
Prescriber – sign + print	14													
	18													
	22													

Medicine (Approved Name)	6													
Dose / Route	8													
Notes / Start Date	12													
Prescriber – sign + print	14													
	18													
	22													

Medicine (Approved Name)	6													
Dose / Route	8													
Notes / Start Date	12													
Prescriber – sign + print	14													
	18													
	22													

Fig. 9.16 Prescription and administration record (regular therapy) for Charlie Manning.

Additional Important Scenarios

10

Ali B.A.K. Al-Hadithi

Chapter Outline

Station 10.1: Discharge Prescribing
Station 10.2: Analgesia
Station 10.3: Dealing With a Medication Error
Station 10.4: Reporting an Adverse Drug Reaction
Station 10.5: Blood Product Prescribing
Station 10.6: Anaphylaxis
Station 10.7: Alcohol Withdrawal
Station 10.8: Vancomycin and Gentamicin Prescribing

STATION 10.1: DISCHARGE PRESCRIBING

Mr Smith is a 50-year-old man who was admitted to your hospital recently with right lower lobe pneumonia. He is now fit for discharge but requires 'to take out' (TTO) prescriptions of his medications.

- The best source of information for prescribers in the UK is the British National Formulary (BNF), which also has information on the prescribing of controlled drugs.
- Familiarise yourself with the common medicines that you will be asked to prescribe.

PRESCRIBING REGULAR MEDICATIONS

- Look at the regular medications section of the drug chart. The patient will need to continue many of these drugs once they leave hospital.
- Take special care not to represcribe drugs that may have been started as short-term measures in hospital (e.g. thromboprophylaxis, analgesics, hypnotics).
- Antibiotics should only be given for the prescribed course (e.g. for three more days). If you do have to prescribe antibiotics on a TTO (Table 10.1), you should know how long they need to be continued and, if unsure, check with a senior colleague.

Do not fill in the pharmacy box because it is for pharmacy staff when they dispense the drugs.

PRESCRIBING PRN (AS REQUIRED) MEDICATION

- Often a patient will only need to be sent home with PRN analgesia.
- It is your job to decide which of these drugs the patient needs to be sent home with.
- PRN medication is usually prescribed for up to 7 days after discharge.
- In order to decide which medications to prescribe, you need to determine how many times these drugs have been administered in the time leading up to discharge and use your common sense.
- If the drug has not been given for a number of days, you may not even need to prescribe it.

EXAMPLE

- Mr AC has been requiring 20 to 30 mg of Oramorph every day as breakthrough analgesia.
- Assuming his pain is improving, you would want to send him home with, for example, 7 days' worth of 20 mg Oramorph per day (Table 10.2). Oramorph is distributed as 10 mg/5 mL strength (of morphine) in 100 and 300 mL bottles (concentrated forms are also available (100 mg/5 mL)):
  - The daily dose of 20 mg = 10 mL.
  - 7 days × 10 mL = 70 mL.
  - Therefore, you would prescribe a 100-mL bottle, which would leave slightly extra in case this patient needs more analgesia.

These types of calculations are mostly done on the basis of common sense. Oramorph is a controlled drug and therefore has a couple of extra requirements with its prescription, which are covered in more detail in the next section.

PRESCRIBING CONTROLLED DRUGS

These drugs often cause the most confusion, but if you follow the following simple rules and are sensible, you should not go wrong!

When prescribing controlled drugs, the prescription must state:

- The name and address of the patient
- The form and strength of the drug (as appropriate)
- Either the total quantity or the number of dosage units of drug written in **both words and figures**
- The dose of the drug

Table 10.1 Examples of Regular Medications Prescribed on a TTO

DRUG	DOSE AND FREQUENCY	ROUTE	DAYS (N)	PHARMACY
Aspirin	75 mg OD	PO	7	
Omeprazole	40 mg OD	PO	7	
Levothyroxine	125 micrograms OD	PO	7	
Ramipril	5 mg OD	PO	7	

OD, Omni die (once daily); *PO*, per oram (orally); *TTO*, 'to take out'.

Table 10.2 Mr AC's PRN Medications on a TTO

DRUG	DOSE AND FREQUENCY	ROUTE	NUMBER OF DAYS	PHARMACY
Oramorph oral solution (morphine) 10 mg/5 mL. Supply 100 mL (one hundred millilitres)	20 mg 2 hourly as required	PO	7	

PO, Per oram (orally); *PRN*, pro re nata (when required); *TTO*, 'to take out'.

Table 10.3 Prescription for Morphine Modified-Release 5 mg BD

DRUG	DOSE AND FREQUENCY	ROUTE	NUMBER OF DAYS	PHARMACY
Morphine modified-release 5 mg tablets. Oral. Supply 56 (fifty-six) tablets	5 mg BD	PO	28	

BD, Bis die (twice daily); *PO*, per oram (orally).

The prescription must then be signed, dated and also contain the prescriber's hospital address. Without such information, the pharmacy will not dispense the controlled drug.

For example, if a patient has been receiving morphine MR modified-release 5 mg oral BD in the hospital, you would prescribe it as shown in Table 10.3.

STATION 10.2: ANALGESIA

Mr Smith is a 45-year-old surgical inpatient who has been diagnosed with appendicitis and is awaiting theatre. He has severe right iliac fossa pain and has not yet received any analgesia. Please prescribe appropriate medication and indicate how you might proceed if the pain were to persist despite initial treatment.

MANAGEMENT OF PAIN

Pain can be difficult to manage. Furthermore, the side effects of analgesics can be more damaging than the pain itself. A simple, structured approach to analgesia will help address these issues in the majority of cases.

Analgesia should be prescribed using the World Health Organization (WHO) analgesic ladder (Fig. 10.1) as a guide. Two general rules to note when using the WHO analgesic ladder are:

1. Start at the step most appropriate for the patient's pain, e.g. if the patient has suffered a fractured femur and is complaining of severe pain, you should move straight to step 3 rather than trying step 1 and waiting to see if the pain settles.
2. If the pain is not controlled, avoid changing one drug for another of equal potency in the same class, e.g. do not change codeine to dihydrocodeine. Instead move up the ladder until adequate analgesia is reached.

NON-OPIOIDS

Paracetamol (1 g PO QDS) is an effective pain killer and should be prescribed regularly to every patient who has pain.

WEAK OPIOIDS

If the pain is not controlled with regular paracetamol alone, a weak opioid should be added. Options include codeine phosphate (30–60 mg up to 4 hourly PO, max 240 mg/24 hours) and dihydrocodeine (30 mg up to 4 hourly PO/SC/IM).

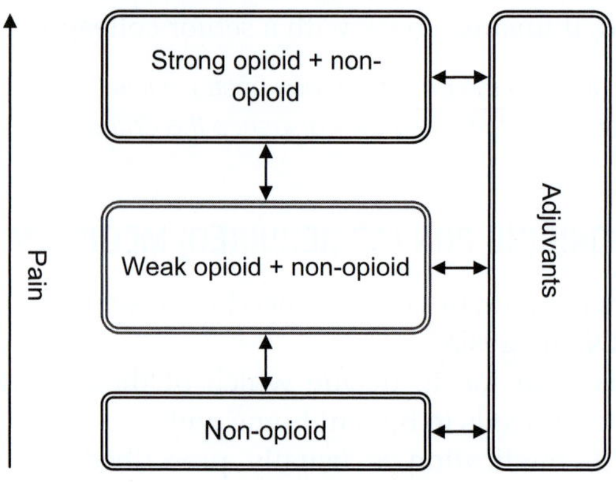

Fig. 10.1 WHO analgesic ladder.

STRONG OPIOIDS

If pain continues despite maximum doses of nonopioids and weak opioids, the weak opioid should be stopped and a trial of strong opioids (e.g. morphine, oxycodone, fentanyl) commenced (Table 10.4). Morphine has serious side effects and needs to be prescribed with care.

ADJUVANTS

These include non-steroidal antiinflammatory drugs (NSAIDs) (for bony metastases, liver pain), corticosteroids (for nerve compression, liver pain, raised intracranial pressure), gabapentin and amitriptyline (for neuropathic pain). The nature of the pain will determine which adjuvant is appropriate and these should be considered with any step in the analgesic ladder. It is best to discuss the use of these drugs with a senior and/or the pain team.

PRESCRIBING MORPHINE

- Morphine can be either a standard (immediate-release) form acting for around 4 hours or a modified-release form acting for between 12 and 24 hours.
- It can be administered orally, IV, IM, SC or PR. In most acute scenarios, the oral route is the most appropriate. If this is not available other routes such as IM, IV and SC can be considered. One should be aware of the dosing differences when using these different routes (see below)
- Most patients with continuous, acute, severe pain should initially be prescribed immediate-release morphine (Oramorph/Sevredol). This takes about 20 minutes to work and acts for approximately 4 hours.
- It is difficult to know how much morphine a patient will need. Therefore, it is best to prescribe it initially as an 'as required' medication (e.g. morphine, 5 mg PO PRN, maximum frequency 4 hourly).
- The dose and frequency of the morphine can be adjusted according to the pain and degree of side effects (e.g. increasing to 5 mg PO PRN, maximum frequency 2 hourly, if the patient continues to be in pain).
- Modified-release morphine (MST Continus/Zomorph/Morphgesic SR) takes longer to have an effect but lasts 12 hours. It is prescribed twice a day after titration with immediate-release morphine has achieved adequate analgesia. The dose of modified-release morphine is calculated by taking the total amount of immediate-release morphine used in 24 hours and dividing by 2.
- Breakthrough immediate-release morphine will also be required and is one-sixth of the total amount of immediate-release morphine used in 24 hours.

For example, if a patient had used 6 × 10 mg PRN doses of Oramorph in 24 hours (i.e. 60 mg), 30 mg (60/2 = 30) of modified-release morphine could be prescribed BD in addition to Oramorph 10 mg PRN 4 hourly (60/6 = 10).

It should be noted that MST should be used when Oramorph is the PRN opioid, whereas Oxycontin should be prescribed when Oxynorm is the breakthrough opioid.

Side effects and cautions of commonly prescribed analgesics are shown in Table 10.5.

In those with renal impairment, instead of morphine or oxycodone, consider alternatives such as alfentanil or fentanyl.

For the majority of patients, the WHO analgesic ladder will provide sufficient analgesia. However, it will not be possible to control every patient's pain with the earlier strategy. In these cases, discussion with your seniors and the pain team would be a useful next step.

Table 10.4 Equivalent Doses of Opioids

PO morphine 5 mg	≈ PO codeine 60 mg
	≈ PO dihydrocodeine 60 mg
	≈ SC morphine 2.5 mg
	≈ PO oxycodone 2.5 mg

PO, Per oram (orally); *SC*, subcutaneous.

Table 10.5 Side Effects of Analgesics

DRUG	SIDE EFFECTS	CAUTIONS
Paracetamol	Rare but may include: Rashes Thrombocytopaenia Neutropenia	Hepatic impairment—avoid large doses Renal impairment—max rate 6 hourly if creatinine clearance (CrCl) <30 mL/min
Codeine phosphate, dihydrocodeine, morphine, oxycodone	Nausea and vomiting Constipation Respiratory depression Dry mouth Difficulty micturating Sedation	Hepatic or renal impairment—reduce dose Respiratory depression, asthma attack Prostatic hypertrophy Elderly

STATION 10.3: DEALING WITH A MEDICATION ERROR

Mr Sanderson was admitted to the cardiology ward last night and you are reviewing him on the ward round. You are asked to review him because he is noted to have a new rash. You find out that he is penicillin allergic and yet was started on penicillin for a presumed chest infection. Please explain how you would go about managing the situation.

1. **Ensure patient safety:** Assess the patient using the ABCDE approach outlined in this book. Medication errors can potentially make patients critically unwell, so your first priority is ensuring no harm has been done.
2. **Verify the information:** Check the prescription chart to see what medications have been prescribed and what has been given. Check for any documented allergies (a) on the drug chart, (b) in the medical notes and (c) with the patient, e.g. a wrist band, GP letter and verbally.
3. **Escalate to senior colleagues:** Any medication errors like this need to be discussed with the consultant and the nurse in charge. It should not happen and therefore needs to be looked into.
4. **Admit error to patient:** Healthcare professionals have a duty of candour, so the patient needs to be told early and directly that an error has been made due to a mistake made by the hospital and is the responsibility of the hospital. Emphasise that you have assessed them and tell them if any direct harm has come of it. Emphasise as well that you take the error very seriously and that you and the hospital will thoroughly investigate why it happened. It should generally be the case that the consultant looking after the patient will want to meet with the patient and discuss what has happened as well.
5. **Identify why the error may have happened (root cause analysis):** There are two aspects to this. First, identify the circumstances of this specific case. Who was the doctor that prescribed the drug? In what circumstance was it prescribed? Were they working beyond their hours? Were they following direct instructions from a consultant/registrar on a ward round without double checking allergies? Had they had adequate prescribing training? Had the original drug chart been filled out correctly: was the drug allergy clearly documented? Which nursing staff gave the medication? What checks were taken to ensure the medication was safe to give?
   Second, what could be done generally to reduce the likelihood of such an event happening again? This can be done by you and the team looking after the patient. In the earlier scenario, it became apparent that the ward did not use allergy bracelets for patients and therefore this was changed. However, it must be escalated higher and a critical incident form would need to be filled in to investigate this at the hospital level.
6. **Report the error:** All hospitals have reporting systems to capture and analyse common errors so that lessons can be learned by staff to provide a safer environment for all patients. These efforts are thwarted if the errors that occur go unreported. Most hospitals now operate a 'no blame' culture that encourages more frequent reporting.

STATION 10.4: REPORTING AN ADVERSE DRUG REACTION

Mr McMillan was started on a new antiplatelet agent, 'Sementy', and within 1 week was noted to have a reduced neutrophil count (Table 10.6). He has been reviewed by the haematologists who felt the low neutrophil count was due to the new drug and, after discussion with cardiology, Sementy was changed to clopidogrel and the neutrophil count recovered. Your consultant has asked you to fill in a Yellow Card to report this adverse drug reaction.

Suspected adverse drug reactions are a common cause of hospital admission (7% of acute admissions) and affect up to 15% of inpatients. It is the duty of hospital prescribers to report them to a national agency that can pool the reports from around the country and begin to identify signals of previously unrecognised reactions. Reports are required not just for medicines but also for blood products, vaccines, herbal or complementary medicine products.

Table 10.6 Mr McMillan's Blood Results 07/12/24

PARAMETER	VALUE	NORMAL RANGE (UNITS)
Haemoglobin	140 g/L	Men: 135–177 (g/L) Women: 115–155 (g/L)
Neutrophil	**0.9 × 10^9/L**	**2.0–7.5 (×10^9/L)**
WCC	8.2 × 10^9/L	3.2–11 (×10^9/L)
Platelet	270 × 10^9/L	150–400 (×10^9/L)
PT	12 seconds	11.5–13.5 seconds
APTT	35 seconds	26–37 seconds
Urea	4.5 mmol/L	2.5–6.7 (mmol/L)
Creatinine	95 µmol/L	79–118 (µmol/L)
eGFR	>60 mL/min	>60 (mL/min)
Sodium	140 mmol/L	135–146 (mmol/L)
Potassium	4.2 mmol/L	3.5–5.0 (mmol/L)
CRP	2 mg/L	0–5 (mg/L)
Bilirubin	10 µmol/L	<17 (µmol/L)
ALT	27 IU/L	<40 (IU/L)
ALP	84 IU/L	39–117 (IU/L)

Data in bold signifies results that are outside the normal laboratory range.
ALP, Alkaline phosphatase; *ALT,* alanine transaminase; *APTT,* activated partial thromboplastin time; *CRP,* C-reactive protein; *eGFR,* estimated glomerular filtration rate; *PT,* prothrombin time; *WCC,* white cell count.

The more information provided the better, but this should not significantly delay the reporting of the reaction (or error).

The Yellow Card system is a voluntary reporting system in the UK used to make reports to the Medicines and Healthcare Products Regulatory Agency (MHRA). Reports can be sent by healthcare professionals as well as patients and carers. Most reports are provided online at http://yellowcard.mhra.gov.uk. Similar pharmacovigilance schemes exist in other countries.

MEDICINES AND HEALTHCARE PRODUCTS REGULATORY AGENCY

The minimum information required for a Yellow Card is:

- Patient information should ideally include age, sex, weight, initials, height and local identification number
- The name of the drug(s) suspected of causing the reaction as well as any other drugs that the patient may be taking
- A brief description of the adverse drug reaction
- Contact details of the reporter (which should be your work contact information)

'MM, a 60-kg, 52-year-old male, 5 foot 10 inches, has had a reported adverse reaction to Sementy 1 week after it was started. The neutrophil count significantly dropped with other parameters remaining normal.'

Further information (though not essential) is of considerable value about:

- The drug:
  - Start and stop date
  - Route of administration
  - Dose
  - Indication
  - Batch number
- The adverse reaction:
  - Start and stop date
  - The outcome
  - Any treatment required
- The patient:
  - Additional medications being taken (including over-the-counter medication, and any medication stopped in the preceding 3 months). Should include dose, route of administration and indication
  - Relevant medical history
  - Relevant recent blood test
- Information on the outcome of any rechallenge with the suspect drug(s)
- Indication of the seriousness of the reaction

'He was started on Sementy 30 mg orally once daily on 01/12/2024, for ischaemic heart disease after having had a STEMI with single vessel disease treated with percutaneous coronary intervention. The batch number of his first packet was 23839273. It was stopped on 07/12/2024 due to the low neutrophil count. No treatment was necessary. He has been on aspirin 75 mg orally once daily, bisoprolol 1.25 mg orally once daily and ramipril 2.5 mg orally once daily since 01/12/24 for ischaemic heart disease. He has no other medical history.

On 07/12/24 he was noted to have a neutrophil count of 0.9 × 10^9/L having had bloods done because his GP was concerned that he looked anaemic. The haemoglobin, platelet, lymphocyte, clotting, renal and liver function were all normal. Two weeks later, after stopping Sementy, on 21/12/24 the neutrophil count was 7 × 10^9/L.'

If no further information is available, it is best to mention this so that the person reading the report will not need to follow it up.

STATION 10.5: BLOOD PRODUCT PRESCRIBING

As an orthopaedic junior doctor, you see Mr McDonald, a 67-year-old man, with a past medical history of angina, heart failure and peptic ulcer disease who is day 1 postop for a left total hemiarthroplasty for a left neck of femur fracture. Intraoperative blood loss was estimated at 1500 mL. His preoperative Hb was 101 g/L and platelets 60 × 10^9/L. He feels lethargic, dizzy and short of breath and reports indigestion but no PR bleeding.

Patient Details

Name:	Graham McDonald
DOB:	09/08/57
Hospital number:	0908472977
Weight:	63 kg
Height:	1.58 m
Consultant:	P Blair
Hospital/Ward:	WGH Ortho Ward
Current medications:	Dalteparin 5000 units SC OD (started this admission: thromboprophylaxis) Cocodamol 30/500 2 tablets PO QDS (started this admission: for postoperative pain) Lansoprazole 30 mg PO OD (for peptic ulcer disease) Aspirin 75 mg PO OD and bisoprolol 10 mg PO OD (for ischaemic heart disease) Simvastatin 40 mg PO OD (for high cholesterol)
Allergies:	Ramipril (anaphylaxis)
Admission date:	11/10/24

INITIAL ASSESSMENT

AIRWAY, BREATHING, CIRCULATION, DISABILITY, EXPOSURE

- Assess patency of the airway. Check respiratory rate, oximetry and auscultate chest. Assess blood pressure (BP), heart rate (HR) and capillary refill time (CRT). Assess conscious level and blood glucose. Expose the patient, where appropriate, to reveal clues (melaena, haematoma).

'The airway is patent. RR 22/min, oxygen saturations 97% on room air and chest auscultation is normal. Heart sounds are normal, HR 80 bpm, BP 123/72 mmHg lying and 120/65 mmHg standing. There is conjunctival pallor. Patient is alert and orientated. Blood glucose is 5.5 mol/L.

Temperature 36.9°C. Exposure reveals a clean left hip wound, rosy urine in catheter and soft nontender abdomen. Gum bleeding is noted. PR examination revealed mild haemorrhoids with no melaena. Faecal occult blood (FOB) is negative.'

The patient has clinical symptoms and signs of anaemia with evidence of external bleeding from haematuria and gum bleeding. He is haemodynamically stable.

Tip: Where possible, anticipate when patients need blood transfusion samples, e.g. preoperatively in potential surgical cases (acute abdomen, hip fractures, etc.).

INITIAL INVESTIGATIONS

- **Bloods:** Group and save, full blood count (FBC). Check anaemia severity by measuring haemoglobin and, at the same time, a platelet count will help assess if thrombocytopaenia is contributory. In this case, the reduced haemoglobin is most likely due to operative and postoperative blood loss, so additional tests may not be necessary (Table 10.7).

Blood Transfusion Samples

Sample and request forms MUST comply with Mandatory Data Set requirements, including hospital ID number, surname, first name, DOB, signatures (prescriber, person taking sample). Any missing/mismatching information means samples will NOT be accepted.

Tip 1: Always HANDWRITTEN (no sticky labels).

Tip 2: NEVER write on sample tube BEFORE drawing sample.

Tip 3: Seek POSITIVE identification of patients at bedside. LABEL tubes immediately.

Indications for Red Cell Transfusion

- Symptomatic anaemia, which can generally occur with a Hb <100 g/L (dyspnoea, angina, syncope, ST depression on ECG)
- Hb <80 g/L or potentially higher target if cardiovascular disease is present
  However, in general:

- Check MCV to determine whether it is a microcytic, macrocytic or normocytic anaemia.
- Check B_{12}, folate, iron levels and TFTs as deficiency in all of the above may cause anaemia.
- Check LFTs and clotting to ensure a coagulation disorder is not contributory.
- Check urea as this is raised acutely in gastrointestinal bleeding.
- If haemolysis is suspected, LDH and haptoglobin are useful markers of the degree of red blood cell break down. Reticulocyte count will allow a measure of how quickly red cells are being reproduced. Coombs' test will help determine if there are antibodies to red cells in the blood stream causing haemolysis.

'Hb 77 g/L, MCV 63 fL, platelets 15 × 10^9/L, normal LFTs and coagulation screen, eGFR >60 mL/min. Your differential diagnosis is symptomatic postoperative microcytic anaemia secondary to ≈1500 mL intraoperative blood loss with peptic ulcer disease, haematuria and haemorrhoids as contributors. The cause of the low platelets is unclear but it may be related to heparin.'

You arrange a blood transfusion and, after discussion with haematology, a platelet transfusion. You give furosemide cover due to the history of heart failure. You stop heparin and aspirin since they may be causing the low platelet count and they are also increasing the risk of bleeding directly. The next dose of bisoprolol is due in the morning so you ask the morning team to

Table 10.7 Mr McDonald's Blood Results

PARAMETER	VALUE	NORMAL RANGE (UNITS)
Haemoglobin	**77 g/L**	**Men: 135–177 (g/L) Women: 115–155 (g/L)**
MCV	83 fL	80–96 (fL)
WCC	7.2 × 10^9/L	3.2–11 (×10^9/L)
Neutrophil	4 × 10^9/L	2–7.5 (×10^9/L)
Lymphocyte	2 × 10^9/L	1.4–4 (×10^9/L)
Platelet	**15 × 10^9/L**	**120–400 (×10^9/L)**
Urea	3.7 mmol/L	2.5–6.7 (mmol/L)
Creatinine	90 µmol/L	70–130 (µmol/L)
Sodium	142 mmol/L	135–145 (mmol/L)
Potassium	3.9 mmol/L	3.5–5.0 (mmol/L)
eGFR	>60 mL/min	>60 (mL/min)
ALT	23 IU/L	5–35 (IU/L)
ALP	45 IU/L	39–117 (IU/L)
Bilirubin	13 µmol/L	3–17 (µmol/L)
PT	12 seconds	11.5–13.5 seconds
APTT	30 seconds	26–37 seconds

Data in bold signifies results that are outside the normal laboratory range.
ALP, Alkaline phosphatase; *ALT,* alanine transaminase; *APTT,* activated partial thromboplastin time; *eGFR,* estimated glomerular filtration rate; *MCV,* mean cell volume; *PT,* prothrombin time; *WCC,* white cell count.

review this. As well as anaemia, hypotension (exacerbated by bisoprolol) could be contributory to the initial symptoms of light headedness and shortness of breath, especially given active bleeding.

Types of Red Cell Concentrates

- ORhD negative 'O neg' (emergency)*
- Group specific ≈15–25 minutes
- Cross-matched ≈40–60 minutes

If red cell antibodies present, allow more time, ask blood bank if specific tests/more samples needed.

*'O neg' (O Rh–ve) blood:

- Use in extreme emergencies only.
- Blood fridges in: theatres, recovery, obstetrics and gynaecology/labour ward, emergency department, HDU/ICU, blood transfusion service.

Prescribe (Figs 10.2–10.4)

Red cell transfusion:

- 1 unit of RED CELL CONCENTRATE (over 4 hours) followed by 1 unit of RED CELL CONCENTRATE (over 4 hours)

Platelet transfusion:

- 1 pool of PLATELETS (over 30 minutes) follow by 1 pool of PLATELETS (over 30 minutes)

Diuretic cover for blood transfusion:

- FUROSEMIDE 20 mg PO (before the second unit of blood)

STOP

Aspirin and dalteparin (due to bleeding, and possible association with low platelets) and consider withholding bisoprolol the following morning

INITIAL MANAGEMENT FOR BLEEDING PATIENTS

- **Call for help:** Involve seniors in the management of the patient. If there is evidence of massive bleeding, put out a peri-arrest/arrest call (dial 2222 in UK hospitals) and activate the major haemorrhage protocol.
- **Inform blood transfusion service (or whoever deals with blood products in your hospital) early:** Discuss with the haematologist if needed. Be aware of issues surrounding transfusion for Jehovah's witnesses and discuss with the patient regarding their preferences.
- **Stop bleeding:** This will depend on the suspected cause—if the patient is suspected of having a gastrointestinal (GI) bleed from the peptic ulcer, or bleeding from the hip wound, gastroenterology or surgical input would be required urgently.
- **Consider high-dependency or intensive care:** Patients with significant blood loss can become unstable very quickly. They may require more intensive monitoring (central lines, arterial lines), or inotropic BP support.

Major Haemorrhage Protocol: 2222, e.g. surgery, trauma, GI, obstetrics. Brings 'blood' in rapid focused approach (porters, blood bank, emergency team).

- **Consider reversal of anticoagulation:** Consider reversal agents if the patient is taking anticoagulation. For example, warfarin can be reversed with vitamin K and prothrombin complex concentrate, while heparin can be reversed using protamine sulfate. Direct oral anticoagulants can generally be reversed with prothrombin complex concentrate, although dabigatran has a specific reversal agent (idarucizumab).
- **Stop potentiating medications:** Both aspirin and prophylactic low-molecular-weight heparin (LMWH) should be stopped in view of thrombocytopaenia with active bleeding. Consider heparin-induced thrombocytopaenia and discuss with haematology. Antihypertensive medications may be causing or exacerbating hypotension and contributing to current symptoms.
- **Counselling:** Discuss the benefits (improve symptoms) and risks (reactions, transmission of blood borne viruses, IV access) of transfusion with the patient. Provide information leaflets on blood transfusion.
- **Logistics:** Obtain IV access, avoid transfusions out-of-hours where possible (less staff available for monitoring and administration), but this patient would require an urgent transfusion regardless of the time. Do NOT transfuse blood through lines used for solutions containing glucose (causes red cells to clump). Use blood warmer for larger or rapid transfusions.

Transfusion decision: Factors to consider include onset (acute/chronic), on-going blood loss, severity, comorbidity and symptoms. 'Right blood, right patient, right time'.

BLOOD PRODUCTS THAT CAN BE PRESCRIBED

- **Red cell concentrate (RCC):** One unit raises Hb by 10 to 15 g/L. **Must be ABO-compatible.** Usually prescribed over 2 to 4 hours (note expiry time outside fridge is shortly beyond 4 hours) unless emergency where it is given 'stat'. Consider diuretic 'cover' if limited cardiac reserve (risk of fluid overload)—furosemide 20 to 40 mg prior to RCC or with alternate bags.
- **Platelets:** Given if platelets <10 × 10^9/L. Consider if no bleeding and platelets <20 × 10^9/L, or if bleeding and platelets <50 × 10^9/L. Recheck FBC for platelet 'increment' 1 hour after transfusing (i.e. if preprocedure). Four units/pools of platelets can be given over 30 to 60 minutes. One unit should raise platelet count by >20 × 10^9/L. Platelet clumping can lead to erroneously low counts; confirm by manual differentiation.

- **Fresh frozen plasma:** Used in reversal of warfarin and treatment of specific factor deficiencies, e.g. II, V, VII, IX, XI. Must be blood group compatible. Usual dose is 10 to 15 mL/kg. Infuse over 30 to 60 minutes and use immediately preprocedure.

LESS COMMONLY PRESCRIBED BLOOD PRODUCTS

- **Cryoprecipitate:** Particularly useful to replace fibrinogen
- **Coagulation factor concentrates factor VIII and IX:** Treatments of haemophilia and von Willebrand disease
- **Human albumin solution (4.5%/20%):** In hypoproteinaemia and hypervolaemic states. Used also following abdominal paracentesis
- **Immunoglobulins:** Hypogammaglobulinaemia and idiopathic thrombocytopaenic purpura; also used as a specific medical treatment, e.g. Kawasaki disease
- In special cases (e.g. bone marrow transplant, leukaemia, renal patients), cytomegalovirus (CMV) negative, irradiated, genotyped, filtered blood may be required

Acute Transfusion Reactions

- Bacterial contamination (and septic shock)
- Anaphylaxis, hypersensitivity
- ABO incompatibility
- Febrile nonhaemolytic transfusion reactions
- Acute intravascular haemolysis
- Fluid/circulatory overload
- Transfusion-related acute lung injury (TRALI)
- Transfusion-associated graft vs host disease (TA-GvHD)

REASSESSMENT

- Following his first unit of RCC, his dyspnoea and dizziness improved. In view of his past medical history of heart failure, furosemide 20 mg oral was prescribed prior to administering his second unit of RCC late that afternoon. A posttransfusion FBC was taken the following day (day 2 postop).
- If more transfusions are needed or time elapsed is >72 hours since the last group and save sample, a new blood sample may need to be sent to the blood bank.
- In acute blood loss, the Hb level may lag behind the actual red cell loss by 12 to 24 hours.

'Posttransfusion Hb improved at 99 g/L, platelets at 85 × 10^9/L and clinically improved with no further symptoms.'

Given this, you give the bisoprolol as normal and prescribe no further blood products.

Patients With Heart Failure

Pulmonary oedema could be precipitated by significant anaemia (causes high-output state) in heart failure. Therefore, you should have a lower threshold for transfusing in these patients. Slow down transfusion to 3–4 h/unit of RCC and consider IV/PO furosemide 10–40 mg before each unit/with alternate units to avoid precipitating fluid overload.

HANDING OVER THE PATIENT

'Mr McDonald is a 67-year-old gentleman who fell and sustained a left neck of femur fracture and is day 2 postop after a left total hip replacement. Postoperatively he dropped his Hb from 101 to 77 g/L with associated dizziness and dyspnoea. He was transfused 2 units of RCC with furosemide cover. Haematology recommended transfusing 2 pools of platelets in view of thrombocytopaenia of 15 × 10^9/L and evidence of external bleeding with haematuria and bleeding gums. His posttransfusion Hb is 99 g/L, platelets 85 × 10^9/L with symptom resolution. Heparin and aspirin have both been withheld.

Symptoms have now completely resolved and observations are normal.

Haematology will review later this evening in view of thrombocytopaenia, which may be related to heparin or aspirin, but we are not clear on the cause so far. Please consider input from urology in view of haematuria and continue monitoring his FBC.'

STATION 10.6: ANAPHYLAXIS

As the emergency department junior doctor, you assess a new arrival into the emergency department. Ms White, a 42-year-old asthmatic woman with multiple allergies, has been brought in by a blue light ambulance from a seafood restaurant where she rapidly started to feel unwell and itchy and developed a rash.

Patient Details

Name:	Joan White
DOB:	15/08/82
Hospital number:	1508723719
Weight:	60 kg
Height:	1.65 m
Consultant:	J Murphy
Hospital/Ward:	LGH emergency department
Current medications:	Nil
Allergies:	Seafood (anaphylaxis) and beta-blockers (anaphylaxis)
Admission date:	12/10/24

Anaphylaxis

- Sudden and rapidly progressing symptoms
- Life-threatening airway and/or breathing and/or circulation problems
- Skin and/or mucosal changes

Some Common Triggers

- Food: Nuts, seafood
- Drugs: Antibiotics (penicillin), muscle relaxants, NSAIDs, ACE inhibitors, vaccines
- Radiopaque dyes/contrast, latex
- Idiopathic

Complications of Anaphylaxis

- Respiratory arrest/airway obstruction
- Cardiac arrest
- Anaphylactic shock

INITIAL ASSESSMENT

AIRWAY

- Assess patency of the airway. Is there any stridor, hoarseness or foreign bodies?

'The airway is patent with mild lip swelling but no stridor or hoarseness.'

No airway adjunct needed at present but call anaesthetist early.

Note: Know where emergency equipment/expertise is available: resus trolley, defibrillator, endotracheal intubation and emergency cricothyrotomy kit.

BREATHING

- Assess respiratory rate, oxygen saturations and work of breathing. Is there any cyanosis? Auscultate for air entry and additional sounds of wheeze and crepitations.

'RR 28/min, oxygen saturations 95% on room air, wheezy and fatiguing. There is no evidence of cyanosis.'

The patient has evidence of anaphylaxis with respiratory compromise. Give IM adrenaline and establish IV access. In addition, it would be reasonable to give nebulised salbutamol in view of her history of asthma.

Prescribe (Figs 10.5–10.7)

Adrenaline:
- ADRENALINE (1:1000) 500 micrograms IM (0.5 mL) STAT

Bronchodilator:
- SALBUTAMOL 5 mg NEB STAT

CIRCULATION

- Check BP and HR. Assess haemodynamic status.

'HR 112 bpm, BP 87/59 mmHg, appears pale and clammy, CRT 3 seconds and has warm peripheries.'

The patient is in anaphylactic shock. Give a fluid bolus of sodium chloride 0.9% and reassess. Perform an electrocardiogram (ECG). Restoration of BP will be aided by laying the patient flat and raising the legs. If patients are unconscious or at risk of vomiting, place in the recovery position.

DISABILITY

- Assess the patient's conscious level. Is there agitation or confusion? Check glucose levels.

'She is slightly drowsy with a GCS 14 (E3, V5, M6) but remains orientated to time, place and person. Blood glucose is 6.4 mmol/L.'

EXPOSURE

- Expose the patient where reasonable. Are there skin and mucosal changes? Is there angioedema (deeper swelling of tissues)?
- Do not forget anaphylaxis can also present with GI symptoms (abdominal pain, incontinence, vomiting).

'She has a widespread urticarial rash all over her body. Her lips and tongue are swollen. Her medic alert bracelet says "Allergic to seafood and beta-blockers". Temperature is 36.5°C. Examination is otherwise normal.'

Prescribe (see Figs 10.5–10.7)

Fluid bolus:
- SODIUM CHLORIDE 0.9% 500 mL (over 15 minutes)

Good Prescribing Practice

- Be aware of agents in similar drug classes/cross-allergies: Penicillin for example with co-amoxiclav, piperacillin + tazobactam, flucloxacillin, benzylpenicillin, with caution for other beta-lactams (cephalosporins, meropenem)—seek microbiology advice if there are concerns about allergies to antibiotics.
- Always document ALLERGIES clearly on prescription chart.
- Where possible, clarify the nature of 'allergy' vs 'intolerance' instead.
- If unsure, clarify with GP, previous hospital notes or family.

Anaphylactic or Anaphylactoid Reaction?

Anaphylaxis refers to IgE-mediated reactions while anaphylactoid reactions are similar in presentation but are non-IgE-mediated. Common IgE-mediated triggers are drugs (e.g. beta-lactam antibiotics), foods or stings. Non-IgE-mediated causes include compounds that act directly on the mast cell membranes (e.g. vancomycin, quinolone antibiotics or radiographic contrast media).

INITIAL INVESTIGATIONS

- **Bloods:** Baseline FBC, urea and electrolyte (U&E), C-reactive protein (CRP), mast cell tryptase. Respiratory distress may be due to infection or anaemia. Renal function is important in a shocked patient. Mast cell tryptase can help confirm diagnosis of anaphylactic reaction, especially in a first presentation. Timing of blood samples is very important; levels peak 1 to 2 hours after onset. Ideally, three timed

Table 10.8 **Ms White's Blood Test and ABG Results**

PARAMETER	VALUE	NORMAL RANGE (UNITS)
WCC	10 × 10^9/L	4–11 (×10^9/L)
Neutrophil	5 × 10^9/L	2–7.5 (×10^9/L)
Lymphocyte	4 × 10^9/L	1.4–4 (×10^9/L)
Platelet	200 × 10^9/L	150–400 (×10^9/L)
Haemoglobin	150 g/L	Men: 135–177 (g/L) Women: 115–155 (g/L)
CRP	3 mg/L	0–5 (mg/L)
Urea	5 mmol/L	2.5–6.7 (mmol/L)
Creatinine	100 μmol/L	79–118 (μmol/L)
Sodium	140 mmol/L	135–146 (mmol/L)
Potassium	4 mmol/L	3.5–5.0 (mmol/L)
eGFR	>60 mL/min	>60 (mL/min)
pH	7.4	7.35–7.45
PaO_2	11.0 kPa on air	10.6–13.3 (kPa) on air
$PaCO_2$	5.0 kPa	4.8–6.1 (kPa)
HCO_3	24 mmol/L	22–26 (mmol/L)

ABG, Arterial blood gas; *CRP*, C-reactive protein; *eGFR*, estimated glomerular filtration rate; *WCC*, white cell count.

samples (onset, 1–2 hours, 24 hours/convalescence) should be collected. However, do not delay treatment for sampling (Table 10.8).

- **Arterial blood gas (ABG):** To assess the degree of hypoxia and any hypercapnia.
- **12-Lead ECG:** An arrhythmia may be causing respiratory distress.
- **Chest radiography (CXR):** To look for other causes such as pneumonia, or a pneumothorax.

'Blood and ABG results are unremarkable. 12-lead ECG shows sinus tachycardia 110 bpm.'

INITIAL MANAGEMENT

 Management Summary: Anaphylaxis

- Resuscitate using an ABCDE approach
- IM adrenaline
- IV fluids
- Identify and eliminate precipitant

- **Call for help: Emergency** response team. Get a senior/consultant anaesthetist; high dependency unit (HDU)/intensive therapy unit (ITU)/ear, nose and throat (ENT) input may be necessary.
- **Discontinue** the suspected agent responsible (e.g. scrape insect sting off skin carefully).
- **Airway:** Airway is patent in this case, so no intervention is required.
- **Continuous cardiac monitor:** Shock (and giving adrenaline) predisposes to arrhythmias.
- **Supplementary oxygen (give as soon as available):** If saturations <94%. Administer high-flow oxygen and give salbutamol nebulisers if there is suspected bronchoconstriction.
- **Position:** Lie flat and raise legs to maximise circulatory return.
- **Adrenaline:** Given via the IM route. Administer as soon as anaphylaxis is suspected (Box 10.1).
- **Gain IV access (alternative: intraosseous route):** To start IV fluids.
- **IV fluid resuscitation (give as soon as available):** 'Anaphylactic shock' causes vasodilatation causing warm peripheries, capillary leak and hypotension. Use crystalloid fluids to resuscitate. Stop ongoing IV colloid in case they might be the case of anaphylaxis.
- **Bronchodilators:** If wheezy or asthma-like features, consider nebulised salbutamol.
- **Special circumstances (beta-blockers):** Adrenaline can fail to reverse anaphylaxis in patients taking beta-blockers and, in such cases, glucagon may be useful.
- **Thromboprophylaxis:** The inflammatory response driven by anaphylaxis promotes a prothrombotic state, so consider starting pharmacological thromboprophylaxis.

REASSESSMENT

- The patient is reassessed clinically and repeat observations are taken. Continuous ECG monitoring, pulse oximetry and frequent noninvasive BP measurements are carried out.

Box 10.1 **Adrenaline (Epinephrine)**

Acts as an α-receptor agonist (reverses peripheral vasodilatation) and β-receptor agonist (dilates bronchial airways, increases myocardial contractility, suppresses histamine and leukotriene release, inhibits mast cell activation).

- Administration: IM, injected into anterolateral thigh (through trousers if needed in emergencies). Standard blue needle (25 mm and 23 G) is best for all ages.
- Familiarise yourself with equipment (available in resuscitation trolleys).
- Different concentration and doses in:
  - Anaphylaxis (1:1000 adrenaline)
    - Adult and child >12 years: 500 micrograms IM (0.5 mL)
    - Child 6–12 years: 300 micrograms IM (0.3 mL)
    - Child <6 years: 150 micrograms IM (0.15 mL)
  - Cardiac arrest (1:10,000 adrenaline)
    - 1 mg IV (10 mL)
- Tip: If only a partial volume of adrenaline is required, first discard the volume not needed then administer the remaining volume to avoid inadvertent overdosing.
- Keep autoinjector handy, i.e. on person
- Repeat if no improvement in 5-minute intervals.
- IV adrenaline should be used only under expert guidance in cases of refractory anaphylaxis (no improvement after two IM adrenaline doses).

'Following treatment, the patient's wheeze, lip swelling and rash are resolving and the patient is less anxious. BP improved to 105/70 mmHg and HR 90 bpm with a urine output of 0.8 mL/kg/h.'

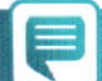

Prescribe (see Figs 10.5–10.7)

Further fluids:
- 1 L SODIUM CHLORIDE 0.9% IV 500 mL/h

Thromboprophylaxis:
- DALTEPARIN SC 5000 units OD

HANDING OVER THE PATIENT

'Ms White is a 42-year-old asthmatic female with multiple allergies who presented in anaphylactic shock presumed to be secondary to seafood ingestion. On examination, her airway was patent but she was tachypnoeic, wheezy, tachycardic and hypotensive.

Emergency IM adrenaline was administered, after which a fluid bolus was given followed by further IV fluids.

The plan is to admit her for a period of observation for 24 hours. She is on a continuous ECG monitor and is getting observations repeated every 2 hours.'

Follow-up Considerations

- Over 60% of patients have repeated attacks!
- Be aware of biphasic reactions. These tend to occur 12 hours after the initial reaction.
- Patients should consider wearing a medic alert bracelet or talisman.
- Prescribe adrenaline autoinjectors on discharge for emergency use by the patient.
- Education on the recognition of anaphylaxis and avoidance of triggers to patients and their families/friends. Signpost them to sources of further information, e.g. Allergy UK, Anaphylaxis Campaign.
- Refer to allergy specialist services.
- Clearly document ALLERGIES on DRUG CHART and MEDICAL NOTES and inform GP.
- If adverse drug reaction, complete Yellow Card scheme (MHRA).

STATION 10.7: ALCOHOL WITHDRAWAL

You are the hospital-at-night medical junior doctor reviewing Mr Johnson, a 48-year-old man admitted yesterday who has become delirious, increasingly tremulous, sweaty and irritable since admission. He drinks 50+ units of alcohol weekly and has a history of previous alcohol withdrawal seizures and delirium tremens.

Patient Details

Name:	Jack Johnson
DOB:	02/11/75
Hospital number:	0211652957
Weight:	78 kg
Height:	1.75 m
Consultant:	A Brown
Hospital/Ward:	LGH Medicine
Current medications:	Nil
Allergies:	Penicillin (rash)
Admission date:	12/10/24

Alcohol Withdrawal Symptoms: (10–72 Hours After Last Drink)

- **Mild:** Tense, irritable, poor concentration
- **Moderate:** Tachycardia, nausea, tremor, sweats, anxious, headache, irritable, flu-like symptoms, seizures
- **Severe:** Confusion, visual/auditory hallucinations, irrational thought/fears, bizarre, aggressive or uncooperative

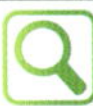

DELIRIUM TREMENS

- Coarse tremor
- Change in mental function, e.g. hallucinations (visual, auditory, tactile), delirium, agitation
- Seizures
- Symptoms of alcohol withdrawal

WERNICKE'S ENCEPHALOPATHY TRIAD

- Cerebellar signs
- Ophthalmoplegia
- Confusion

KORSAKOFF'S PSYCHOSIS

- Amnesia (anterograde and retrograde)
- Confabulation
- Loss of insight
- Apathy
- Meagre content in conversation

Differential Diagnosis: Alcohol Withdrawal

- Acute liver failure
- Severe acute kidney injury
- Hepatic/hypertensive/uraemic encephalopathy
- Hypoglycaemia or other electrolyte disturbance
- Head trauma
- Sepsis
- Meningitis/encephalitis
- Hypoxia
- Neoplasm
- Drug intoxication/withdrawal

INITIAL ASSESSMENT

AIRWAY

- Assess patency of the airway. Is there any vomit obstructing?

'The airway is patent with no obstruction.'

BREATHING

- Assess RR, oxygen saturation, work of breathing and auscultate the chest.

'RR 16/min, oxygen saturations 98% on air and chest is clear.'

CIRCULATION

- Assess BP, HR, CRT and hydration status.

'HR 90 bpm, BP 101/75 mmHg, CRT 2 seconds and there is reduced skin turgor. Heart sounds normal.'

IV access will be required but not urgently and the initial ABCDE assessment can continue.

DISABILITY

- Assess conscious level and evidence of acute intoxication.
- Assess cognition, memory and orientation (abbreviated mental test (AMT) or Mini-Mental State Examination (MMSE), confabulation).
- Any other neurological signs (cerebellar signs from alcohol excess, withdrawal tremor).
- Check glucose levels (hypoglycaemia).
- Examine pupils, range of eye movements and coordination.

'The patient is alert and orientated but anxious and sweaty. He does not seem delirious or to have hallucinations. His blood glucose is 5.9 mmol/L. There is bilateral tremor of both hands but no hepatic flap. There is mild past pointing and dysdiadochokinesis bilaterally and horizontal nystagmus in both directions. Extraocular eye movements are intact with no diplopia reported.'

EXPOSURE

- Examine for signs of malnourishment, self-care, injuries sustained if intoxicated (head injury may coexist), tongue-biting (alcohol withdrawal seizures) and incontinence.
- Check for foetor hepaticus (smell associated with severe liver disease), signs of chronic liver disease and decompensation (ascites, jaundice, encephalopathy).

'Temperature is 36.8°C. Patient appears unkempt and sweaty. Examination reveals alcoholic foetor, spider naevi and palmar erythema.'

INITIAL INVESTIGATIONS

- **Alcohol levels:** Breathalyser, serum ethanol level.
- **Bloods:** FBC (if microcytic anaemia, consider iron deficiency and GI bleeding; if macrocytic anaemia, check for B_{12}/folate deficiency), U&E (electrolyte imbalance may cause a confusional state), liver function tests (LFTs) (raised gamma-glutamyl transferase (GGT) suggests alcohol excess and more broadly alcohol can cause liver dysfunction), coagulation screen (liver damage resulting in coagulopathy), CRP (underlying infection), amylase (if any concerns re: pancreatitis). Check glucose (Table 10.9).

'Bloods show macrocytic anaemia and raised GGT consistent with excessive alcohol intake. Electrolyte levels and coagulation screen are normal.'

Complications of Chronic Alcohol Excess

- Pancreatitis
- Hypertension
- Cardiac arrhythmias
- Iron deficiency anaemia
- GI bleeds, impaired clotting
- Cancer of the oropharynx, oesophagus, pancreas, liver and lungs
- Fetal alcohol syndrome
- Cerebellar degeneration and myopathy

Management Summary: Alcohol Withdrawal

- Benzodiazepines
- Thiamine replacement
- Counselling for alcohol excess

Environmental changes can make a huge difference, e.g. quiet private single room, presence of relatives, supportive and nonthreatening staff, good lighting.

Table 10.9 Mr Johnson's Blood Results

PARAMETER	VALUE	NORMAL RANGE (UNITS)
WCC	10.5×10^9/L	4–11 ($\times 10^9$/L)
Neutrophil	5.2×10^9/L	2–7.5 ($\times 10^9$/L)
Lymphocyte	3.5×10^9/L	1.4–4 ($\times 10^9$/L)
Platelet	200×10^9/L	150–400 ($\times 10^9$/L)
Haemoglobin	**100 g/L**	**Men: 135–177 (g/L)** **Women: 115–155 (g/L)**
MCV	**110 fL**	**80–96 (fL)**
B_{12}	622 ng/L	160–925 (ng/L)
Folate	15 µg/L	4–18 (µg/L)
Urea	5.3 mmol/L	2.5–6.7 (mmol/L)
Creatinine	82 µmol/L	79–118 (µmol/L)
eGFR	>60 mL/min	>60 (mL/min)
Sodium	138 mmol/L	135–146 (mmol/L)
Potassium	4.2 mmol/L	3.5–5.0 (mmol/L)
CRP	3 mg/L	0–5 (mg/L)
PT	12 seconds	11.5–13.5 seconds
APTT	30 seconds	26–37 seconds
ALT	17 IU/L	5–35 (IU/L)
ALP	82 IU/L	39–117 (IU/L)
GGT	**72 IU/L**	**11–58 (IU/L)**
Bilirubin	14 µmol/L	3–17 (µmol/L)
Amylase	85 IU/L	25–125 (IU/L)
Glucose	5 mmol/L	4.5–5.6 (mmol/L) (fasting)

Data in bold signifies results that are outside the normal laboratory range. *ALP,* Alkaline phosphatase; *ALT,* alanine transaminase; *APTT,* activated partial thromboplastin time; *CRP,* C-reactive protein; *eGFR,* estimated glomerular filtration rate; *GGT,* gamma-glutamyl transferase; *MCV,* mean cell volume; *PT,* prothrombin time; *WCC,* white cell count.

INITIAL MANAGEMENT

- **Benzodiazepines (oral):** Diazepam (10–20 mg), chlordiazepoxide (10–50 mg), lorazepam (1–2 mg). Clomethiazole is a second-line option in those who do not tolerate benzodiazepines. Benzodiazepines can be prescribed on a symptom-triggered protocol on ward with the required nurse training. Otherwise, a fixed-dosing regimen can be used, as has been done in this case. The exact dosing protocols vary according to local guidelines.
- **Severe cases (risk to self/others):** In these circumstances, intravenous benzodiazepines might be considered or antipsychotics such as haloperidol.
- **Thiamine (vitamin B_1) replacement:** Pabrinex IV High Potency Injection (Ampoules 1 and 2) 2 pairs then later oral thiamine 100 mg TDS. Treatment duration varies depending on risk factors and severity but it is important to replace thiamine in patients with chronic alcoholism who are often deplete.
- **Thromboprophylaxis:** Benefits and risks should be judged on an individual basis (mobility of patient, risk of trauma, any existing abnormalities in clotting or platelet count).

Prescribe (Figs 10.8–10.10)

Benzodiazepines:

- DIAZEPAM 20 mg PO STAT, 20 mg QDS DAY 1, 15 mg QDS, DAY 2, 10 mg QDS DAY 3, 5 mg QDS DAYS 4 and 5. (Make sure it is prescribed on the as required prescription as well—higher doses may be required—dosing depends on symptoms.)

Thiamine replacement:

- PABRINEX IV (HIGH POTENCY) (Ampoules 1 and 2) 2 pairs STAT, then TDS for 3 DAYS, followed by THIAMINE 100 mg PO TDS

Thromboprophylaxis:

- DALTEPARIN 5000 units SC OD

- **Note:** In cases where IV glucose will be administered, give thiamine BEFORE IV glucose to avoid precipitating Wernicke's syndrome.

REASSESSMENT

- Hours after diazepam, the patient appears more settled and less tremulous.

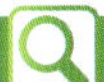

Benzodiazepines

- Reduce dose in elderly, liver disease, significant comorbidity (respiratory disease, cerebrovascular disease, reduced conscious level). Consider oral lorazepam instead in these groups (slower onset peak effect, quicker elimination).
- Sedation may mask encephalopathy/hepatic coma.
- Avoid abrupt withdrawal of benzodiazepines.
- Dependence may occur after ≈9 days.

'The patient has responded to benzodiazepines. The regular and PRN dose should be frequently reviewed and gradually weaned (frequency and dose) over the next few days and titrated to symptoms. His observations (HR, oximetry, RR, GCS) will be monitored closely.'

Alcohol withdrawal tools such as the CIWA-Ar (Clinical Institute Withdrawal Assessment for Alcohol, Revised) and more recently GMAWS (Glasgow Modified Alcohol Withdrawal Scale) help guide symptom-triggered treatment.

HANDING OVER THE PATIENT

'Mr Johnson is a 48-year-old man with a background of alcohol excess who is being treated for mild to moderate alcohol withdrawal, having increasing tremors, agitation and sweats since admission a day ago.

Examination reveals signs of chronic liver disease and some mild cerebellar signs. His conscious level and orientation appear normal. Blood tests reveal macrocytic anaemia as well as raised GGT but are otherwise normal.

His symptoms have improved with commencement of benzodiazepines. Thiamine has been commenced to prevent Wernicke–Korsakoff's syndrome.

The plan is to wean him off the diazepam gradually, continue with IV Pabrinex for 3 days then to switch this to oral thiamine 100 mg TDS. We have referred him on to the dietitian to optimise his nutritional status. Please chase his vitamin B_{12} and folate result in view of his macrocytic anaemia. He has been admitted to the general medical ward.

He has insight into the negative effects excessive alcohol consumption is causing and is keen for abstinence. He wishes to attend Alcoholics Anonymous after discharge. He might benefit from input from local alcohol liaison services and specialist psychiatry.'

Pabrinex High Potency by IV infusion should be given over at least 30 minutes. There is a risk of anaphylaxis, so resuscitation facilities should be available. The dose for the treatment of Wernicke's encephalopathy is 2–3 pairs TDS while for prophylaxis 1 pair daily is sufficient.

STATION 10.8: VANCOMYCIN AND GENTAMICIN PRESCRIBING

You are the junior doctor covering the general medical ward at the weekend. At handover, you are asked by the team to review the antibiotic dosing of two patients:

1. Mrs O'Neill, a 74-year-old lady, is on vancomycin for a methicillin-resistant *Staphylococcus aureus* (MRSA)-positive leg ulcer. She is 58 kg and has a creatinine clearance (CrCl) of 62 mL/min.

2. Mr Donaldson, a 70-year-old gentleman, is on gentamicin for acute pyelonephritis. His body weight is 75 kg and he has a CrCl of 74 mL/min.

Patient Details (Vancomycin)

Name:	Georgina O'Neill
DOB:	11/04/50
Hospital number:	1104402148
Weight:	58 kg
Height:	1.56 m
Consultant:	Mr Horn
Hospital/Ward:	BFG Gen med
Current medications:	Vancomycin IV (started on admission: for leg ulcer) Paracetamol 1 g PO QDS (started on admission: for pain) Enoxaparin 40 mg SC OD (started on admission) Omeprazole 40 mg PO OD (for peptic ulcer disease)
Allergies:	No known drug allergies
Admission date:	22/10/24

Patient Details (Gentamicin)

Name:	Andrew Donaldson
DOB:	12/07/54
Hospital number:	1207442158
Weight:	75 kg
Height:	1.56 m
Consultant:	Dr Kahn
Hospital/Ward:	FGH Gen med
Current medications:	Gentamicin IV (started on admission: for acute pyelonephritis) Paracetamol 1 g PO QDS (started on admission: for abdominal pain) Enoxaparin 40 mg SC OD (started on admission)
Allergies:	No known drug allergies
Admission date:	22/10/24

There are three main challenges in prescribing vancomycin and gentamicin:

1. Loading vancomycin/gentamicin
2. Monitoring the treatment regimen
3. Making subsequent dosage adjustments based on serum levels and kidney function

In calculating both vancomycin and gentamicin dosages, CrCl is required and can be calculated from the Cockcroft–Gault equation:

$$eC_{Cr} = \frac{(140 - \text{Age}) \times \text{Weight (in kilograms)} \times Constant}{\text{Creatinine } (\mu\text{mol/L})}$$

Note that the use of actual body weight in this equation may not hold for patients with a significantly raised body mass index (BMI): in such scenarios, 'ideal body weights' (giving a predicted weight based on height) may need to be used instead. The constant is 1.23 (male) or 1.04 (female).

Accurate documentation of blood samples taken and time of doses are essential. Both vancomycin and gentamicin tend to have local guidelines on dosing and sample testing; examples regimens are provided in the below cases.

VANCOMYCIN

BACKGROUND INFORMATION

- Mainly given by intravenous route but can be given orally, e.g. for *Clostridium difficile* GI infection.
- Commonly used in MRSA-related infections.
- Largely renally excreted.
- Concentration and time of trough sample taken must be accurately documented to guide subsequent dosage adjustments.
- Daily monitoring of renal function is required.

1. INITIATING VANCOMYCIN

Before prescribing the loading and the maintenance dose of vancomycin, check:

a. Body weight (58 kg)
b. CrCl (62 mL/min)

The loading dose (Table 10.10) is purely based on body weight. The initial maintenance dose (Table 10.11) is purely based on CrCl.

'Based on the dosage tables above, her loading dose is 1000 mg. Her first maintenance dose is 750 mg given at 12 hourly intervals after her loading dose.'

Table 10.10 Loading Dose of Vancomycin

BODY WEIGHT	LOADING DOSE	DURATION OF INFUSION
<40 kg	750 mg	1.5 hours
40–59 kg	1000 mg	2 hours
60–90 kg	1500 mg	3 hours
>90 kg	2000 mg	4 hours

Table 10.11 Initial Predicted Maintenance Dose for Vancomycin

CRCL (ML/MIN)	MAINTENANCE DOSE	DOSE INTERVAL
<20	500 mg over 1 hour	48 hours
20–29	500 mg over 1 hour	24 hours
30–39	750 mg over 1.5 hours	24 hours
40–54	500 mg over 1 hour	12 hours
55–74	750 mg over 1.5 hours	12 hours
75–89	1000 mg over 2 hours	12 hours
90–110	1250 mg over 2.5 hours	12 hours
>110	1500 mg over 3 hours	12 hours

CrCl, Creatinine clearance.

Table 10.12 Subsequent Dose Adjustment

TROUGH CONCENTRATION (MG/L)	RECOMMENDED DOSE CHANGE
<10	Move up one dosing band in table.
10–20	Maintain the present dose.
>20	Withhold. Recheck prior to when next dose is due, and withhold until <20 mg/L. Seek advice.

2. MONITORING REGIMEN

Trough concentration check for patients should be done at:

- 30 minutes before the first maintenance dose (if on 48-hour regimen)
- 30 minutes before the second maintenance dose (if on 12- or 24-hour regimen)

Target trough concentration is usually 10 to 20 mg/L.

Note: In deep-seated infection, e.g. bone or joints, endocarditis, hospital-acquired pneumonia and meningitis, target trough may need to be on higher end of the range—consult local policies.

3. SUBSEQUENT DOSE ADJUSTMENTS

Table 10.12 can help guide dose adjustment.

'Mrs O'Neill is on a 12-hourly regimen. The nurse on the ward has taken a trough level prior to her second maintenance dose. Her trough level (pre-second dose) returns as 8 mg/L. You are asked to review her subsequent dose.'

'Her trough level of 8 mg/L is subtherapeutic. Based on the dosage table, her next maintenance dose will need to be increased to a band higher, which is 1000 mg 12 hourly. There has been a dose change and therefore the levels need to be rechecked. This is done using the same guideline as checking the first vancomycin level as explained above. Since she is still on a 12-hourly regimen, her next trough level should be checked before the second subsequent dose, i.e. before the fourth maintenance dose.'

When the vancomycin levels and renal function are stable, it is sufficient to check levels twice weekly.

Prescribe (see Figs 10.12–10.13)

VANCOMYCIN 1000 mg IV (over 2 hours) BD

STOP
Previous vancomycin prescription

GENTAMICIN

Note: This regimen is different to that used in the paediatrics section. Policies vary when comparing adults and children and when comparing different local guidelines.

Table 10.13 Importance of Assessing Creatinine Clearance in Gentamicin Prescription

CREATININE CLEARANCE	INITIAL DOSAGE
>20 mL/min	7 mg/kg
<20 mL/min	Seek microbiology advice to ensure gentamicin is a suitable choice 2.5 mg/kg

How to Give Gentamicin

Dilute the gentamicin dose in 100 mL sodium chloride 0.9% and give IV infusion over 1 hour.

BACKGROUND INFORMATION

- Administrated mainly intravenously, occasionally intramuscularly.
- Largely renally excreted.
- Monitor for nephrotoxicity and ototoxicity, especially in prolonged treatment.
- Prescribed as (i) once-daily regimen, (ii) multiple-daily regimen or (iii) a one-off single dose (e.g. for a catheter change). The once-daily regimen is described here.

You are asked to review Mr Donaldson's serum gentamicin level and his subsequent doses. Your local intranet provides Hartford policy as the guideline for gentamicin use. As a means of good clinical practice, you take the opportunity to review the gentamicin dosage regimen.

1. INITIATING GENTAMICIN

Before prescribing the gentamicin dose, check the CrCl. In this case, it is 74 mL/min. For a creatine clearance >20 mL/min, 7 mg/kg of gentamicin can be prescribed as an initial once daily dose. If the creatine clearance is <20 mL/min, seek specialist advice (Table 10.13). Some centres implement a maximum dose of gentamicin (e.g. 400 mg or 600 mg).

'Mr Donaldson's initial gentamicin dose had been prescribed as 525 mg IV and was given 6 hours ago.'

2. MONITORING REGIMEN

- CrCl >20 mL/min: Check serum concentration 6 to 14 hours after the first infusion, and plot on the Hartford nomogram. Alternatively, check predose levels and consult local guidelines.
- CrCl <20 mL/min: Check level 24 hours after the first dose, and do not plot it onto the Hartford nomogram.

3. SUBSEQUENT DOSE ADJUSTMENTS

'His serum gentamicin concentration, which was taken at 7 hours postdose, returned as 6 mg/L. Renal function remains normal. This is plotted onto the normogram as in Fig. 10.11.'

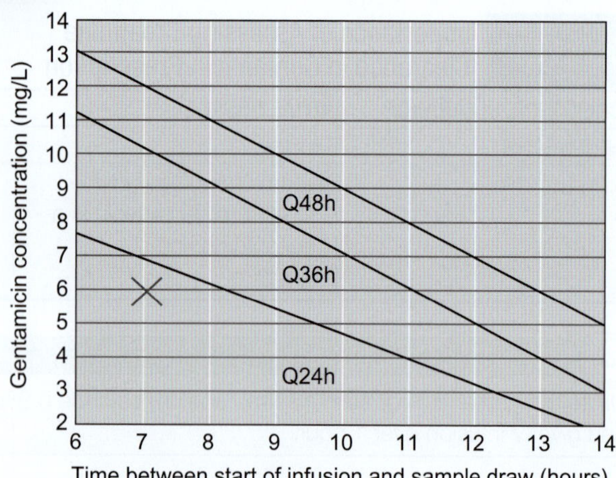

Fig. 10.11 Hartford nomogram. Plot the concentration between 6 and 14 hours on the nomogram. If the level falls in the area designated 24h, 36h or 48h, then dosing interval is 24 hours, 36 hours or 48 hours, respectively. If the level falls on the line between dosing intervals choose the longer interval. If the level is above the 48h line, then stop the treatment and seek microbiology advice.

'As his level falls within the range for 24 hour interval dosing, his current dose can be given once daily.'

For patients who are on a 24-hourly regimen, provided the renal function is stable, a further serum sampling can be checked at 6 to 14 hours postdose every 2 to 3 days. For patients who are on a 36- to 48-hourly regimen, serum concentration check is recommended after each dose.

- In patients with CrCl <20 mL/min, it is recommended to give the next dose if the serum concentration taken at 24 hours postdose is <1 mg/L. Therefore, the levels in these cases are not plotted. If the gentamicin level is >1 mg/L, it should be repeated 24 hours later.
- If renal function is unstable or concentration levels are unexpectedly high, seek microbiology advice.

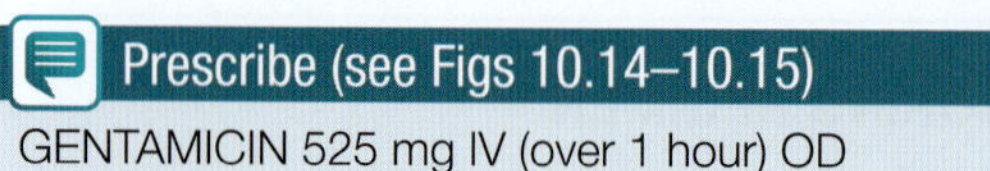

GENTAMICIN 525 mg IV (over 1 hour) OD

'Mr Donaldson is prescribed a daily dose of 525 mg gentamicin IV. A "level check" is inserted into the drug chart for gentamicin levels to be checked again 6–14 hours post dose after 2 days.'

FURTHER READING

Resuscitation Council UK, 2021. Emergency treatment of anaphylactic reactions. https://www.resus.org.uk/library/additional-guidance/guidance-anaphylaxis/emergency-treatment (Last accessed 12.09.24).

Scottish Antimicrobial Prescribing Group, 2019. Guidance on gentamicin and vancomycin. https://www.sapg.scot/guidance-qi-tools/antimicrobial-specific-guidance/(Last accessed 12.09.24).

PRESCRIPTION CHARTS

PRESCRIPTION AND ADMINISTRATION RECORD

Standard Chart

Hospital/Ward: WGH ORTHO WARD **Consultant:** MR BLAIR	**Name of Patient:** GRAHAM MCDONALD
Weight: 63 kg **Height:** 158 cm	**Hospital Number:** 0908472977
If re-written, date:	**D.O.B:** 09/08/1957
DISCHARGE PRESCRIPTION **Date completed:-** **Completed by:-**	

OTHER MEDICINE CHARTS IN USE		PREVIOUS ADVERSE REACTIONS This section must be completed before any medicine is given		Completed by (sign & print)	Date
Date	Type of Chart	None known ☐			
		Medicine/Agent	Description of Reaction		
		RAMIPRIL	ANAPHYLAXIS	P. Smith PAUL SMITH	11/10/24

CODES FOR NON-ADMINISTRATION OF PRESCRIBED MEDICINE

If a dose is not administered as prescribed, initial and enter a code in the column with a circle drawn round the code according to the reason as shown below. **Inform the responsible doctor in the appropriate timescale.**

1. Patient refuses
2. Patient not present
3. Medicines not available – CHECK ORDERED
4. Asleep/drowsy
5. Administration route not available – CHECK FOR ALTERNATIVE
6. Vomiting/nausea
7. Time varied on doctor's instructions
8. Once only/as required medicine given
9. Dose withheld on doctor's instructions
10. Possible adverse reaction/side effect

ONCE-ONLY

Date	Time	Medicine (Approved Name)	Dose	Route	Prescriber – Sign + Print	Time Given	Given By
12/10/24	14.00	FUROSEMIDE (give before 2nd unit of red cell concentrate)	20 mg	ORAL	P. Smith PAUL SMITH	14.00	FG

OXYGEN	Start Date	Start Time	Route Mask (%)	Route Prongs (L/min)	Prescriber – Sign + Print	Administered by	Stop Date	Stop Time

Fig. 10.2 Prescription and administration record (standard chart) for Graham McDonald.

Name: GRAHAM MCDONALD
Date of Birth: 09/08/1957

REGULAR THERAPY

PRESCRIPTION	Date → / Time ↓	11/10/24	12/10/24	13/10/24
Medicine (Approved Name): DALTEPARIN (crossed out); **Dose:** 5000 units; **Route:** SC; **Notes:**; **Start Date:** 11/10/24; **Prescriber – sign + print:** P. Smith PAUL SMITH	6			
	8			
	12			
	14			
	(18)	FD		
	22			

Stopped 12/10/24 due to bleeding and low platelets P. Smith PAUL SMITH

PRESCRIPTION	Time	11/10/24	12/10/24	13/10/24
Medicine (Approved Name): CO-CODAMOL 30/500; **Dose:** 2 tablets; **Route:** ORAL; **Notes:**; **Start Date:** 11/10/24; **Prescriber – sign + print:** P. Smith PAUL SMITH	(6)	FD	FD	FD
	8			
	(12)	FD	FD	FD
	14			
	(18)	FD	FD	FD
	22 (24)	FD	FD	FD

PRESCRIPTION	Time	11/10/24	12/10/24	13/10/24
Medicine (Approved Name): LANSOPRAZOLE; **Dose:** 30 mg; **Route:** ORAL; **Notes:**; **Start Date:** 11/10/24; **Prescriber – sign + print:** P. Smith PAUL SMITH	6			
	(8)	FD	FD	FD
	12			
	14			
	18			
	22			

PRESCRIPTION	Time	11/10/24	12/10/24	13/10/24
Medicine (Approved Name): ASPIRIN (crossed out); **Dose:** 75 mg; **Route:** ORAL; **Notes:**; **Start Date:** 11/10/24; **Prescriber – sign + print:** P. Smith PAUL SMITH	6			
	(8)	FD	FD	
	12			
	14			
	18			
	22			

Stopped 12/10/24 due to bleeding and low platelets P. Smith PAUL SMITH

PRESCRIPTION	Time	11/10/24	12/10/24	13/10/24
Medicine (Approved Name): SIMVASTATIN; **Dose:** 40 mg; **Route:** ORAL; **Notes:**; **Start Date:** 11/10/24; **Prescriber – sign + print:** P. Smith PAUL SMITH	6			
	8			
	12			
	14			
	18			
	(22)	FD	FD	

PRESCRIPTION	Time	11/10/24	12/10/24	13/10/24
Medicine (Approved Name): BISOPROLOL; **Dose:** 10 mg; **Route:** ORAL; **Notes:** Review 13/10/24; **Start Date:** 11/10/24; **Prescriber – sign + print:** P. Smith PAUL SMITH	6			Review
	(8)	FD	FD	FD
	12			
	14			
	18			
	22			

Fig. 10.3 Prescription and administration record (regular therapy) for Graham McDonald.

FLUID PRESCRIPTION CHART

Hospital/Ward: WGH ORTHO WARD	Consultant: MR BLAIR	Name of Patient: GRAHAM MCDONALD
		Hospital Number: 0908472977
Weight: 63 kg	Height: 158 cm	D.O.B: 09/08/1957

Date/ Time	FLUID / ADDED DRUGS	VOLUME / DOSE	ROUTE	RATE	PRESCRIBER – SIGN AND PRINT
12/10/24 10.00	RED CELL CONCENTRATE	1 unit	IV	Over 4 h	P. Smith PAUL SMITH
12/10/24 14.00	RED CELL CONCENTRATE	1 unit	IV	Over 4 h	P. Smith PAUL SMITH
12/10/24 10.00	PLATELETS	1 pool	IV	Over 30 min	P. Smith PAUL SMITH
12/10/24 10.30	PLATELETS	1 pool	IV	Over 30 min	P. Smith PAUL SMITH

Fig. 10.4 **Fluid prescription chart for Graham McDonald.** Note blood prescriptions are often done on a separate prescription chart.

PRESCRIPTION AND ADMINISTRATION RECORD

Standard Chart

Hospital/Ward: LGH A&E **Consultant:** J. MURPHY	**Name of Patient:** JOAN WHITE
Weight: 60 kg **Height:** 165 cm	**Hospital Number:** 1508723719
If re-written, date:	**D.O.B:** 15/08/1982
DISCHARGE PRESCRIPTION **Date completed:-** **Completed by:-**	

OTHER MEDICINE CHARTS IN USE		PREVIOUS ADVERSE REACTIONS This section must be completed before any medicine is given		Completed by (sign & print)	Date
Date	Type of Chart	None known ☐			
		Medicine/Agent	Description of Reaction		
		SEAFOOD	ANAPHYLAXIS	P. Smith PAUL SMITH	12/10/24
		BETA-BLOCKERS	ANAPHYLAXIS	P. Smith PAUL SMITH	12/10/24

CODES FOR NON-ADMINISTRATION OF PRESCRIBED MEDICINE

If a dose is not administered as prescribed, initial and enter a code in the column with a circle drawn round the code according to the reason as shown below. **Inform the responsible doctor in the appropriate timescale.**

1. Patient refuses
2. Patient not present
3. Medicines not available – CHECK ORDERED
4. Asleep/drowsy
5. Administration route not available – CHECK FOR ALTERNATIVE
6. Vomiting/nausea
7. Time varied on doctor's instructions
8. Once only/as required medicine given
9. Dose withheld on doctor's instructions
10. Possible adverse reaction/side effect

ONCE-ONLY

Date	Time	Medicine (Approved Name)	Dose	Route	Prescriber – Sign + Print	Time Given	Given By
12/10/24	10.00	ADRENALINE (1:1000)	500 micrograms	IM	P. Smith PAUL SMITH	10.00	FR
12/10/24	10.05	HYDROCORTISONE	200 mg	IV	P. Smith PAUL SMITH	10.05	FR
12/10/24	10.05	CHLORPHENAMINE	10 mg	IV	P. Smith PAUL SMITH	10.05	FR
12/10/24	10.05	SALBUTAMOL	5 mg	NEB	P. Smith PAUL SMITH	10.05	FR

OXYGEN	Start		Route		Prescriber – Sign + Print	Administered by	Stop	
	Date	Time	Mask (%)	Prongs (L/min)			Date	Time

Fig. 10.5 Prescription and administration record (standard chart) for Joan White.

Name: JOAN WHITE

Date of Birth: 15/08/1982

REGULAR THERAPY

PRESCRIPTION

Date → Time ↓		12/10/24											

Medicine (Approved Name): HYDROCORTISONE
Dose: 200 mg | Route: IV
Notes: | Start Date: 12/10/24
Prescriber – sign + print: P. Smith PAUL SMITH

Time		12/10/24											
6													
(8)													
(12)		X											
14													
(18)		DF											
(22)		DF											

Medicine (Approved Name): CHLORPHENAMINE
Dose: 10 mg | Route: IV
Notes: | Start Date: 12/10/24
Prescriber – sign + print: P. Smith PAUL SMITH

Time		12/10/24											
6													
(8)													
(12)		X											
14													
(18)		DF											
(22)		DF											

Medicine (Approved Name): DALTEPARIN
Dose: 5000 units | Route: SC
Notes: | Start Date: 12/10/24
Prescriber – sign + print: P. Smith PAUL SMITH

Time		12/10/24											
6													
8													
12													
14													
(18)		DF											
22													

Medicine (Approved Name):
Dose: | Route:
Notes: | Start Date:
Prescriber – sign + print:

Time													
6													
8													
12													
14													
18													
22													

Medicine (Approved Name):
Dose: | Route:
Notes: | Start Date:
Prescriber – sign + print:

Time													
6													
8													
12													
14													
18													
22													

Medicine (Approved Name):
Dose: | Route:
Notes: | Start Date:
Prescriber – sign + print:

Time													
6													
8													
12													
14													
18													
22													

Fig. 10.6 Prescription and administration record (regular therapy) for Joan White.

FLUID PRESCRIPTION CHART

Hospital/Ward: LGH A&E	**Consultant:** J. MURPHY
Weight: 60 kg	**Height:** 165 cm

Name of Patient: JOAN WHITE

Hospital Number: 1508723719

D.O.B: 15/08/1982

Date/ Time	FLUID / ADDED DRUGS	VOLUME / DOSE	ROUTE	RATE	PRESCRIBER – SIGN AND PRINT
12/10/24 10.00	SODIUM CHLORIDE 0.9%	500 mL	IV	Over 15 min	P. Smith PAUL SMITH
12/10/24 11.00	SODIUM CHLORIDE 0.9%	1000 mL	IV	500 mL/h	P. Smith PAUL SMITH

Fig. 10.7 Fluid prescription chart for Joan White.

PRESCRIPTION AND ADMINISTRATION RECORD

Standard Chart

Hospital/Ward: LGH MEDICINE **Consultant:** A BROWN	**Name of Patient:** JACK JOHNSON
Weight: 78 kg **Height:** 175 cm	**Hospital Number:** 0211652957
If re-written, date:	**D.O.B:** 02/11/1975
DISCHARGE PRESCRIPTION Date completed:- Completed by:-	

OTHER MEDICINE CHARTS IN USE		PREVIOUS ADVERSE REACTIONS This section must be completed before any medicine is given		Completed by (sign & print)	Date
Date	Type of Chart	None known ☒			
		Medicine/Agent	Description of Reaction		
		PENICILLIN	RASH	P. Smith PAUL SMITH	12/10/24

CODES FOR NON-ADMINISTRATION OF PRESCRIBED MEDICINE

If a dose is not administered as prescribed, initial and enter a code in the column with a circle drawn round the code according to the reason as shown below. **Inform the responsible doctor in the appropriate timescale.**

1. Patient refuses
2. Patient not present
3. Medicines not available – CHECK ORDERED
4. Asleep/drowsy
5. Administration route not available – CHECK FOR ALTERNATIVE
6. Vomiting/nausea
7. Time varied on doctor's instructions
8. Once only/as required medicine given
9. Dose withheld on doctor's instructions
10. Possible adverse reaction/side effect

ONCE-ONLY

Date	Time	Medicine (Approved Name)	Dose	Route	Prescriber – Sign + Print	Time Given	Given By
12/10/24	00.00	DIAZEPAM	20 mg	ORAL	P. Smith PAUL SMITH	00.00	FD
12/10/24	00.05	PABRINEX (HIGH POTENCY) (over 30 mins)	(Ampoules 1 and 2) 2 pairs	IV	P. Smith PAUL SMITH	00.05	FD

OXYGEN	Start		Route		Prescriber – Sign + Print	Administered by	Stop	
	Date	Time	Mask (%)	Prongs (L/min)			Date	Time

Fig. 10.8 Prescription and administration record (standard chart) for Jack Johnson.

Name: JACK JOHNSON

Date of Birth: 02/11/1975

REGULAR THERAPY

PRESCRIPTION

Medicine (Approved Name): DIAZEPAM
Dose: 20 mg | Route: ORAL
Notes: Alcohol withdrawal reducing regimen (day 1) | Start Date: 12/10/24
Prescriber – sign + print: P. Smith PAUL SMITH

Time		12/10/24	13/10/24	14/10/24	15/10/24	16/10/24	17/10/24	18/10/24					
6													
(8)		GH	X	X	X	X	X	X	X	X	X	X	X
(12)		GH	X	X	X	X	X	X	X	X	X	X	X
14													
(18)		GH	X	X	X	X	X	X	X	X	X	X	X
(22)		GH	X	X	X	X	X	X	X	X	X	X	X

Medicine (Approved Name): DIAZEPAM
Dose: 15 mg | Route: ORAL
Notes: Day 2 | Start Date: 13/10/24
Prescriber – sign + print: P. Smith PAUL SMITH

Time		12/10/24	13/10/24	14/10/24	15/10/24	16/10/24	17/10/24	18/10/24					
6													
(8)		X	GH	X	X	X	X	X	X	X	X	X	X
(12)		X	GH	X	X	X	X	X	X	X	X	X	X
14													
(18)		X	GH	X	X	X	X	X	X	X	X	X	X
(22)		X	GH	X	X	X	X	X	X	X	X	X	X

Medicine (Approved Name): DIAZEPAM
Dose: 10 mg | Route: ORAL
Notes: Day 3 | Start Date: 14/10/24
Prescriber – sign + print: P. Smith PAUL SMITH

Time		12/10/24	13/10/24	14/10/24	15/10/24	16/10/24	17/10/24	18/10/24					
6													
(8)		X	X		X	X	X	X	X	X	X	X	X
(12)		X	X		X	X	X	X	X	X	X	X	X
14													
(18)		X	X		X	X	X	X	X	X	X	X	X
(22)		X	X		X	X	X	X	X	X	X	X	X

Medicine (Approved Name): DIAZEPAM
Dose: 5 mg | Route: ORAL
Notes: Day 4 and day 5 | Start Date: 15/10/24
Prescriber – sign + print: P. Smith PAUL SMITH

Time		12/10/24	13/10/24	14/10/24	15/10/24	16/10/24	17/10/24	18/10/24					
6													
(8)		X	X	X			X	X	X	X	X	X	X
(12)		X	X	X			X	X	X	X	X	X	X
14													
(18)		X	X	X			X	X	X	X	X	X	X
(22)		X	X	X			X	X	X	X	X	X	X

Medicine (Approved Name): PABRINEX (HIGH POTENCY)
Dose: (Ampoules 1 and 2) 2 pairs | Route: IV
Notes: For 3 days. Give over 30 mins | Start Date: 12/10/24
Prescriber – sign + print: P. Smith PAUL SMITH

Time		12/10/24	13/10/24	14/10/24	15/10/24	16/10/24	17/10/24	18/10/24					
6													
(8)		GH	GH		X	X	X	X	X	X	X	X	X
12													
(14)		GH	GH		X	X	X	X	X	X	X	X	X
18													
(22)		GH	GH		X	X	X	X	X	X	X	X	X

Medicine (Approved Name): THIAMINE
Dose: 100 mg | Route: ORAL
Notes: | Start Date: 15/10/24
Prescriber – sign + print: P. Smith PAUL SMITH

Time		12/10/24	13/10/24	14/10/24	15/10/24	16/10/24	17/10/24	18/10/24					
6													
(8)		X	X	X									
12													
(14)		X	X	X									
18													
(22)		X	X	X									

Fig. 10.9 Prescription and administration record (regular therapy) for Jack Johnson (part 1).

Name: *JACK JOHNSON*

Date of Birth: *02/11/1975*

REGULAR THERAPY

PRESCRIPTION

Medicine (Approved Name)	
DALTEPARIN	
Dose: *5000 units*	Route: *SC*
Notes:	Start Date: *12/10/24*
Prescriber – sign + print: *P. Smith PAUL SMITH*	

Date → / Time ↓		12/10/24	13/10/24										
6													
8													
12													
14													
(18)		*GH*	*GH*										
22													

Medicine (Approved Name)	
Dose	Route
Notes	Start Date
Prescriber – sign + print	

Time													
6													
8													
12													
14													
18													
22													

Medicine (Approved Name)	
Dose	Route
Notes	Start Date
Prescriber – sign + print	

Time													
6													
8													
12													
14													
18													
22													

Medicine (Approved Name)	
Dose	Route
Notes	Start Date
Prescriber – sign + print	

Time													
6													
8													
12													
14													
18													
22													

Medicine (Approved Name)	
Dose	Route
Notes	Start Date
Prescriber – sign + print	

Time													
6													
8													
12													
14													
18													
22													

Medicine (Approved Name)	
Dose	Route
Notes	Start Date
Prescriber – sign + print	

Time													
6													
8													
12													
14													
18													
22													

Fig. 10.10 Prescription and administration record (regular therapy) for Jack Johnson (part 2).

PRESCRIPTION AND ADMINISTRATION RECORD

Standard Chart

Hospital/Ward: BFG GEN MED **Consultant:** MR HORN	**Name of Patient:** GEORGINA O'NEILL
Weight: 58 kg **Height:** 1.56 m	**Hospital Number:** 1104402148
If re-written, date:	**D.O.B:** 11/04/1950
DISCHARGE PRESCRIPTION **Date completed:-** **Completed by:-**	

OTHER MEDICINE CHARTS IN USE		PREVIOUS ADVERSE REACTIONS This section must be completed before any medicine is given		Completed by (sign & print)	Date
Date	Type of Chart	None known ☒		JM JOHN MALIK	22/10/24
		Medicine/Agent	Description of Reaction		

CODES FOR NON-ADMINISTRATION OF PRESCRIBED MEDICINE

If a dose is not administered as prescribed, initial and enter a code in the column with a circle drawn round the code according to the reason as shown below. **Inform the responsible doctor in the appropriate timescale.**

1. Patient refuses
2. Patient not present
3. Medicines not available – CHECK ORDERED
4. Asleep/drowsy
5. Administration route not available – CHECK FOR ALTERNATIVE
6. Vomiting/nausea
7. Time varied on doctor's instructions
8. Once only/as required medicine given
9. Dose withheld on doctor's instructions
10. Possible adverse reaction/side effect

ONCE-ONLY

Date	Time	Medicine (Approved Name)	Dose	Route	Prescriber – Sign + Print	Time Given	Given By
22/10/24	08.00	VANCOMYCIN (give over 2 hours)	1000 mg	IV	JM JOHN MALIK	08.00	JK

OXYGEN	Start Date	Start Time	Route Mask (%)	Route Prongs (L/min)	Prescriber – Sign + Print	Administered by	Stop Date	Stop Time

Fig. 10.12 Prescription and administration record (standard chart) for Georgina O'Neill.

Name: *GEORGINA O'NEILL*

Date of Birth: *11/04/1950*

REGULAR THERAPY

PRESCRIPTION

Medicine (Approved Name)		Date → / Time ↓		22/10/24	23/10/24	24/10/24									
VANCOMYCIN (crossed through)		6		Check level pre-dose											
Dose: 750 mg	Route: IV	(8)		X	JK										
Notes: Leg ulcer. Review in 48H. Give over 90 minutes.	Start Date: 22/10/24	12													
		14													
Prescriber – sign + print: JM JOHN MALIK		18													
		~~22~~	(20)	JK											

Trough level at 07.30, 23/10/24 prior to second maintenance dose = 8 mg/L: therefore dose increased
JM JOHN MALIK 23/10/24

Medicine (Approved Name)		Time		22/10/24	23/10/24	24/10/24									
PARACETAMOL		6													
Dose: 1 g	Route: ORAL	(8)		GF											
		(12)		GF											
Notes	Start Date: 22/10/24	14													
		(18)		GF											
Prescriber – sign + print: JM JOHN MALIK		(22)		GF											

Medicine (Approved Name)		Time		22/10/24	23/10/24	24/10/24									
OMEPRAZOLE		6													
Dose: 40 mg	Route: ORAL	(8)		GF											
		12													
Notes	Start Date: 22/10/24	14													
		18													
Prescriber – sign + print: JM JOHN MALIK		22													

Medicine (Approved Name)		Time		22/10/24	23/10/24	24/10/24									
ENOXAPARIN		6													
Dose: 40 mg	Route: SC	8													
		12													
Notes	Start Date: 22/10/24	14													
		(18)		JK	JK										
Prescriber – sign + print: JM JOHN MALIK		22													

Medicine (Approved Name)		Time		22/10/24	23/10/24	24/10/24									
VANCOMYCIN		6				Check level pre-dose									
Dose: 1000 mg	Route: IV	(8)													
		12													
Notes: Leg ulcer. Review in 48H. Dose increase 23/10/24. Give over 2 hours	Start Date: 23/10/24	14													
		18													
Prescriber – sign + print: JM JOHN MALIK		22	(20)		JK										

Medicine (Approved Name)		Time													
		6													
Dose	Route	8													
		12													
Notes	Start Date	14													
		18													
Prescriber – sign + print		22													

Fig. 10.13 **Prescription and administration record (regular therapy) for Georgina O'Neill.**

PRESCRIPTION AND ADMINISTRATION RECORD

Standard Chart

Hospital/Ward: FGH GEN MED **Consultant:** DR KAHN	**Name of Patient:** ANDREW DONALDSON
Weight: 75kg **Height:** 1.56m	**Hospital Number:** 1207442158
If re-written, date:	**D.O.B:** 12/07/1954
DISCHARGE PRESCRIPTION **Date completed:-** **Completed by:-**	

OTHER MEDICINE CHARTS IN USE		PREVIOUS ADVERSE REACTIONS This section must be completed before any medicine is given		Completed by (sign & print)	Date
Date	Type of Chart	None known ☒		Jeremy Smith JEREMY SMITH	22/10/24
		Medicine/Agent	Description of Reaction		

CODES FOR NON-ADMINISTRATION OF PRESCRIBED MEDICINE

If a dose is not administered as prescribed, initial and enter a code in the column with a circle drawn round the code according to the reason as shown below. **Inform the responsible doctor in the appropriate timescale.**

1. Patient refuses
2. Patient not present
3. Medicines not available – CHECK ORDERED
4. Asleep/drowsy
5. Administration route not available – CHECK FOR ALTERNATIVE
6. Vomiting/nausea
7. Time varied on doctor's instructions
8. Once only/as required medicine given
9. Dose withheld on doctor's instructions
10. Possible adverse reaction/side effect

ONCE-ONLY

Date	Time	Medicine (Approved Name)	Dose	Route	Prescriber – Sign + Print	Time Given	Given By
22/10/24	08.00	GENTAMICIN (over 1 hour)	525mg	IV	Jeremy Smith JEREMY SMITH	08.00	RK

OXYGEN	Start Date	Start Time	Route Mask (%)	Route Prongs (L/min)	Prescriber – Sign + Print	Administered by	Stop Date	Stop Time

Fig. 10.14 Prescription and administration record (standard chart) for Andrew Donaldson

Name: ANDREW DONALDSON

Date of Birth: 12/07/1954

REGULAR THERAPY

PRESCRIPTION

Medicine (Approved Name)	
GENTAMICIN	
Dose: 525 mg	Route: IV
Notes: For pyelonephritis. Review after 48 hour. Level after first dose 6 mg/L therfore on 24 hour regimen. Give over 1 hour.	Start Date: 22/10/24
Prescriber – sign + print: Jeremy Smith JEREMY SMITH	

Date → / Time ↓		22/10/24	23/10/24	24/10/24	25/10/24								
6													
(8)			SD	[boxed]									
12													
14													
18													
22													

Check level 6–14H post-dose

Medicine (Approved Name)	
PARACETAMOL	
Dose: 1g	Route: ORAL
Notes	Start Date: 22/10/24
Prescriber – sign + print: Jeremy Smith JEREMY SMITH	

Time		22/10/24	23/10/24	24/10/24	25/10/24								
6													
(8)		SD											
(12)		SD											
14													
(18)		SD											
(22)		SD											

Medicine (Approved Name)	
ENOXAPARIN	
Dose: 40 mg	Route: SC
Notes	Start Date: 22/10/24
Prescriber – sign + print: Jeremy Smith JEREMY SMITH	

Time		22/10/24	23/10/24	24/10/24	25/10/24								
6													
8													
12													
14													
(18)		SD											
22													

Medicine (Approved Name)	
Dose	Route
Notes	Start Date
Prescriber – sign + print	

Time													
6													
8													
12													
14													
18													
22													

Medicine (Approved Name)	
Dose	Route
Notes	Start Date
Prescriber – sign + print	

Time													
6													
8													
12													
14													
18													
22													

Medicine (Approved Name)	
Dose	Route
Notes	Start Date
Prescriber – sign + print	

Time													
6													
8													
12													
14													
18													
22													

Fig. 10.15 Prescription and administration record (regular therapy) for Andrew Donaldson.

Index

Note: Page numbers followed by 'b', 'f' and 't' refer to boxes, figures and tables, respectively.

A

Abbreviated mental test score (AMTS), 183*b*
Abdominal pain, differential diagnosis of, in pregnancy, 209*b*, 223*b*
Abdominal sepsis, 99
  handing over the patient, 102
  initial assessment of, 100
  initial differential diagnosis of, 100*b*
  initial investigations of, 100
  initial management of, 101
  management of, 102
  patient details, 99*t*
  patient's blood results, 101*t*
  prescription and, 100*b*, 101*b*–102*b*
    administration record, 115*f*
    fluid prescription chart, 117*f*
  reassessment of, 102
  regular therapy for, 116*f*
Abdominal X-ray (AXR)
  for abdominal sepsis, 101
  for intestinal obstruction, 245
  for ulcerative colitis, 92
Actrapid, 158–159, 159*b*, 171*b*
Acute breathless and wheeze, initial differential diagnosis of, 66*b*
Acute bronchiolitis, 269
  blood test results, 270*t*, 270
  calculating 24-hour volume requirements, 271*b*
  complications of, 269*b*
  handing over the patient, 271
  initial assessment of, 269
  initial investigations of, 270
  initial management of, 271
  management of, 271*b*
  patient details, 269*t*
  prescription, 270*b*, 290*f*, 291*f*
  reassessment of, 271
  respiratory distress, initial differential diagnosis, 269*b*
Acute coronary syndrome, 37
  complications of, 40*b*
  handing over patient, 40
  initial assessment of, 38
  initial investigations of, 39
  initial management of, 38*b*, 39
  management of, 41
  patient details, 37*t*
  prescription for, 41*b*, 56*f*, 57*f*
  reassessment of, 40
Acute diarrhoea, differential diagnosis of, 280*b*
Acute dyspnoea
  and chest pain, initial differential diagnosis of, 75*b*
Acute dyspnoea *(Continued)*
  differential diagnosis of, 34*b*
  initial differential diagnosis of, 63*b*
Acute headache, differential diagnosis of, 129*b*
Acute left ventricular failure, 33, 34*b*
  handing over patient to intensive therapy unit (ITU), 36
  initial assessment of, 34
  initial investigations of, 35
  initial management of, 35
  management of, 37
  patient details, 33*t*
  prescription for, 34*b*, 35*t*, 36*b*, 37*b*, 53*f*–55*f*
  reassessment of, 36
Acute pancreatitis, 241
  causes of, 241*b*
  complications of, 241*b*
  handing over patient, 244
  initial assessment, 241
  initial investigations, 242
  initial management, 242
  management summary, 242*b*
  patient details, 241*t*
  prescription, 242*b*–244*b*, 255*f*–257*f*
  reassessment, 243
Acute pericarditis, 31
  causes of, 32*b*
  complications of, 33*b*
  handing over patient, 33
  initial assessment of, 31
  initial investigations of, 32
  management of, 31*b*, 32
  patient details, 31*t*
  prescription for, 33*b*, 51*f*, 52*f*
  reassessment of, 33
  treatment of, 33
Acute stroke, care of a patient following an, 136
Acute transfusion reactions, 314*b*
Acute upper GI bleed, 102
  complications of, 102*b*
  handing over the patient, 105
  initial assessment of, 102
  initial differential diagnosis of, 102*b*
  initial investigations of, 103
  initial management for, 103
  management of, 102*b*, 105
  patient details, 102*t*
  patient's blood test results, 103, 105*t*
  prescription and, 103*b*, 105*b*
    administration record, 118*f*, 119*f*
    fluid prescription chart, 120*f*
  reassessment of, 105
Acute upper GI bleed *(Continued)*
  regular therapy for, 119*f*
Addisonian crisis, 177
  complications of, 177*b*
  differential diagnosis of, 177*b*
  handing over the patient, 179
  initial assessment of, 177
  initial investigations of, 178
  initial management of, 178
  management of, 179
  management summary of, 178*b*
  patient details, 177*t*
  prescription, 177*b*, 178*b*, 201*f*–204*f*
  reassessment of, 178
Adenosine, 43*b*
Adjuvants, 309
Adrenaline (epinephrine), 316*b*, 316
Adverse drug reactions (ADRs), 9
  causes of, 11*t*
  classification, 9
  detecting, 11
  frequency of, 9
  prevalence of, 9, 11*b*
    common causes of drugs, 11*t*
  prevention, 12
  reporting of, 310
    medicines and healthcare products regulatory agency, 310*t*, 311
  reproductive, 11
  risk factors for, 12*b*
  suspecting, 12
Age, in prescribing, 10*t*
Agonists, 3
Airway
  in abdominal sepsis, 100
  in acute bronchiolitis, 269, 271
  in acute exacerbation of asthma, 63, 275
  in acute pancreatitis, 241
  in acute upper GI bleed, 102
  in Addisonian crisis, 177
  in alcohol withdrawal, 317
  in anaphylaxis, 315
  in bacterial peritonitis, 94
  bleeding in pregnancy, 212
  in community-acquired pneumonia (CAP), 70
  in diabetes in surgical patient, 247, 248
  in diabetic ketoacidosis (DKA), 157
  in exacerbation of COPD, 67
  in gastroenteritis, 280, 281
  in hospital-acquired pneumonia, 72, 73

Airway *(Continued)*
in hypercalcaemia, 172
in hyperkalaemia, 169
in hyperosmolar hyperglycaemic state (HHS), 160
in hyperthyroid crisis, 180
in hypoglycaemia, 164, 165
in hyponatraemia, 174
in hypothyroidism, 182
in idiopathic nephrotic syndrome, 286
in infective exacerbation of cystic fibrosis, 277
in intestinal obstruction, 244, 246
in ischaemic stroke, 133, 136
in meningitis, 121, 123
in myasthenia gravis, 138, 139
in paracetamol overdose, 97
in postoperative fluid loss, 250, 251
in preeclampsia, 215
in preterm labour, 209
in pulmonary embolism, 75, 76
in respiratory distress in the newborn, 272
in seizures, 125, 127
in sickle cell chest crisis, 283, 284
in subarachnoid haemorrhage, 129, 131
in ulcerative colitis, 91
Albumin infusion, in bacterial peritonitis, 96
Alcohol, 5*t*, 18*t*
in prescribing, 10*t*
Alcohol breathalyzer, in hypoglycaemia, 165
Alcohol withdrawal, 317
differential diagnosis of, 317*b*
handing over the patient, 319
initial assessments of, 317
initial investigations of, 318
initial management of, 319
management summary of, 318*b*
patient details, 317*t*
prescription for, 319*b*, 329*f*, 330*f*, 331*f*
reassessment of, 319
symptoms of, 317*b*
Allopurinol, 18*t*
Aminoglycosides, 18*t*
Amoxicillin, for urinary tract infection, 224
AMTS. *See* Abbreviated mental test score (AMTS)
Analgesia, 308
in abdominal sepsis, 101
adjuvants, 309
in diabetes in surgical patient, 249
in meningitis, 124
non-opioids, 308
in postoperative fluid loss, 251
in pregnancy, 224*t*
prescribing morphine, 309
in pulmonary embolism, 77
in sickle cell chest crisis, 284
strong opioids, 309, 309*t*
in subarachnoid haemorrhage, 131
weak opioids, 308
World Health Organization (WHO) analgesic ladder, 308*f*, 308
Analgesics, side effects of, 309*t*
Anaphylaxis, 314*b*, 314
complications of, 315*b*
follow-up considerations, 317*b*
handing over the patient, 317
initial assessment of, 315
initial investigations of, 315
initial management of, 316
management summary of, 316*b*
patient details, 314*t*
prescription for, 315*b*, 317*b*, 326*f*, 327*f*, 328*f*
reassessment of, 316
some common triggers of, 315*b*
Angiotensin-converting enzyme (ACE) inhibitors, 11*t*, 18*t*
Angiotensin II receptor blockers (ARBs) inhibitors, 18*t*
Antagonists, 3
competitive, 3
noncompetitive, 3–4
Antenatal corticosteroids, in preeclampsia, 218
Antibiotics, 11*t*
for abdominal sepsis, 101
for acute exacerbation of asthma, 65
for acute GI bleed, 104
for community-acquired pneumonia (CAP), 71
for exacerbation of COPD, 71
for hospital-acquired pneumonia, 74
in infective exacerbation of cystic fibrosis, 279
for meningitis, 124
for respiratory distress in the newborn, 273
in sickle cell chest crisis, 284
Anticholinesterase therapy, for myasthenia gravis, 139–140
Anticoagulants, 11*t*
Antiemetics
for abdominal sepsis, 101
for hyperemesis gravidarum, 221*b*, 221, 222*t*
for subarachnoid haemorrhage, 131–132
Antiepileptics, 18*t*
Antihypertensive drugs, 18*t*
Antipsychotics, 11*t*
Antipyretics
for community-acquired pneumonia (CAP), 71
for hospital-acquired pneumonia, 74
for hyperthyroid crisis, 181
for sickle cell chest crisis, 284
Antiviral treatment for meningitis, 124
Arterial blood gas (ABG)
in abdominal sepsis, 100
in acute coronary syndrome, 39
in acute exacerbation of asthma, 64, 65*t*, 276*t*
in acute left ventricular failure, 34, 35*t*, 35
in acute pancreatitis, 242
in acute upper GI bleed, 103
in Addisonian crisis, 178*t*, 178
in anaphylaxis, 316*t*, 316
in bacterial peritonitis, 95
in community-acquired pneumonia (CAP), 70
Arterial blood gas (ABG) *(Continued)*
in diabetes in surgical patient, 248*t*, 248
in diabetic ketoacidosis (DKA), 158*b*
in exacerbation of COPD, 67, 68*t*
in hyperemesis gravidarum, 220
in hyperkalaemia, 170*t*, 170
in hypoglycaemia, 165, 166*t*
in intestinal obstruction, 245, 246*t*
in myasthenia gravis, 139
in paracetamol overdose, 97
postoperative fluid loss and, 251*t*, 251
in pulmonary embolism, 75, 76*t*
in respiratory distress in the newborn, 273*t*
in seizures, 127, 128*t*
in ulcerative colitis, 92
Aspirin, 11*t*
Asthma, acute exacerbation of, 63, 274
assessment of severity of, 65*t*
complications of, 63*b*, 274*b*
handing over the patient, 66, 277
initial assessment of, 63, 275
initial investigations of, 64, 275
initial management of, 64, 275
management of, 66, 275*b*
patient details in, 63*t*, 274*t*
prescription, 64*b*, 79*f*, 80*f*, 275*b*, 276*b*, 296*f*, 297*f*
reassessment of, 65, 277
Atenolol, 18*t*
Atrial fibrillation, causes of, in hyperthyroid crisis, 179*b*
Autoimmune conditions, in hypothyroidism, 184

B

Bacterial meningitis, 123*b*, 124
Bamford classification, 134*b*
Bed rest, for subarachnoid haemorrhage, 131
Bedside spirometry, for myasthenia gravis, 139
Benzodiazepines, 5*t*, 11*t*, 18*t*, 319*b*
alcohol withdrawal, 319
Beta-adrenergic blockade, in hyperthyroid crisis, 181
Beta-blockers, 11*t*, 18*t*
Bicarbonate, in diabetic ketoacidosis (DKA), 158
Bioavailability, 5
Biphasic insulin, 168
Bisphosphonates, in hypercalcaemia, 173*b*, 173, 174
Blatchford score, in GI bleed, 103, 104*t*
Bleeding in pregnancy, 211
differential diagnosis, 212*b*
handing over the patient, 214
holistic practice, 212*b*
initial assessment of, 212*b*, 212
initial investigation of, 213
initial management of, 212*b*, 213
patient details, 211*t*
prescription for, 212*b*, 214*b*, 229*f*, 230*f*, 231*f*
Blood culture
for community-acquired pneumonia (CAP), 70

Blood culture *(Continued)*
for diabetic ketoacidosis (DKA), 158
for exacerbation of COPD, 67
for hospital-acquired pneumonia, 73
for hyperosmolar hyperglycaemic state (HHS), 161
for hyperthyroid crisis, 180
for meningitis, 122
and meningococcal PCR for subarachnoid haemorrhage
for myasthenia gravis, 139
for seizures, 126–127
for subarachnoid haemorrhage, 130
Blood gases
in diabetic ketoacidosis (DKA), 158*b*
in hyperkalaemia, 170*b*
Blood glucose
capillary, in hyperthyroid crisis, 180
derangements of, 167*b*
in diabetes in surgical patient, 249
for hyperosmolar hyperglycaemic state (HHS), 163
in hypoglycaemia, 164
Blood pressure control, for ischaemic stroke, 136
Blood product prescribing, 311
blood products that can be prescribed, 313
handing over the patient, 314
initial assessment of, 312
airway, breathing, circulation, disability, and exposure, 312
initial investigations of, 312
initial management, 313
less common prescribed blood product, 314
patient details, 311*t*
prescription for, 313*b*, 323*f*–325*f*
reassessment of, 314
Blood test
Blood tests
for abdominal sepsis, 100, 101*t*
in acute bronchiolitis, 270*t*, 270
for acute coronary syndrome, 39*t*, 39
in acute exacerbation of asthma, 275, 276*t*
for acute exacerbation of asthma, 64, 65*t*
for acute left ventricular failure, 35*t*, 35
for acute pancreatitis, 242
for acute pericarditis, 32*t*, 32
for acute upper GI bleed, 103, 105*t*
for Addisonian crisis, 178*t*, 178, 179*t*
in alcohol withdrawal, 318*t*, 318
in anaphylaxis, 315–316, 316*t*
for bacterial peritonitis, 95*t*, 95
bleeding in pregnancy, 213*t*, 213
blood product prescribing, 312*t*, 312
for bradycardia, 42*t*, 42
for community-acquired pneumonia (CAP), 70, 71*t*
for diabetes in surgical patient, 248*t*, 248
for exacerbation of COPD, 67, 68*t*
in gastroenteritis, 281
for hospital-acquired pneumonia, 73*t*, 73
for hypercalcaemia, 173*t*, 173

Blood tests *(Continued)*
for hyperemesis gravidarum, 220*t*, 220
for hyperkalaemia, 170*t*, 170
for hyperosmolar hyperglycaemic state (HHS), 161, 162*t*
for hyperthyroid crisis, 180, 181*t*
for hypoglycaemia, 165, 166*t*
for hyponatraemia, 175*t*, 175
for hypothyroidism, 183
in idiopathic nephrotic syndrome, 287*t*, 287
in infective exacerbation of cystic fibrosis, 278*t*, 278
for intestinal obstruction, 245, 246*t*
for ischaemic stroke, 135*t*, 135
for meningitis, 122, 123*t*
for myasthenia gravis, 139*t*, 139
for paracetamol overdose, 97, 98*t*
in postoperative fluid loss, 251*t*, 251
for preeclampsia, 216*t*, 216
for preterm labour, 210*t*, 210
for pulmonary embolism, 75–76, 76*t*
in respiratory distress in the newborn, 273*t*, 273
for seizures, 126, 128*t*
in sickle cell chest crisis, 283, 284*t*
for subarachnoid haemorrhage, 130, 131*t*
for tachycardia, 44*t*, 44
for ulcerative colitis, 92, 93*t*
for urinary tract infection, 224
BNF. *See* British National Formulary (BNF)
Body weight, in prescribing, 10*t*
Bone protection, in ulcerative colitis, 93
Bowel obstruction, complications of, 244*b*
Bradycardia, 41
differential diagnosis of, 41*b*
handing over patient, 43
initial assessment of, 41
initial investigations of, 42
initial management of, 42
management of, 41*b*, 43
patients details, 41*t*
potential complications of, 43*b*
prescription for, 42*b*, 59*f*
reassessment of, 43
Breathing
in abdominal sepsis, 100
in acute bronchiolitis, 269
in acute exacerbation of asthma, 275
in acute pancreatitis, 241
in acute upper GI bleed, 103
in Addisonian crisis, 177
in alcohol withdrawal, 317
in anaphylaxis, 315
in bacterial peritonitis, 94
in bleeding in pregnancy, 212
in community-acquired pneumonia (CAP), 67
in diabetes in surgical patient, 247
in diabetic ketoacidosis (DKA), 157
in exacerbation of COPD, 67
in gastroenteritis, 280
in hospital-acquired pneumonia, 72
in hypercalcaemia, 172
in hyperkalaemia, 169

Breathing *(Continued)*
in hyperosmolar hyperglycaemic state (HHS), 161
in hyperthyroid crisis, 180
in hypoglycaemia, 164
in hyponatraemia, 175
in hypothyroidism, 182
in idiopathic nephrotic syndrome, 286
in infective exacerbation of cystic fibrosis, 277
in intestinal obstruction, 244
in ischaemic stroke, 134
in meningitis, 121
in myasthenia gravis, 138
in paracetamol overdose, 97
in postoperative fluid loss, 250
in preeclampsia, 215
in preterm labour, 209
in pulmonary embolism, 75
in respiratory distress in the newborn, 272
in seizures, 126
in sickle cell chest crisis, 283
in subarachnoid haemorrhage, 130
in ulcerative colitis, 91
British National Formulary (BNF), 19
Bronchiolitis, acute, 269
Bronchodilators
anaphylaxis, 316
in exacerbation of COPD, 68
in sickle cell chest crisis, 284

C

Calcium
in hypercalcaemia, 171*b*
in hyperthyroid crisis, 180
Calcium-channel blockers, 11*t*
Calcium gluconate, 218
Cannabinoids, 5*t*
Capillary blood gas (CBG)
in acute bronchiolitis, 270
in acute exacerbation of asthma, 275
in respiratory distress in the newborn, 273
in sickle cell chest crisis, 283
Capillary blood glucose, hyperthyroid crisis, 180
Capillary ketones
for diabetic ketoacidosis (DKA), 158
for hyperosmolar hyperglycaemic state (HHS), 161
Carbimazole, 181
Carboprost, 214
Cardiac stabilisation, in hyperkalaemia, 170
Cardiology, 31
acute coronary syndrome, 37
acute left ventricular failure, 33
acute pericarditis, 31
bradycardia, 41
tachycardia, 43
warfarin prescribing, 45
Cardiomegaly, 35*b*
Cardiotocography (CTG)
in preeclampsia, 216
in preterm labour, 210
Carotid endarterectomy, for ischaemic stroke, 137

Catheter, in abdominal sepsis, 101
Cefalexin, for urinary tract infection, 224–225
Central nervous system depressant drugs, 18*t*
Cephalosporins, 18*t*
Cerebral oedema, 159*b*
Channel-linked receptors, 3*t*
Check blood glucose, for seizures, 127
Chest pain, differential diagnosis of
  for acute coronary syndrome, 37*b*
  in acute pericarditis, 31*b*
Chest radiography/chest X-ray (CXR)
  for abdominal sepsis, 100–101
  for acute bronchiolitis, 270
  for acute coronary syndrome, 39
  for acute exacerbation of asthma, 64, 275
  for acute left ventricular failure, 35
  for acute pancreatitis, 242
  for acute pericarditis, 32
  for acute upper GI bleed, 103
  for Addisonian crisis, 178
  for anaphylaxis, 316
  for bacterial peritonitis, 95
  for bradycardia, 42
  for community-acquired pneumonia (CAP), 70
  for diabetes in surgical patient, 248
  for diabetic ketoacidosis (DKA), 158
  for exacerbation of COPD, 67
  and foot/leg X-rays, for diabetes in surgical patient, 248
  for hospital-acquired pneumonia, 73
  for hypercalcaemia, 173
  for hyperemesis gravidarum, 220
  for hyperkalaemia, 170
  for hyperosmolar hyperglycaemic state (HHS), 161
  for hyperthyroid crisis, 180
  for hyponatraemia, 175
  for hypothyroidism, 183
  for idiopathic nephrotic syndrome, 287
  for infective exacerbation of cystic fibrosis, 278
  for intestinal obstruction, 245
  for ischaemic stroke, 135
  for myasthenia gravis, 139
  for postoperative fluid loss, 251
  for pulmonary embolism, 76
  for respiratory distress in the newborn, 273
  for sickle cell chest crisis, 283
  for ulcerative colitis, 92
Children, 17
Chloramphenicol, 18*t*
Chloride, in diabetic ketoacidosis (DKA), 158
Chronic alcohol excess, complications of, 318*b*
Chronic liver disease
  complications of, 94*b*
  management of, 94*b*
Chronic obstructive pulmonary disease (COPD), exacerbation of, 66
  handing over the patient, 69
  initial assessment of, 67
Chronic obstructive pulmonary disease (COPD), exacerbation of *(Continued)*
  initial investigations of, 67
  initial management of, 68
  long-term complications of, 67*b*
  management of, 67*b*, 69
  patient details, 66*t*
  prescriptions, 67*b*–69*b*, 81*f*, 82*f*
  reassessment of, 68
Ciprofloxacin, 225
Circulation
  in abdominal sepsis, 100
  in acute bronchiolitis, 270
  in acute exacerbation of asthma, 64, 275
  in acute pancreatitis, 241
  in acute upper GI bleed, 103
  in Addisonian crisis, 177
  in alcohol withdrawal, 318
  in anaphylaxis, 315
  in bacterial peritonitis, 94
  bleeding in pregnancy, 212
  in community-acquired pneumonia (CAP), 67
  in diabetes in surgical patient, 247
  in diabetic ketoacidosis (DKA), 157
  in exacerbation of COPD, 67
  in gastroenteritis, 280
  in hospital-acquired pneumonia, 73
  in hypercalcaemia, 172
  in hyperkalaemia, 169
  in hyperosmolar hyperglycaemic state (HHS), 161
  in hyperthyroid crisis, 180
  in hypoglycaemia, 164
  in hyponatraemia, 175
  in hypothyroidism, 182
  in idiopathic nephrotic syndrome, 286
  in infective exacerbation of cystic fibrosis, 278
  in intestinal obstruction, 245
  in ischaemic stroke, 134
  in meningitis, 121
  in myasthenia gravis, 138
  in paracetamol overdose, 97
  in postoperative fluid loss, 250
  in preeclampsia, 215
  in preterm labour, 209
  in pulmonary embolism, 75
  in respiratory distress in the newborn, 272
  in seizures, 126
  in sickle cell chest crisis, 283
  in subarachnoid haemorrhage, 130
  in ulcerative colitis, 91
Clarithromycin, 163*b*
Clinical pharmacology
  basic principles of, 1
  pharmacodynamics, 1
  pharmacokinetics, 5*f*, 5
Clonidine, 5*t*
Clotting
  bleeding in pregnancy, 213
  in preeclampsia, 216
Coagulopathy, for subarachnoid haemorrhage, 131
Co-amoxiclav, 158*b*, 159*b*, 171*b*, 225*b*
Codeine phosphate, 224*t*
Cognitive impairment, differential diagnosis for, in hypothyroidism, 182*b*
Coma, differential diagnosis of, in hypoglycaemia, 164*b*
Community-acquired pneumonia (CAP), 69
  handing over the patient, 72
  initial assessment of, 70
  initial investigations of, 70
  initial management of, 71
  management of, 69*b*, 71
  patient details, 69*t*
  prescription, 71*b*, 83*f*, 84*f*–86*f*
  reassessment of, 71
  severity assessment, 70*b*
Competitive antagonists, 3
Computed tomographic pulmonary angiography (CTPA), in pulmonary embolism, 76
Concentration–time relationships, 7
  first-order kinetics, 8*f*
Corticosteroids, 5*t*, 18*t*, 33*b*
  in acute exacerbation of asthma, 65, 276
  in exacerbation of COPD, 68
  in hyperthyroid crisis, 181
  in idiopathic nephrotic syndrome, 287–288
  in infective exacerbation of cystic fibrosis, 279
  IV, for ulcerative colitis, 93
  in meningitis, 124
  in myasthenia gravis, 140
  in preeclampsia, 218
  in sickle cell chest crisis, 285
Cough swab, in infective exacerbation of cystic fibrosis, 278
Cough, with sputum, initial differential diagnosis of, 69*b*
C-reactive protein (CRP), in diabetic ketoacidosis (DKA), 158
Creatinine, 210*t*
CT scan
  in abdominal sepsis, 101
  of brain, in hypothyroidism, 183
  of head
    in hyponatraemia, 175–176
    for ischaemic stroke, 135
    for meningitis, 123
    for subarachnoid haemorrhage, 130
Cystic fibrosis, infective exacerbation of, 277
Cystic fibrosis transmembrane conductance regulator (CFTR) modulators, 279
Cytotoxic drugs, 18*t*

D

Dalteparin, 159*b*, 163*b*, 171*b*, 171, 173*b*, 176*b*, 178*b*, 181*b*
Decompression, in intestinal obstruction, 246
Deep vein thrombosis (DVT) prophylaxis treatment, 124
Delirium
  differential diagnosis of, in hyponatraemia, 174*b*
  screen for causes of, 175–176
Delirium tremens, 317
Desensitisation, 4

Diabetes
complications of, 157*b*
in surgical patient, 247
airway assessment of, 247
breathing in, 247
circulation in, 247
complications of, 247*b*
disability in, 247
exposure in, 247
handing over patient, 249
initial assessment of, 247
initial investigations of, 248
initial management of, 248
management summary, 248*b*
patient details, 247*t*
prescriptions, 247*b*, 249*b*, 261*f*, 262*f*, 263*f*
reassessment of, 249
symptoms of, 247*b*
type I, causes of hypoglycaemia in, 165*b*
Diabetes mellitus, complications of, 247*b*
Diabetic ketoacidosis (DKA), 157
blood gases, 158*b*
blood tests, 158, 159*t*, 159
complications of, 157*b*
definition of, 158*b*
handing over the patient, 160
initial assessment of, 157
initial investigations of, 158
initial management of, 158
management of, 160
management summary of, 158*b*
patient details, 157*t*
prescription for, 158*b*, 159*b*, 185*f*–187*f*
triggers of, 157*b*
Diagnostic paracentesis, in bacterial peritonitis, 95
Diazepam, 18*t*
Digoxin, 11*t*, 18*t*, 30*t*
Disability
in abdominal sepsis, 100
in acute bronchiolitis, 270
in acute exacerbation of asthma, 64, 275
in acute pancreatitis, 242
in acute upper GI bleed, 103
in Addisonian crisis, 178
in alcohol withdrawal, 318
in anaphylaxis, 315
in bacterial peritonitis, 95
bleeding in pregnancy, 212
in community-acquired pneumonia (CAP), 70
in diabetes in surgical patient, 247
in diabetic ketoacidosis (DKA), 158*b*
in exacerbation of COPD, 67
in gastroenteritis, 280
in hospital-acquired pneumonia, 73
in hypercalcaemia, 172
in hyperkalaemia, 169
in hyperosmolar hyperglycaemic state (HHS), 161
in hyperthyroid crisis, 180
in hypoglycaemia, 164
in hyponatraemia, 175
in hypothyroidism, 183
Disability *(Continued)*
in idiopathic nephrotic syndrome, 286
in infective exacerbation of cystic fibrosis, 278
in intestinal obstruction, 245
in ischaemic stroke, 134
in meningitis, 122
in myasthenia gravis, 138
in paracetamol overdose, 97
in postoperative fluid loss, 250
in preeclampsia, 215
in pulmonary embolism, 75
in respiratory distress in the newborn, 272
in seizures, 126
in sickle cell chest crisis, 283
in subarachnoid haemorrhage, 130
in ulcerative colitis, 92
Discharge prescribing, 307
prescribing controlled drugs, 307, 308*t*
prescribing PRN (as required) medications, 307, 308*t*
prescribing regular medications, 307, 308*t*
Diuretics, 11*t*
Diverticulitis, complications of, 100*b*
DK. *See* Diabetic ketoacidosis (DKA)
DNA-linked receptors, 3*t*
Domperidone, in infective exacerbation of cystic fibrosis, 279*b*, 279
Dose–response
curve, 4*f*
relationships, 2
Doxycycline, 225
Drugs
absorption, 6
distribution, 6
excretion, 7
interactions, 11*b*, 12, 13*t*
pharmacodynamics, 12
pharmacokinetics, 12
risk of, 13
metabolism, 7
in prescribing, 10*t*
therapy
clinical and surrogate endpoints, 29
monitoring, 29
plasma drug concentration, 29, 30*t*

E

Early senior review, in community-acquired pneumonia (CAP), 71
Early specialist input, in ulcerative colitis, 93
Echocardiogram
in acute left ventricular failure, 35
for acute pericarditis, 32
E. coli, 225
EEG and MRI, for meningitis, 123
Efficacy, 4
Elderly, 17, 18*t*
Electrocardiogram (ECG)
of abdominal sepsis, 101
of acute coronary syndrome, 39, 40*b*
of acute exacerbation of asthma, 64
Electrocardiogram (ECG) *(Continued)*
of acute left ventricular failure, 35
of acute pericarditis, 32
of acute upper GI bleed, 103
of Addisonian crisis, 178
of bacterial peritonitis, 95
of bradycardia, 42
of community-acquired pneumonia (CAP), 70–71
of diabetes in surgical patient, 248
of exacerbation of COPD, 67
of hyperemesis gravidarum, 220
of hyperkalaemia, 170
of hyperosmolar hyperglycaemic state (HHS), 161–162
of hyponatraemia, 175
of ischaemic stroke, 135
of paracetamol overdose, 97
of postoperative fluid loss, 251
of pulmonary embolism, 76
of subarachnoid haemorrhage, 131
of tachycardia, 44
of ulcerative colitis, 92
Embolism, pulmonary, 74
Empirical antibiotics, diabetes in surgical patient, 249
Encourage oral intake, in hyperemesis gravidarum, 222
Endocrinology
Addisonian crisis, 177
diabetic ketoacidosis (DKA), 157
hypercalcaemia, 172
hyperkalaemia, 168
hyperosmolar hyperglycaemic state (HHS), 160
hyperthyroid crisis, 179
hypoglycaemia, 164
hyponatraemia, 174
hypothyroidism, 182
insulin prescribing, 166
Endoscopy, in hyperemesis gravidarum, 220
Entero-hepatic circulation, 7
Environmental changes, 318*b*
Enzyme inducers, 46*b*
Enzyme inhibitors, 46*b*
Enzymes, 3*t*
Epigastric pain, differential diagnosis of, 241*b*
Epinephrine, 316*b*
Exacerbation
acute, of asthma, 63, 274
assessment of severity of, 65*t*
complications of, 63*b*, 274*b*
handing over the patient, 66, 277
initial assessment of, 63, 275
initial investigations of, 64, 275
initial management of, 64, 275
management of, 66, 275*b*
patient details in, 63*t*, 274*t*
prescription, 64*b*, 79*f*, 80*f*, 275*b*, 276*b*, 296*f*, 297*f*
reassessment of, 65, 277
of chronic obstructive pulmonary disease (COPD), 66
handing over the patient, 69
initial assessment of, 67
initial investigations of, 67
initial management of, 68

Exacerbation *(Continued)*
long-term complications of, 67*b*
management of, 67*b*, 69
patient details, 66*t*
prescriptions, 67*b*–69*b*, 81*f*, 82*f*
reassessment of, 68
Exposure
in abdominal sepsis, 100
in acute bronchiolitis, 270
in acute exacerbation of asthma, 64, 275
in acute pancreatitis, 242
in acute upper GI bleed, 103
in Addisonian crisis, 178
in alcohol withdrawal, 318
in anaphylaxis, 315
in bacterial peritonitis, 95
bleeding in pregnancy, 212
in community-acquired pneumonia (CAP), 70
in diabetes in surgical patient, 247
in diabetic ketoacidosis (DKA), 158*b*
in exacerbation of COPD, 67
in gastroenteritis, 280
in hospital-acquired pneumonia, 73
in hypercalcaemia, 172
in hyperkalaemia, 169
in hyperosmolar hyperglycaemic state (HHS), 161
in hyperthyroid crisis, 180
in hypoglycaemia, 165
in hyponatraemia, 175
in hypothyroidism, 183
in idiopathic nephrotic syndrome, 286
in infective exacerbation of cystic fibrosis, 278
in intestinal obstruction, 245
in ischaemic stroke, 134
in meningitis, 122
in myasthenia gravis, 138
in paracetamol overdose, 97
in postoperative fluid loss, 251
in preeclampsia, 215
in pulmonary embolism, 75
in respiratory distress in the newborn, 272
in seizures, 126
in sickle cell chest crisis, 283
in subarachnoid haemorrhage, 130
in ulcerative colitis, 92

F
Feeding advice, in gastroenteritis, 281
Fetal fibronectin, 210*b*
Fetal monitoring, in preeclampsia, 218
First-order kinetics, pharmacokinetics, 7, 8*f*
Fixed rate IV insulin infusion
in diabetic ketoacidosis (DKA), 158–159
in hyperosmolar hyperglycaemic state (HHS), 163
Flexible sigmoidoscopy, in ulcerative colitis, 92
Fludrocortisone, in Addisonian crisis, 179
Fluid balance, in hyperthyroid crisis, 181
Fluid loss, postoperative, 250
Fluid management, in idiopathic nephrotic syndrome, 288
Fluid prescription chart
in abdominal sepsis, 117*f*
in acute bronchiolitis, 291*f*
in acute exacerbation of asthma, 297*f*
in acute left ventricular failure, 55*f*
in acute pancreatitis, 257*f*
in acute upper GI bleed, 120*f*
in Addisonian crisis, 204*f*
in anaphylaxis, 328*f*
bleeding in pregnancy, 231*f*
in blood product prescribing, 325*f*
in community-acquired pneumonia (CAP), 85*f*
diabetes in surgical patient, 263*f*
in diabetic ketoacidosis (DKA), 187*f*
in hospital-acquired pneumonia, 88*f*
in hypercalcaemia, 198*f*
in hyperemesis gravidarum, 235*f*
in hyperkalaemia, 196*f*
in hyperosmolar hyperglycaemic state (HHS), 190*f*
in hypoglycaemia, 191*f*
in hyponatraemia, 200*f*
in intestinal obstruction, 260*f*
in ischaemic stroke, 153*f*
in meningitis, 144*f*
in myasthenia gravis, 156*f*
in paracetamol overdose, 114*f*
in postoperative fluid loss, 267*f*
in respiratory distress in the newborn, 294*f*
in seizures, 147*f*
in severe ulcerative colitis, 109*f*
in sickle cell chest crisis, 304*f*
in spontaneous bacterial peritonitis, 112*f*
in subarachnoid haemorrhage, 150*f*
Fluid resuscitation
in intestinal obstruction, 246
in preterm labour, 213, 214*b*
Fluids, in sickle cell chest crisis, 284
Fluid support
in acute bronchiolitis, 271
in acute exacerbation of asthma, 276
in acute pancreatitis, 242–243
in diabetes in surgical patient, 248
in hospital-acquired pneumonia, 74
and inotropes, in pulmonary embolism, 77
in respiratory distress in the newborn, 274
Fluid therapy
monitoring, 29
potential complications of, 29
Folate antagonist, 225
Folate, in hypothyroidism, 183
Food, in prescribing, 10*t*
Full blood count (FBC), in diabetic ketoacidosis (DKA), 158
Furosemide, 180*b*

G
Gastric protection
acute coronary syndrome, 39
acute pericarditis, 33
postoperative fluid loss, 251
Gastroenteritis, 280
case of, 281
complications of, 280*b*
differential diagnosis of acute diarrhoea, 280*b*
handing over the patient, 282
initial assessment of, 280
initial investigations of, 281
initial management of, 281
management of, 281*b*
patient details, 280*t*
prescription, 282*b*, 301*f*
reassessment of, 282
Gastroenterology
abdominal sepsis, 99
acute upper GI bleed, 102
paracetamol overdose, 96
severe ulcerative colitis, 91
spontaneous bacterial peritonitis, 94
Gastrointestinal function, in prescribing, 10*t*
Gastro-oesophageal reflux, 221, 222
Gentamicin, 30*t*, 158*b*, 170*b*, 321
background information for, 321
initiating, 321
creatinine clearance in, 321*t*
monitoring regimen, 321
patient details, 320*t*
prescription for, 322*b*, 334*f*, 335*f*
subsequent dose adjustments, 321, 322*f*
Global Registry of Acute Cardiac Events (GRACE) score, 39–40
Glucagon, 165
Glucose, 165*b*, 180
in hyperkalaemia, 171*b*, 171
in hyperthyroidism, 181*b*
in hyponatraemia, 175
monitoring
in Addisonian crisis, 179
in diabetic ketoacidosis, 160
prescription, in hyperkalaemia, 171
replacement, in hyperosmolar hyperglycaemic state (HHS), 163
Glucose bolus, in respiratory distress in the newborn, 274
Glycaemic control, for ischaemic stroke, 136–137
Good prescriber
characteristics of, 1
subcomponents of, 2*f*
G-protein-coupled receptors (GPCRs), 3*t*
GRACE score. *See* Global Registry of Acute Cardiac Events (GRACE) score
Group and save, in preeclampsia, 216
Gynaecology, obstetrics and
bleeding in pregnancy, 211
hyperemesis gravidarum, 219
preeclampsia, 215
preterm labour, 209
urinary tract infection in pregnancy, 223

H
Haemodialysis, in hyperkalaemia, 171
Haemoglobin
level, postoperative fluid loss and, 251
spontaneous bacterial peritonitis, 95

Haemorrhage protocol, in acute GI bleed, 104
Half-life, 7
Hand-held doppler, in urinary tract infection, 223
HDU environment
  in Addisonian crisis, 179
  in hyperthyroid crisis, 182
Headache, differential diagnosis of, in pregnancy, 215*b*
Heart failure, 314*b*
  New York Heart Association (NYHA) functional classification of, 37*b*
Height
  in idiopathic nephrotic syndrome, 287
  in infective exacerbation of cystic fibrosis, 278
Heparin, in pulmonary embolism, 76–77
Hepatic disease, 18*t*
  prescribing for patients with, 17
Hepatic function, in prescribing, 10*t*
HHS. *See* Hyperosmolar hyperglycaemic state (HHS)
High-dose corticosteroids, for myasthenia gravis, 140
High-flow oxygen, 161*b*
  for community-acquired pneumonia (CAP), 71
  in exacerbation of COPD, 68
  for seizures, 127
High vaginal swab (HVS), 210
History, in hypoglycaemia, 165
Holistic practice, 212*b*
Hospital-acquired pneumonia, 72
  handling over the patient, 74
  initial assessment of, 72
  initial investigations of, 73
  initial management of, 73
  management of, 72*b*
  patient details, 72*t*
  prescription, 72*b*, 74*b*, 86*f*–88*f*
  reassessment of, 74
Human chorionic gonadotrophin (HCG), 219
Humulin M3, 168*b*, 168
Hydralazine, 217
Hydrocortisone, 181*b*
  Addisonian crisis, 178, 179
Hypercalcaemia, 172
  calcium adjustment, 172*b*
  complications of, 172*b*
  differential diagnosis of, 172*b*
  handing over the patient, 174
  initial assessment of, 172
  initial investigations of, 173
  management summary of, 173*b*
  patient details, 172*t*
  prescription, 172*b*, 197*f*, 198*f*
  reassessment of, 174
Hypercoagulability, in idiopathic nephrotic syndrome, 288
Hyperemesis gravidarum, 219
  diagnosis of, 220
  differential diagnosis of, 219*b*
  handing over, 222
  initial assessment of, 219
Hyperemesis gravidarum *(Continued)*
  initial investigation of, 220
  initial management of, 220
  management, 220*b*
  patient details, 219*t*
  prescription, 221*b*, 222*b*, 234*f*–236*f*
Hyperkalaemia, 168
  causes of, 169*b*
  complications of renal failure with, 169*b*
  differential diagnosis of, 170*b*
  handing over the patient, 171
  initial assessment of, 169
  initial investigations of, 170
  initial management of, 170
  management of, 171
  management summary, 170*b*
  patient details, 168*t*
  prescription, 169*b*, 170*b*, 171*b*, 194*f*–196*f*
  reassessment of, 171
  treatment of, 170*b*
Hyperosmolar hyperglycaemic state (HHS), 160
  complications of, 160*b*
  definition of, 161*b*
  differential diagnosis of presenting complaint, 160*b*
  handing over the patient, 163
  initial assessment of, 161
  initial investigations of, 161
  initial management of, 162
  management of, 163
  management summary of, 162*b*
  patient details, 160*t*
  prescription, 161*b*, 163*b*, 188*f*–190*f*
  reassessment of, 163
Hypersusceptibility, 4*f*
Hypertension, in pregnancy, 215*b*
  differential diagnosis of, 215*b*
  drugs to control, 217*t*
Hyperthyroid crisis, 179
  causes of atrial fibrillation in, 179*b*
  complications of, 180*b*
  handing over the patient, 182
  initial assessment of, 180
  initial differential diagnosis of, 180*b*
  initial investigations of, 180
  initial management of, 181
  management of, 182
  management summary of, 181*b*
  patient details, 179*t*
  prescription, 180*b*–182*b*, 205*f*, 206*f*
  reassessment of, 181
Hypoglycaemia, 164
  causes of, in type I diabetes, 165*b*
  complications of, 164*b*
  differential diagnosis of coma in, 164*b*
  handing over the patient, 166
  initial assessment of, 164
  initial investigations of, 165
  initial management of, 165
  management of, 165
  normal values in, 166*t*
  patient details, 164*t*
Hypoglycaemia *(Continued)*
  prescription, 164*b*, 191*f*
  reassessment of, 165
  symptoms of, 165*b*
  treatment, 165
Hyponatraemia, 174
  causes of, 174*b*, 175*b*
  complications of, 174*b*
  differential diagnosis of delirium in, 174*b*
  handing over the patient, 177
  initial assessment of, 174
  initial investigations of, 175
  initial management of, 176
  management of, 176
  management summary of, 175*b*
  patient details, 174*t*
  prescription, 176*b*, 199*f*, 200*f*
  reassessment of, 176
Hypothyroidism, 182
  complications of, 182*b*
  differential diagnosis for cognitive impairment in, 182*b*
  initial assessment of, 182
  initial investigations of, 183
  initial management of, 183
  management of, 184
  management summary of, 183*b*
  patient details, 182*t*
  prescription, 183*b*, 207*f*
  reassessing patient in clinic, 184
  reassessment of, 183
  short letter to the patient's GP, 184

I

Idiopathic nephrotic syndrome, 285
  acute complications of, 286*b*
  atypical features, 287*b*
  bloods, 287*t*, 287
  definitions in, 288*b*
  diagnostic criteria for, 286*b*
  handing over the patient, 288
  initial assessment of, 286
  initial differential diagnosis of oedema, 286*b*
  initial investigations of, 287
  initial management of, 287
  management summary, 287*b*
  patient details, 285*t*
  prescription, 288*b*, 305*f*
  reassessment of, 288
Immunosuppressive agents, for myasthenia gravis, 139
Incentive spirometry, in sickle cell chest crisis, 284
Infection, in idiopathic nephrotic syndrome, 288
Infective exacerbation of cystic fibrosis, 277
  blood test results, 278*t*, 278
  complications of, 277*b*
  differential diagnosis of, 277*b*
  handing over the patient, 279
  initial assessment of, 277
  initial investigations of, 278
  initial management of, 279
  management of, 279*b*
  patient details, 277*t*

Infective exacerbation of cystic fibrosis *(Continued)*
- prescription, 279*b*, 298*f*–300*f*
- reassessment of, 279

Inhaled bronchodilators
- in acute exacerbation of asthma, 276
- in infective exacerbation of cystic fibrosis, 279
- in respiratory distress in the newborn, 276

Insulin, 11*t*, 18*t*
- in hyperkalaemia, 171*b*, 171
- in hyperosmolar hyperglycaemic state (HHS), 163
- in infective exacerbation of cystic fibrosis, 279
- infusion
  - in diabetic ketoacidosis, 158–159, 159*b*, 171*b*
  - in hyperosmolar hyperglycaemic state, 163
- prescribing, 166
  - adjusting short-acting insulin, 167
  - biphasic insulin, 168
  - general guide to, 166*b*
  - long-acting insulin, 168
  - prescribed, 167*b*, 168*b*, 192*f*, 193*f*
  - starting a basal-bolus, 166
- types of, 167*t*

Intensive care, in sickle cell chest crisis, 285

Interindividual variation, 8
- pharmacodynamic, 8–9
- pharmacogenetic, 9
- pharmacokinetic, 9

Interventions, in acute GI bleed, 105

Intestinal obstruction, 244
- cardinal features of, 244*b*
- differential diagnosis of causes of, 244*b*
- handing over patient, 246
- indications for operative intervention of, 246*b*
- initial assessment of, 244
- initial investigations of, 245
- initial management of, 245
- management of, 245*b*
- patient details, 244*t*
- prescription, 245*b*, 246*b*, 258*f*–260*f*
- reassessment of, 246

Intraindividual variation, 10*t*

Intravenous (IV) antibiotics
- for bacterial peritonitis, 96
- for sickle cell chest crisis, 284*b*
- for ulcerative colitis, 93

Intravenous (IV) fluids, 27
- in abdominal sepsis, 101
- in acute GI bleed, 104
- in Addisonian crisis, 178
- in community-acquired pneumonia (CAP), 71
- in diabetic ketoacidosis (DKA), 158, 160
- in exacerbation of COPD, 68
- in gastroenteritis, 281
- in hospital parenteral drug administration chart, 27, 28*f*

Intravenous (IV) fluids *(Continued)*
- in hyperosmolar hyperglycaemic state (HHS), 162, 163
- making assessment of fluid requirements, 26
- for meningitis, 124
- monitoring fluid therapy, 29
- in myasthenia gravis, 140
- normal fluid requirements, 26
- ongoing, in diabetic ketoacidosis, 160
- potential complications, 29
- prescribing, 26
- in respiratory distress in the newborn, 274
- types of, 27, 27*t*
- in ulcerative colitis, 92

Intravenous immunoglobulins, for myasthenia gravis, 140

Iodine solution, 181, 182

Ipratropium bromide, in acute exacerbation of asthma, 65, 275, 277

Ischaemia, myocardial, 39*b*

Ischaemic stroke, 133*b*, 133
- causes of, 133*b*
- complications of, 133*b*
- handing over the patient of, 137
- initial assessment of, 133
- initial investigations of, 135
- initial management of, 135
- management of, 136
- Oxford Stroke Classification, 134*b*
- patient details of, 133*t*
- prescription, 136*b*, 151*f*–153*f*
- for thrombolysis, 137*b*

ITU, in hyperthyroid crisis, 182

J

Joint X-ray, in sickle cell chest crisis, 283

Jugular venous pressure (JVP), 31

K

Ketones, 216
- in diabetic ketoacidosis, 160

Kinase-linked receptors, 3*t*

Korsakoff's psychosis, 317

L

Lactulose, in bacterial peritonitis, 96

Lantus, 159*b*, 159, 167*b*, 167

Left ventricular failure, acute, 33

Leucocytes, 216

Level 2/HDU monitoring, in preeclampsia, 217

Levemir, 168*b*, 168, 193*f*

Levothyroxine, in hypothyroidism, 183*b*, 183, 184

Lithium, 18*t*, 30*t*

Liver failure, in paracetamol overdose, 99

Long-acting insulin, 168
- analogues, in diabetic ketoacidosis (DKA), 159

Lower serum potassium, in hyperkalaemia, 171

Lumbar puncture
- for meningitis, 123

Lumbar puncture *(Continued)*
- for respiratory distress in the newborn, 274
- results of, 124, 125*t*
- for subarachnoid haemorrhage, 130–131

M

Magnesium, 218

Medication errors, 13
- dealing with, 310
- prevention of, 14
- responding to, 14
- types and causes, 13, 14*b*, 14*t*

Meningitis, 121
- complications of, 121*b*
- handing over the patient of, 125
- headache with a fever, differential diagnosis of, 121*b*
- initial assessment of, 121
- initial investigations of, 122
- initial management of, 123
- management summary of, 123*b*
- patient details of, 121*t*
- prescription, 124*b*, 142*f*–144*f*
- reassessment after investigation results of, 124
  - interpreting lumbar puncture results, 124, 125*t*

Metformin, 18*t*

Methotrexate, 18*t*

Metoclopramide, 221

Metronidazole, 225*b*

Miscarriage, 212*b*

Modified Glasgow score (Imrie), for acute pancreatitis, 243*b*, 243

Monitoring drug therapy, 29

Monitoring, in acute GI bleed, 104

Morning sickness, 219

Morphine, 224*t*
- prescribing, 309

Mucolytics, in infective exacerbation of cystic fibrosis, 279

Multivitamins, in infective exacerbation of cystic fibrosis, 279

Myasthenia gravis, 137
- causes of relapse of, 138*b*
- complications of, 138*b*
- features of a relapse of, 138*b*
- handing over the patient of, 141
- initial assessment of, 138
- initial investigations of, 139
- initial management of, 139
- management of, 139*b*, 139
- medications that worsen, 140*b*
- patient details of, 137*t*
- prescription, 140*b*, 154*f*–156*f*

Myocardial ischaemia, 39*b*

N

N-Acetylcysteine (NAC), 98
- NAC doses, 99*t*
- prescribing, 98, 99*t*

Nasogastric (NG) tube, in hyperthyroid crisis, 181

Nasopharyngeal aspirate, in acute bronchiolitis, 270

Neonatal team, 218*b*

Nephrotic syndrome, 288*b*
management summary of, 287*b*
Nephrotoxic drugs, withhold, in hyperkalaemia, 171
Neurology
ischaemic stroke, 133
meningitis, 121
myasthenia gravis, 137
seizures, 125
Newborn, respiratory distress in, 271
New York Heart Association (NYHA) functional classification, of heart failure symptoms, 37*b*
Nitrates, 5*t*
Nitrites, 216
Nitrofurantoin, 225*b*
for urinary tract infection, 224
Noncompetitive antagonists, 3–4
Non-opioids, 308
Non-ST elevation (NSTEMI) acute coronary syndrome, management of, 38*b*
Nonsteroidal anti-inflammatory drug (NSAID), 9, 11*t*, 18*t*, 224*t*
Normal metabolism, in hyperemesis gravidarum, 222
NovoRapid, 166*b*, 167*b*, 167
Nutrition
for acute pancreatitis, 243
for infective exacerbation of cystic fibrosis, 279
for ischaemic stroke, 137

O
Obstetrics and gynaecology
bleeding in pregnancy, 211
hyperemesis gravidarum, 219
preeclampsia, 215
preterm labour, 209
urinary tract infection in pregnancy, 223
Obstruction, intestinal, 244
Oculogyric crisis, 221
Oedema, pulmonary, 314*b*
Oesophageal variceal bleeding, management for, 105–106
Opioids, 5*t*, 18*t*
analgesics, 11*t*, 18*t*
equivalent doses of, 309*t*
Oral corticosteroids
in acute exacerbation of asthma, 276
in respiratory distress in the newborn, 276
Osmolality, in hyponatraemia, 176
Outcome, in preterm labour, 211
Oxford Stroke Classification, 134*b*
Oxygen
in acute exacerbation of asthma, 64, 276
in acute GI bleed, 104
in bacterial peritonitis, 96
high flow, 180
in sickle cell chest crisis, 284
via a venturi mask, 163*b*

P
Pabrinex, IV, in bacterial peritonitis, 96
Paediatrics
acute bronchiolitis, 269
Paediatrics *(Continued)*
acute exacerbation of asthma, 274
gastroenteritis, 280
infective exacerbation of cystic fibrosis, 277
respiratory distress in the newborn, 271
sickle cell chest crisis, 282
Palpitations, in tachycardia, differential diagnosis of, 43*b*
Pamidronate, 173*b*, 173, 174
Pancreatic enzyme supplements (Creon), in infective cystic fibrosis, 279
Pancreatitis
acute, 241
complications of, 241*b*
Paracetamol, 158*b*, 161*b*, 224*t*
Paracetamol overdose, 96
amount of overdose, 97
common overdoses, 99*t*
complications of, 97*b*
handing over the patient, 99
high-risk groups, 98*b*
initial assessment of, 97
initial investigations of, 97
initial management of, 98
monitoring for liver failure, 99
N-acetylcysteine (NAC) commencement, 98, 99*t*
management summary, 97*b*
patient details, 96*t*
patient's blood results, 98*t*
prescription, 98*b*
fluid prescription chart, 114*f*
reassessment of, 99
treatment nomogram, 113*f*
Partial exchange transfusion, in sickle cell chest crisis, 285
Patient stabilisation, in preeclampsia, 216–217
Peak flow, in acute exacerbation of asthma, 64, 65*t*, 275
Penicillin, 18*t*
Pericardial friction rub, 31
Pericarditis, acute. *See* Acute pericarditis
Pharmacodynamics, 1
agonists and antagonists, 3
desensitisation and withdrawal, 4, 5*t*
dose–response relationships, 2, 4*f*
drug targets, 3*t*
efficacy and potency, 4
handling, 10*t*
interactions, 12, 13*t*
interindividual variation, 8–9
intraindividual variation, 10*t*
and pharmacokinetics, 2*f*
response, 10*t*
therapeutic index, 4
Pharmacogenetics
interindividual variation, 9
intraindividual variation, 10*t*
Pharmacokinetics, 5*f*, 5
concentration–time relationships, 7
drug absorption, 6
drug distribution, 6
drug excretion, 7
drug metabolism, 7
Pharmacokinetics *(Continued)*
first-order kinetics, 7, 8*f*
interactions, 12, 13*t*
interindividual variation, 9
intraindividual variation, 10*t*
pharmacodynamics and, 2*f*
repeated doses, 7, 8*f*
summary, 5*f*
volume of distribution, 6
Pharmacovigilance, 11
Phenytoin, 18*t*, 30*t*
example prescription of, 127*b*
therapy, 128
Phosphate, in hypercalcaemia, 173
Physiotherapy, in infective exacerbation of cystic fibrosis, 279
Plasma exchange, for myasthenia gravis, 140
Plasma glucose
in diabetic ketoacidosis (DKA), 158
in hyperosmolar hyperglycaemic state (HHS), 162, 163
Plasma osmolality, in hyponatraemia, 176
Plasma sodium monitoring, in hyponatraemia, 176
Pneumonia
acute complications of, 69*b*, 72*b*
community-acquired, 69
hospital-acquired, 72
Postoperative fluid loss, 250
handing over patient, 252
initial assessment of, 250
initial investigations of, 251
initial management of, 251
patient details, 250*t*
prescription, 250*b*, 252*b*, 264*f*, 265*f*–267*f*
reassessment of, 252
Potassium
elimination, in hyperkalaemia, 171
faecal excretion, in hyperkalaemia, 171
monitoring, diabetes in surgical patient, 249
Potassium replacement
in diabetic ketoacidosis (DKA), 159
for hyperosmolar hyperglycaemic state (HHS), 162
Potency, 4
Precipitant identification
in hyperosmolar hyperglycaemic state, 162
in hypoglycaemia, 166
Preeclampsia, 215
diagnosis of, 216
initial assessment of, 215
initial investigation of, 216
management of, 216
obstetric consultant, 218
outcome, 219
patient details, 215*t*
prescription, 217*b*, 232*f*, 233*f*
risk factors for, 215*b*
Pregnancy, 18*t*
analgesia in, 224*t*
bleeding in, 211
differential diagnosis of

Pregnancy *(Continued)*
abdominal pain in, 209*b*, 223*b*
headache in, 215*b*
hypertension in, 215*b*
urinary tract infection in, 223
Pregnancy test, in diabetic ketoacidosis (DKA), 158
Prescribing
additional important scenarios
alcohol withdrawal, 317
analgesia, 308
anaphylaxis, 314
blood product prescribing, 311
dealing with medication error, 310
discharge prescribing, 307
reporting adverse drug reaction, 310
vancomycin and gentamicin prescribing, 319
British National Formulary (BNF), 19
characteristics of, 1
drug interactions, 12
errors
causes of, 13, 14*b*
prevention, 14
responding to error, 14
types of, 13, 14*t*
general practice, 26
getting information about medicines, 19
high-risk, 24*t*
hospital, 20
discharge medicines, 25
electronic, 25
intravenous (IV) fluids, 26, 27
hospital parenteral drug administration chart, 27, 28*f*
making assessment of fluid requirements, 26
normal fluid requirements, 26
potential complications, 29
types of, 27, 27*t*
medication errors, 13
monitoring fluid therapy, 29
other considerations, 25
for patients, 18*t*
children, 17
elderly, 17
with hepatic disease, 17
pregnant women or breast-feeding, 17
race and ethnicity, 19
with renal disease, 16
with special requirements, 16
rational, 15
Prescribing practice, 315*b*
Prescription
and administration record
in Addisonian crisis, 201*f*
in diabetic ketoacidosis, 185*f*
in hyperkalaemia, 194*f*
in hyperosmolar hyperglycaemic state, 188*f*
in hyperthyroid crisis, 205*f*
errors, 23*f*
example, 21*f*–22*f*
general considerations, 21
in phenytoin, 127*b*
Prescription *(Continued)*
in preeclampsia, 217*b*, 232*f*, 233*f*
in preterm labour, 211*b*, 227*f*, 228*f*
in urinary tract infection, 224, 225*b*, 237*f*, 238*f*
writing, 20, 23
Preterm labour, 209
handing over, 211
initial assessment of, 209
initial investigation of, 210
initial management of, 210
management of, 210*b*
patient details, 209*t*
prescription for, 211*b*, 227*f*, 228*f*
Prolonged seizures, 127
Propranolol, 18*t*
Prostaglandin F. *See* Carboprost
Proteinuria, 216
Proton pump inhibitors (PPIs)
for acute coronary syndrome, 39
for acute GI bleed, 104
for acute pancreatitis, 243*b*
for meningitis, 124
for postoperative fluid loss, 251
Pulmonary embolism, 74
clinical decision rules for, 76*b*
complications of, 75*b*
in haemodynamically unstable patients, 77*b*
handing over the patient, 77
initial assessment of, 75
initial investigations of, 75
initial management of, 76
management of, 77
patient details, 74*t*
prescription, 75*b*, 77*b*, 89*f*
reassessment of, 77
revised Geneva score for, 76*t*
Pulmonary oedema, 314*b*
Pyrexia, in a hospitalised patient, initial differential diagnosis, 72*b*

Q

Quinolones, 225

R

Raised intracranial pressure, suggestive signs of, 122*b*
Ranitidine, in infective exacerbation of cystic fibrosis, 279
Rational prescribing, 15. *See also* Prescribing
choosing dosage regimen, 15
choosing drug, 15
choosing therapeutic approach, 15
diagnosis, 15
establishing therapeutic goal, 15
informing patient, 16
monitoring treatment effects, 16
stopping drug therapy, 16
writing prescription, 16
Red blood cell
concentrates, types of, 313*b*
transfusion, indications for, 312*b*
Reduced sensitivity to drug action, in prescribing, 10*t*
Refeeding complications, in hyperemesis gravidarum, 221
Regular fluid reviews, importance of, 36*b*
Regular therapy
in abdominal sepsis, 116*f*
in acute coronary syndrome, 57*f*
in acute exacerbation of asthma, 80*f*
in acute left ventricular failure, 54*f*
in acute pancreatitis, 256*f*
in acute pericarditis, 52*f*
in acute upper GI bleed, 119*f*
in Addisonian crisis, 202*f*, 203*f*
in alcohol withdrawal, 330*f*, 331*f*
in anaphylaxis, 327*f*
bleeding in pregnancy, 230*f*
in blood product prescribing, 324*f*
in community-acquired pneumonia (CAP), 84*f*
diabetes in surgical patient, 262*f*
in diabetic ketoacidosis (DKA), 186*f*
in exacerbation of COPD, 82*f*
in gentamicin, 335*f*
in hospital-acquired pneumonia, 87*f*
in hypercalcaemia, 197*f*
in hyperemesis gravidarum, 234*f*
in hyperkalaemia, 195*f*
in hyperosmolar hyperglycaemic state (HHS), 189*f*
in hyperthyroid crisis, 206*f*
in hyponatraemia, 199*f*
in hypothyroidism, 207*f*
in infective exacerbation of cystic fibrosis, 298*f*
in intestinal obstruction, 259*f*
in ischaemic stroke, 152*f*
in meningitis, 143*f*
in myasthenia gravis, 155*f*
in postoperative fluid loss, 265*f*, 266*f*
in preeclampsia, 228*f*, 233*f*
in preterm labour, 228*f*
in respiratory distress in the newborn, 293*f*
in seizures, 146*f*
in severe ulcerative colitis, 108*f*
in sickle cell chest crisis, 303*f*
in spontaneous bacterial peritonitis, 111*f*
in subarachnoid haemorrhage, 149*f*
in vancomycin, 333*f*
Rehydration
in hyperemesis gravidarum, 220
and maintenance fluids, in gastroenteritis, 281
Renal disease, 18*t*
prescribing for patients with, 16
Renal failure, complications of, with hyperkalaemia, 169*b*
Renal function, in prescribing, 10*t*
Renal ultrasound (USS)
in diabetic ketoacidosis (DKA), 158
in hyperkalaemia, 170
Repeated drug doses, 7, 8*f*
Reproductive adverse drug reactions (ADRs), 11
Respiratory distress in the newborn, 271
blood test results and ABG, 273*t*
calculating 24-hour volume requirements in neonates, 274*b*
complications of, 272*b*
congenital pneumonia management, 273*b*

Respiratory distress in the newborn *(Continued)*
differential diagnosis of, 272*b*
handing over the patient, 274
initial assessment of, 272
initial differential diagnosis of, 269*b*
initial investigations of, 273
initial management of, 273
management summary, 273*b*
patient details, 272*t*
prescription, 272*b*, 274*b*, 292*f*–295*f*
reassessment of, 274
Respiratory medicine
acute exacerbation of asthma, 63
community-acquired pneumonia (CAP), 69
exacerbation of COPD, 66
hospital-acquired pneumonia, 72
pulmonary embolism, 74
Retinoids, 18*t*
Rifampicin, 18*t*
Risk assessment scores, in acute GI bleed, 103
Rockall score, in GI bleed, 103, 104*t*

S
Salbutamol
for acute exacerbation of asthma, 64, 275, 277
for hyperkalaemia, 171*b*, 171
Secondary prevention
in hypothyroidism, 184
in ischaemic stroke, 137
Seizures, 125
causes of, 125*b*
complications of, 125*b*
handing over the patient of, 129
initial assessment of, 125
initial investigations of, 126
initial management of, 127
management of, 127*b*
patient details of, 125*t*
prescription, 126*b*, 128*b*, 145*f*–147*f*
reassessment of, 128
Selective serotonin reuptake inhibitors, 5*t*
Senna, 173*b*, 173
Sepsis
in gastroenteritis, 281
in hyperkalaemia, 171
Septic screen, for meningitis, 123
Serum level, in paracetamol overdose, 97
Severe ulcerative colitis, 91
complications of, 91*b*
differential diagnosis of, 91*b*
handing over the patient, 93
initial assessment of, 91
initial investigations of, 92
initial management of, 92
management of, 93
patient details, 91*t*
patient's blood results, 93*t*
prescription and, 92*b*, 93*b*
administration record, 107*f*, 108*f*
fluid prescription chart, 109*f*
reassessment of, 93
regular therapy for, 108*f*
Witts' criteria and truelove definition of, 91*b*
Sex, in prescribing, 10*t*
Short-acting insulin, 167
Sickle cell chest crisis, 282
acute chest syndrome management, 284*b*
causes of chest pain in a child, 282*b*
complications of, 282*b*
diagnostic criteria for, 282*b*
handing over the patient, 285
initial assessment of, 283
initial investigations of, 283
initial management of, 284
IV antibiotics for, 284*b*
management summary, 284*b*
patient details, 282*t*
prescription, 283*b*, 285*b*, 302*f*–304*f*
reassessment of, 285
Sodium chloride, 160, 161*b*, 163, 176*b*, 176
Sodium, in hyponatraemia
osmolality of urine, 176
prescription of, 176*b*
Spirometry
incentive, in sickle cell chest crisis, 284
in infective exacerbation of cystic fibrosis, 278
for myasthenia gravis, 139
Spironolactone, 18*t*
Spontaneous bacterial peritonitis, 94
differential diagnosis of, 94*b*
handing over the patient, 96
initial assessment of, 94
initial investigations of, 95
initial management of, 96
patient details, 94*t*
patient's blood results, 95*t*
prescription for, 94*b*, 96*b*
administration record, 110*f*, 111*f*
fluid prescription chart, 112*f*
reassessment of, 96
regular therapy for, 111*f*
Sputum culture
in community-acquired pneumonia (CAP), 70
in exacerbation of COPD, 70
in hospital-acquired pneumonia, 73
in infective exacerbation of cystic fibrosis, 278
Statins, 11*t*
Statin therapy
for acute coronary syndrome, 41
for ischaemic stroke, 137
Status epilepticus, 127*b*
ST elevation (STEMI) acute coronary syndrome, management of, 38*b*
Steroids
in acute exacerbation of asthma, 276
in exacerbation of COPD, 68
in hyperthyroid crisis, 181
in idiopathic nephrotic syndrome, 287–288
in infective exacerbation of cystic fibrosis, 279
IV, for ulcerative colitis, 93
in meningitis, 124
Steroids *(Continued)*
in myasthenia gravis, 140
in preeclampsia, 218
in sickle cell chest crisis, 285
Stool chart, in ulcerative colitis, 93
Stool culture, in hospital-acquired pneumonia, 73
Stool sample
for microscopy, in gastroenteritis, 281
in ulcerative colitis, 92
Stroke unit, for ischaemic stroke, 136
Strong opioids, 309
Subarachnoid haemorrhage, 129
complications of, 129*b*, 132
fluid prescribing in patients with, 132
handing over the patient of, 133
Hunt and Hess scale, 130, 130*t*
initial assessment of, 129
initial investigations of, 130
initial management of, 131
management of, 131*b*, 132
patient details of, 129*t*
prescription, 132*b*, 133*b*, 148*f*–150*f*
Subcutaneous heparin, in ulcerative colitis, 93
Sulfonylureas, 18*t*
Supplementary oxygen
for acute bronchiolitis, 271
for acute exacerbation of asthma, 276
for diabetes in surgical patient, 248
for hospital-acquired pneumonia, 74
for infective exacerbation of cystic fibrosis, 279
for intestinal obstruction, 246
for ischaemic stroke, 136
for meningitis, 124
for myasthenia gravis, 139
for postoperative fluid loss, 251
for pulmonary embolism, 76
for respiratory distress in the newborn, 273
Surgery, general
for acute pancreatitis, 241
for diabetes in surgical patient with osteomyelitis, 247
for intestinal obstruction, 244
postoperative fluid loss in, 250
venous thromboembolism (VTE) prophylaxis, 239
Surgical input, in ulcerative colitis, 93
Symptom control, in hypercalcaemia, 173
Symptom management, in preeclampsia, 218
Syndrome of inappropriate antidiuretic hormone (SIADH), 271*b*, 271
Systemic inflammatory response syndrome (SIRS), 100*b*, 101, 121

T
Tachycardia, 43
handing over patient, 45
initial assessment of, 43
initial investigations of, 44
initial management of, 44

Tachycardia *(Continued)*
management of, 43*b*, 45
patient details, 43*t*
potential complications of, 45*b*
prescription for, 45*b*, 60*f*
reassessment of, 45
Tachyphylaxis, 4
Terlipressin, in acute GI bleed, 105
Tetracyclines, 18*t*
Theophylline, 30*t*
Therapeutic efficacy, 4
Therapeutic index, 4*f*, 4
Thiamine (vitamin B_1), 221
alcohol withdrawal, 319
Throat swab, for meningitis, 123
Thrombolysis
contraindications to, 137*b*
in pulmonary embolism, 77
Thromboprophylaxis, 222*b*, 239
in Addisonian crisis, 178
in alcohol withdrawal, 319
in anaphylaxis, 316
in bacterial peritonitis, 96
in diabetic ketoacidosis (DKA), 159
in hypercalcaemia, 173
in hyperkalaemia, 171*b*
in hyperthyroid crisis, 181
in hyponatraemia, 176
in ischaemic stroke, 136
mechanical, 240
pharmacological, 240
prescribing pharmacological, 240*b*, 240, 253*f*, 254*f*
Thyroid autoantibodies, 183
Thyroid function tests (TFTs)
in hypercalcaemia, 173
in hyperthyroid crisis, 180, 181*t*
in hyponatraemia, 175
in hypothyroidism, 183, 184
Thyroid hormone, in hyperthyroid crisis
inhibition, 182
production, 181
Thyroid storm. *See* Hyperthyroid crisis
Tolerance, 4
Toxic megacolon, in ulcerative colitis, 93
Tramadol, 224*t*
Transfusion, in sickle cell chest crisis, 284
Transfusion reactions, acute, 314*b*
Transporter proteins, 3*t*
Trimethoprim, 225
Troponin
in acute coronary syndrome, 39
in hyponatraemia, 175

U
Ultrasound scan
for hyperemesis gravidarum, 220
for preeclampsia, 216
Urea and electrolytes (U&Es)
in diabetic ketoacidosis (DKA), 158
Urinalysis
in abdominal sepsis, 100
in hospital-acquired pneumonia, 73
in hyperemesis gravidarum, 220
in idiopathic nephrotic syndrome, 287
in preeclampsia, 216
in preterm labour, 210
in urinary tract infection, 223
Urinary ketone measurement, in diabetic ketoacidosis (DKA), 158
Urinary pregnancy test, in hyperemesis gravidarum, 220
Urinary tract infection, 223
initial assessment of, 223
investigations of, 223
management of, 224
patient details, 223*t*
prescription, 224, 225*b*, 237*f*, 238*f*
Urine dipstick
in Addisonian crisis, 178
in bacterial peritonitis, 95
in diabetes in surgical patient, 248
in diabetic ketoacidosis (DKA), 158
in hypercalcaemia, 173
in hyperosmolar hyperglycaemic state (HHS), 161
in hyperthyroid crisis, 180
in hyponatraemia, 175
in hypothyroidism, 183
in intestinal obstruction, 245
in ulcerative colitis, 92
Urine drug screen, in hypoglycaemia, 165
Urine, in community-acquired pneumonia (CAP), 70
Urine sodium osmolality, in hyponatraemia, 176

V
Vancomycin, 18*t*, 30*t*, 320
background information for, 320
initiating, 320, 320*t*
loading dose of, 320*t*
maintenance dose of, 320*t*
monitoring regimen, 321
patient details, 320*t*
prescription for, 321*b*, 332*f*, 333*f*
subsequent dose adjustments of, 321, 321*t*
Venous blood gas (VBG)
in diabetic ketoacidosis (DKA), 158*b*, 158, 159*t*, 159, 160
in hyperosmolar hyperglycaemic state (HHS), 161
in hypoglycaemia, 165
in meningitis, 122–123
monitoring, in diabetic ketoacidosis, 160
Venous thromboembolism (VTE) prophylaxis, 239
additional examples, 241*b*, 241
assessment of risk factors, 239
in community-acquired pneumonia (CAP), 71
in diabetes in surgical patient, 249
in exacerbation of COPD, 68
general measures to reduce, 239
in hyperemesis gravidarum, 222
in hyperosmolar hyperglycaemic state (HHS), 162
in intestinal obstruction, 246
in myasthenia gravis, 140
patient details, 239*t*
patient risk factors and bleeding risk, 240
in preeclampsia, 217
in preterm labour, 214
for subarachnoid haemorrhage, 132
thromboprophylaxis, 239
mechanical, 240
pharmacological, 240
prescription, 240*b*, 240, 253*f*, 254*f*
Vitamin B_1 (thiamine), 221
alcohol withdrawal, 319
Vitamin K, in respiratory distress in the newborn, 274
Voltage-sensitive ion channels, 3*t*
Volume of distribution, 6

W
Warfarin, 18*t*
side effects of, 48*b*
stopping, 50*b*
Warfarin prescribing, 45. *See also* Prescribing
additional example scenarios, 50
adjusting warfarin dose, 48
background information for, 46
in community, 48
Fennerty regimen for, 47*t*
in hospitalised patient, 48
initiating warfarin, 46, 47*t*
management of overcoagulation, 49
patient details, 45*t*
patient taking with bleeding, 49
prescription for, 46*b*, 49*t*, 61*f*
warfarin counselling, 46
Weak opioids, 308
Weight
in gastroenteritis, 281
in idiopathic nephrotic syndrome, 287
Wernicke's encephalopathy, 221, 317
Withdrawal, 4, 5*t*
World Health Organization (WHO) analgesic ladder, 308*f*, 308
Wound swab
in diabetes in surgical patient, 248
in hospital-acquired pneumonia, 73